FUNDAMENTALS OF
MUSCULOSKELETAL ULTRASOUND

EDITION 3

FUNDAMENTALS OF
MUSCULOSKELETAL ULTRASOUND

JON A. JACOBSON, MD

Professor of Radiology
University of Michigan
Ann Arbor, Michigan

ELSEVIER

ELSEVIER

1600 John F. Kennedy Blvd.
Ste 1800
Philadelphia, PA 19103-2899

FUNDAMENTALS OF MUSCULOSKELETAL ULTRASOUND, THIRD EDITION

ISBN: 978-0-323-44525-2

Notices

Knowledge and best practice in this field are constantly changing. As new research and experience broaden our understanding, changes in research methods, professional practices, or medical treatment may become necessary.

Practitioners and researchers must always rely on their own experience and knowledge in evaluating and using any information, methods, compounds, or experiments described herein. In using such information or methods they should be mindful of their own safety and the safety of others, including parties for whom they have a professional responsibility.

With respect to any drug or pharmaceutical products identified, readers are advised to check the most current information provided (i) on procedures featured or (ii) by the manufacturer of each product to be administered, to verify the recommended dose or formula, the method and duration of administration, and contraindications. It is the responsibility of practitioners, relying on their own experience and knowledge of their patients, to make diagnoses, to determine dosages and the best treatment for each individual patient, and to take all appropriate safety precautions.

To the fullest extent of the law, neither the Publisher nor the authors, contributors, or editors, assume any liability for any injury and/or damage to persons or property as a matter of products liability, negligence or otherwise, or from any use or operation of any methods, products, instructions, or ideas contained in the material herein.

Previous editions copyrighted 2013 and 2007.

Library of Congress Cataloging-in-Publication Data

Names: Jacobson, Jon A. (Jon Arthur), author.
Title: Fundamentals of musculoskeletal ultrasound / Jon A. Jacobson.
Description: Third edition. | Philadelphia, PA : Elsevier, [2018] | Includes bibliographical references and index.
Identifiers: LCCN 2017014007 | ISBN 9780323445252 (hardcover : alk. paper)
Subjects: | MESH: Musculoskeletal Diseases–diagnostic imaging | Ultrasonography–methods | Musculoskeletal System–diagnostic imaging
Classification: LCC RC925.7 | NLM WE 141 | DDC 616.7/07543–dc23 LC record available at https://lccn.loc.gov/2017014007

International Standard Book Number: 978-0-323-44525-2

Content Strategist: Robin Carter
Content Development Specialist: Lisa M. Barnes
Publishing Services Manager: Catherine Jackson
Senior Project Manager: Rachel E. McMullen
Design Direction: Ashley Miner

Printed in India

Last digit is the print number: 9   8   7

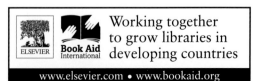

*This book is dedicated to my wife, Karen, and our daughters,
Erica and Marie, for their continued support.*

*To my parents, Ken and Dorothy, who showed
me the value of hard work.*

*To my students, residents, fellows, and technologists,
who are a joy to teach.*

*And to my mentors, Marnix van Holsbeeck and Donald Resnick,
who continue to amaze me with their knowledge
and dedication.*

PREFACE

It is my pleasure to present the third edition of the textbook, *Fundamentals of Musculoskeletal Ultrasound*. Since the last edition, there have been further advances in the clinical applications of musculoskeletal ultrasound and related research. Scanning techniques and protocols have also been refined with improved knowledge of anatomy as seen with ultrasound. This revision provides an update of important clinical applications and scanning techniques, based on progress in the field and relevant peer-reviewed publications. This third edition includes nearly 400 new images, including color photographs and color illustrations.

The organization of the textbook is similar to prior editions. New to this edition is the inclusion of Chapters 1 and 2 in hard copy form, which provides an introduction to musculoskeletal ultrasound and basic pathology concepts, respectively. Chapters 3 through 8 review anatomy, scanning technique, and common pathology of each specific joint and regional anatomy, including the shoulder; elbow; wrist and hand; hip and thigh; knee; and ankle, foot, and lower leg, respectively. To illustrate scanning technique, photographs show transducer placement and corresponding ultrasound images show resulting anatomy. Scanning protocols and sample reports are also included. In addition to common pathology of tendons, muscle, and ligaments, other topics include ultrasound evaluation of masses, peripheral nerves, and inflammatory arthritis. Chapter 9 provides an overview of ultrasound-guided musculoskeletal procedures, which is a very popular application of musculoskeletal ultrasound. Photographs show simulated needle and ultrasound transducer placement on a model to illustrate guidance techniques.

A new feature of the third edition are the updated online videos showing ultrasound cine clips, which simulate real-time scanning. Each of the over 200 videos are now individually narrated, where I describe the pertinent imaging findings using a pointer, similar to a lecture format. This enhanced feature will help emphasize the specific teaching points for each video. In addition to the videos, a complete electronic version of the textbook is available online via www. Expertconsult.com.

It has been exciting to see the popularity and clinical applications of musculoskeletal ultrasound continue to increase. With knowledge of anatomy and pathology as seen with ultrasound and proper scanning technique, musculoskeletal ultrasound can play an important role in the evaluation of the musculoskeletal system.

Jon A. Jacobson, MD

ACKNOWLEDGMENT

I would like to thank Philips Healthcare for use of their ultrasound equipment.

CONTENTS

VIDEOS
Videos are included in the ebook. To access the ebook, go to expertconsult.inkling.com.

EXAMINATION CHECKLISTS

TABLE 3.1 Shoulder Ultrasound Examination Checklist

Step	Structures/Pathologic Features of Interest
1	Biceps brachii long head
2	Subscapularis, biceps tendon dislocation
3	Supraspinatus, infraspinatus
4	Acromioclavicular joint, subacromial-subdeltoid bursa, dynamic evaluation
5	Posterior glenohumeral joint, labrum, teres minor, infraspinatus, atrophy

TABLE 4.1 Elbow Ultrasound Examination Checklist

Location	Structures of Interest
Anterior	Brachialis
	Biceps brachii
	Median nerve
	Anterior joint recess
Medial	Ulnar collateral ligament
	Common flexor tendon and pronator teres
	Ulnar nerve
Lateral	Common extensor tendon
	Lateral collateral ligament complex
	Radial head and annular recess
	Capitellum
	Radial nerve
Posterior	Posterior joint recess
	Triceps brachii
	Olecranon bursa

TABLE 5.1 Wrist and Hand Ultrasound Examination Checklist

Location	Structures of Interest/Pathologic Features
Volar (1)	Median nerve
	Flexor tendons
	Volar joint recesses
Volar (2)	Scaphoid
	Flexor carpi radialis
	Radial artery
	Volar ganglion cyst
Volar (3)	Ulnar nerve and artery
Dorsal (1)	Extensor tendons
	Dorsal joint recesses
Dorsal (2)	Scapholunate ligament
	Dorsal ganglion cyst
Dorsal (3)	Triangular fibrocartilage complex

TABLE 5.2 Finger Ultrasound Examination Checklist

Location	Structures of Interest
Volar	Flexor tendons
	Pulleys
	Volar plate
	Joint recesses
Dorsal	Extensor tendon
	Joint recesses
Other	Collateral ligaments

TABLE 6.1 Hip and Thigh Ultrasound Examination Checklist

Location	Structures of Interest
Hip: anterior	Hip joint, iliopsoas, rectus femoris, sartorius, pubic symphysis
Hip: lateral	Greater trochanter, gluteal tendons, bursae, iliotibial tract, tensor fascia latae
Hip: posterior	Sacroiliac joints, piriformis, and other external rotators of the hip
Inguinal region	Deep inguinal ring, Hesselbach triangle, femoral artery region
Thigh: anterior	Rectus femoris, vastus medialis, vastus intermedius, vastus lateralis
Thigh: medial	Femoral artery and nerve, sartorius, gracilis, adductors
Thigh: posterior	Semimembranosus, semitendinosus, biceps femoris, sciatic nerve

TABLE 7.1 Knee Ultrasound Examination Checklist

Location of Interest	Structures/Pathologic Features
Anterior	Quadriceps tendon Patella Patellar tendon Patellar retinaculum Suprapatellar recess Medial and lateral recesses Anterior knee bursae Femoral articular cartilage
Medial	Medial collateral ligament Medial meniscus: body and anterior horn Pes anserinus
Lateral	Iliotibial tract Lateral collateral ligament Biceps femoris Common peroneal nerve Anterolateral ligament Popliteus Lateral meniscus: body and anterior horn
Posterior	Baker cyst Menisci: posterior horns Posterior cruciate ligament Anterior cruciate ligament Neurovascular structures

TABLE 8.1 Ankle, Calf, and Forefoot Ultrasound Examination Checklist

Location	Structures of Interest
Ankle: anterior	Anterior tibiotalar joint recess Tibialis anterior Extensor hallucis longus Dorsal pedis artery Superficial peroneal nerve Extensor digitorum longus
Ankle: medial	Tibialis posterior Flexor digitorum longus Tibial nerve Flexor hallucis longus Deltoid ligament
Ankle: lateral	Peroneus longus and brevis Anterior talofibular ligament Calcaneofibular ligament Anterior tibiofibular ligament
Ankle: posterior	Achilles tendon Posterior bursae Plantar fascia
Calf	Soleus Medial and lateral heads of gastrocnemius Plantaris Achilles tendon
Forefoot	Dorsal joint recesses Morton neuroma Tendons and plantar plate

INTRODUCTION

■ EQUIPMENT CONSIDERATIONS AND IMAGE FORMATION

One of the primary physical components of an ultrasound machine is the transducer, which is connected by a cable to the other components, including the image screen or monitor and the computer processing unit. The transducer is placed on the skin surface and determines the imaging plane and structures that are imaged. Ultrasound is a unique imaging method in that sound waves are used rather than ionizing radiation for image production. An essential principle of ultrasound imaging relates to the piezoelectric effect of the ultrasound transducer crystal, which allows electrical signal to be changed to ultrasonic energy and vice versa. An ultrasound machine sends the electrical signal to the transducer, which results in the production of sound waves. The transducer is coupled to the soft tissues with acoustic transmission gel, which allows transmission of the sound waves into the soft tissues. These sound waves interact with soft tissue interfaces, some of which reflect back toward the skin surface and the transducer, where they are converted to an electrical current used to produce the ultrasound image. At soft tissue interfaces between tissues that have significant differences in impedance, there is sound wave reflection, which produces a bright echo that is proportional to the impedance

difference. A sound wave that is perpendicular to the surface of an object being imaged will be reflected more than if it is not perpendicular. In addition to reflection, sound waves can be absorbed and refracted by the soft tissue interfaces. The absorption of a sound wave is enhanced with increasing frequency of the transducer and greater tissue viscosity.[1]

An important consideration in ultrasound imaging is the frequency of the transducer because this determines image quality. A transducer is designated by the range of sound wave frequencies it can produce, described in megahertz (MHz). The higher the frequency, the higher the resolution of the image; however, this is at the expense of sound beam penetration as a result of sound wave absorption.[1] In contrast, a low-frequency transducer optimally assesses deeper structures, but it has relatively lower resolution. Transducers may also be designated as linear or curvilinear (Fig. 1.1). With a linear transducer, the sound wave is propagated in a linear fashion parallel to the transducer surface (Video 1.1). This is optimum in evaluation of the musculoskeletal system to assess linear structures, such as tendons, to avoid artifact. A curvilinear transducer may be used in evaluation of deeper structures because this increases the field of view (Video 1.2). A small footprint linear probe is ideal for imaging the hand, ankle, and foot given the contours of these body parts that allow only limited contact with the probe surface (Fig. 1.1C). A small footprint transducer with an offset is helpful when performing procedures on the distal extremities.

The physical size, power, resolution, and cost of ultrasound units vary, and these factors are all related. For example, an ultrasound machine that is approximately 3 × 3 × 4 feet high will likely be very powerful, have many imaging applications, and be able to support multiple transducers, including high-frequency transducers that result in exquisite high-resolution images. Smaller, portable machines are also available, some of which are smaller than a notebook computer. Although these machines cost less than the larger units, there may be tradeoffs related to image resolution and applications. Ultrasound units as small as a handheld electronic device have been introduced, although transducer options may be limited at

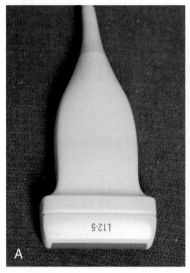
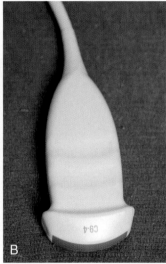
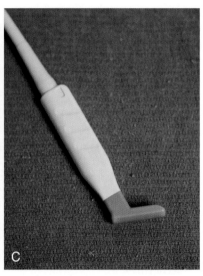

■ **FIGURE 1.1 Transducers.** Photographs show linear 12-5 MHz (A), curvilinear 9-4 MHz (B), and compact linear 15-7 MHz (C) transducers.

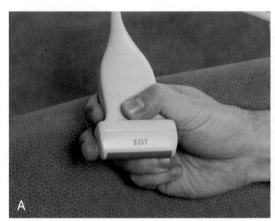
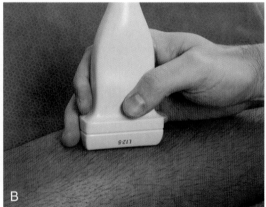

■ **FIGURE 1.2 Transducer Positioning.** A and B, Photographs show that the transducer is stabilized with simultaneous contact of the transducer, the skin surface, and the examiner's hand.

this time. As technology advances, these differences have been minimized as the portable ultrasound machines have become more powerful and the larger units have become smaller. It is therefore essential in the selection of a proper ultrasound unit to consider how an ultrasound machine will be used, the size of the structures that need to be imaged, the need for machine portability, and the capabilities of the ultrasound machine.

■ SCANNING TECHNIQUE

To produce an ultrasound image, the transducer is held on the surface of the skin to image the underlying structures. Ample acoustic transmission gel should be used to enable the sound beam to

be transmitted from the transducer to the soft tissues and to allow the returning echoes to be converted to the ultrasound image. I prefer a layer of thick transmission gel over a more cumbersome gel standoff pad. Gel that is more like liquid consistency is also less ideal because the gel tends not to stay localized at the imaging site. The transducer should be held between the thumb and fingers of the examiner's dominant hand, with the end of the transducer near the ulnar aspect of the hand (Fig. 1.2A). The transducer should be stabilized or anchored on the patient with either the small finger or the heel of the imaging hand (Fig. 1.2B). This technique is essential to maintain proper pressure of the transducer on the skin, to avoid involuntary movement of the transducer, and to allow fine adjustments in transducer positioning. Remember that the sound beam

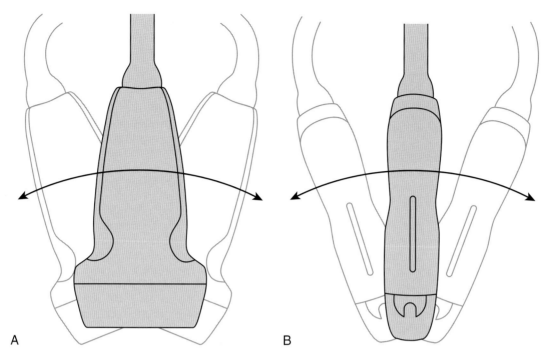

■ **FIGURE 1.3 Transducer Movements.** A, Heel-toe maneuver. B, Toggle maneuver. *(Modified from an illustration by Carolyn Nowak, Ann Arbor, Michigan; http://www.carolyncnowak.com/medtech.html.)*

emitted from the transducer is focused relative to the short end of the transducer, and side-to-side movement of the transducer should only be a millimeter at a time.

Various terms describe manual movements of the transducer during scanning. The term *heel-toe* is used when the transducer is rocked or angled along the long axis of the transducer (Fig. 1.3A). The term *toggle* is used when the transducer is angled from side to side (Fig. 1.3B). With both the heel-toe and toggle maneuvers, the transducer is not moved from its location, but rather the transducer is angled. The term *translate* is used when the transducer is moved to a new location while maintaining a perpendicular angle with the skin surface. The term *sweep* is used when the transducer is slid from side to side while maintaining a stable hand position, similar to sweeping a broom.

With regard to ergonomics, proper ultrasound scanning technique can help minimize fatigue and work-related injuries. Anchoring of the transducer to the patient by making contact between the scanning hand and the patient as described earlier decreases muscle fatigue of the examining arm. In addition, making sure that the scanning hand is lower than the ipsilateral shoulder with the elbow close to the body also decreases fatigue of the shoulder. If the examiner uses a chair, one at the appropriate height, preferably with wheels and with some type of back support, will improve

comfort and maneuverability. Last, the ultrasound monitor should be near the patient's area being scanned so that visualization of both the patient and the monitor can occur while minimizing turning of the head or spine.

There are three basic steps when performing musculoskeletal ultrasound, and these steps are also similar to obtaining an adequate image with magnetic resonance imaging (MRI). The first step is to image the structure of interest in long axis and short axis (if applicable), which depends on knowledge of anatomy. Identification of bone landmarks is helpful for orientation. The second step is to eliminate artifacts, more specifically anisotropy (see later discussion in this chapter) when considering ultrasound. When imaging a structure over bone, the cortex will appear hyperechoic and well defined when the sound beam is perpendicular, which indicates that the tissues over that segment of bone are free of anisotropy. The last step is characterization of pathology. Note the use of bone in two of the previous steps to understand anatomy and the proper imaging plane and to indicate that the sound beam is directed correctly to eliminate anisotropy.

■ IMAGE APPEARANCE

Once the transducer is placed on the patient's skin with intervening gel, a rectangular image

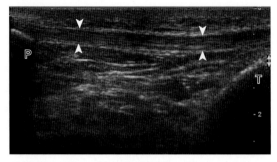

■ **FIGURE 1.4 Normal Patellar Tendon.** Ultrasound image of patellar tendon in long axis *(arrowheads)* shows hyperechoic fibrillar echotexture. *P,* Patella; *T,* tibia.

(when using a linear transducer) appears on the monitor. The top of the image represents the superficial soft tissues that are in contact with the transducer, and the deeper structures appear toward the lower aspect of the image (Fig. 1.4). To understand the resulting ultrasound image, consider the sound beam as a plane or slice that extends down from the transducer along its long axis. It is this plane that is portrayed on the image. The left and right sides of the image can represent either end of the transducer, and this can usually be switched by using the left-to-right invert button on the ultrasound machine or by simply rotating the transducer 180 degrees. When imaging a structure in long axis, it is common to have the proximal aspect on the left side of the image and the distal aspect on the right.

Image optimization is essential to maximize resolution and clarity. The first step is to select the proper transducer and frequency. Higher-frequency transducers (10 MHz or greater) optimally evaluate superficial structures, whereas lower-frequency transducers are used for deep structures. Linear transducers are typically used, unless the area of interest is deep, such as the hip region, where a curvilinear transducer may be chosen. After the proper transducer is selected and placed on the patient, the next step is to adjust the depth of the sound beam; this is accomplished by a button or dial on the ultrasound machine. The depth of the sound beam is adjusted until the structure of interest is visible and centered in the image (Fig. 1.5A and B). The next step in optimization is to adjust the focal zones of the ultrasound beam, if present on the ultrasound machine. This feature is typically displayed on the side of the image as a number of cursors or other symbols. It is optimum to reduce the number of focal zones to span the area of interest because increased focal zones will decrease the frame rate that produces a windshield-wiper effect. It is also important to move the depth of the focal zones to the depth where the structure is to be imaged

to optimize resolution (Fig. 1.5C). Some ultrasound machines have a broad focal zone that may not have to be moved. Finally, the overall gain can be adjusted by a knob on the ultrasound machine to increase or decrease the overall brightness of the echoes, which is in part determined by the ambient light in the examination room (Fig. 1.5D). The gain should ideally be set where one can appreciate the ultrasound characteristics of normal soft tissues (as described later in this chapter).

The ultrasound image is produced when the sound beam interacts with the tissues beneath the transducer and this information returns to the transducer. At an interface between tissues where there is a large difference in impedance, the sound beam is strongly reflected, and this produces a very bright echo on the image, which is described as *hyperechoic.* Examples include interfaces between bone and soft tissues, where the area beneath the interface is completely black from shadowing because no echoes extend beyond the interface. An area on the image that has no echo and is black is termed *anechoic,* whereas an area with a weak or low echo is termed *hypoechoic.* If a structure is of equal echogenicity to the adjacent soft tissues, it may be described as *isoechoic.*

■ SONOGRAPHIC APPEARANCES OF NORMAL STRUCTURES

Musculoskeletal structures have characteristic appearances on ultrasound imaging.[2] Normal tendons appear hyperechoic with a fiber-like or fibrillar echotexture (see Fig. 1.4).[3] At close inspection, the linear fibrillar echoes within a tendon represent the endotendineum septa, which contain connective tissue, elastic fibers, nerve endings, blood, and lymph vessels.[3] Continuous tendon fibers are best appreciated when they are imaged long axis to the tendon. On such a long axis image, by convention the proximal aspect is on the left side of the image, with the distal aspect on the right. In short axis, normal hyperechoic tendon fibers appear as bristles of a brush seen on end (see Fig. 1.9A). Normal muscle tissue appears relatively hypoechoic (Fig. 1.6). At closer inspection, the hypoechoic muscle tissue is separated by fine hyperechoic fibroadipose septa or perimysium, which surrounds the hypoechoic muscle bundles. The surface of bone or calcification is typically very hyperechoic, with posterior acoustic shadowing and possibly posterior reverberation if the surface of the bone is smooth and flat (Fig. 1.6). The hyaline cartilage covering the articular surface of bone is hypoechoic and uniform (Fig. 1.7A and B), whereas the fibrocartilage, such as the

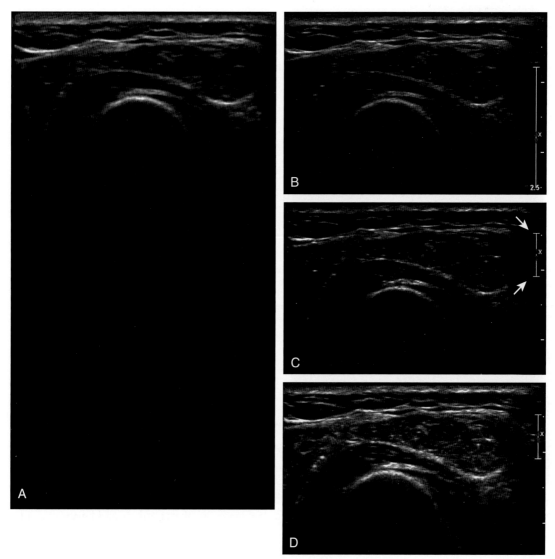

■ FIGURE 1.5 **Optimizing the Ultrasound Image.** A, Ultrasound image of forearm musculature shows improper depth, focal zone, and gain. B, Depth is corrected as area of interest is centered in image. C, Focal zone width is decreased and centered at area of interest *(arrows)*. D, Gain is increased.

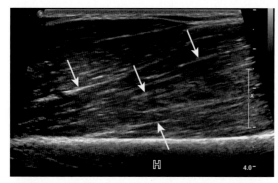

■ FIGURE 1.6 **Muscle.** Ultrasound image of brachialis and biceps brachii muscles in long axis shows hypoechoic muscle and hyperechoic fibroadipose septa *(arrows)*. *H,* Humerus.

labrum of the hip and shoulder, and the knee menisci are hyperechoic (Fig. 1.7B). Ligaments have a hyperechoic, striated appearance that is more compact compared with tendons (Fig. 1.8). In addition, ligaments are also identified in that they connect two osseous structures. Often normal ligaments may appear relatively hypoechoic when surrounded by hyperechoic subcutaneous fat; however, a compact linear hyperechoic ligament can be appreciated when imaged in long axis perpendicular to the ultrasound beam.

Normal peripheral nerves have a fascicular appearance in which the individual nerve fascicles are hypoechoic, surrounded by hyperechoic connective tissue epineurium (Fig. 1.9).[4] Hyperechoic fat is typically seen around larger peripheral nerves.

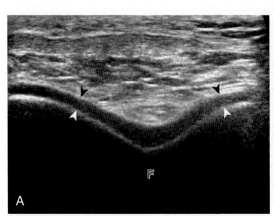

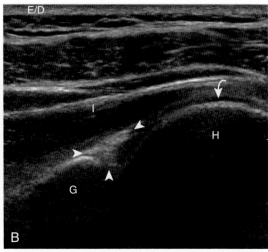

■ **FIGURE 1.7 Cartilage.** A, Ultrasound image transverse over the distal anterior femur shows hypoechoic hyaline cartilage *(arrowheads)*. *F*, Femur. B, Ultrasound image of infraspinatus in long axis (I) shows a hyperechoic fibrocartilage glenoid labrum *(arrowheads)* and hypoechoic hyaline cartilage *(curved arrow)*. Note hyperechoic epidermis and dermis (E/D), and adjacent deeper hypoechoic hypodermis with hyperechoic septa. *G*, Glenoid; *H*, humerus.

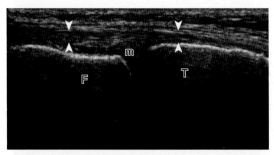

■ **FIGURE 1.8 Tibial Collateral Ligament.** Ultrasound image of tibial collateral ligament of the knee in long axis shows compact fibrillar echotexture *(arrowheads)*. *F*, Femur; *m*, meniscus; *T*, tibia.

In short axis, peripheral nerves display a honeycomb or speckled appearance, which assists in their identification. Because peripheral nerves have a relatively mixed hyperechoic and hypoechoic echotexture, their appearance changes relative to the adjacent tissues. For example, the median nerve in the forearm, when surrounded by hypoechoic muscle, appears relatively hyperechoic; in contrast, more distally in the carpal tunnel, when it is surrounded by hyperechoic tendon, the median nerve appears relatively hypoechoic (see Fig. 5.4D). The epidermis and dermis collectively appear hyperechoic, whereas the hypodermis shows hypoechoic fat and hyperechoic fibrous septa (see Fig. 1.7).

■ SONOGRAPHIC ARTIFACTS

One should be familiar with several artifacts common to musculoskeletal ultrasound.[5] One

such artifact is *anisotropy*.[6] When a tendon is imaged perpendicular to the ultrasound beam, the characteristic hyperechoic fibrillar appearance is displayed. However, when the ultrasound beam is angled as little as 2 to 3 degrees relative to the long axis of such a structure, the normal hyperechoic appearance is lost; the tendon becomes more hypoechoic with increased insonation angle (Figs. 1.10 to 1.13). A tissue is anisotropic if its properties change when measured from different directions. This variation of ultrasound interaction with fibrillar tissues involves tendons and ligaments and, to a lesser extent, muscle. Because abnormal tendons and ligaments may also appear hypoechoic, it is important to focus on that segment of tendon or ligament that is perpendicular to the ultrasound beam, to exclude anisotropy. With a curved structure, such as the distal aspect of the supraspinatus tendon, the transducer is continually repositioned or angled to exclude anisotropy as the cause of a hypoechoic tendon segment (Fig. 1.11 and Video 1.3). Anisotropy is noted both in long axis and short axis of ligaments and tendons (Video 1.4), but it occurs when the sound beam is angled relative to the long axis of a structure (Fig. 1.12). Therefore, to correct for anisotropy, the transducer is angled along the long axis of the imaged tendon or ligament; when imaging a tendon in long axis, the transducer is angled as a heel-toe maneuver (see Fig. 1.3A and Video 1.5), whereas in short axis, the transducer is toggled (see Fig. 1.3B and Video 1.6). Anisotropy can be used to one's advantage in identification of a hyperechoic tendon or ligament in close proximity to hyperechoic soft tissues, such as

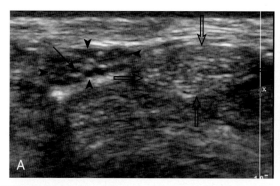 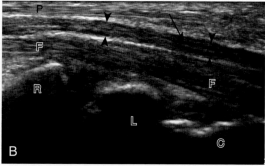

■ **FIGURE 1.9** **Median Nerve.** A, Ultrasound image of median nerve in short axis *(arrowheads)* shows individual hypoechoic nerve fascicles *(arrow)* and the adjacent hyperechoic flexor carpi radialis tendon *(open arrows)*. B, Ultrasound image of median nerve in long axis *(arrowheads)* shows hypoechoic nerve fascicles *(arrow)*. Note the adjacent fibrillar flexor digitorum (F) and palmaris longus (P) tendons. *C*, Capitate; *L*, lunate; *R*, radius.

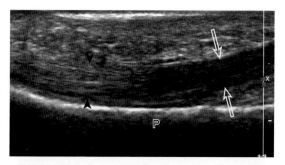

■ **FIGURE 1.10** **Anisotropy.** Ultrasound image of flexor tendons of the finger in long axis shows normal tendon hyperechogenicity *(arrowheads)* becoming more hypoechoic as the tendon becomes oblique relative to the sound beam *(open arrows)*. *P*, Proximal phalanx.

in the ankle and wrist. When imaging a tendon in short axis, toggling the transducer will cause the tendon to become hypoechoic, thus allowing its distinction from the adjacent hyperechoic fat that does not demonstrate anisotropy (Fig. 1.12). Once the tendon is identified, anisotropy must be corrected to exclude pathology. Anisotropy is also helpful in identification of some ligaments, such as in the ankle, because they are often adjacent to hyperechoic fat (Fig. 1.13). In addition, hyperechoic tendon calcifications can be made more conspicuous when they are surrounded by hypoechoic tendon from anisotropy with angulation of the transducer (see Fig. 3.63). When performing an interventional procedure, it is anisotropy that causes the needle to become less conspicuous when the needle is not perpendicular to the sound beam (see Fig. 9.8).

Another important artifact is *shadowing*. This occurs when the ultrasound beam is reflected, absorbed, or refracted.[7] The resulting image shows an anechoic area that extends deep from the involved interface. Examples of structures that produce shadowing include interfaces with bone or calcification (Fig. 1.14), some foreign bodies (see Chapter 2), and gas. An object with a small radius of curvature or a rough surface will display a clean shadow, whereas an object with a large radius of curvature and a smooth surface will display a dirty shadow (resulting from superimposed reverberation echoes).[8] Refractile shadowing may also occur at the edge of some structures, such as a foreign body or the end of a torn Achilles or patellar tendon (Fig. 1.15).[9]

Another type of artifact is *posterior acoustic enhancement* or *increased through-transmission*. This occurs during imaging of fluid (Figs. 1.16 and 1.17) and some solid soft tissue tumors, such as peripheral nerve sheath tumors (see Fig. 2.59) and pigmented villonodular tenosynovitis (giant cell tumors of tendon sheath) (Fig. 1.18).[10] In these situations, the sound beam is relatively less attenuated compared with the adjacent tissues; therefore, the deeper soft tissues will appear relatively hyperechoic compared with the adjacent soft tissues.[7]

Another artifact with musculoskeletal implications is *posterior reverberation*. This occurs when the surface of an object is smooth and flat, such as a metal object or the surface of bone. In this situation, the sound beam reflects back and forth between the smooth surface and the transducer and produces a series of linear reflective echoes that extend deep to the structure.[7] If the series of reflective echoes is more continuous deep to the structure, the term *ring-down artifact* is used, as may be seen with metal surfaces (Fig. 1.19). Ultrasound is ideal in evaluation of structures immediately overlying metal hardware because this reverberation artifact occurs deep to the hardware without obscuring the superficial soft tissues. Related to posterior reverberation is the

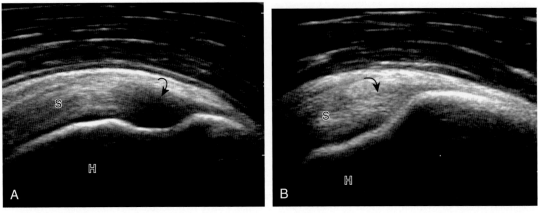

■ **FIGURE 1.11 Anisotropy.** Ultrasound images of distal supraspinatus tendon in long axis *(S)* shows an area of hypoechoic anisotropy *(curved arrow)* (A), where the tendon fibers become oblique to the sound beam, which is eliminated (B) when the transducer is repositioned so that the tendon fibers are perpendicular to the sound beam. *H,* Humerus.

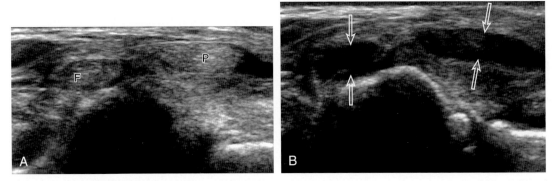

■ **FIGURE 1.12 Anisotropy.** Ultrasound images of tibialis posterior (P) and flexor digitorum longus (F) tendons in short axis at the ankle show normal tendon hyperechogenicity (A) and hypoechoic anisotropy *(open arrows)* (B), when angling or toggling the transducer along the long axis of the tendons, thus aiding in identification of tendons relative to surrounding hyperechoic fat.

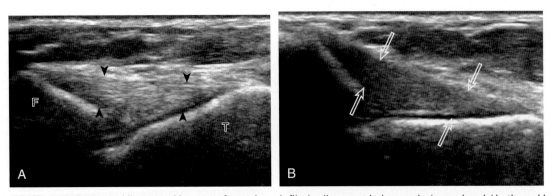

■ **FIGURE 1.13 Anisotropy.** Ultrasound images of anterior talofibular ligament in long axis *(arrowheads)* in the ankle show normal ligament hyperechogenicity (A) and hypoechoic anisotropy *(open arrows)* (B), when angling the transducer along the long axis of the ligament, thus aiding in identification of ligament relative to surrounding hyperechoic fat. *F,* Fibula; *T,* talus.

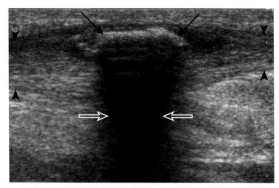

■ **FIGURE 1.14 Shadowing.** Ultrasound image of Achilles tendon in long axis *(arrowheads)* shows hyperechoic ossification *(arrows)* with posterior acoustic shadowing *(open arrows)*.

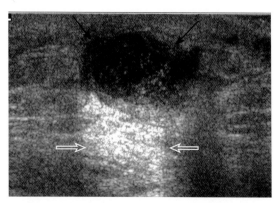

■ **FIGURE 1.17 Increased Through-Transmission.** Ultrasound image of a soft tissue abscess *(arrows)* in the shoulder shows increased through-transmission *(open arrows)*.

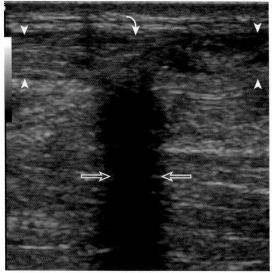

■ **FIGURE 1.15 Refractile Shadowing.** Ultrasound image of Achilles tendon in long axis *(arrowheads)* shows shadowing *(open arrows)* at the site of a full-thickness tear *(curved arrow)*.

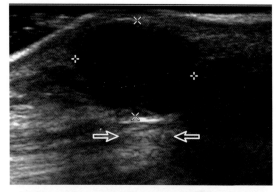

■ **FIGURE 1.18 Increased Through-Transmission.** Ultrasound image of a pigmented villonodular tenosynovitis (giant cell tumor of the tendon sheath) *(between × and + cursors)* shows increased through-transmission *(open arrows)*.

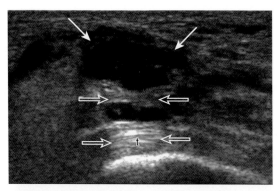

■ **FIGURE 1.16 Increased Through-Transmission.** Ultrasound image of a ganglion cyst *(arrows)* in the ankle shows increased through-transmission *(open arrows)*. *t,* Flexor hallucis longus tendon.

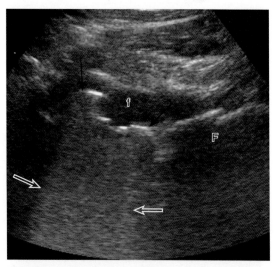

■ **FIGURE 1.19 Ring-Down Artifact.** Ultrasound image in long axis to the femoral component of a total hip arthroplasty shows the hyperechoic metal surface of the arthroplasty *(arrows)* and posterior ring-down artifact *(open arrows)*. Note the overlying joint fluid (f) and adjacent native femur (F).

comet-tail artifact, such as that seen with soft tissue gas (Fig. 1.20), which appears as a short segment of posterior bright echoes that narrows further from the source of the artifact.

One additional artifact to consider is *beam-width artifact*. This is essentially analogous to volume averaging and occurs if the ultrasound beam is too wide relative to the object being imaged. An example is imaging of a small calcification in which the relatively large beam width may eliminate shadowing. This effect can be reduced by adjusting the focal zone to the level of the object of interest.[7]

■ MISCELLANEOUS ULTRASOUND TECHNIQUES

Several ultrasound techniques or applications available with some ultrasound machines can enhance scanning and diagnostic capabilities. One such method is *spatial compound sonography*.[11] Unlike conventional ultrasound, sound beams with spatial compound sonography are produced at several different angles, with information combined to form a single ultrasound image. This improves tissue plane definition, but it has a smoothing effect, and motion blur is more likely because frames are compounded (Fig. 1.21). The use of spatial compounding may alter the artifact produced by a foreign body, which may change its conspicuity (see Fig. 2.47).

Another ultrasound technique is *tissue harmonic imaging*. Unlike conventional ultrasound, which receives only the fundamental or transmitted frequency to produce the image, with tissue harmonic imaging, harmonic frequencies produced during ultrasound beam propagation through tissues are used to produce the image. This technique assists in evaluation of deep structures and also improves joint and tendon surface visibility.[12,13] The technique may more clearly delineate the edge of a soft tissue mass (Fig. 1.22) or a fluid-filled tendon tear (Fig. 1.23). One pitfall is that hypoechoic tendinosis may appear more anechoic with tissue harmonic imaging and simulate a tendon tear.

One helpful technique available on some ultrasound machines is *extended field of view*. With this technique, an ultrasound image is produced by combining image information obtained during real-time scanning. This allows imaging of an entire muscle from origin to insertion; it is helpful in measuring large abnormalities (e.g., tumor or tendon tear) and in displaying and communicating ultrasound findings (Figs. 1.24 and 1.25).[14] An alternative to extended field of view imaging that is available on some ultrasound equipment is the split-screen function, which essentially joins two images on the display screen that doubles the field of view.

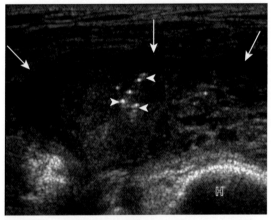

■ FIGURE 1.20 **Comet-Tail Artifact.** Ultrasound over an infected subacromial-subdeltoid bursa *(arrows)* shows hyperechoic foci of gas with comet-tail artifact *(arrowheads)*. H, Greater tuberosity of the humerus.

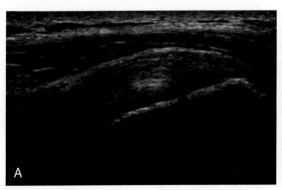 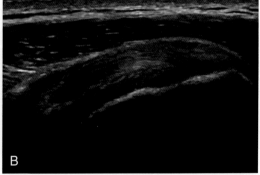

■ FIGURE 1.21 **Spatial Compounding.** Ultrasound images of the supraspinatus tendon without (A) and with (B) spatial compounding show softening of the image in B.

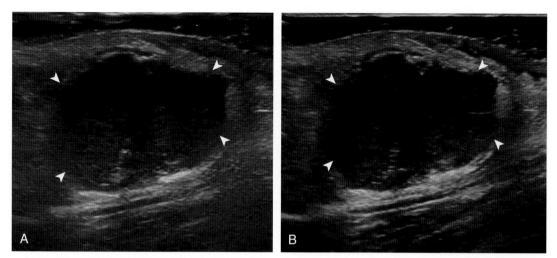

■ FIGURE 1.22 **Tissue Harmonic Imaging.** Ultrasound images of a recurrent giant cell tumor *(arrowheads)* without (A) and with (B) tissue harmonic imaging show increased definition of the mass borders in B. Note posterior increased through-transmission.

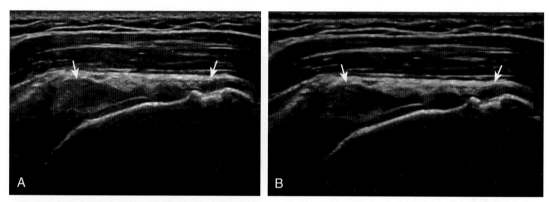

■ FIGURE 1.23 **Tissue Harmonic Imaging.** Ultrasound images of full-thickness supraspinatus tendon tear in long axis *(arrows)* without (A) and with (B) tissue harmonic imaging show clearer distinction of retracted tendon stump *(left arrow)* because intervening fluid is more hypoechoic.

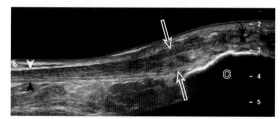

■ FIGURE 1.24 **Extended Field of View.** Ultrasound image of the Achilles tendon in long axis shows hypoechoic and enlarged tendinosis *(open arrows)* and retro-Achilles bursitis *(curved arrow).* Note the normal Achilles thickness proximally *(arrowheads). C,* Calcaneus.

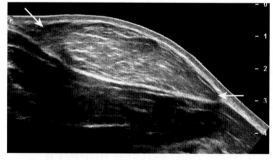

■ FIGURE 1.25 **Extended Field of View.** Ultrasound image shows full extent of a lipoma *(between arrows).*

A number of ultrasound techniques are relatively new, and their practical musculoskeletal applications are still being defined. One such technique is *three-dimensional ultrasound,* which acquires data as a volume (either mechanically or freehand) and thus enables reconstruction at any imaging plane (Fig. 1.26). This technique has been used to characterize rotator cuff tears and to quantify a volume of tissue such as tumor or synovial hypertrophy.[15,16] An additional technique

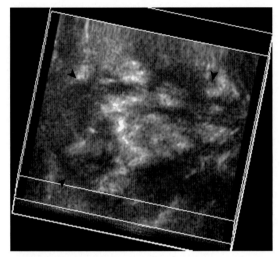

■ FIGURE 1.26 **Three-Dimensional Imaging.** Ultrasound image reconstructed in the coronal plane shows a heterogeneous thigh sarcoma *(arrowheads).*

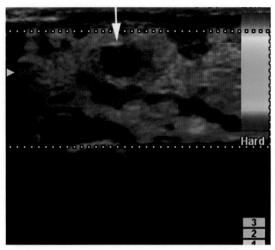

■ FIGURE 1.27 **Ultrasound Elastography: Foreign Body Granuloma.** Ultrasound image of common extensor tendon elbow shows suture granuloma *(blue mass-like area below white arrow).* Note that hard tissues are displayed in blue and soft tissues in red. *(Courtesy Y. Morag, Ann Arbor, Michigan.)*

is *fusion imaging*, in which real-time ultrasound imaging can be superimposed on computed tomography (CT) or MRI; this has been used to assist with needle guidance for sacroiliac joint injections.[17] One last technique is *sonoelastography*, which is used to assess the elastic properties of tissue. The three types of sonoelastography include compression elastography (using manual compression), shear wave elastography (using a directional shear wave), and transient elastography (using a short pulse).[18] With compression elastography, manual compression of tissue produces strain or displacement within the tissue. Displacement is less when tissue is hard; it is displayed as blue on the ultrasound image, whereas soft tissue is displayed as red (Fig. 1.27). With regard to musculoskeletal applications, normal tendons appear as blue, whereas areas of tendinopathy, such as of the Achilles tendon or common extensor tendon of the elbow, appear as red.[16,19-22] With shear wave and transient elastography, the velocity of the shear wave is measured to determine elasticity and has the advantage of less operator dependence and ability to produce qualitative and quantitative information.[18,23]

■ COLOR AND POWER DOPPLER

Most ultrasound machines include color and power Doppler imaging capabilities, with possible spectral waveform analysis. Ultrasound uses the *Doppler effect*, in which the sound frequency of an object changes as the object travels toward or away from a point of reference, to obtain information about blood flow. *Color flow imaging* shows

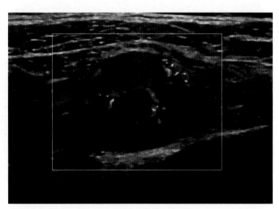

■ FIGURE 1.28 **Color Doppler: Schwannoma.** Color Doppler ultrasound image shows increased blood flow in hypoechoic peripheral nerve sheath tumor.

colored blood flow superimposed on a gray-scale image, in which two colors such as red and blue represent flow toward and away from the transducer, respectively (Fig. 1.28).[24] *Pulsed-wave* or *duplex Doppler ultrasound* displays an ultrasound image and waveform (Fig. 1.29). There are important considerations to optimize the Doppler ultrasound. Reducing the width of the field of view and increasing the frame rate are helpful. To correct for aliasing (when the Doppler shift frequency of blood is greater than the detected frequency, which causes an error in frequency measurement), one can increase the pulse repetition frequency, lower the ultrasound frequency, or increase the angle between the sound beam

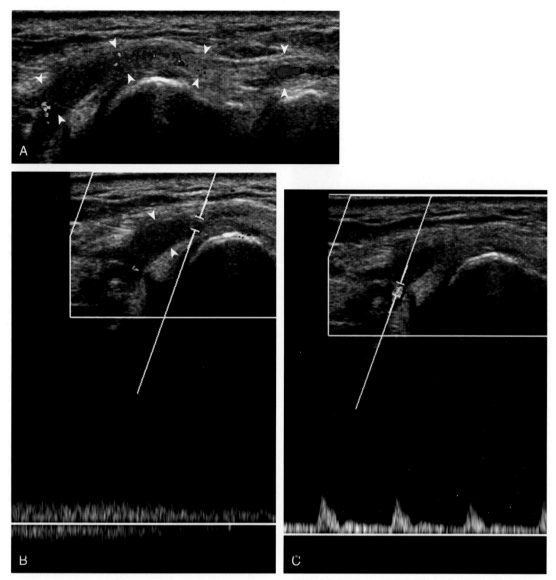

■ **FIGURE 1.29 Color Doppler: Radial Artery Thrombosis.** A, Color Doppler ultrasound image in long axis to the radial artery *(arrowheads)* at the wrist shows hypoechoic thrombus and diminished blood flow. B, Pulsed-wave Doppler shows the loss of normal arterial flow at the site of thrombus (B) and distal reconstitution from the deep palmar arch (C).

and the flow direction toward perpendicular. *Power Doppler* is another method of color Doppler ultrasound that is generally considered more sensitive to blood flow (it shows small vessels and slow flow rates) compared with conventional color Doppler, although significant variability exists depending on the ultrasound machine.[25] Unlike conventional color Doppler, power Doppler assigns a color to blood flow regardless of direction (Fig. 1.30) and is extremely sensitive to movement of the transducer, which produces a flash artifact. The color gain should be optimally adjusted for Doppler imaging to avoid artifact if the setting

is too sensitive and for false-negative flow if sensitivity is too low. To optimize power Doppler imaging, set the color background (without the gray-scale displayed) so that the lowest level of color nearly uniformly is present, with only minimal presence of the next highest color level.[26]

Increased blood flow on color or power Doppler imaging may occur with increased perfusion, inflammation, and neovascularity. In imaging soft tissues, color and power Doppler imaging are used to confirm that an anechoic tubular structure is a blood vessel and to confirm blood flow. When a mass is identified, increased blood

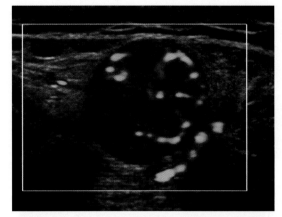

■ **FIGURE 1.30** **Power Doppler: Schwannoma**. Power Doppler ultrasound image shows increased blood flow in hypoechoic peripheral nerve sheath tumor.

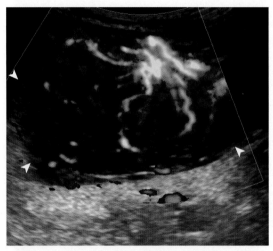

■ **FIGURE 1.31** **Power Doppler: B-Cell Lymphoma**. Power Doppler ultrasound image shows increased blood flow in hypoechoic lymphoma *(arrowheads)*. Note posterior increased through-transmission.

flow may suggest neovascularity, possibly from malignancy (Fig. 1.31).[27] Although the finding is nonspecific, a tumor without flow is more likely to be benign, and malignant tumors usually demonstrate increased flow and irregular vessels.[28] With regard to superficial lymph nodes, either no flow or hilar flow is more common with benign lymph node enlargement, and spotted, peripheral, or mixed patterns of flow are more common with malignant lymph node enlargement (see Chapter 2).[29] Color or power Doppler imaging is also helpful in the differentiation between complex fluid and a mass or synovitis; the former typically has no internal flow, and the latter may show increased flow.[30] After treatment for inflammatory

arthritis, color and power Doppler imaging can show interval decrease in flow, which would indicate a positive response.[31] It is also important to use color Doppler imaging during a biopsy to ensure that major vessels are avoided.

■ DYNAMIC IMAGING

One significant advantage of ultrasound over other static imaging methods, such as radiography, CT, and conventional MRI, is the *dynamic capability*. On a basic level, ultrasound evaluation can be directly guided by a patient's history, symptoms, and findings at physical examination. In fact, regardless of the protocol followed for imaging a joint, it is essential that ultrasound is focused during one aspect of the examination over any area of point tenderness or focal symptoms.[32] Once ultrasound examination is begun, the patient can directly provide feedback with regard to pain or other symptoms with transducer pressure over an ultrasound abnormality. When a patient has a palpable abnormality, direct palpation under ultrasound visualization will ensure that the imaged abnormality corresponds to the abnormality. Graded compression also provides additional information about soft tissue masses; lipomas are often soft and pliable (see Video 2.7).

In the setting of a rotator cuff tear, compression can help demonstrate the volume loss associated with a full-thickness tear (see Video 3.23). With regard to peripheral nerves, transducer pressure over a nerve at the site of entrapment can reproduce symptoms and help to guide the examination. Transducer pressure over a stump neuroma is also used to determine if a neuroma is causing symptoms. If during examination there is question of a complex fluid collection, variable transducer pressure can demonstrate swirling of internal debris and displacement, which indicates a fluid component (see Videos 6.14 to 6.16). In contrast, synovial hypertrophy would show only minimal compression without internal movement of echoes, with possible additional findings of flow on color and power Doppler imaging (see Video 8.5).

Dynamic imaging is also important in evaluation of complete full-thickness muscle, tendon, or ligament tear. When a full-thickness muscle or tendon tear is suspected, the muscle-tendon unit may be actively contracted or passively moved during imaging in long axis (see Videos 7.15 and 8.46). Demonstration of muscle or tendon stumps that move away from each other during this dynamic maneuver at the site of the tear indicates full-thickness extent. With regard to ligament tear, a joint can be stressed while imaging in long axis to the ligament to evaluate for ligament disruption and abnormal joint space widening. One example of this is applying valgus stress to the elbow when evaluating for ulnar collateral ligament tear (see Videos 4.15 to 4.17).

One last application of dynamic imaging is in evaluation of an abnormality that is present only when an extremity is moved or positioned in a particular manner. Examples of this include evaluation of the long head of biceps brachii tendon for subluxation or dislocation with shoulder external rotation (see Video 3.43), the ulnar nerve (see Video 4.21) and snapping triceps syndrome with elbow flexion (see Video 4.22), the peroneal tendon with dorsiflexion and eversion of the ankle (see Videos 8.30 to 8.33), and snapping hip syndrome (see Videos 6.18 to 6.21). Muscle contraction is often required for the diagnosis of muscle hernia (see Videos 8.40 to 8.42). Dynamic imaging of a patient during Valsalva maneuver is an essential component in evaluation for inguinal region hernia (see Videos 6.26 to 6.31). In addition to the foregoing examples, if the patient has any complaints that occur with a specific movement or position, the ultrasound transducer can be placed over the abnormal area, and the patient can be asked to re-create the symptom.

SELECT REFERENCES

  5. Gimber LH, Melville DM, Klauser AS, et al: Artifacts at musculoskeletal US: resident and fellow education feature. *Radiographics* 36(2):479–480, 2016.
 12. Anvari A, Forsberg F, Samir AE: A primer on the physical principles of tissue harmonic imaging. *Radiographics* 35(7):1955–1964, 2015.
 16. Klauser AS, Peetrons P: Developments in musculoskeletal ultrasound and clinical applications. *Skeletal Radiol* (Sep 3), 2009.
 18. Klauser AS, Miyamoto H, Bellmann-Weiler R, et al: Sonoelastography: musculoskeletal applications. *Radiology* 272(3):622–633, 2014.
 24. Boote EJ: AAPM/RSNA physics tutorial for residents: topics in US: Doppler US techniques: concepts of blood flow detection and flow dynamics. *Radiographics* 23(5):1315–1327, 2003.

The complete references for this chapter can be found on *www.expertconsult.com.*

BASIC PATHOLOGY CONCEPTS

■ MUSCLE AND TENDON INJURY

Muscle and tendon injuries may be categorized as acute and chronic. Acute injuries tend to take the form of direct impact injury, stretch injury during contraction (strain), or penetrating injury. Acute muscle injury can be clinically categorized as grade 1 (no appreciable fiber disruption), grade 2 (partial tear or moderate fiber disruption with compromised strength), and grade 3 (complete fiber disruption).[1] At sonography, muscle contusion and hemorrhage acutely appear hyperechoic (Fig. 2.1).[2,3] Excessive and intense muscle activity may produce diffuse muscle hyperechogenicity if imaged acutely from transient muscle edema, termed *delayed onset muscle soreness* (Fig. 2.2).[4] Muscle tears will appear as an abnormal hypoechoic or mixed echogenicity area or muscle defect.[5] One hallmark of full-thickness tear is muscle or tendon retraction, which is made more obvious with passive movement or active muscle contraction. Hemorrhage will later appear more hypoechoic

(Fig. 2.3), although a heterogeneous appearance with mixed echogenicity is common (Fig. 2.4). As soft tissue hemorrhage resorbs, a hematoma will become smaller and more echogenic, beginning at the periphery (Fig. 2.5). A residual anechoic fluid collection or seroma may remain (Fig. 2.6). Hemorrhage located between the subcutaneous fat and the adjacent hip musculature can occur with trauma as a degloving-type injury, called the *Morel-Lavallée lesion* (Fig. 2.7).[6] Residual scar formation appears hyperechoic (Fig. 2.8). Heterotopic ossification may remain and is hyperechoic with posterior acoustic shadowing (Fig. 2.9). An area of damaged muscle may ossify, termed *myositis ossificans* (Fig. 2.10), and ultrasound can show early mineralization before visualization on radiography.[7] Often, computed tomography (CT) is needed to demonstrate the characteristic peripheral rim of mineralization characteristic of myositis ossificans, given shadowing seen on ultrasound. Prior trauma to muscle or its nerve supply can result in muscle atrophy, which causes increased echogenicity and decreased size of the affected muscle (Fig. 2.11).

With direct impact injury, the belly of a muscle is typically involved with hematoma and variable fiber disruption (Fig. 2.12). In contrast, stretching of a contracting muscle typically results in injury at the musculotendinous junction and is more common with muscles that span two joints, such as the hamstring muscles (Fig. 2.13) and the medial head of the gastrocnemius (Fig. 2.14). The specific type of muscle architecture should be considered when evaluating for myotendinous injury. For example, a muscle with a unipennate architecture (e.g., the medial head of the gastrocnemius) shows injury at the myotendinous junction located at its periphery (Fig. 2.14).[8] A muscle with circumpennate or bipennate architecture (e.g., the indirect head of the rectus femoris) may show injury at its distal musculotendinous junction or within the muscle belly as a central aponeurosis tear (see Fig. 6.65A).[9] Musculotendinous injury also demonstrates variable echogenicity from hemorrhage and fluid, depending on the age of the injury and the degree of fiber disruption. Passive joint movement or active muscle contraction can demonstrate retraction at the site of the injury that indicates full-thickness tear. Particularly in children, these types of acute tendon injuries may

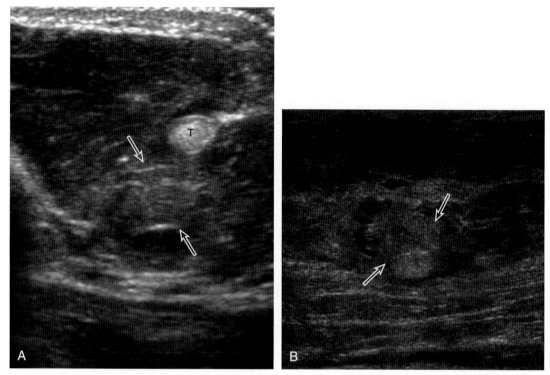

■ **FIGURE 2.1 Acute Muscle Injury.** Ultrasound images of (A) the thenar musculature and (B) the tibialis anterior muscle show areas of hyperechoic hemorrhage *(open arrows)*. *T*, Tendon.

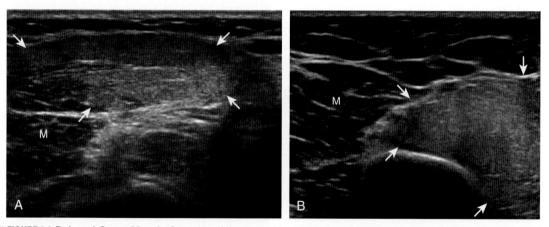

■ **FIGURE 2.2 Delayed Onset Muscle Soreness.** Ultrasound images of (A) brachioradialis and (B) brachialis muscle in short axis from two different patients show diffuse hyperechoic muscle edema *(arrows)* compared with normal muscle (M).

be associated with bone fragment avulsion at the tendon attachments, which appear hyperechoic with possible shadowing.

With penetrating injury or laceration, acute muscle and tendon injury may occur at any site. The obvious physical examination findings usually guide the ultrasound evaluation. Muscle and tendon injuries are again classified as partial-thickness or full-thickness tears. Dynamic imaging is helpful in this distinction because it makes retraction related to full-thickness tears more conspicuous. Gas introduced during the penetrating injury can make evaluation extremely difficult; air appears hyperechoic with heterogeneous posterior shadowing. In addition to muscle or tendon abnormality, penetrating injury may also produce bone and peripheral nerve injury (see Fig. 6.93B).

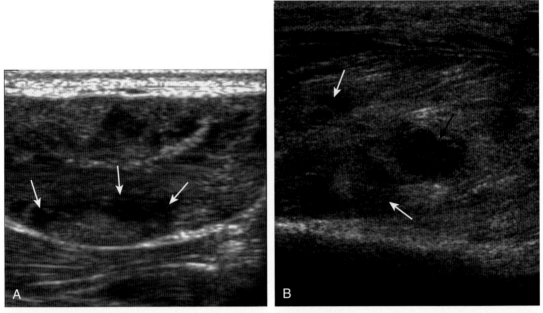

■ **FIGURE 2.3 Subacute Muscle Injury.** Ultrasound images of (A) the thenar musculature and (B) the tibialis anterior muscle show heterogeneous areas of hypoechoic hemorrhage *(arrows)*.

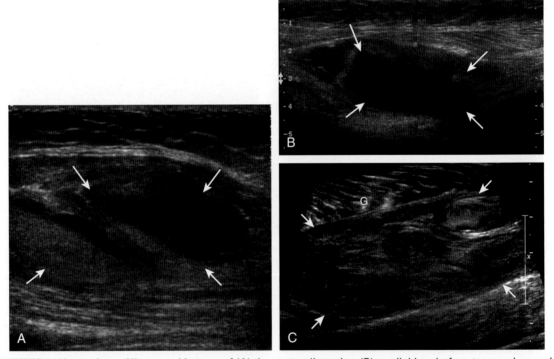

■ **FIGURE 2.4 Hemorrhage.** Ultrasound images of (A) the pectoralis major, (B) medial head of gastrocnemius, and (C) soleus show heterogeneous mixed echogenicity hemorrhage *(arrows)*. *G,* Gastrocnemius.

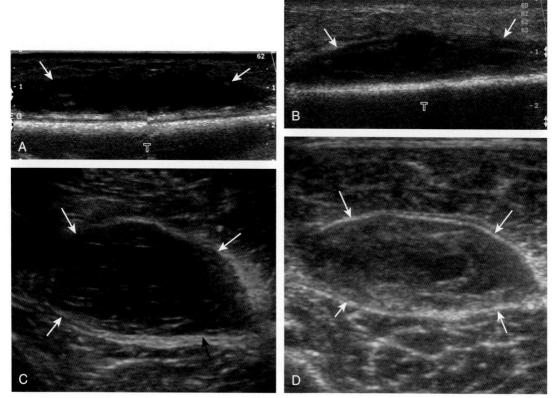

■ **FIGURE 2.5 Organizing Hematoma.** Ultrasound images (A and B) anterior to the tibia and (C and D) within the calf show interval decrease in size of hematoma *(arrows)* (A to B, C to D) with increased echogenicity at the periphery. *T,* Tibia.

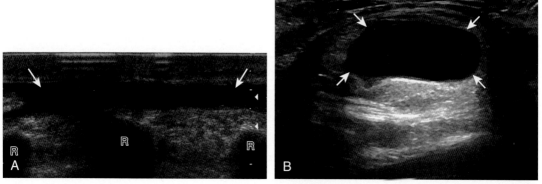

■ **FIGURE 2.6 Seroma.** Ultrasound images (A and B) from two different patients show anechoic fluid collection *(arrows)* at site of prior hemorrhage. *R,* Ribs in A.

Chronic muscle and tendon injuries are usually the result of overuse, with tendon degeneration and possible tear. It has been shown that such involved tendons show eosinophilic, fibrillar, and mucoid degeneration but do not contain acute inflammatory cells; therefore, the term *tendinosis* is used rather than *tendinitis*.[10-12] At sonography,

tendinosis appears as hypoechoic enlargement of the involved tendon, but without tendon fiber disruption (see later chapters). Several tendons may commonly show increased blood flow on color or power Doppler imaging in the setting of tendinosis, such as the patellar tendon, Achilles tendon, and common extensor tendon of the

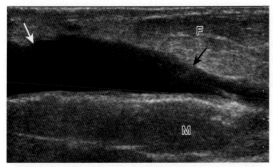

■ FIGURE 2.7 **Morel-Lavallée Lesion.** Ultrasound image over lateral hip shows anechoic fluid *(arrows)* at the site of prior hemorrhage between subcutaneous fat (F) and musculature (M).

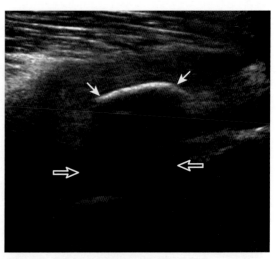

■ FIGURE 2.9 **Heterotopic Ossification.** Ultrasound image shows hyperechoic surface of heterotopic ossification *(arrows)* with posterior acoustic shadowing *(open arrows)*.

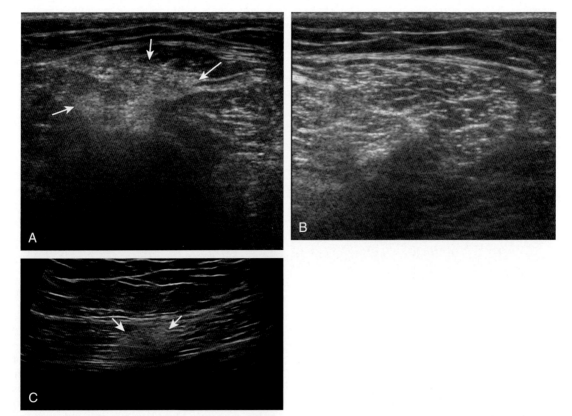

■ FIGURE 2.8 **Muscle Scar.** Ultrasound images of (A) the symptomatic semimembranosus and (B) the contralateral asymptomatic side show hyperechoic scar formation *(arrows)* and decreased size of affected muscle. Ultrasound image of (C) rectus femoris in long axis shows focal increased echogenicity *(arrows)*.

elbow. This increase in blood flow is not due to inflammation but rather represents neovascularity. Tendinosis may progress to partial-thickness and full-thickness tendon tear. Chronic muscle and tendon injuries that result in tear can be associated with atrophy of the muscle, which appears hyperechoic and decreased in size. After surgery, misplaced hardware or screw-tip penetration beyond the bone cortex may cause excessive wear of an adjacent tendon (Fig. 2.15). Ultrasound

is helpful in this diagnosis because artifact from metal hardware does not obscure overlying soft tissues. In addition, dynamic imaging with joint movement or muscle contraction can determine whether a tendon is in contact with metal hardware with specific positions (Video 2.1).

■ BONE INJURY

The normal osseous surfaces are smooth and echogenic with posterior shadowing and possibly reverberation when imaged perpendicular

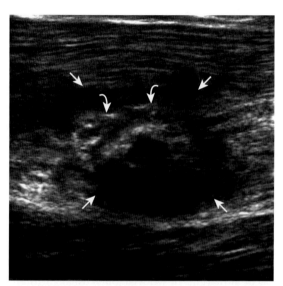

■ FIGURE 2.10 **Myositis Ossificans.** Ultrasound image shows hypoechoic hemorrhage *(arrows)* with echogenic mineralization *(curved arrows)*.

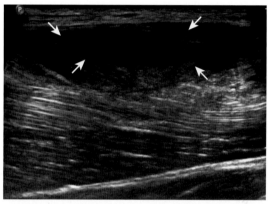

■ FIGURE 2.12 **Muscle Tear and Hematoma.** Ultrasound image of triceps brachii tendon in long axis shows heterogeneous but predominantly hypoechoic intramuscular hematoma *(arrows)* with partial muscle fiber disruption.

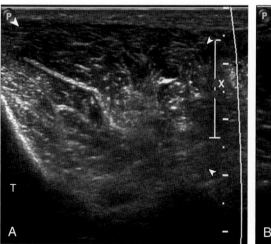
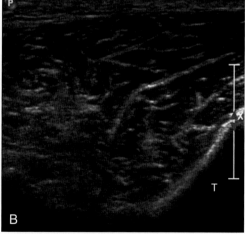

■ FIGURE 2.11 **Muscle Atrophy.** Ultrasound images of (A) the symptomatic tibialis anterior muscle and (B) the contralateral asymptomatic side show decreased size and increased echogenicity of the affected muscle *(arrowheads)*. *T,* Tibia.

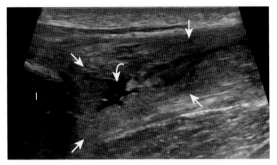

■ **FIGURE 2.13 Proximal Semimembranosus Injury.** Ultrasound image of semimembranosus tendon origin in long axis shows abnormal heterogeneous hypoechoic enlargement of the tendon *(arrows)* with anechoic interstitial tears *(curved arrow)*. *I*, Ischium.

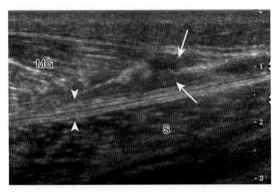

■ **FIGURE 2.14 Medial Head of Gastrocnemius Tear.** Ultrasound image of distal medial head of gastrocnemius in long axis shows hypoechoic disruption at the musculotendinous junction *(arrows)*. Note intact plantaris tendon *(arrowheads)*. *MG*, Medial head of gastrocnemius; *S*, soleus.

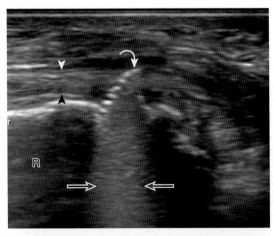

■ **FIGURE 2.15 Screw Impingement of Extensor Carpi Radialis Tendon.** Ultrasound image of extensor carpi radialis tendon in long axis *(arrowheads)* shows a metal screw with reverberation artifact *(open arrows)*, with the tip protruding into the tendon *(curved arrow)*. Note associated tenosynovitis. *R*, Radius.

to the sound beam. The hallmark of an acute fracture is discontinuity of the bone cortex with possible step-off deformity (Fig. 2.16).[13] Adjacent mixed echogenicity hemorrhage may also be present. A stress fracture, for example involving a metatarsal, may initially appear as an abnormal focal hypoechoic area adjacent to bone, which may progress to fracture step-off deformity or hyperechoic callus formation (see Fig. 8.145).[14] This is typically associated with point tenderness induced by pressure from the transducer. A patient also commonly indicates focal pain in the area. At the completion of any ultrasound examination a focused evaluation at location of symptoms often reveals underlying pathology that may not be otherwise evaluated.

Other types of bone injuries involve avulsion at tendon and ligament attachments. In these situations, a small fragment of bone with variable shadowing is seen attached to the involved tendon or ligament (see Fig. 8.140). Asymmetrical widening and irregularity of an open growth plate with adjacent hypoechogenicity and point tenderness can indicate a physeal injury (Fig. 2.17).[15] While ultrasound is sensitive in the identification of abnormalities involving the surfaces of bone, the findings are often not specific for one diagnosis. When cortical irregularity is identified at ultrasound, true bone injury must be differentiated from other etiologies such as osteophytes. This differentiation is possible because osteophytes occur at margins of synovial joints usually without point tenderness, whereas a fracture shows a cortical step-off deformity. Correlation with radiography should always be considered to assist with this differentiation.

In many situations in which a fracture is identified at ultrasound, the fracture is unsuspected. The indication for the examination is often to evaluate a soft tissue or joint abnormality after a "negative" radiograph. This is not uncommon in the foot and ankle, where multiple overlapping osseous structures may make radiographic diagnosis of fracture difficult. The other situation is the greater tuberosity fracture of the proximal humerus, which can be overlooked at radiography because of suboptimal patient positioning or suboptimal radiographic technique (see Fig. 3.103).[16] It has been shown that ultrasound is more effective than radiography in the diagnosis of rib fracture (see Fig. 2.16A).[17,18] As a fracture begins to heal, early hypoechoic callus becomes hyperechoic hard callus, which can eventually bridge the fracture gap or step-off deformity.[13] This can also be applied to limb-lengthening procedures, in which ultrasound can detect new bone prior to being seen at radiography. Ultrasound has also been shown to be effective in

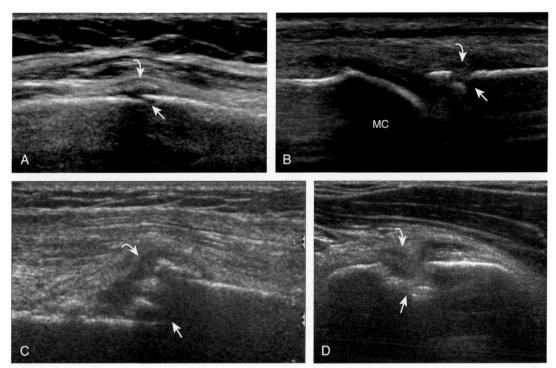

■ **FIGURE 2.16 Fractures.** Ultrasound images from four different patients show fractures as cortical discontinuity and step-off deformity *(arrows)* with variable hemorrhage *(curved arrows)* involving (A) rib, (B) proximal phalanx, (C) humerus, and (D) coracoid process. *MC,* Metacarpal head.

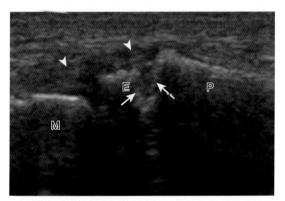

■ **FIGURE 2.17 Growth Plate Injury.** Ultrasound image of first metacarpophalangeal joint in long axis shows bone irregularity, widening, and offset at the physeal plate *(arrows)*. *E,* Epiphysis; *M,* metacarpal; *P,* proximal phalanx. Note the collateral ligament *(arrowheads)*.

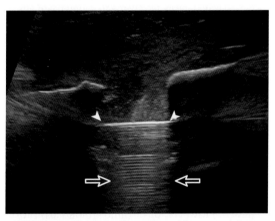

■ **FIGURE 2.18 Fracture Nonunion.** Ultrasound image shows hyperechoic intramedullary nail *(arrowheads)* with posterior reverberation artifact indicating incomplete healing of the tibial fracture *(open arrows)*.

diagnosis of tibial fracture nonunion with static interlocked nail placement; ultrasound can detect healing before radiography, whereas visualization of the hyperechoic nail indicates no overlying callus formation (Fig. 2.18).[13] Another advantage of ultrasound is in the evaluation of nonossified structures, such as the distal humeral epiphyses in children and the anterior costocartilage.[19,20]

■ INFECTION

The imaging appearances of soft tissue infection are largely predicted by the route of infection spread. For example, in adults, infection commonly occurs through a puncture wound or skin ulcer. This produces infection of the soft tissues or cellulitis, which may have several appearances

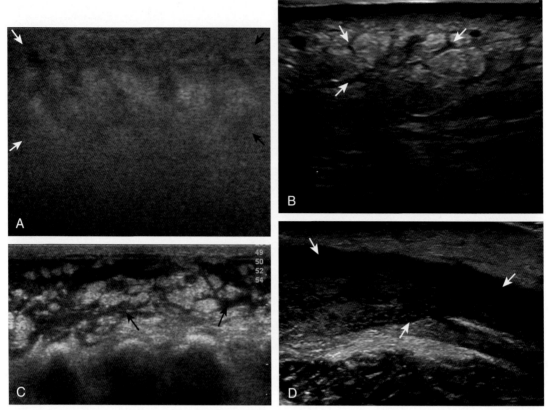

■ **FIGURE 2.19 Cellulitis: Progressive Findings.** Ultrasound images from four different patients show (A) diffuse increased echogenicity *(arrows)* with sound beam attenuation, (B) increased echogenicity with intervening hypoechoic channels *(arrows)*, (C) confluent hypoechoic fluid channels *(arrows)*, and (D) hypoechoic infected fluid collection *(arrows)*.

(Fig. 2.19). Acutely, cellulitis appears as hyperechoic and thickened subcutaneous tissue.[21,22] Later, hypoechoic or anechoic branching channels are visualized, with distortion of the soft tissues and possibly increased flow on color or power Doppler imaging.[21] Such branching channels can coalesce as purulent fluid and can progress to frank abscess, where ultrasound-guided aspiration may be of benefit.[21] However, ultrasound-guided aspiration may be less effective in the setting of methicillin-resistant *Staphylococcus aureus* infection.[23] When evaluating for cellulitis, the findings of anechoic perifascial fluid and gas (appearing as hyperechoic foci with comet-tail artifact or dirty shadowing) at the deep fascia can indicate necrotizing fasciitis.[24] The differential diagnosis for ultrasound findings of hyperechoic subcutaneous fat, as seen with acute cellulitis, includes fat necrosis (Fig. 2.20); however, the latter condition is usually more focal, may be multiple, and is without physical examination findings of infection.[25]

The ultrasound appearance of abscess is variable (Fig. 2.21) but commonly appears as well-defined

hypoechoic heterogeneous fluid collection with posterior through-transmission and peripheral hyperemia on color or power Doppler imaging.[26] A thick hyperechoic and hyperemic wall may also be seen, as may soft tissue gas.[27] Uncommonly, an abscess may be isoechoic or hyperechoic relative to the adjacent soft tissues (Fig. 2.21D). In this situation, in which it may be difficult to identify an abscess, increased through-transmission and swirling of echoes within the abscess with transducer pressure are helpful features to indicate the presence of a fluid component (Videos 2.2 and 2.3).[28] Increasing the depth and field of view around a possible abscess will often make the increased through-transmission more conspicuous relative to the surrounding tissues.

Some infections occur after surgery and may be located immediately adjacent to metal hardware (see Fig. 2.21E). Ultrasound is ideal for evaluation in this situation because the reverberation artifact from the hardware occurs deep to the metal and does not obscure the overlying soft tissues.[29] Soft tissue infection may also involve a bursa, which

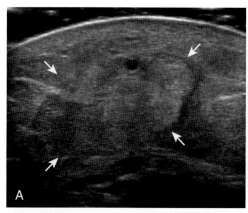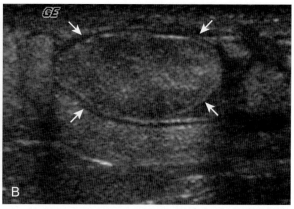

■ **FIGURE 2.20 Fat Necrosis.** Ultrasound images from two different patients show (A) hyperechoic subcutaneous area *(arrows)* and (B) focal hyperechoic nodule *(arrows)* representing fat necrosis. *(From Walsh M, Jacobson JA, Kim SM, et al: Sonography of fat necrosis involving the extremity and torso with magnetic resonance imaging and histologic correlation. J Ultrasound Med 27:1751–1757, 2008. Reproduced with permission from the American Institute of Ultrasound in Medicine.)*

can produce complex fluid and synovitis, and possibly gas, which appears hyperechoic with comet-tail artifact (Fig. 2.22; Video 2.4). Unlike a nonspecific abscess, a bursal fluid collection tends to be more defined and, more importantly, occurs where bursae reside. If an area of soft tissue infection is identified adjacent to bone, then osteomyelitis should be considered (Fig. 2.23). In the presence of cortical irregularity resulting from erosions or destruction, osteomyelitis is likely, although confirmation with magnetic resonance imaging (MRI) is typically required to fully assess the extent of infection.

Another route of infection is hematogenous, which may manifest as a muscle abscess, septic arthritis, or osteomyelitis. This mode of infection is more common in children, intravenous drug abusers, or patients with sepsis. In the correct clinical scenario, septic arthritis is suspected when there is fluid distention of a joint recess, which may range from anechoic to hyperechoic, with possible hypoechoic or isoechoic synovial hypertrophy (see later in this chapter). The echogenicity of fluid or the presence of flow on color or power Doppler imaging cannot predict the presence of infection, and therefore ultrasound-guided percutaneous fluid aspiration should be considered if there is concern for infection. When distention of a joint recess is not anechoic, the possibility of complex fluid versus synovial hypertrophy must be considered. To help in this distinction, compressibility of the recess, redistribution of the contents with joint positions, and lack of internal flow on color Doppler imaging suggest complex fluid rather than synovial hypertrophy. It is often difficult to predict if fluid is amenable to aspiration in this setting so ultrasound-guided aspiration

should always be considered if any joint recess distention is present when there is concern for infection, with possible lavage and aspiration if fluid is not initially aspirated. Joint aspiration can utilize ultrasound guidance to target the joint recess and avoid overlying cellulitis. If using fluoroscopy for guidance, ultrasound should be considered to evaluate the soft tissues for pathology thereby avoiding theoretical contamination of a sterile joint if a needle were passed through an abscess or infected bursa.[30] When synovial hypertrophy related to a septic joint is present, discontinuity or irregularity of the adjacent bone cortex suggests erosions and possible osteomyelitis (Fig. 2.24). Joint inflammation and synovitis from infection are indistinguishable from other inflammatory conditions, such as rheumatoid arthritis. In children, hematogenous spread of infection may also directly infect the bone. In this situation, a subperiosteal abscess may be identified because the periosteum is loosely adherent in children when compared with adults (Fig. 2.25).

■ ARTHRITIS

The foregoing descriptions relate to infection of soft tissues and bone. However, inflammation may have noninfective causes. Other inflammatory conditions, such as rheumatoid arthritis, can produce joint findings (effusion, synovial hypertrophy, and erosions), which can resemble infection.[31] Often, the distribution of the abnormalities and the clinical history assist with the differential diagnosis. Infection more commonly causes abnormalities at one site, and this diagnosis must be excluded before considering single-site involvement of a

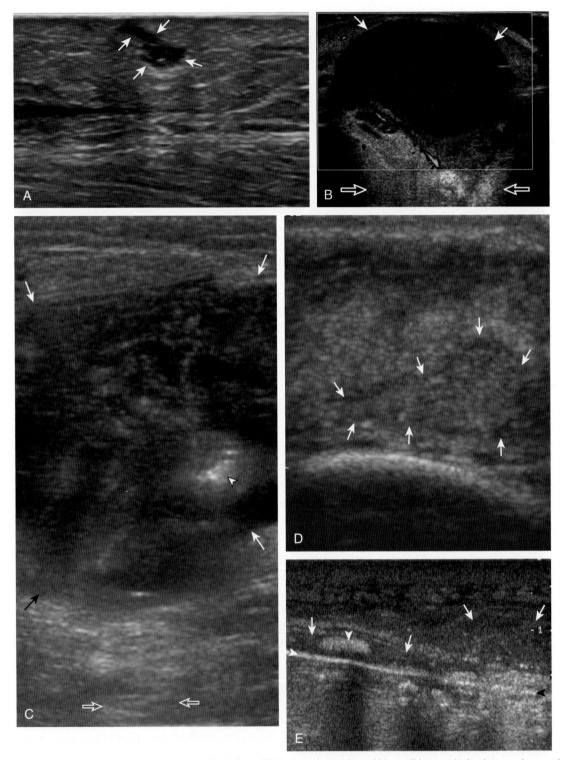

■ **FIGURE 2.21 Abscess.** Ultrasound images from five different patients show (A) small hypoechoic abscess *(arrows)* (methicillin-resistant *Staphylococcus aureus*) with surrounding cellulitis, (B) predominantly hypoechoic but heterogeneous abscess *(arrows)*, (C) heterogeneous abscess *(arrows)*, and (D) isoechoic abscess *(arrows)*. Note increased through-transmission *(open arrows)* in B and C and gas *(arrowhead)* in C. E, Ultrasound image shows isoechoic abscess *(arrows)* adjacent to metal side plate and screws *(arrowheads)*.

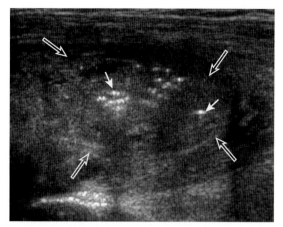

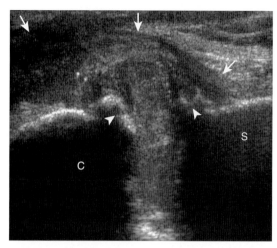

■ FIGURE 2.22 **Septic Bursitis With Gas.** Ultrasound image shows hyperechoic foci of gas *(arrows)* with comet-tail artifacts within a mixed hypoechoic and isoechoic septic subacromial-subdeltoid bursitis *(open arrows).*

■ FIGURE 2.24 **Septic Sternoclavicular Joint.** Ultrasound image shows heterogeneous distention of the sterno-clavicular joint capsule *(arrows).* Note erosions *(arrowheads)* of the sternum (S) and clavicle (C). *(From Johnson M, Jacobson JA, Fessell DP, et al: The sterno-clavicular joint: can imaging differentiate infection from degenerative change? Skeletal Radiol 39:551–558, 2010.)*

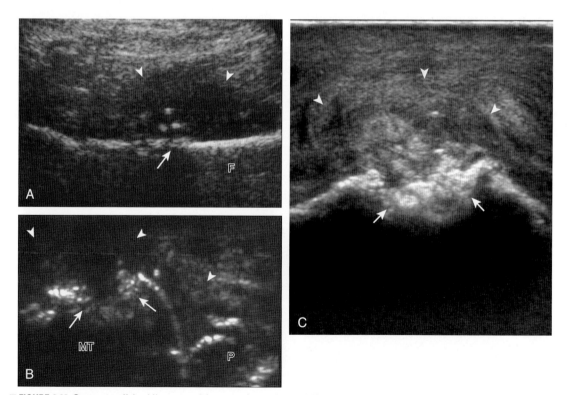

■ FIGURE 2.23 **Osteomyelitis.** Ultrasound images from three different patients show (A) bone destruction *(arrow)* and hypoechoic abscess *(arrowheads)* of the femur (F), (B) cortical destruction *(arrows)* with adjacent hypoechoic infection *(arrowheads)* of the metatarsal head (MT), and (C) bone destruction *(arrows)* at tibial amputation site with adjacent inflammation *(arrowheads).* P, Proximal phalanx.

systemic inflammatory arthritis. The following represents general concepts of some inflammatory conditions with additional examples and text found in later chapters.

Rheumatoid Arthritis

The characteristic features of rheumatoid arthritis at ultrasound include synovial hypertrophy and erosions.[32] Ultrasound can be used for early diagnosis, assessment of response to therapy, and can guide injections or aspirations.[33] Synovial hypertrophy appears as hypoechoic (Figs. 2.26 and 2.27) or, less commonly, isoechoic or hyperechoic relative to subdermal fat, poorly compressible tissue within a joint or a joint recess.[34] Synovial hypertrophy may also involve other synovial spaces, such as a bursa or tendon sheath (Fig. 2.28). Flow may be seen on color or power Doppler imaging, depending on the inflammatory activity of the synovitis. When assessing for hyperemia of synovial hypertrophy, transducer pressure should be minimized to avoid occluding

or dampening flow (Fig. 2.29; Video 2.5). Synovial hypertrophy may be seen in the dorsal recesses of the wrist, the volar and dorsal recesses of the metacarpophalangeal and interphalangeal joints of the hand, and the metatarsophalangeal and interphalangeal joints of the feet.[35,36] In the diagnosis of synovial hypertrophy related to rheumatoid arthritis, both ultrasound and MRI perform similarly.[37] However, minimal synovial hypertrophy is not specific for one disease and is often seen in normal asymptomatic wrists.[38] Erosions appear as discontinuity of the bone cortex seen in two orthogonal planes as seen with ultrasound (Fig. 2.30).[34] Such erosions begin in the marginal regions of a joint, where the bone cortex is not covered with hyaline cartilage and is directly exposed to joint inflammation.[32] Ultrasound is sensitive to bone cortex abnormalities but is not specific for erosions, with a reported false-positive rate of 29% for diagnosis of true

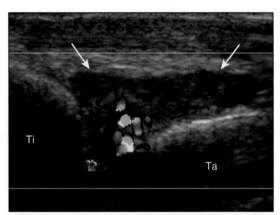

■ FIGURE 2.27 **Rheumatoid Arthritis: Synovial Hypertrophy.** Ultrasound image in the sagittal plane over the anterior ankle shows hypoechoic synovial hypertrophy *(arrows)* distending the dorsal ankle joint recess with hyperemia. *Ti,* Tibia; *Ta,* talus.

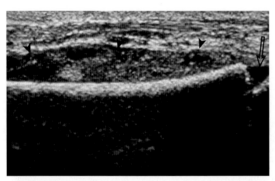

■ FIGURE 2.25 **Subperiosteal Abscess.** Ultrasound image shows isoechoic subperiosteal abscess *(arrowheads)* *(open arrow,* physis). *(Courtesy P. Strouse, MD, Ann Arbor, Michigan.)*

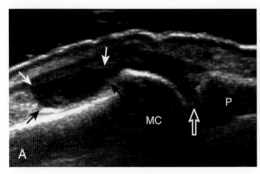

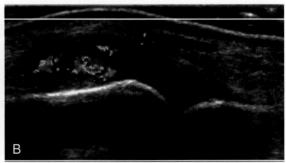

■ FIGURE 2.26 **Rheumatoid Arthritis: Hypoechoic Synovial Hypertrophy.** Ultrasound images in the sagittal plane show hypoechoic synovial hypertrophy *(arrows)* and hyperemia distending the dorsal (A) second and (B) third metacarpophalangeal joint recesses, which extend from the metacarpophalangeal joint articulation *(open arrow).* *MC,* Metacarpal head; *P,* proximal phalanx.

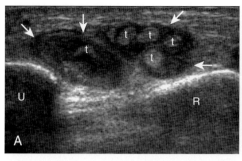 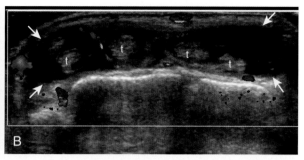

■ **FIGURE 2.28 Rheumatoid Arthritis: Tenosynovitis.** Ultrasound images in short axis to the extensor tendons of the wrist in two different patients show (A) hypoechoic synovial hypertrophy *(arrows)* and (B) anechoic fluid *(arrows)* and hyperemia. *t,* Tendons; *R,* radius; *U,* ulna.

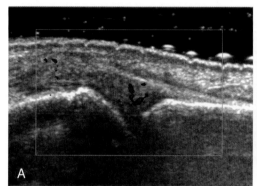 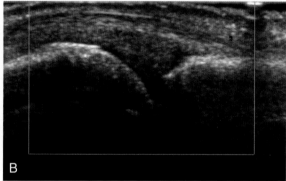

■ **FIGURE 2.29 Hyperemia: Effects of Compression (Rheumatoid Arthritis).** Ultrasound images in the sagittal plane of the third metacarpophalangeal joint dorsal recess (A) without and (B) with minimal transducer pressure show hyperemia of dorsal triangular connective tissue that is obliterated with transducer pressure. Note intervening thick gel layer between the transducer and skin surface in A.

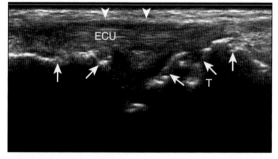

■ **FIGURE 2.30 Rheumatoid Arthritis: Erosions.** Ultrasound image over the lateral wrist in the coronal plane shows osseous erosions *(arrows)* and extensor carpi ulnaris (ECU) tenosynovitis *(arrowheads).* *T,* Triquetrum.

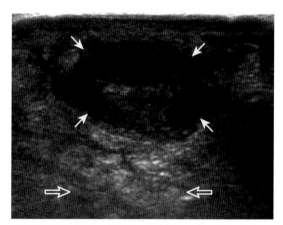

■ **FIGURE 2.31 Rheumatoid Nodule.** Ultrasound image shows hypoechoic rheumatoid nodule *(arrows).* Note posterior increased through-transmission *(open arrows).*

erosions.[39] The finding of synovial hypertrophy directly over a cortical irregularity also increases the likelihood that an erosion is present. Correlation with radiographic and clinical findings remains important, in addition to the distribution of imaging findings. For example, rheumatoid arthritis commonly involves the metacarpophalangeal joints of the hands (especially the second),

the metatarsophalangeal joints of the feet (usually at least the fifth), and the wrist joints (especially the distal ulna).[40] A rheumatoid nodule typically appears as a hypoechoic nodule at ultrasound (Fig. 2.31).[41]

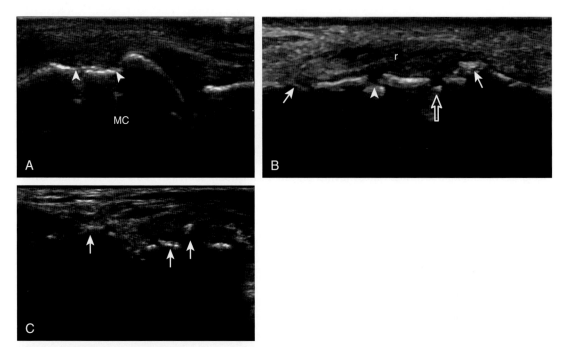

■ **FIGURE 2.32 Psoriatic Arthritis.** Ultrasound image shows (A) metacarpal head (MC) erosion *(arrowheads)*, (B) radial collateral ligament (r) of a proximal interphalangeal joint *(open arrow)* with areas of bone proliferation at the ligament attachments *(arrows)* and an erosion *(arrowhead)* with adjacent hypoechoic soft tissue swelling, and (C) dorsal wrist in the transverse plane with diffuse areas of bone proliferation *(arrows)* and overlying hypoechoic soft tissue swelling.

Psoriatic Arthritis

Psoriatic arthritis also involves synovial articulations, which can cause joint effusion, synovial hypertrophy, and erosions (Fig. 2.32A).[42] One distinguishing feature of psoriatic arthritis, similar to other seronegative spondyloarthropathies, is the presence of bone proliferation at tendon and ligament attachments (Fig. 2.32B and C).[43] Such sites, such as the collateral ligaments of the digits, should be included when evaluating for psoriatic arthritis, often directed by patient symptoms or physical examination findings. Because bone proliferation of psoriatic arthritis may at times appear similar to other forms of bone proliferation, such as osteophytes with osteoarthritis, it is critical to correlate with radiography to assist in this distinction. The presence of hyperemia, often seen in psoriatic arthritis, is another feature. Similarly, a degenerative enthesophyte must be differentiated from true inflammatory enthesopathy at a tendon attachment, with the latter showing hyperemia and adjacent tendon abnormality at ultrasound and indistinct cortical margins on radiography. The soft tissues over a joint or tendon may also show abnormal swelling and hyperemia.[44]

Gout

The ultrasound findings of gout include joint effusion (with possible visualization of hyperechoic crystals), erosions, and tophi.[45] Joint distention may range from anechoic to heterogeneous, especially in the presence of crystals, tophi, and synovial hypertrophy (Fig. 2.33A). In addition, crystal deposition on the surface of the cartilage (urate icing) will appear hyperechoic, also called the *double contour sign* (Fig. 2.33B). This finding is differentiated from the normal hyperechoic cartilage interface in that the latter is only seen when the sound beam is perpendicular to the cartilage surface and is uniform. The double contour sign is also different from chondrocalcinosis, in which reflective echoes from crystals are located within the cartilage rather than on the surface, as seen with calcium pyrophosphate deposition disease.[46] Monosodium urate tophi characteristically appear as an amorphous but fairly well-defined echogenic area with internal foci of hyperechoic foci surrounded by a hypoechoic inflammatory halo (Fig. 2.34). A tophus may be associated with adjacent cortical erosion, especially at the medial aspect of the distal first metatarsal (Fig. 2.35). Tendon and

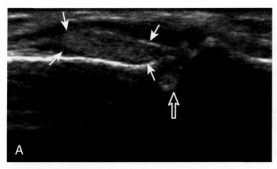 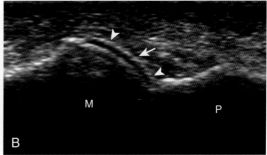

■ **FIGURE 2.33 Gout.** Ultrasound images show (A) hyperechoic joint effusion *(arrows)* distending dorsal recess of the first metatarsophalangeal joint *(open arrow)*, (B) urate crystal deposition on the hyaline cartilage *(arrowheads)* (double contour sign). *M*, Metatarsal head; *P*, proximal phalanx. *(B, Courtesy Ralf Thiele, MD, Rochester, New York.)*

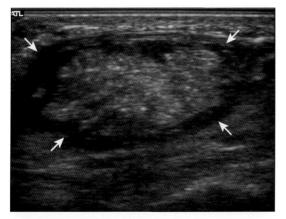

■ **FIGURE 2.34 Gout: Tophus.** Ultrasound image shows hyperechoic soft tissue tophus with hypoechoic rim *(arrows)*.

tendon sheath involvement are also possible (Fig. 2.36). Other common sites for tophi include the olecranon region at the elbow (see Fig. 4.31), as well as the patellar tendon (see Fig. 7.57) and the popliteus tendon (see Fig. 7.58) at the knee.

Osteoarthritis

The hallmark of osteoarthritis is cartilage loss and osteophyte formation, typically in a predictable distribution related primarily to wear-and-tear of a joint. Synovial hypertrophy is often secondary and relatively mild without pronounced hyperemia compared with other conditions, such as rheumatoid arthritis.[47] Ultrasound can detect findings of osteoarthritis, especially in accessible peripheral joints.[48] Osteophytes appear as a well-defined bone excrescence at a margin of an involved joint. Joint effusion may also be present. Common sites of involvement include the first metatarsophalangeal joint (Fig. 2.37), the interphalangeal and first carpometacarpal joints of the hand and wrist (Fig. 2.38), and the acromioclavicular joint.[49] First metatarsophalangeal joint fluid and acromiocla-

vicular joint involvement are commonly asymptomatic with preclinical osteoarthritis. Synovial hypertrophy may also be seen as hypoechoic, minimally compressible tissue distending a joint recess, although such minimal findings are also commonly seen in asymptomatic joints such as the interphalangeal joints of the hand.[49] In addition, increased flow on color or power Doppler imaging is uncommon, and the presence of synovial hypertrophy does not necessarily correlate with patient symptoms.[47]

■ MYOSITIS AND DIABETIC MUSCLE INFARCTION

Inflammatory myositis, such as polymyositis, appears hyperechoic with possible increased flow on color or power Doppler imaging (Fig. 2.39).[50] In later stages, increased muscle echogenicity and diminished volume are characteristic of muscle atrophy. Sarcoidosis may also involve muscle, where the nodular type of sarcoidosis produces hypoechoic masses or nodules.[51]

In the evaluation of inflammation or infection around the thigh or calf, one condition in the differential diagnosis is *diabetic muscle infarction*. In this condition, the involved thigh musculature is hypoechoic and enlarged, although the hyperechoic fibroadipose septum or epimysium are still identified throughout, a feature that helps to exclude soft tissue abscess or tumor (Fig. 2.40).[52] Subfascial fluid may also be seen. Diabetic muscle infarction most commonly involves the thigh or calf musculature, it may be bilateral, and it occurs in patients with longstanding diabetes and without laboratory findings to support infection.

■ SOFT TISSUE FOREIGN BODIES

Another cause of soft tissue infection is a soft tissue foreign body. At sonography, all foreign

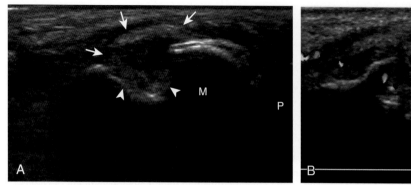

■ **FIGURE 2.35 Gout: Tophus and Erosion.** Ultrasound images in axial plane over medial distal first metatarsal show (A and B) cortical erosion *(arrowheads)* and adjacent echogenic tophus *(arrows)* with increased flow on color Doppler imaging. *M*, Metatarsal; *P*, proximal phalanx.

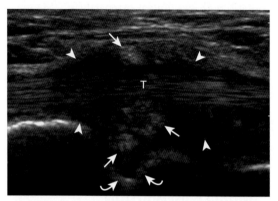

■ **FIGURE 2.36 Gout: Tophus and Tenosynovitis.** Ultrasound image shows hyperechoic tophus *(arrows)* surrounding the tibialis posterior tendon (T) causing osseous erosion *(curved arrows)* and surrounding hypoechoic tenosynovitis *(arrowheads)*.

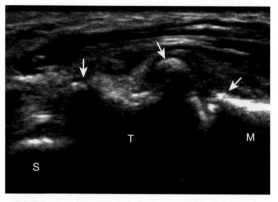

■ **FIGURE 2.38 Osteoarthritis: Trapezium.** Ultrasound image over thumb base shows trapezium (T) osteophytes *(arrows)* at articulations with scaphoid (S) and first metacarpal (M).

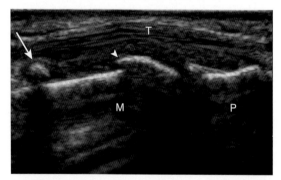

■ **FIGURE 2.37 Osteoarthritis: First Metacarpophalangeal Joint.** Ultrasound image dorsally over first metacarpophalangeal joint shows osteophytes *(arrowhead)* an intra-articular body *(arrow)*. *M*, Metacarpal; *P*, proximal phalanx; *T*, extensor tendon.

bodies are initially hyperechoic (Fig. 2.41), although organic or plant material may become less echogenic over time.[53] The surface of the foreign body is more echogenic and conspicuous when the sound beam is perpendicular to the

surface of the foreign body (Fig. 2.42). Therefore, in addition to directly imaging over the entry site, the involved soft tissues should also be interrogated at various angles in order to direct the sound beam perpendicular to the surface of the foreign body and eliminate anisotropy. It is often helpful to use a thick layer of gel to float the transducer above the skin surface so as not to overlook any superficial foreign bodies and to optimize the sound beam angulation (Fig. 2.42D).

Conspicuity of a soft tissue foreign body is additionally enhanced by the soft tissue reaction around the foreign body and the foreign body artifact if present.[54] A hypoechoic halo with possible hyperemia may be present, representing hemorrhage, granulation tissue, or abscess. This produces a halo appearance as the hypoechoic reaction surrounds the hyperechoic foreign body (Fig. 2.43). Some foreign bodies, such as metal, may have little if any foreign body response (Fig. 2.44).

Foreign body artifact depends on the surface attributes of the foreign body rather than its

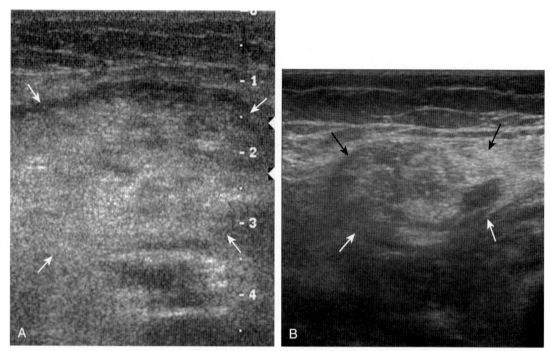

■ FIGURE 2.39 **Myositis.** Ultrasound images show (A) increased echogenicity and size of the sartorius *(arrows)* representing inflammatory myositis and (B) increased echogenicity of the rectus femoris *(arrows)* representing post-chemotherapy and radiation recall myositis.

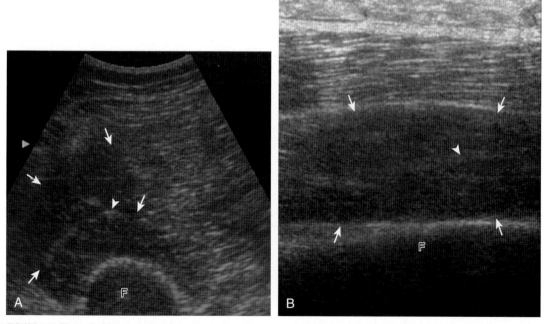

■ FIGURE 2.40 **Diabetic Muscle Infarction.** Ultrasound images in (A) short axis and (B) long axis to the rectus femoris show hypoechoic swelling of the vastus intermedius muscle *(arrows)*. Note visible hyperechoic fibroadipose septa or epimysium *(arrowheads)*. F, Femur.

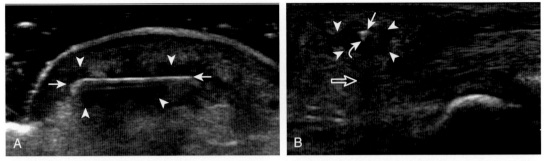

■ **FIGURE 2.41 Wooden Foreign Body.** Ultrasound images in (A) long axis and (B) short axis to a hyperechoic wooden foreign body *(arrows)* show hypoechoic halo *(arrowheads)* with mild shadowing *(open arrow)* and posterior reverberation *(curved arrow)* artifact.

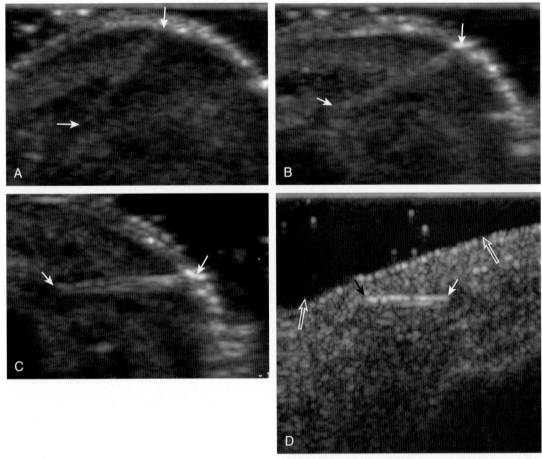

■ **FIGURE 2.42 Wooden Foreign Body.** A to C, Ultrasound images show hyperechoic wooden splinter *(arrows)*, which becomes more echogenic and conspicuous when imaged perpendicular to the sound beam. D, Ultrasound image shows thick layer of gel *(open arrows)* used to allow the wooden foreign body *(arrows)* to be imaged perpendicular to the sound beam.

internal composition.[53] For example, a foreign body with a smooth and flat surface, such as glass, produces posterior reverberation artifact (Fig. 2.45). A foreign body with an irregular surface and small radius of curvature usually shows posterior shadowing (Fig. 2.46). Many foreign bodies show both shadowing and reverberation artifact (see Figs. 2.41 and 2.44). Evaluation of a foreign body should include a field of view that includes soft tissues deep to the foreign body to recognize any posterior artifact. The use of spatial compound sonography may smooth out the image

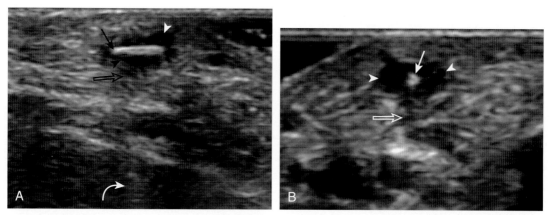

■ **FIGURE 2.43 Wooden Foreign Body.** Ultrasound images in (A) long axis and (B) short axis to a hyperechoic rose thorn *(arrow)* show hypoechoic halo *(arrowheads)* with mild shadowing *(open arrow)* and posterior reverberation *(curved arrow)* artifact.

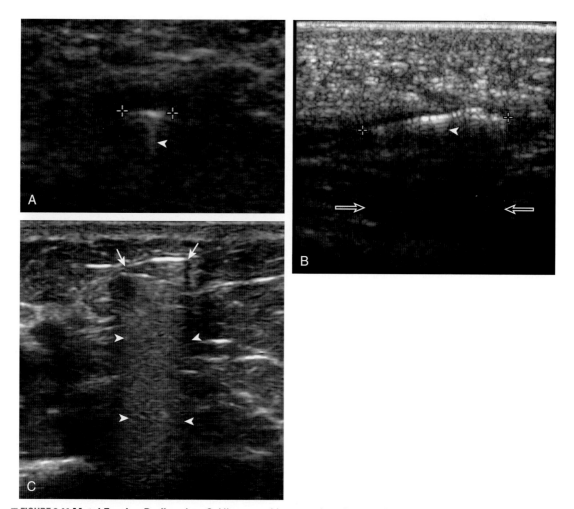

■ **FIGURE 2.44 Metal Foreign Bodies.** A to C, Ultrasound images show hyperechoic needles *(calipers* or *arrows)* and variable posterior reverberation artifact *(arrowheads)* and heterogeneous shadowing *(open arrows)*. Note little foreign body response.

that may affect the appearance of the foreign body and associated artifacts (Fig. 2.47).

Although ultrasound can accurately identify and localize soft tissue foreign bodies, ultrasound has an essential role in evaluation of foreign bodies that are not radiopaque on radiography, such as those composed of wood or plastic (Fig. 2.48).[53] All glass is opaque on radiographs regardless of color or tint if large enough to be resolved, if projected off adjacent osseous structures, and if

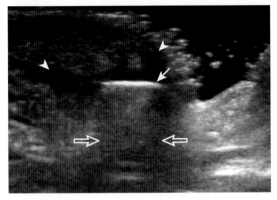

■ FIGURE 2.45 **Glass Foreign Body.** Ultrasound image shows hyperechoic glass foreign body *(arrow)*, adjacent hypoechoic inflammation *(arrowheads)*, and central posterior reverberation artifact and peripheral shadowing *(open arrows)*.

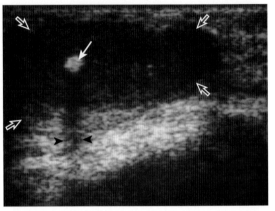

■ FIGURE 2.46 **Wooden Foreign Body.** Ultrasound image shows a hyperechoic wooden splinter *(arrow)* with posterior acoustic shadowing *(arrowheads)* and a surrounding hypoechoic abscess *(open arrows)*. Note increased through-transmission deep to the abscess.

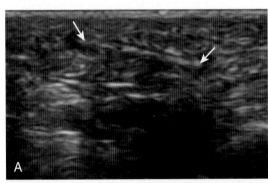

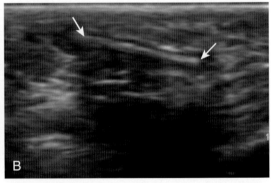

■ FIGURE 2.47 **Spatial Compound Sonography.** Ultrasound images (A) without and (B) with spatial compounding show the hyperechoic wooden foreign body *(arrows)* and mild hypoechoic halo.

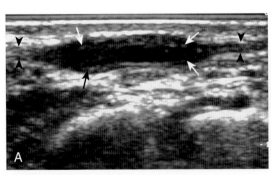

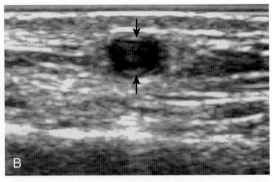

■ FIGURE 2.48 **Plastic Catheter Foreign Body.** Ultrasound images in (A) long axis and (B) short axis to a superficial foot vein show the hyperechoic walls *(arrows)* of the plastic catheter within the collapsed vein *(arrowheads)*. *(From Fessell DP, Jamadar DA, Jacobson JA, et al: Sonography of dorsal ankle and foot abnormalities.* AJR Am J Roentgenol *181:1571–1573, 2003.)*

imaged with proper radiographic technique.[53] One potential pitfall in sonography of soft tissue of foreign bodies is the presence of soft tissue gas, usually the result of prior attempted removal or, less likely, infection, which in itself may simulate a foreign body and alter the sonographic characteristics of a foreign body (Fig. 2.49; Video 2.6).[55]

Ultrasound can also assess for related complications, such as adjacent tenosynovitis (Fig. 2.50), periostitis (Fig. 2.51), and abscess (Fig. 2.52).[54] Ultrasound can aid removal by accurately marking the skin surface over the foreign body before removal, by guiding a localization wire, or by directly guiding percutaneous removal.[56,57] A chronic foreign body reaction may simulate a soft tissue mass at imaging.

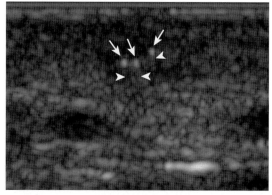

■ FIGURE 2.49 **Soft Tissue Gas.** Ultrasound image shows hyperechoic gas foci *(arrows)* with comet-tail artifacts *(arrowheads)*. No foreign body was present.

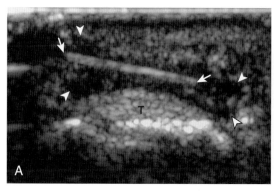

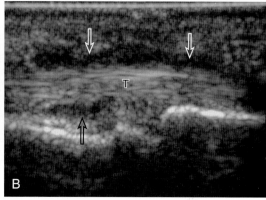

■ FIGURE 2.50 **Foreign Body: Septic Tenosynovitis.** Ultrasound images (A and B) show a hyperechoic wooden splinter *(arrows)* with a hypoechoic halo *(arrowheads)* and more proximal septic tenosynovitis *(open arrows).* *T,* Flexor digitorum profundus tendon.

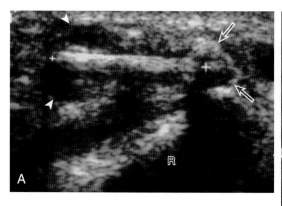

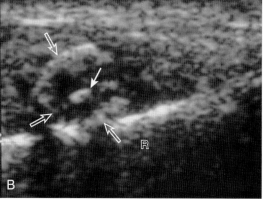

■ FIGURE 2.51 **Foreign Body: Periostitis.** Ultrasound images (A to C) show a hyperechoic wooden splinter *(calipers and arrow)* with a hypoechoic halo *(arrowheads)* and hyperechoic periostitis *(open arrows).* *R,* Radius.

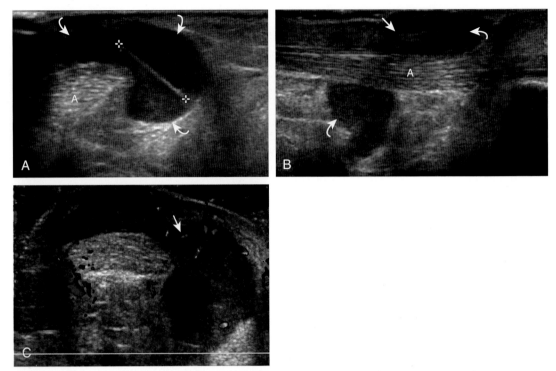

■ **FIGURE 2.52 Foreign Body: Abscess**. Ultrasound images (A and B) show hyperechoic wooden foreign body *(calipers and arrow)* with surrounding hypoechoic abscess *(curved arrows)* and hyperemia. *A*, Achilles tendon.

■ PERIPHERAL NERVE ENTRAPMENT

There are specific anatomic sites where a peripheral nerve may be entrapped, typically when a nerve traverses a confined space as a result of osseous, ligamentous, or fibrous constraints.[58-60] Examples in the upper extremity include the median nerve in the carpal tunnel (carpal tunnel syndrome) (see Fig. 5.62), the ulnar nerve in the Guyon canal (ulnar canal syndrome) (see Fig. 5.72), the ulnar nerve in the cubital tunnel of the elbow (cubital tunnel syndrome) (see Fig. 4.55), and the deep branch of the radial nerve at the level of the supinator muscle (see Fig. 4.67). Examples in the lower extremity include the tibial nerve at the ankle (tarsal tunnel syndrome) (see Fig. 8.152) and the common plantar digital nerve in the distal foot (Morton neuroma) (see Fig. 8.149). Common sonographic features of each of these conditions are hypoechoic enlargement of the involved nerve at and proximal to the entrapment site with possible compression distally. Transducer pressure on the involved nerve segment often elicits symptoms. Evaluation for denervation and muscle atrophy is also a clue to peripheral nerve entrapment and chronicity, where ultrasound shows increased echogenicity of the involved muscle. Knowledge of peripheral nerve anatomy and sites prone to nerve compression is essential for an accurate diagnosis.

■ SOFT TISSUE MASSES

Although the etiology of some soft tissue tumors may be suggested based on anatomic location, physical examination findings, and the patient's history and age, many masses remain nonspecific by ultrasound. The primary roles of ultrasound in this situation are to differentiate cyst versus solid mass, and to guide biopsy for definitive histologic diagnosis when required. Ultrasound does play an important role in the assessment of benign subcutaneous masses by improving diagnostic accuracy.[61] In the following chapters, soft tissue masses that are specific or common to each anatomic region are discussed. Some masses occur throughout the body and have similar sonographic features regardless, and several of these are discussed here.

Lipoma

Soft tissue lipomas can occur anywhere in the body and may be multiple, although many lipomas involve the shoulder region, upper extremity, trunk, and back. Soft tissue lipomas may be located within

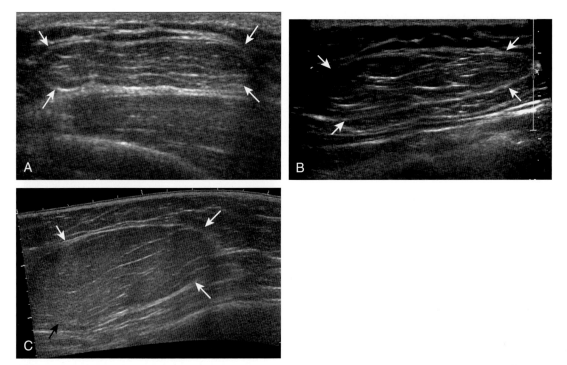

■ **FIGURE 2.53 Subcutaneous Lipomas.** Ultrasound images from three different patients show well-defined oval isoechoic to minimally hyperechoic subcutaneous lipomas *(arrows)*.

the subcutaneous fat, within muscle, or within tissue planes. When present in the subcutaneous tissues, the findings of a homogeneous, oval, isoechoic to minimally hyperechoic mass, with little or no flow on color or power Doppler imaging, that is soft and pliable with transducer pressure are compatible with lipoma (Fig. 2.53; Video 2.7). If any clinical findings are worrisome, such as associated pain or enlarging mass, MRI is recommended for confirmation. When a lipoma is located in an intramuscular location, the appearance is somewhat nonspecific but often is relatively hyperechoic (Fig. 2.54).[62] Because a lipoma in a deep or intramuscular location is more difficult to characterize by ultrasound and assess clinically, MRI is indicated to evaluate any intramuscular mass.

The echogenicity of a lipoma may be variable related to the amount of fat and connective tissue in the tumor as well as to the surrounding tissue echogenicity. For example, a homogeneous fatty mass is hypoechoic; as the amount of fibrous tissue within the lipoma increases, the lipoma will appear more hyperechoic owing to the reflective soft tissue interfaces (Fig. 2.55).[62] In addition, a lipoma that is isoechoic to the surrounding subcutaneous fat appears relatively hyperechoic when located in muscle. Subcutaneous lipomas that are isoechoic to the surrounding tissues may not be immediately apparent on ultrasound. Imaging findings should be directly correlated with physical examination

findings, with direct palpation of the mass under ultrasound visualization (Video 2.8), or by placing an opened paper clip or other similar marker over the edge of the palpable mass and then scanning the region.[56]

The sensitivity and specificity of ultrasound in the diagnosis of a subcutaneous lipoma are 88% and 99%, respectively.[61] In the correct clinical setting, sonography may determine that a soft tissue mass is compatible with a lipoma; however, a mass that is enlarging or painful or not in a subcutaneous location requires MRI or histologic evaluation for confirmation as ultrasound cannot reliably differentiate lipoma from well-differentiated liposarcoma. The ultrasound appearance of a low-grade well-differentiated liposarcoma is variable but often appears hyperechoic, related to the amount of soft tissue stranding or nodules within the predominantly fatty tumor (Fig. 2.56). A high-grade or poorly differentiated liposarcoma is heterogeneous but predominantly hypoechoic, similar to other sarcomas (see later section in this chapter).

If a small hyperechoic mass is seen in the subcutaneous tissues, additional diagnoses should be considered. With this appearance, one possibility would be an angiolipoma, which is considered a vascular variant of a lipoma or hamartoma, and is often multiple (Fig. 2.57).[63] Subcutaneous fat necrosis (as part of panniculitis or after trauma)

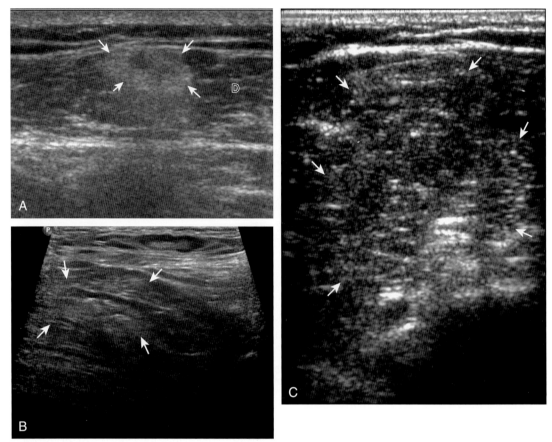

■ **FIGURE 2.54 Intramuscular Lipomas.** Ultrasound images from three different patients show hyperechoic intramuscular lipomas *(arrows)*. *D*, Deltoid muscle.

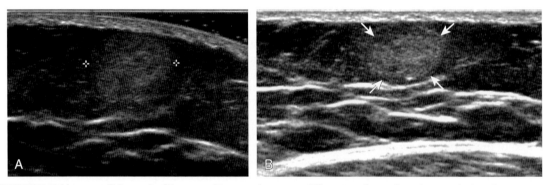

■ **FIGURE 2.55 Lipomas: Echogenic.** Ultrasound images from two different patients show hyperechoic subcutaneous lipomas *(between cursors and arrows)*.

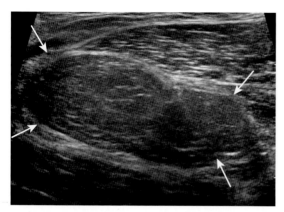

■ FIGURE 2.56 **Liposarcoma (Well Differentiated, Low Grade).** Ultrasound image shows hyperechoic mass that cannot be differentiated from a lipoma *(arrows).*

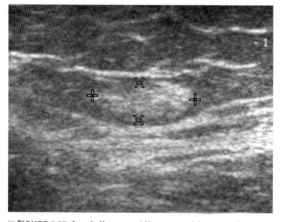

■ FIGURE 2.57 **Angiolipoma.** Ultrasound image shows a hyperechoic angiolipoma (calipers).

has a variable appearance but may look like a focal hyperechoic mass or nodule (see Fig. 2.20B).[25] Dermatofibrosarcoma protuberans may appear as either a hypoechoic (discussed later in Malignant Soft Tissue Tumors) or uncommonly a hyperechoic subcutaneous mass; the latter appearance is different from a lipoma, given a wide base contact with the skin with possible ill-defined borders and hyperemia.[64]

Peripheral Nerve Sheath Tumors

A solid soft tissue mass that is in continuity with a peripheral nerve is diagnostic for a peripheral nerve sheath tumor (PNST). Ultrasound is often used to demonstrate peripheral nerve continuity given its high resolution. At ultrasound, a PNST is hypoechoic with a low level of homogeneous internal echoes, round or oval, and appears well defined (Fig. 2.58). Increased through-transmission is usually seen deep to the mass, which may cause the hypoechoic mass to be mistaken for a complex cyst; however, the presence of flow on color or power Doppler imaging confirms the solid nature of the mass (Fig. 2.59; Video 2.9).[65] Transducer pressure over a PNST usually elicits symptoms.

A solitary PNST that is eccentric to the peripheral nerve is characteristic of a schwannoma (or neurilemmoma) (see Fig. 8.154), whereas neurofibromas tend to be central relative to the nerve, although differentiation between the two is often difficult with ultrasound.[66] The three ultrasound features that predict that a PNST is a neurofibroma include lobulated contour, hypovascularity, and fusiform shape.[67] In addition, a

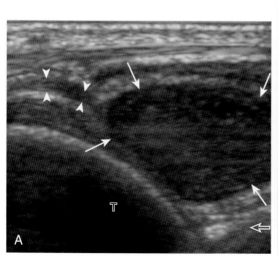

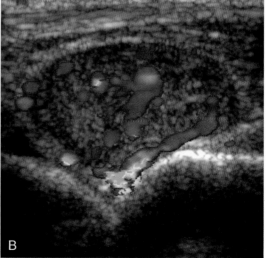

■ FIGURE 2.58 **Schwannoma.** Ultrasound images show (A and B) a hypoechoic schwannoma *(arrows)* with homogeneous diffuse internal echoes. Note flow on color Doppler imaging, continuity with a branch of the deep peroneal nerve *(arrowheads),* and increased through-transmission *(open arrow).* T, Talus.

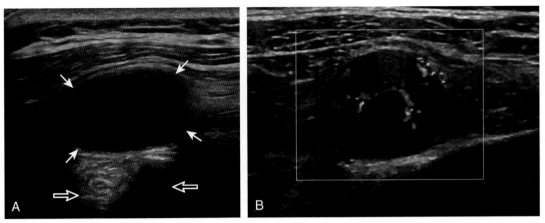

■ **FIGURE 2.59 Schwannoma: Pseudocyst Appearance.** A, Ultrasound image shows a hypoechoic schwannoma *(arrows)* with increased posterior through-transmission *(open arrows)* that may simulate a cyst. B, Note flow on color Doppler imaging that indicates that the abnormality is a solid mass and not a cyst.

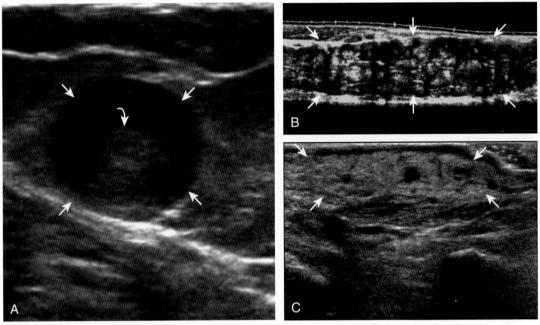

■ **FIGURE 2.60 Forms of Neurofibromas.** Ultrasound images from three different patients show (A) solitary neurofibroma appearing hypoechoic *(arrows)* with hyperechoic center *(curved arrow)* creating a target appearance, (B) plexiform neurofibroma *(arrows)*, and (C) diffuse subcutaneous neurofibroma *(arrows)*.

target appearance has also been described in neurofibromas, which appears as an echogenic fibrous center surrounded by a hypoechoic myxoid periphery, reported as a possible indicator of a benign PNST (Fig. 2.60A).[68] Neurofibromas may have three different forms: localized (Fig. 2.60A), plexiform, and diffuse.[69] Plexiform neurofibroma is described as a "bag of worms" appearance (Fig. 2.60B), whereas the diffuse form appears as diffuse echogenic subcutaneous tissues with hypoechoic tubules (Fig. 2.60C), most commonly involving the head, neck, and trunk regions. Peripheral

nerve sheath tumors may have internal cystic areas (Fig. 2.61) and calcification (such as in a longstanding or ancient schwannoma). Ultrasound cannot accurately differentiate benign from malignant peripheral nerve sheath tumors; the latter often appear similar to other soft tissue malignancies (Fig. 2.62).

Vascular Anomalies

Based on clinical and histologic findings, soft tissue vascular anomalies can be categorized into vascular

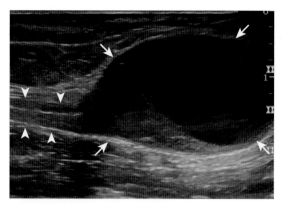

■ **FIGURE 2.61 Schwannoma: Cystic.** Ultrasound image shows peripheral nerve continuity *(arrowheads)* with a predominantly cystic schwannoma *(arrows)*. Note increased through-transmission.

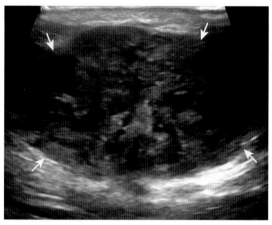

■ **FIGURE 2.62 Malignant Peripheral Nerve Sheath Tumor.** Ultrasound image shows heterogeneous but predominantly hypoechoic mass *(arrows)* with increased through-transmission.

tumors and vascular malformations.[70,71] A common childhood vascular tumor is an infantile hemangioma, which undergoes spontaneous involution in most cases. Vascular malformations are subcategorized as low flow (capillary, venous, lymphatic, or a combination of each) and high flow (arteriovenous fistula and arteriovenous malformation).[70] Although this is one described classification system, focal and well-defined intramuscular vascular lesions commonly presenting in an adult may also be called *hemangiomas*, subdivided by their dominant vascularity.[72]

At ultrasound, an infantile hemangioma is characterized by a mixed hyperechoic and hypoechoic mass with few or no visible vessels but with increased flow on color or power Doppler imaging.[70] Intramuscular vascular malformations have a heterogeneous appearance, with a variable echogenicity, ranging from hypoechoic to isoechoic to hyperechoic, which often infiltrates the involved soft tissue (Figs. 2.63 and 2.64).[70,73] Anechoic or hypoechoic channels that demonstrate flow on color or power Doppler imaging are typical, although flow may be very slow and difficult to identify without augmenting flow with manual compression. The hyperechoic areas represent the interfaces with the vascular structures, associated fatty tissue, and adjacent soft tissues. Focal hyperechoic and shadowing phleboliths, which represent dystrophic calcification in an organizing thrombus, may also be seen. When evaluating a vascular anomaly with ultrasound, the presence of an area of abnormal vascular channels without an associated soft tissue mass suggests the diagnosis of a vascular malformation, such as an arteriovenous malformation having the appearance of a tangle of vessels (Fig. 2.65).[70,74] Both infantile hemangiomas and arteriovenous malformations tend to have a greater vessel density than other vascular

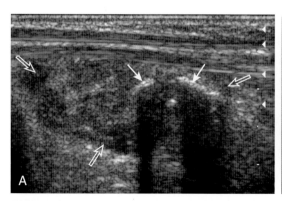
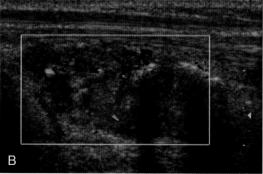

■ **FIGURE 2.63 Vascular Malformation (Intramuscular).** A and B, Ultrasound images show a heterogeneous hypoechoic and isoechoic vascular malformation *(open arrows)* with hyperemia and hyperechoic and shadowing calcifications *(arrows)*.

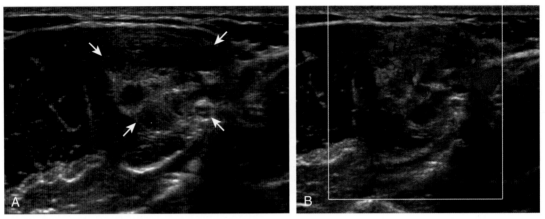

■ **FIGURE 2.64 Vascular Malformation (Intramuscular).** A and B, Ultrasound images show a heterogeneous hypoechoic and isoechoic vascular malformation *(arrows)* with hyperemia.

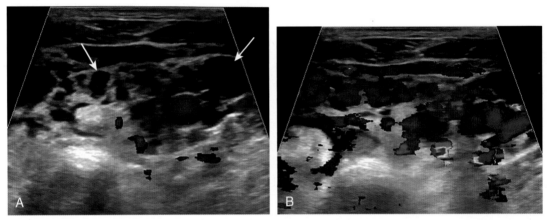

■ **FIGURE 2.65 Vascular Malformation.** A and B, Ultrasound images show blood flow within compressible anechoic channels *(arrows)* without a soft tissue mass representing a vascular malformation.

malformations.[74] It is important to distinguish the foregoing features of vascular anomalies from more nonspecific neovascularity and possible dystrophic calcification of a malignant soft tissue neoplasm. Demonstration of the characteristic features of phleboliths on radiography is helpful; however, percutaneous biopsy may be required if an associated soft tissue mass is present.

Ganglion Cysts

Ganglion cysts have several appearances at ultrasound. The most common appearance is that of a hypoechoic or anechoic, multilocular or multilobular, noncompressible cyst that may look complex.[75,76] Smaller ganglion cysts are more likely hypoechoic and may show only limited increased through-transmission.[76] The multilocular appearance of a cyst is specific to both ganglion cysts and fibrocartilage cysts (parameniscal and paralabral); the location of the multilocular cyst assists

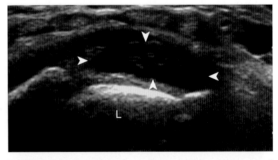

■ **FIGURE 2.66 Ganglion Cyst: Dorsal Wrist.** Ultrasound image in axial plane over dorsal wrist shows ganglion cyst *(arrowheads)* as hypoechoic and multilobular. *L,* Lunate.

in this diagnosis. If in contact with fibrocartilage, then parameniscal or paralabral cyst is likely. If located superficial to the scapholunate ligament (Fig. 2.66), near the radial artery at the wrist (a very common site) (Fig. 2.67), at the sinus tarsi

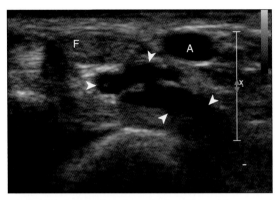

■ **FIGURE 2.67 Ganglion Cyst: Volar Wrist**. Ultrasound image in short axis to the radial artery (A) shows an anechoic multilocular ganglion cyst *(arrowheads)*. F, Flexor carpi radialis tendon.

of the ankle (see Fig. 8.160), or within the Hoffa infrapatellar fat pad or at the gastrocnemius tendon origin at the knee (see Figs. 7.75 and 7.76), ganglion cyst is likely. The other appearance of a ganglion cyst is a unilocular fluid collection, which can be associated with wrist, hand, ankle, and foot tendons.[75] Unlike a bursal fluid collection, such unilocular ganglion cysts are usually not compressible and not in a location of an expected bursa. Aspiration should only be attempted with a larger diameter needle (such as a 16- or 18-gauge needle), given the high viscosity of the gel-like fluid.

Lymph Nodes

A normal lymph node will appear oval, with a central hyperechoic hilum and a variable-thickness hypoechoic peripheral cortex rim (Fig. 2.68A).[77] The central echogenicity is not from fat but rather interfaces with sinuses and lymphatic cords.[77] The peripheral hypoechoic cortex will be of variable thickness but should be uniform. Flow on color or power Doppler imaging, if present, should have a hilar pattern. With age and after repeated inflammation, the outer cortex of the node will thin, whereas the central aspect becomes more hyperechoic but may decrease or increase in size. A hyperplastic lymph node will be enlarged but maintain the essential sonographic features of a lymph node as described (Fig. 2.68B; Video 2.10). When a lymph node is malignant (primary or metastatic), the echogenic hilum will narrow and could disappear, whereas the outer hypoechoic cortex will enlarge or become asymmetric, and the lymph node will lose its oval shape and become round (Fig. 2.68C). Flow on color or power Doppler imaging will become heterogeneous,

mixed, and peripheral (Fig. 2.68D). Although size criteria are used throughout the body to determine when a lymph node has enlarged, it is critical not to rely solely on size criteria but rather to evaluate the sonographic characteristics for early malignancy, taking into account patient history (Fig. 2.68E). Increased posterior through-transmission is often present with abnormal lymph nodes.

Malignant Soft Tissue Tumors

The precise diagnosis of a malignant soft tissue tumor typically cannot be made with ultrasound; however, a large soft tissue mass that does not originate from a joint or synovial space (bursa or tendon sheath) and that is hypoechoic with hypervascularity suggests a possible malignant origin, although biopsy is required for confirmation. Soft tissue sarcomas are predominantly hypoechoic (Fig. 2.69), with possible heterogeneous hyperechoic and hypervascular regions and anechoic necrotic regions as they enlarge, especially when high grade. Increased posterior through-transmission is often present, as with many solid soft tissue masses. An important teaching point is that a mass that originates within a joint or synovial space is related to a synovial process (proliferation or inflammation) and rarely malignancy; synovial sarcoma is similar to other sarcomas and appears as a hypoechoic mass near but outside of a joint (Fig. 2.69C). Granulocytic or myeloid sarcoma (also called *chloroma*), as a complication of myelogenous leukemia, may also appear as a hypoechoic mass (Fig. 2.70).[78] Lymphoma also presents as a hypoechoic mass with increased through-transmission or an infiltrating hypoechoic mass (Fig. 2.71).[79] A soft tissue tumor that is calcified or ossified will require further evaluation with MRI or CT because shadowing may obscure much of the mass (Fig. 2.72). Radiography is also indicated for further characterization.

Common diagnoses can be suggested based on the patient's age and the location of the tumor, but percutaneous biopsy with use of ultrasound guidance is usually needed.[80] With ultrasound guidance, a needle can be accurately placed into the soft tissue component of the tumor, while avoiding the necrotic center and adjacent neurovascular structures and thus increasing diagnostic yield. Soft tissue metastases are commonly hypoechoic with possible hypervascularity (Fig. 2.73).[81] Ultrasound is also effective in evaluation for recurrence of soft tissue malignancy after treatment (Fig. 2.74).[82] With melanoma, ultrasound can detect soft tissue recurrence or metastasis before findings at clinical examination (Fig. 2.74A).[83] It has been shown that ultrasound is as effective as MRI in evaluation for soft tissue

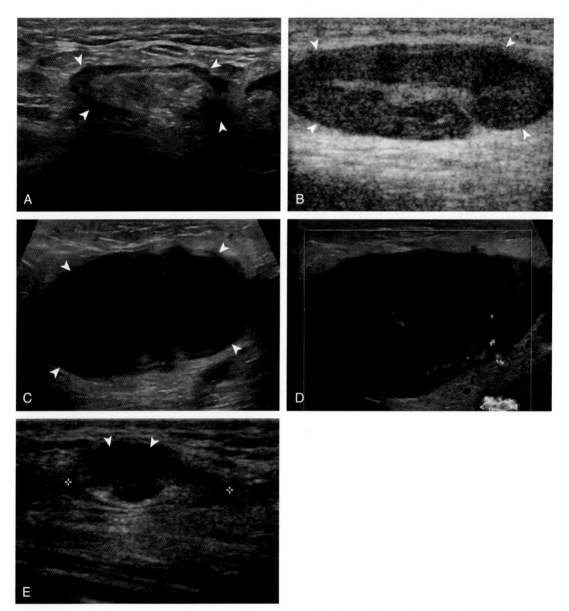

■ **FIGURE 2.68 Lymph Nodes.** Ultrasound images show (A) normal lymph node *(arrowheads)* (groin), (B) hyperplastic lymph node *(arrowheads)* (groin), (C and D) malignant lymph node *(arrowheads)* (lymphoma), and (E) focal lymph node metastasis *(arrowheads)* (angiosarcoma) *(cursors* denote lymph node borders). Note increased through-transmission with abnormal lymph nodes.

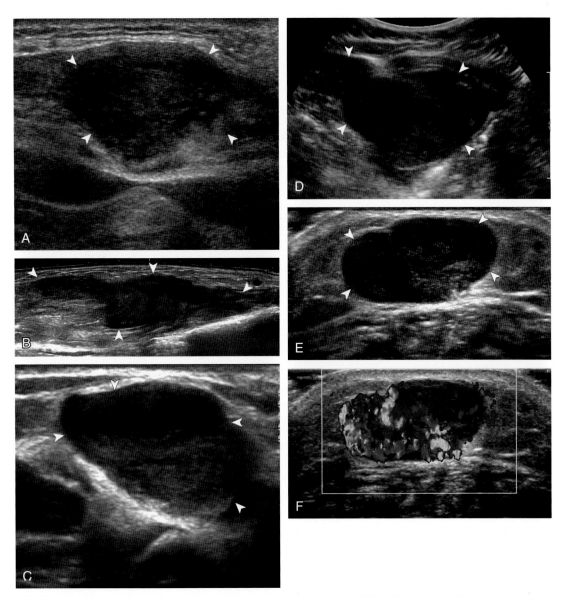

■ FIGURE 2.69 **Soft Tissue Sarcoma.** Ultrasound images show *(arrowheads)* (A) undifferentiated pleomorphic sarcoma, (B) high-grade leiomyosarcoma, (C) synovial sarcoma, (D) Ewing sarcoma, and (E and F) dermatofibrosarcoma protuberans. Note increased through-transmission in several of the examples.

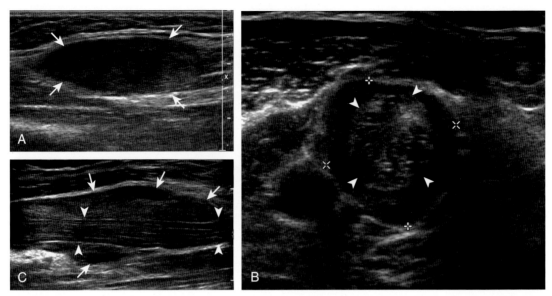

■ **FIGURE 2.70 Granulocytic or Myeloid Sarcoma (Chloroma).** Ultrasound images from two different patients show (A) soft tissue chloroma *(arrows)* and (B and C) chloroma *(cursors and arrowheads)* surrounding median nerve *(arrows)* proximal to the elbow.

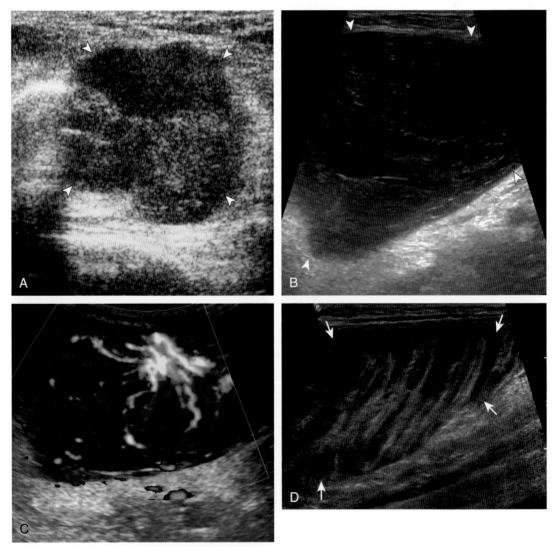

■ **FIGURE 2.71 Lymphoma.** Ultrasound images from four different patients show (A and B) hypoechoic lymphoma *(arrowheads)* with increased through-transmission, (C) irregular hypervascularity with power Doppler within hypoechoic lymphoma, and (D) infiltrating intramuscular lymphoma *(arrows)*.

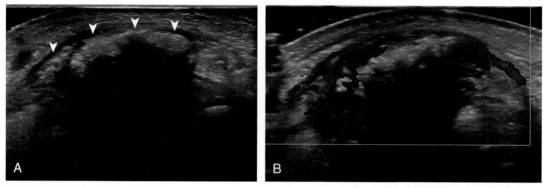

■ **FIGURE 2.72 Soft Tissue Chondroma.** A and B, Ultrasound images show hyperechoic surface of the mineralized chondroma *(arrowheads)* with significant shadowing, which obscures the soft tissue mass. Note hyperemia in B.

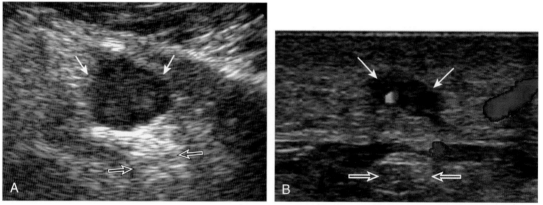

■ **FIGURE 2.73 Soft Tissue Metastases.** Ultrasound images show *(arrows)* (A) hypoechoic metastatic lung cancer and (B) epithelioid sarcoma. Note increased through-transmission *(open arrows)*.

sarcoma recurrence after treatment (Fig. 2.74B and C).[84]

■ BONE MASSES

In evaluation for bone involvement from a soft tissue tumor, or a primary benign or malignant osseous tumor, radiography is an important initial imaging method. Ultrasound is limited with regard to osseous abnormalities when compared with MRI; however, a bone process that creates cortical irregularity, destruction, or periosteal reaction may be identified at ultrasound. When using ultrasound to evaluate the soft tissues, one must consider and evaluate the underlying osseous structures as the possible primary pathologic process. Correlation with radiography is always essential, and further evaluation with MRI should always be a consideration.

One primary benign bone abnormality that may be visible at ultrasound is an osteochondroma (or exostosis) (Fig. 2.75; Video 2.11), which appears as a well-demarcated osseous excrescence that typically points away from the adjacent joint. Correlation with radiography is essential to identify both cortical and medullary continuity with the underlying bone to ensure the correct diagnosis. Ultrasound can also identify complications related to an enchondroma, such as fracture, bursa formation (Fig. 2.76), pseudoaneurysm, and malignant degeneration to chondrosarcoma. Other benign bone lesions that may be visible at ultrasound include aneurysmal bone cysts (Fig. 2.77).

When there is destruction of the bone cortex, an aggressive process is present, and considerations include both primary and secondary bone malignancy. Correlation with patient age, history, radiography, and distribution of pathology can suggest primary versus secondary processes. Considerations for primary bone tumor include osteosarcoma (Fig. 2.78), undifferentiated pleomorphic sarcoma (Fig. 2.79), chondrosarcoma, lymphoma, and Ewing sarcoma (Fig. 2.80).

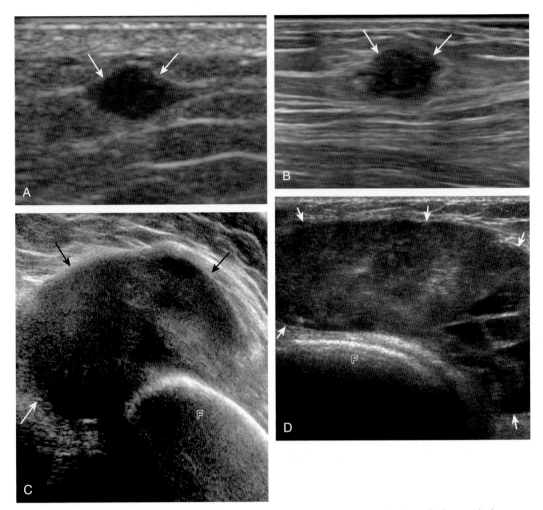

■ **FIGURE 2.74 Soft Tissue Recurrence.** Ultrasound images show *(arrows)* predominantly hypoechoic recurrent (A) melanoma, (B) sarcoma, (C) lymphoma, and (D) sarcoma. Note increased heterogeneity with larger tumor size. *F*, Femur.

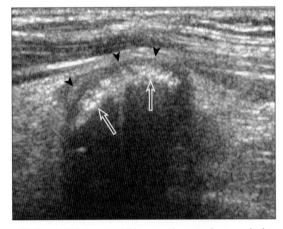

■ **FIGURE 2.75 Osteochondroma (Exostosis).** Ultrasound image shows a hyperechoic ossified surface *(open arrows)* and an overlying hypoechoic cartilage cap *(arrowheads)* of osteochondroma.

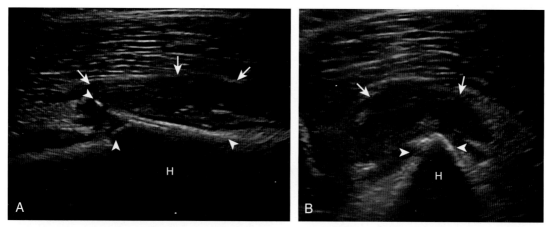

■ FIGURE 2.76 **Osteochondroma (Exostosis): Bursa Formation**. Ultrasound images in (A) short axis and (B) long axis to humerus (H) show osteochondroma *(arrowheads)* and overlying complex hypoechoic bursa *(arrows)*.

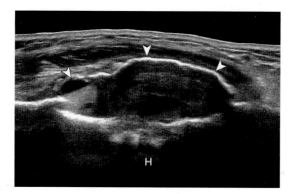

■ FIGURE 2.77 **Aneurysmal Bone Cyst**. Ultrasound images show expansile nature of aneurysmal bone cyst *(arrowheads)*. *H*, Humerus.

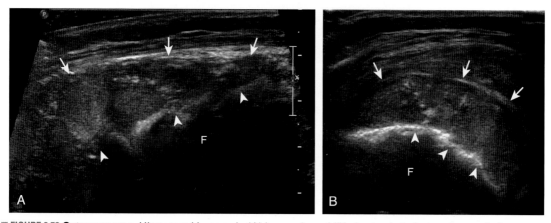

■ FIGURE 2.78 **Osteosarcoma**. Ultrasound images in (A) long axis and (B) short axis to femur show soft tissue mass *(arrows)* extending from femur (F). Note significant cortical irregularity of the femur *(arrowheads)*.

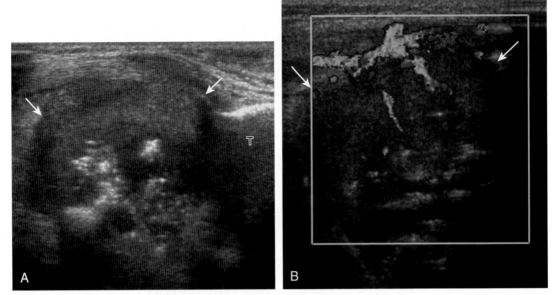

■ FIGURE 2.79 **Undifferentiated Pleomorphic Sarcoma of Bone**. Ultrasound images show (A and B) a mixed-echogenicity mass *(arrows)* arising from the tibia (T).

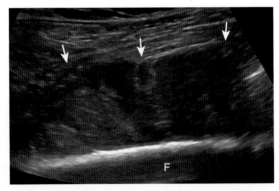

■ FIGURE 2.80 **Ewing Sarcoma**. Ultrasound image shows hypoechoic soft tissue Ewing sarcoma *(arrows)* originating from the fibula (F). Note absence of gross cortical destruction.

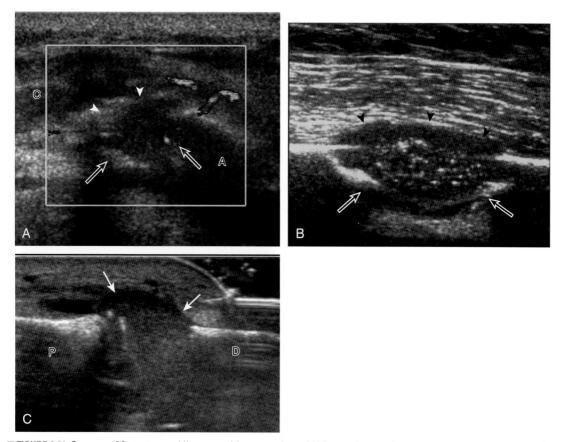

■ **FIGURE 2.81 Osseous Metastases.** Ultrasound images show (A) bone destruction *(open arrows)* with hyperemic soft tissue mass *(arrowheads)* representing a renal cell carcinoma metastasis, (B) bone destruction *(open arrows)* centered at the humeral cortex with a soft tissue mass *(arrowheads)* characteristic of a lung cancer metastasis (termed a *cookie-bite lesion*), and (C) a lung cancer metastasis *(arrows)* to the distal phalanx of the first toe. *A,* Acromion; *C,* clavicle; *D,* distal phalanx; *P,* proximal phalanx.

Osseous metastasis may also produce bone destruction (Fig. 2.81; Video 2.12).[85] A cortically based destructive process suggests lung cancer metastasis (Fig. 2.81B), whereas an expansile hyperemic process could indicate a vascular metastasis, such as from renal cell or thyroid carcinoma.

SELECT REFERENCES

8. Peetrons P: Ultrasound of muscles. *Eur Radiol* 12(1):35–43, 2002.
13. Craig JG, Jacobson JA, Moed BR: Ultrasound of fracture and bone healing. *Radiol Clin North Am* 37(4):737–751, ix, 1999.
27. Turecki MB, Taljanovic MS, Stubbs AY, et al: Imaging of musculoskeletal soft tissue infections. *Skeletal Radiol* 39(10):957–971, 2010.
29. Weiss DB, Jacobson JA, Karunakar MA: The use of ultrasound in evaluating orthopaedic trauma patients. *J Am Acad Orthop Surg* 13(8):525–533, 2005.
30. Hadduck TA, van Holsbeeck MT, Girish G, et al: Value of ultrasound before joint aspiration. *AJR Am J Roentgenol* 201(3):W453–W459, 2013.
32. Taljanovic MS, Melville DM, Gimber LH, et al: High-resolution US of rheumatologic diseases. *Radiographics* 35(7):2026–2048, 2015.
34. Wakefield RJ, Balint PV, Szkudlarek M, et al: Musculoskeletal ultrasound including definitions for ultrasonographic pathology. *J Rheumatol* 32(12): 2485–2487, 2005.
45. Thiele RG: Role of ultrasound and other advanced imaging in the diagnosis and management of gout. *Curr Rheumatol Rep* 13(2):146–153, 2011.
54. Boyse TD, Fessell DP, Jacobson JA, et al: US of soft-tissue foreign bodies and associated complications with surgical correlation. *Radiographics* 21(5): 1251–1256, 2001.
58. Jacobson JA, Fessell DP, Lobo Lda G, et al: Entrapment neuropathies I: upper limb (carpal tunnel excluded). *Semin Musculoskelet Radiol* 14(5): 473–486, 2010.

59. Klauser AS, Faschingbauer R, Bauer T, et al: Entrapment neuropathies II: carpal tunnel syndrome. *Semin Musculoskelet Radiol* 14(5):487–500, 2010.

70. Dubois J, Alison M: Vascular anomalies: what a radiologist needs to know. *Pediatr Radiol* 40(6): 895–905, 2010.

76. Wang G, Jacobson JA, Feng FY, et al: Sonography of wrist ganglion cysts: variable and noncystic appearances. *J Ultrasound Med* 26(10):1323–1328, 2007 [quiz 30–31].

77. Esen G: Ultrasound of superficial lymph nodes. *Eur J Radiol* 58(3):345–359, 2006.

The complete references for this chapter can be found on
www.expertconsult.com.

SHOULDER ULTRASOUND

The rotator cuff is composed of four tendons (Fig. 3.1). Anteriorly, the subscapularis with its tendons converges onto the lesser tuberosity. Superiorly, the supraspinatus inserts on the superior aspect of the greater tuberosity; its footprint or attachment averages 2.25 cm anterior to posterior, which covers the superior facet and the anterior portion of the middle facet of the greater tuberosity (Fig. 3.2).[1,2] Uncommonly, anterior fibers of the supraspinatus may extend anterior to the lesser tuberosity.[3] Posterior to the scapula and inferior to the scapular spine, the infraspinatus tendon inserts on the middle facet of the greater tuberosity, overlapping the posterior aspect of the supraspinatus tendon.[1] The smaller and more inferior teres minor tendon inserts on the inferior facet of the greater tuberosity. Between the lesser and greater tuberosities anteriorly is the bicipital groove, which contains the long head of the biceps brachii tendon; although not a part of the rotator cuff, its proximal intra-articular portion courses through a space between the supraspinatus and subscapularis tendons, called the *rotator interval*. The intra-articular portion of the biceps tendon is stabilized by the biceps reflection pulley comprised of the superior glenohumeral ligament and the coracohumeral ligament, which are essentially thickened reflections of the joint capsule.[4] The glenohumeral joint normally communicates with the biceps brachii long head tendon sheath.[5] Several joint recesses also exist and include the axillary recess, which extends inferiorly, and the subscapularis recess, which extends medially through the rotator interval to be located inferior to the coracoid process at the superior aspect of the subscapularis tendon in an inverted U shape.[6] In contrast, the subcoracoid bursa is located anterior to the subscapularis and does not communicate with the glenohumeral joint.[6] The subacromial-subdeltoid bursa is located between the rotator cuff and the overlying deltoid muscle and acromion (Fig. 3.1).[7] The glenoid labrum represents a rim of fibrocartilage at the periphery of the glenoid.

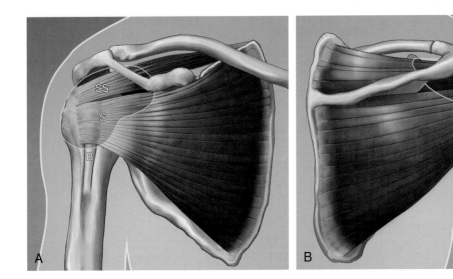

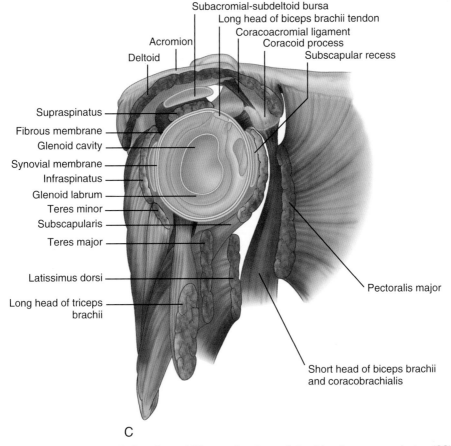

C

■ FIGURE 3.1 Shoulder Anatomy. A, Anterior and (B) posterior views of shoulder show supraspinatus *(SS)*, infraspinatus *(IS)*, subscapularis *(S)*, teres minor *(Tm)*, long head of biceps brachii *(B)*, and subacromial-subdeltoid bursa *(light blue)*. C, Lateral view of right glenohumeral joint and surrounding muscles with humerus removed. *(A and B, Image courtesy Carolyn Nowak, Ann Arbor, Michigan. C, From Drake R, Vogl W, Mitchell A:* Gray's Anatomy for Students, *Philadelphia, 2005, Churchill Livingstone.)*

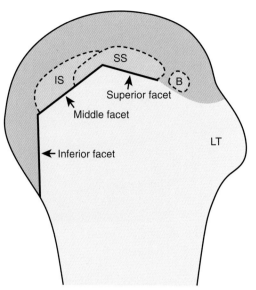

■ FIGURE 3.2 **Greater Tuberosity Facets.** Illustration of lateral humerus shows superior, middle, and inferior facets. *B,* Long head of biceps brachii; *SS,* supraspinatus; *IS,* infraspinatus; *LT,* lesser tuberosity. *(Image courtesy Carolyn Nowak, Ann Arbor, Michigan.)*

 BOX 3.1 Sample Diagnostic Shoulder Ultrasound Report: Normal, Complete

Examination: Ultrasound of the Shoulder
　Date of Study: March 11, 2017
　Patient Name: Juan Atkins
　Registration Number: 8675309
　History: Shoulder pain, evaluate for rotator cuff abnormality
　Findings: No evidence of joint effusion. The biceps brachii long head tendon is normal without tendinosis, tear, tenosynovitis, or subluxation/dislocation. The supraspinatus, infraspinatus, subscapularis, and teres minor tendons are also normal. No subacromial-subdeltoid bursal abnormality and no sonographic evidence for subacromial impingement with dynamic maneuvers. The posterior labrum is unremarkable. Additional focused evaluation at site of maximal symptoms was unrevealing.
　Impression: Unremarkable ultrasound examination of the shoulder. No rotator cuff abnormality.

BOX 3.2 Sample Diagnostic Shoulder Ultrasound Report: Abnormal, Complete

Examination: Ultrasound of the Shoulder
　Date of Study: March 11, 2017
　Patient Name: Chazz Michael Michaels
　Registration Number: 8675309
　History: Shoulder pain, evaluate for rotator cuff abnormality
　Findings: There is a focal anechoic tear of the anterior, distal aspect of the supraspinatus tendon measuring 1 cm short axis by 1.5 cm long axis. The anterior margin of the tear is adjacent to the rotator interval. There is no involvement of the subscapularis, infraspinatus, or rotator interval. A moderate amount of infraspinatus and supraspinatus fatty degeneration is present. There is a small joint effusion distending the biceps brachii tendon sheath and moderate distention of the subacromial-subdeltoid bursa. No biceps brachii long head tendon abnormality and no subluxation/dislocation. Mild osteoarthritis of the acromioclavicular joint. Additional focused evaluation at site of maximal symptoms was unrevealing.
　Impression: Focal or incomplete full-thickness tear of the supraspinatus tendon with infraspinatus and supraspinatus muscle atrophy.

TABLE 3.1 Shoulder Ultrasound Examination Checklist

Step	Structures/Pathologic Features of Interest
1	Biceps brachii long head
2	Subscapularis, biceps tendon dislocation
3	Supraspinatus, infraspinatus
4	Acromioclavicular joint, subacromial-subdeltoid bursa, dynamic evaluation
5	Posterior glenohumeral joint, labrum, teres minor, infraspinatus, atrophy

■ ULTRASOUND EXAMINATION TECHNIQUE

Table 3.1 is a shoulder ultrasound examination checklist. Examples of diagnostic shoulder ultrasound reports are shown in Boxes 3.1 and 3.2.

General Comments

For ultrasound examination of the shoulder, the patient sits on a stool with low back support but without wheels, and the sonographer sits on a stool with wheels to allow easy maneuvering. For examination of the patient's left shoulder when holding the transducer with the right hand, the patient faces the ultrasound machine, with the sonographer sitting somewhat between the patient and ultrasound machine (Fig. 3.3A). For examination of the patient's right shoulder, the patient turns toward the left and faces the sonographer (Fig. 3.3B). The transducer frequency for the shoulder is generally at least 10 to 15 MHz, although one may need to use a lower frequency in evaluation of the deeper structures such as the posterior glenoid labrum or if the patient has a

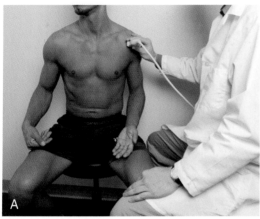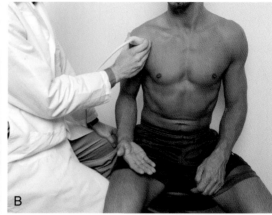

■ **FIGURE 3.3 Shoulder Ultrasound Examination.** A and B, Patient positioning.

large body habitus. Following a sequence of steps will ensure a complete and thorough evaluation.[8] Although a targeted approach is often used in other peripheral joints, this is not recommended with the shoulder because pain is often diffuse or referred. It is recommended, however, that every sonographic evaluation be followed by targeted evaluation over any area with point tenderness or focal symptoms.

Position 1: Long Head of Biceps Brachii Tendon

The patient places the hand on his or her leg (Fig. 3.4A). This position rotates the bicipital groove anteriorly, an important bone landmark. The hand may be in any position as this has no effect on the humerus. The transducer is placed in the transverse plane on the patient, and the long head of the biceps brachii tendon is seen within the bicipital groove in short axis (Fig. 3.4B) (Video 3.1). Because the distal biceps tendon courses deep, tendon obliquity to the transducer sound beam commonly creates anisotropy and an artifactual hypoechoic appearance of the normal tendon (Fig. 3.4C). This is corrected by toggling the transducer to aim the sound beam superiorly (Video 3.2). A hyperechoic and well-defined humeral cortex in the floor of the bicipital groove indicates that the sound beam is perpendicular to the overlying biceps tendon. The biceps brachii tendon is evaluated in short axis from proximal to distal. The proximal aspect of the biceps brachii tendon over the humeral head to the level of biceps reflection pulley is evaluated as this is a common site for pathology.[4,9] Proximal to the bicipital groove, the long head of the biceps brachii tendon normally appears oval in an oblique orientation, which should not be mistaken for tendon subluxation.[10] Evaluation is also continued

inferiorly to the level of the pectoralis tendon (Fig. 3.4D) to assess the pectoralis and biceps because complete biceps brachii long head tendon tears may retract to this level. The transducer is then turned 90 degrees to visualize the tendon in long axis from the humeral head to the pectoralis tendon (Fig. 3.5A) (Video 3.3). Asymmetrical pressure on the distal aspect of the transducer (or heel-toe maneuver) is typically needed to bring the biceps tendon fibers perpendicular to the transducer sound beam to eliminate anisotropy (Fig. 3.5B and C) (Video 3.4). An additional method to visualize the biceps tendon in long axis is to identify the characteristic pyramid shape of the lesser tuberosity (Fig. 3.5D); movement of the transducer laterally from this point will visualize the bicipital groove and biceps brachii long head tendon (Video 3.5).

Position 2: Subscapularis and Biceps Tendon Dislocation

The transducer is placed in the transverse plane, as before, to first visualize the bicipital groove and then the transducer is moved medial over the lesser tuberosity (see Fig. 3.4A). In this neutral position, although the subscapularis tendon can be seen in long axis, there is significant anisotropy (Fig. 3.6A). Ask the patient to rotate the shoulder externally (Fig. 3.6B), and this will bring the subscapularis tendon fibers into view perpendicular to the transducer sound beam and will eliminate anisotropy (Fig. 3.6C) (Video 3.6). The transducer is then moved superiorly and inferiorly over the lesser tuberosity to ensure complete evaluation of the subscapularis tendon. The transducer should also be moved laterally over the bicipital groove to evaluate for potential biceps brachii tendon subluxation or dislocation, which may be present only in external rotation (see Biceps Brachii

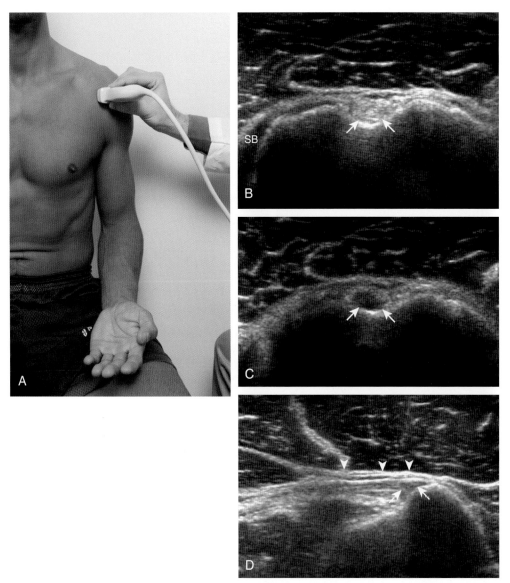

■ FIGURE 3.4 **Biceps Brachii Long Head Tendon Evaluation: Short Axis.** A, Transverse imaging over the bicipital groove shows (B) the hyperechoic biceps brachii long head tendon *(arrows)* within the bicipital groove. Note subscapularis tendon *(SB)* (medial is left side of image). C, Toggling the transducer creates anisotropy of biceps tendon *(arrows)*. D, Distal image shows biceps tendon *(arrows)* and overlying pectoralis major tendon *(arrowheads)*.

Tendon, Subluxation and Dislocation).[11] Center the transducer over the distal subscapularis tendon again, rotate the transducer 90 degrees, and assess the subscapularis tendon in short axis (Fig. 3.7A and B). In this view, it is common to see hypoechoic striations of muscle or interfaces between the several tendon bundles (Fig. 3.7C) (Video 3.7).

Position 3: Supraspinatus and Infraspinatus

The goal and challenge when imaging the supraspinatus is to evaluate the tendon precisely in long and short axis, identifying characteristic bone landmarks. This will avoid numerous diagnostic pitfalls and is an indicator that the operator has a thorough understanding of anatomy and shoulder ultrasound technique. The key to obtaining such images is to understand the anatomy of the greater tuberosity and the effects of various shoulder positioning. If one wanted to assess the supraspinatus tendon in long axis with the shoulder in neutral position, the transducer would be placed in the coronal plane over the greater tuberosity.[12] While the distal supraspinatus and related pathology can be seen, more proximal pathology may

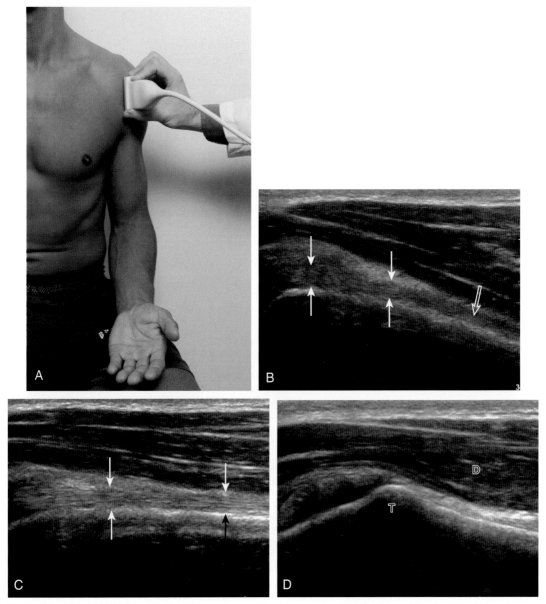

■ FIGURE 3.5 **Biceps Brachii Long Head Tendon Evaluation: Long Axis** A, Sagittal imaging over the bicipital groove shows (B) the biceps tendon *(arrows)* and anisotropy *(open arrow)*. C, Anisotropy is corrected when the transducer is positioned perpendicular to the tendon (distal is right side of image). D, Note the pyramid shape of the lesser tuberosity *(T)* medial to the bicipital groove in the sagittal plane. *D,* Deltoid muscle.

not be visible due to shadowing from the acromion (Fig. 3.8). One way to correct this is to ask the patient to place the back of his or her ipsilateral hand in the lower lumbar region and to keep the elbow close to the body (called the *Crass position*) (Fig. 3.9).[13] In this position, the humerus is rotated internally such that the greater tuberosity is located anteriorly on the patient. By placing the transducer in the sagittal plane anteriorly on the patient over the greater tuberosity, a long axis

view of the supraspinatus tendon is demonstrated. Rotating the transducer 90 degrees (or transverse on the patient) will produce a short axis image of the supraspinatus. The Crass position is helpful when one is first learning shoulder ultrasound technique in that long and short axis views are easily obtained; however, the significant disadvantages of this position include limited view of the rotator interval (see discussion later in chapter) and, often, significant patient discomfort.

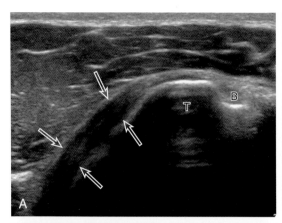

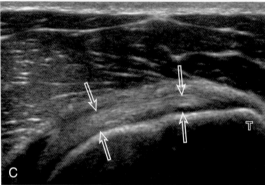

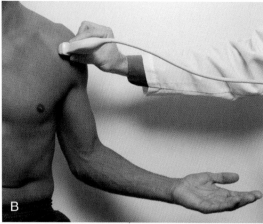

■ FIGURE 3.6 **Subscapularis Tendon Evaluation: Long Axis.** A, Transverse imaging over the lesser tuberosity *(T)* shows the subscapularis tendon *(open arrows)* hypoechoic from anisotropy (left side of image is medial). B, Imaging with external rotation optimally shows (C) the normal hyperechoic subscapularis tendon *(open arrows)*. B, Biceps brachii long head tendon.

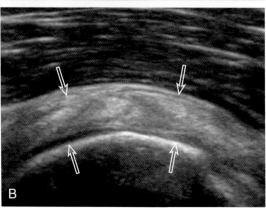

■ FIGURE 3.7 **Subscapularis Tendon Evaluation: Short Axis.** A, Sagittal imaging over anterior shoulder shows (B) the normal hyperechoic tendon *(open arrows)* (left side of image is cephalad). C, Note heterogeneity resulting from visualization of individual hyperechoic tendon bundles *(arrows)* with adjacent hypoechoic muscle and interfaces *(arrowheads)*.

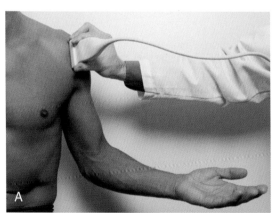

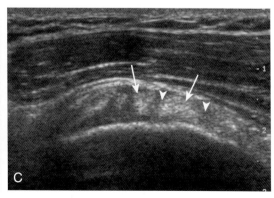

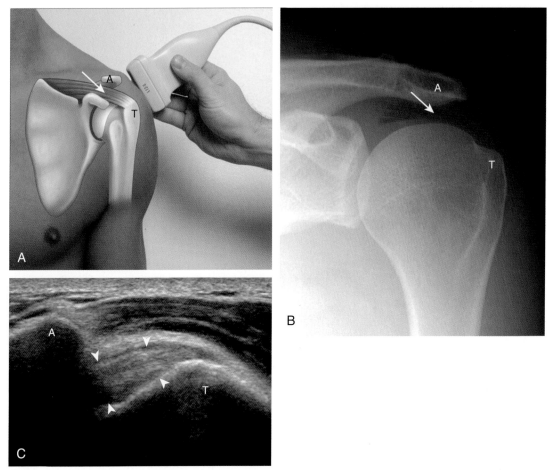

■ **FIGURE 3.8 Supraspinatus Evaluation: Neutral Position.** A, The supraspinatus tendon *(arrow)* inserts laterally on the greater tuberosity *(T)*. B, An anteroposterior shoulder radiograph illustrates that much of the supraspinatus tendon *(arrow)* is hidden beneath the acromion *(A)*. C, Ultrasound image long axis to supraspinatus only shows distal supraspinatus *(arrowheads)*. *T,* Greater tuberosity.

Because of this, the *modified Crass position* is used (I primarily use the modified Crass position and less commonly the Crass position for problem solving).[14]

To obtain the modified Crass position, the patient is asked to place his or her hand on the ipsilateral hip area (Fig. 3.10). The elbow should be pointed posteriorly to ensure some degree of shoulder external rotation compared with the Crass position; otherwise, the rotator interval may not be visible. To obtain a long axis view of the supraspinatus tendon in this position, the transducer is placed on the rounded contour of the anterior shoulder and directed superior and oblique toward the patient's ear (Fig. 3.10). Usually, the axis of the transducer is parallel to the proximal biceps tendon and humeral shaft

regardless of each position when imaging the supraspinatus in long axis.[8] With positioning of the patient in the Crass or modified Crass position, supraspinatus evaluation begins with evaluation in long axis because this important view allows visualization of the three surfaces of the supraspinatus tendon (articular, bursal, greater tuberosity) and allows for initial screening for pathology.[15] In long axis, the normal supraspinatus will appear hyperechoic and fibrillar, with a convex superior margin (Fig. 3.10) (Video 3.8). The thin hypoechoic layer over the curved humeral head represents the hyaline articular cartilage. A thin hypoechoic fibrocartilage layer over the greater tuberosity facets should not be confused with hyaline articular cartilage over the rounded humeral head.[16] One must be aware that the distal

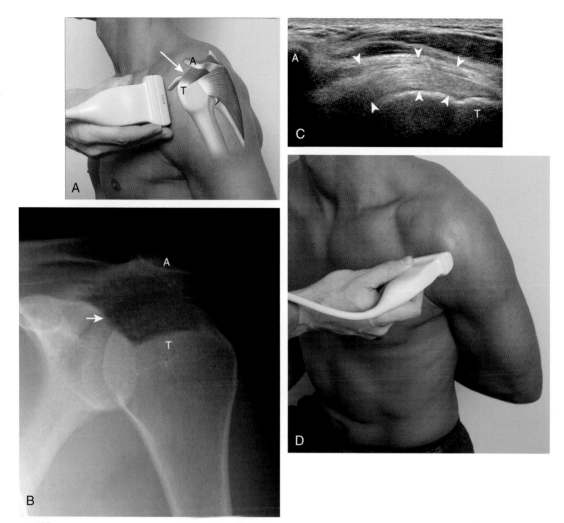

■ **FIGURE 3.9 Supraspinatus Evaluation: Crass Position.** A and B, The greater tuberosity *(T)* rotates anteriorly with the distal supraspinatus tendon *(arrow)* now visible, which was previously hidden beneath the acromion *(A)*. The transducer is placed anteriorly in the sagittal plane on the body (A) for a long axis view and improved visualization of the supraspinatus *(arrowheads)* (C). The transducer is placed transverse (D) for a short axis image of the supraspinatus.

fibers of the tendon curve downward at the greater tuberosity near the articular surface, and the transducer orientation should be adjusted using the heel-toe maneuver to eliminate anisotropy (Fig. 3.11) (Video 3.9).[16] A hyperechoic and well-defined humeral head cortex indicates that the sound beam is perpendicular to the bone and overlying tendon. The footprint of the supraspinatus tendon inserts over approximately 2.25 cm of the greater tuberosity shelf from anterior to posterior, so the transducer should be moved anterior and posterior over the greater tuberosity without changing the long axis imaging plane to ensure complete evaluation.[2] Scanning should be

continued anteriorly along the greater tuberosity until the intra-articular portion of the biceps tendon is identified to ensure that the anterior extent of the supraspinatus was evaluated, a location where supraspinatus tendon tears commonly occur.[17,18] Including a long axis image of the intra-articular portion of the long head biceps brachii tendon will document that the most anterior aspect of the supraspinatus was evaluated (Fig. 3.10C). As the transducer is moved posteriorly over the middle facet of the greater tuberosity, the infraspinatus is also evaluated (Fig. 3.10D).[19] At the middle facet, the angle between the greater tuberosity and the articular surface of the humeral

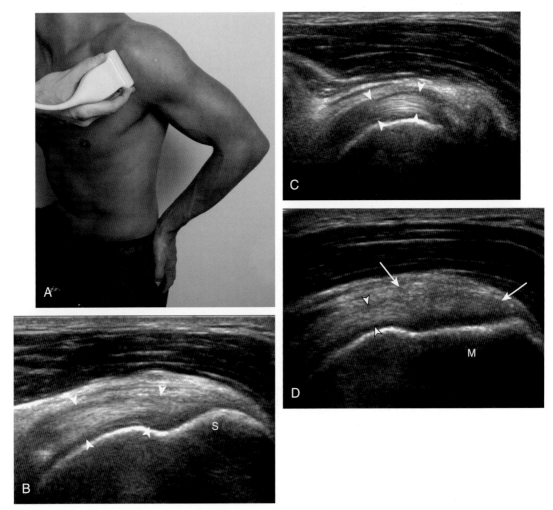

■ **FIGURE 3.10 Supraspinatus Long Axis: Modified Crass Position.** The supraspinatus is evaluated in the long axis (A) with the patient's hand placed near the ipsilateral hip and the elbow directed posteriorly. (B) The normal supraspinatus is hyperechoic and fibrillar with a convex superior margin *(arrowheads)*, shown at the level of the superior facet *(S)*. C, Transducer positioning in the same plane but anterior to (B) over the rotator interval shows the long head of biceps brachii tendon *(arrowheads)*. D, Transducer positioning in the same plane but posterior to (A) over the middle facet *(M)* shows hypoechoic bands from the overlying infraspinatus *(arrows)* superficial to supraspinatus *(arrowheads)*.

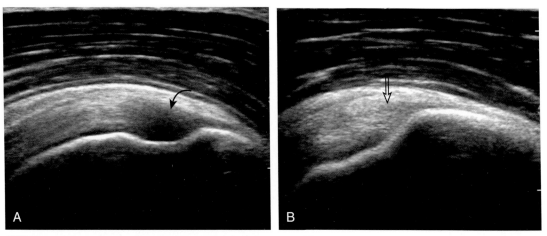

■ **FIGURE 3.11 Supraspinatus Tendon (Long Axis): Anisotropy.** Ultrasound images long axis to the supraspinatus show (A) artifactual hypoechogenicity *(curved arrow)* where the distal tendon fibers curve downward to the greater tuberosity, oblique to the sound beam. With the transducer repositioned (B), the distal tendon fibers appear hyperechoic *(open arrow)* when they are perpendicular to the sound beam.

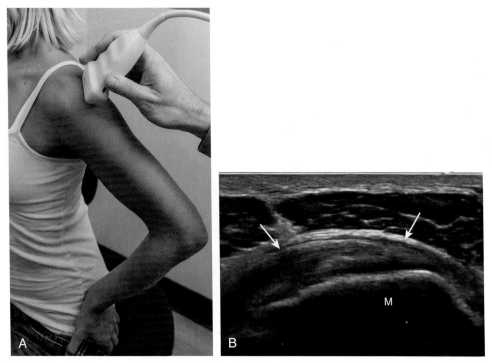

■ **FIGURE 3.12 Infraspinatus Long Axis: Modified Crass Position.** A, When over the middle facet of the greater tuberosity, the transducer is angled posteriorly to visualize (B) long axis of infraspinatus tendon *(arrows)*. *M,* Middle facet of greater tuberosity.

head flattens, and alternating hypoechoic linear areas representing anisotropy of the infraspinatus helps to identify the infraspinatus tendon superficial to the supraspinatus tendon (Video 3.10).[20] The transducer can then be angled more posterior to align the infraspinatus in long axis (Fig. 3.12).

After assessment of the supraspinatus in long axis, the transducer is turned 90 degrees to evaluate the tendon in short axis (Fig. 3.13A) (Video 3.11). First, beginning over the proximal aspect of the supraspinatus, the humeral head should be seen as a round echogenic line with overlying

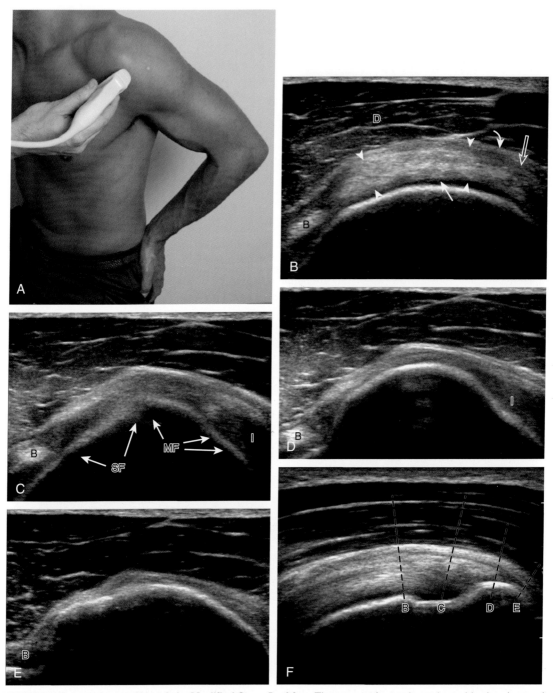

■ **FIGURE 3.13 Supraspinatus Short Axis: Modified Crass Position.** The supraspinatus is evaluated in the short axis (A) with the patient's hand placed near the ipsilateral hip and the elbow directed posteriorly. B, The normal supraspinatus *(arrowheads)* over the humeral head is of uniform thickness and hyperechoic. Note the intra-articular portion of the biceps brachii tendon *(B)* in the rotator interval, supraspinatus-infraspinatus junction *(open arrow)*, hyaline articular cartilage *(arrow)*, collapsed subacromial-subdeltoid bursa *(curved arrow)*, and deltoid muscle *(D)* (left side of image is anterior on the greater tuberosity). Sequential short axis images of the supraspinatus tendon show (C–E) gradual thinning of the tendon beyond the hyaline cartilage and absence of the supraspinatus beyond the greater tuberosity. Note the superior facet *(SF)* and the middle facet *(MF)* of the greater tuberosity. F, Long axis image of the supraspinatus tendon is used as a reference for images B to E. *B,* Biceps tendon; *I,* infraspinatus tendon.

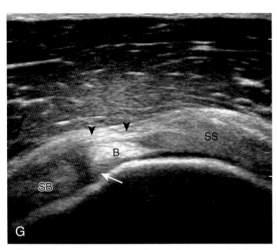

■ FIGURE 3.13, cont'd G, Ultrasound image of the intra-articular portion of the biceps brachii long head in short axis *(B)* at rotator interval shows the coracohumeral ligament and joint capsule *(arrowheads)* and the superior glenohumeral ligament *(arrow)*. *SB,* Subscapularis tendon; *SS,* supraspinatus tendon.

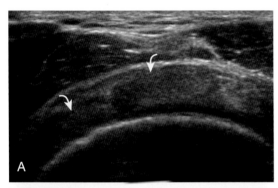

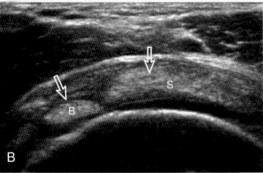

■ FIGURE 3.14 **Supraspinatus Tendon (Short Axis): Anisotropy.** Ultrasound images short axis to the supraspinatus show (A) artifactual hypoechogenicity *(curved arrows)*, which is eliminated with toggling of the transducer to show (B) hyperechoic *(open arrows)* supraspinatus *(S)*, biceps brachii *(B)*, and bone cortex. Note hyperechoic and well-defined cortex in (B).

hypoechoic hyaline cartilage (Fig. 3.13B). The transducer should be toggled until the bone cortex and overlying tendon are hyperechoic and well defined to eliminate anisotropy (Fig. 3.14). At this level, the rotator cuff should be of fairly uniform thickness, similar to a tire on a wheel rim, measuring on average 6 ± 1.1 mm.[21] This appearance indicates that the transducer is in the true short axis plane relative to the supraspinatus tendon and not in an oblique plane. The transducer is then moved distally relative to the supraspinatus tendon (Video 3.12). As the hyaline cartilage disappears from view, the round humeral head surface will be replaced with the angulated surface of the greater tuberosity facets (Fig. 3.13C). At this point, the tendon uniformly becomes thinner, an indication that the transducer position is now beyond the articular surface. The facets of the greater tuberosity from anterior to posterior appear as three flat surfaces: the superior, middle, and inferior facets (see Fig. 3.2).[1] The supraspinatus tendon inserts on the superior facet and the superior half of the middle facet, the infraspinatus inserts on the middle facet (overlapping the supraspinatus tendon superficially), and the teres minor inserts on the inferior facet.[1] At this point, both the distal supraspinatus and infraspinatus are assessed. Similar to long axis imaging, alternating hypoechoic lines are seen over the middle facet, which represent anisotropy of the infraspinatus tendon fibers superficial to the supraspinatus (Video 3.13). As the transducer is moved more distally, the greater tuberosity becomes square or rounded (Fig. 3.13D), and the rotator cuff thins even more and eventually disappears as the transducer moves beyond the greater tuberosity and the rotator cuff (Fig. 3.13E). Similar to evaluation of the supraspinatus tendon in long axis, the intra-articular portion of the biceps tendon (in the rotator interval) should be identified to indicate that the most anterior aspect of the supraspinatus tendon is evaluated (Fig. 3.13G). This is one of the advantages of the modified Crass position because the important landmark of the biceps tendon is well visualized. In addition, the superior glenohumeral ligament is seen at the anterior aspect of the biceps tendon adjacent to the humerus, and the coracohumeral ligament is identified over the biceps tendon as it courses lateral to merge with the supraspinatus tendon.[4]

Another structure of the rotator cuff is the rotator cable, which may be identified by its characteristic shape and position (Fig. 3.15).[22] The rotator cable has a U shape when viewed from above with each limb attaching to the greater tuberosity. The curved aspect of the U is visualized with its fibers perpendicular to the supraspinatus at the articular surface. The rotator cable is more

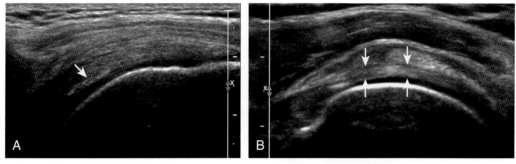

■ FIGURE 3.15 **Rotator Cable.** Ultrasound images (A) long axis and (B) short axis to supraspinatus show the hyperechoic and fibrillar rotator cable *(arrows). (Courtesy Y. Morag, MD, Ann Arbor, Michigan.)*

prominent in some individuals (termed *cable dominant*) and outlines an area of the rotator cuff within the U, termed the *rotator crescent.*

Position 4: Acromioclavicular Joint, Subacromial-Subdeltoid Bursa, and Dynamic Evaluation

The acromioclavicular joint can be located with palpation of the clavicle and placement of the transducer in the coronal-oblique plane over the distal clavicle (Fig. 3.16A) or by moving the transducer superiorly in the transverse plane from the bicipital groove region. The acromioclavicular joint is identified by hypoechoic joint space and bone landmarks; the clavicle is normally seen more superior relative to the acromion. A hyperechoic fibrocartilage disk may be seen between the clavicle and acromion, and the hypoechoic joint capsule is normally less than 3 mm measured superiorly (Fig. 3.16B).[23] If the acromioclavicular joint is widened, the patient can place his or her hand on the opposite shoulder to assess for acromioclavicular joint widening or, conversely, narrowing, which may be associated with pain.[24] The transducer is then moved laterally in the coronal place over the proximal humerus beyond the greater tuberosity to assess for fluid within the dependent portion of the subacromial-subdeltoid bursa (Fig. 3.16C).

To dynamically assess for subacromial impingement, the transducer is positioned in the coronal-oblique plane to visualize the lateral border of the acromion and the adjacent greater tuberosity (Fig. 3.17). The examiner assesses the supraspinatus tendon and subacromial-subdeltoid bursa dynamically first by passively abducting the arm (typically with elbow flexion). This allows the examiner to slow or stop the patient's movement if the bone landmarks are not visualized to allow repositioning of the transducer and also trains the patient to abduct the arm at a particular speed.

The movement is then repeated actively (Fig. 3.17C and D). Subsequent pooling of fluid within or bunching of the subacromial-subdeltoid bursa indicates subacromial impingement, although more advanced cases can show additional upward movement of the humeral head and osseous impingement.[25,26] The finding of incomplete sliding of the supraspinatus beneath the acromion during this dynamic maneuver indicates adhesive capsulitis.[27] When assessing for subacromial impingement, the transducer should also be moved anterior to the acromion to assess the region of the coracoacromial ligament for abnormal distention of the subacromial-subdeltoid bursa.

Position 5: Infraspinatus, Teres Minor, and Posterior Glenoid Labrum

The patient rotates on the stool to permit visualization of the posterior structures of the shoulder; initially, the patient keeps his or her hand on the thigh. Place the transducer in the oblique axial plane angled superiorly toward the humeral head parallel and just inferior to the scapular spine (Fig. 3.18). Position the transducer to visualize the well-defined central tendon of the infraspinatus muscle at the musculotendinous junction posterior to the glenoid to ensure an imaging plane that is long axis to the infraspinatus (Fig. 3.18B). The infraspinatus tendon can then be followed distally to its insertion on the middle facet at the posterior aspect of the greater tuberosity. Evaluation of the distal infraspinatus tendon supplements earlier evaluation from the modified Crass position (see Figs. 3.10D and 3.12). If the infraspinatus tendon is not visible because of shadowing beneath the acromion, then the patient can place the hand on the opposite shoulder to improve visualization; this maneuver is less ideal because the infraspinatus tendon, seen linear and perpendicular to the sound beam in neutral shoulder position, becomes curved, introducing anisotropy. The

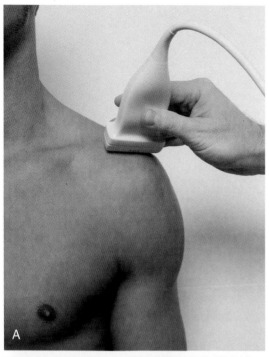

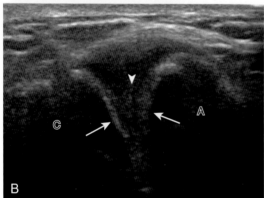

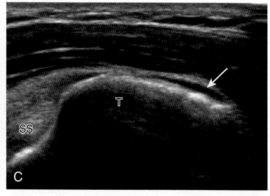

■ FIGURE 3.16 **Acromioclavicular Joint and Subacromial-Subdeltoid Bursa Evaluation.** A, Coronal-oblique imaging over the distal clavicle shows (B) the acromioclavicular joint space *(arrows)* with a hypoechoic joint capsule and a hyperechoic fibrocartilaginous disk *(arrowhead).* C, Imaging more lateral over the greater tuberosity shows minimal anechoic fluid *(arrow)* that distends the most dependent region of the subacromial-subdeltoid bursa. Note the hyperechoic bursal wall and peribursal fat (left side of image is cephalad). *A,* Acromion; *C,* clavicle; *SS,* supraspinatus tendon; *T,* greater tuberosity.

transducer can then be moved inferiorly to visualize the smaller teres minor, with its tendon more superficial over the muscle compared with the infraspinatus tendon (Fig. 3.18C). The transducer is then turned 90 degrees to evaluate the infraspinatus and teres minor in short axis (Fig. 3.19). Note osseous landmarks of scapula spine and osseous ridge of posterior scapula that demarcates the supraspinatus, infraspinatus, and teres minor (Fig. 3.19E).

An alternate approach in identification of the infraspinatus and teres minor is to palpate the scapular spine, place the transducer sagittal on the patient over the scapular spine, and then move the transducer inferiorly. The first structure identified inferior to the scapular spine is the infraspinatus. Once the infraspinatus and teres minor are identified, the transducer is turned long axis to the infraspinatus tendon to evaluate the hyperechoic triangle-shaped posterior glenoid labrum (see Fig. 3.18B).

The area medial to the glenohumeral joint should also be assessed to include the spinoglenoid notch, a site where paralabral cysts may be found.

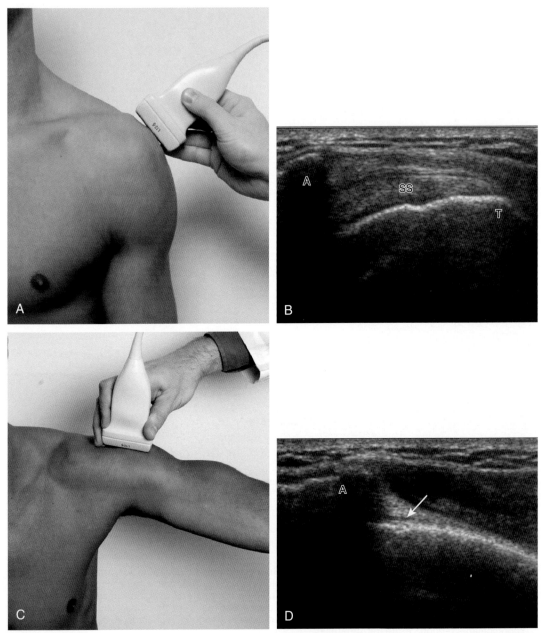

■ **FIGURE 3.17 Dynamic Evaluation for Subacromial Impingement and Adhesive Capsulitis.** A, The transducer is positioned between the greater tuberosity and acromion (B), the patient raises the arm (C) during visualization with ultrasound. D, Normally, the supraspinatus *(SS)* glides beneath the acromion *(A)*. The subacromial-subdeltoid bursa *(arrow)* remains collapsed without pooling of fluid or bunching of bursal tissue at the acromion tip. *T,* Greater tuberosity.

The patient can actively internally and externally rotate the shoulder to assess the infraspinatus tendon and posterior glenoid labrum dynamically (Video 3.14). External rotation improves visualization of joint fluid distention of the posterior recess, which also facilitates evaluation of potential paralabral tears (see Glenoid Labrum and Paralabral Cyst). In shoulder external rotation, the suprascapular vein may dilate, and this can simulate a paralabral cyst (see Glenoid Labrum and Paralabral Cyst) (Video 3.15), especially since blood flow is too slow to be detected at Doppler imaging. Unlike a paralabral cyst, the suprascapular vein collapses with internal rotation.

To complete the posterior shoulder examination, the transducer is turned 90 degrees and moved

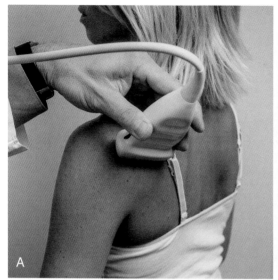

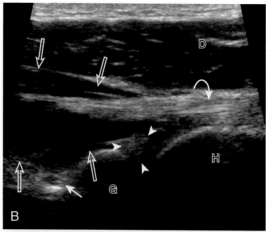

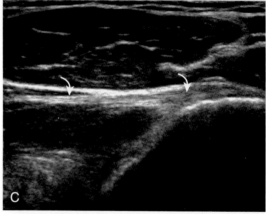

■ **FIGURE 3.18** **Infraspinatus (Long Axis), Teres Minor (Long Axis), and Posterior Labrum Evaluation.** A, Imaging over the posterior shoulder shows (B) the infraspinatus muscle *(open arrows)* and tendon *(curved arrow)*. Note posterior glenoid labrum *(arrowheads)*, spinoglenoid notch *(arrow)*, humeral head *(H)*, glenoid *(G)*, and deltoid muscle *(D)* (right side of image is distal). C, Just inferior to the infraspinatus, the thinner and more superficial hyperechoic teres minor tendon can be seen *(curved arrows)*.

medial to assess the infraspinatus and teres minor in short axis globally at the musculotendinous junctions for fatty degeneration or atrophy; the infraspinatus muscle should be nearly twice the size of the teres minor over the scapular body, with normal muscle appearing relatively hypoechoic compared with hyperechoic tendon (see Fig. 3.19B). At this site, a bony ridge is identified in the scapula, which forms a concave surface beneath each muscle and aids in their identification. The transducer can be moved superiorly to similarly assess the supraspinatus muscle in short axis for fatty infiltration and atrophy. An extended field of view image may be considered (if available on the ultrasound machine) to include the supraspinatus, infraspinatus, and teres minor in one image (see Fig. 3.19E).[28] The transducer is then turned 90 degrees and long axis to the supraspinatus, where the concavity of the superior scapular cortex identifies the suprascapular notch and at times portions of the superior labrum (Fig. 3.19F).

■ ROTATOR CUFF ABNORMALITIES
Supraspinatus Tears and Tendinosis

GENERAL COMMENTS

Most rotator cuff tears involve the supraspinatus tendon, although they may extend posterior to involve the infraspinatus and anterior to involve the biceps reflection pulley and subscapularis tendons.[17] The anterior aspect of the distal supraspinatus is a common site of tear, often near the rotator interval, although a more posterior location near the supraspinatus-infraspinatus junction has been described with degenerative cuff tears.[17,29] Most tendon tears are the result of chronic attrition and possible superimposed injury, and they typically occur after the age of 40 years. Such chronic supraspinatus tears occur distally and are associated with cortical irregularity of the greater tuberosity, an important indirect sign of supraspinatus tendon tear.[30-32] Acute tears may

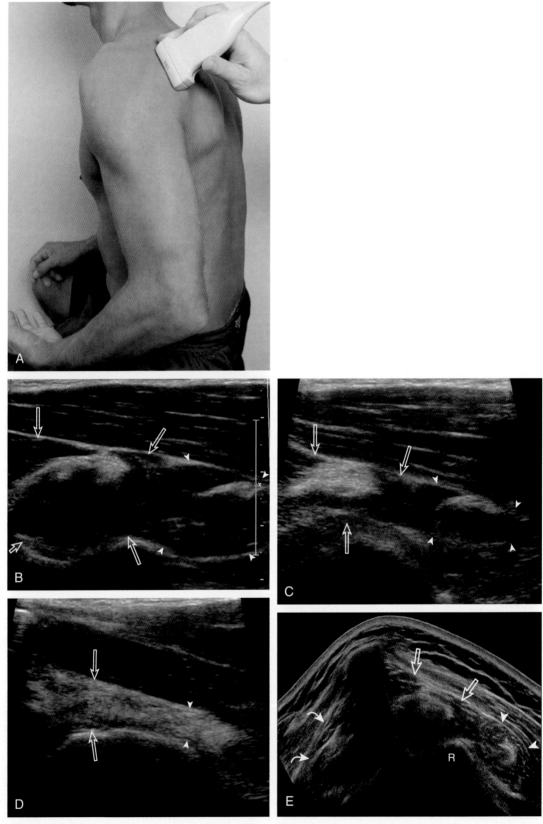

■ **FIGURE 3.19 Infraspinatus (Short Axis) and Teres Minor (Short Axis).** A, Imaging over posterior shoulder shows progressive transition (B–D) from hypoechoic muscle to hyperechoic tendon of the infraspinatus *(open arrows)* and teres minor *(arrowheads)* (left side of image is superior). Extended field of view image (E) shows supraspinatus *(curved arrows),* infraspinatus *(open arrows),* and teres minor *(arrowheads).* Note osseous ridge of posterior scapula *(R)* and spine of scapula *(S).*

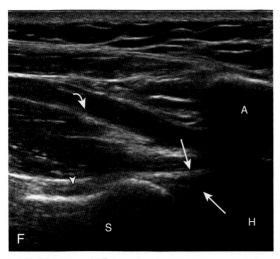

occur more proximally and may or may not have associated cortical irregularity, depending on the age of the patient and the chronicity of the rotator cuff. Accurate localization of a tendon tear is essential to classify the tear properly (Fig. 3.20). For example, partial-thickness tears could involve the articular or bursal surface of the tendon. A tear that is localized within the tendon or that extends only to the greater tuberosity surface (or footprint) of the supraspinatus attachment is called an *interstitial or intra-substance (or concealed interstitial delamination) tear* because it would not be visible at arthroscopy or bursoscopy.[2,17] A tear that extends from articular to bursal surfaces is a full-thickness tear. Correct description and nomenclature are also essential. A full-thickness tear may be focal or incomplete, whereas a full-thickness tear that involves the entire width of a tendon can be termed a *complete* or *full-width* full-thickness tear. Initial evaluation in long axis

■ FIGURE 3.19, cont'd F, Imaging long axis to supraspinatus *(curved arrow)* over supraspinatus fossa shows suprascapular notch *(arrowhead)* and superior labrum *(arrows). S,* Scapula; *A,* acromion; *H,* humeral head.

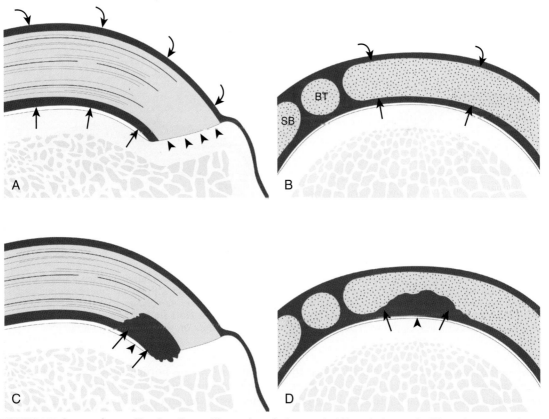

■ FIGURE 3.20 **Supraspinatus Tendon Tears.** Illustrations in long axis (A) and short axis (B) to the supraspinatus tendon show the articular *(arrows),* bursal *(curved arrows),* and greater tuberosity *(arrowheads)* surfaces of the supraspinatus tendon. C and D, Articular-side partial-thickness tears *(black)* contact the articular surface *(arrows)* and hyaline cartilage *(arrowhead).*

Continued

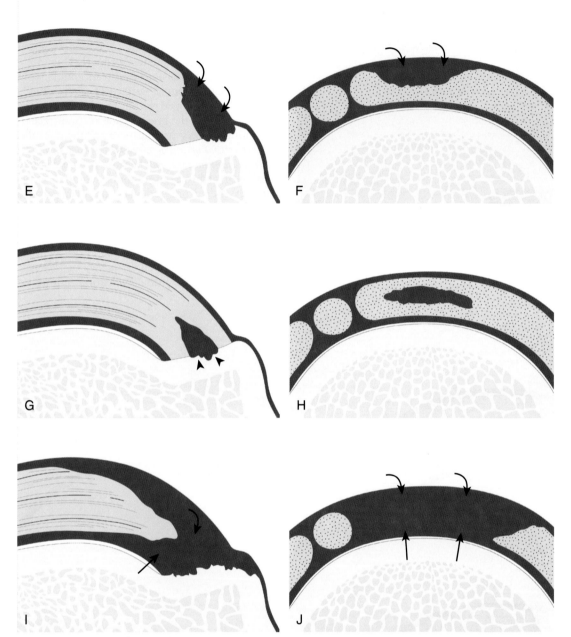

■ **FIGURE 3.20, cont'd** E and F, Bursal-side partial-thickness tears *(black)* contact the bursal surface *(curved arrows)*. G and H, Intra-substance tears *(black)* reside within the tendon not in contact with the articular or bursal surface, although isolated greater tuberosity contact within the tendon may be seen *(arrowheads)*. I and J, Full-thickness tears extend from articular *(arrows)* to bursal *(curved arrows)* surfaces. Note that all types of tears may contact the greater tuberosity, associated with bone irregularity. *BT,* Biceps tendon; *SB,* subscapularis tendon.

of the supraspinatus is recommended in that the three surfaces of the rotator cuff (articular, bursal, greater tuberosity) and characteristic bone contours are visible and easily identified.[15] Most tears are anechoic or hypoechoic, although acute tears will more likely appear anechoic from fluid.[33] As a supraspinatus tendon tear becomes large, tendon retraction and volume loss of the tendon occur,

with loss of the normal superior convex shape. Full-thickness tears located anteriorly are associated with tendon retraction, muscle atrophy, and propagation over time.[34,35] Ultrasound and magnetic resonance imaging (MRI) have comparable accuracies in detection and measurement of rotator cuff tears.[36] A meta-analysis of 65 articles has also shown that ultrasound and MRI are comparable in sensitivity and specificity for the diagnosis of rotator cuff tear.[37] An algorithm approach to diagnostic imaging evaluation of suspected rotator cuff disease has been suggested that incorporates ultrasound.[38]

PARTIAL-THICKNESS TEAR

Partial-thickness supraspinatus tendon tears are characterized by a well-defined hypoechoic or anechoic abnormality that disrupts the tendon fibers, which may be articular-side or bursal-side partial-thickness tears determined by which surface

of the tendon is involved.[30,39] An intra-substance or interstitial tear may also be considered a form of partial-thickness tear, but one that does not extend to the articular or bursal surface.

Articular-side partial-thickness tears most commonly involve the supraspinatus anteriorly and distally at the greater tuberosity and are seen with increased frequency in patients younger than 40 years.[17,18] A mixed hyperechoic-hypoechoic appearance may be present, which represents hypoechoic fluid that surrounds the hyperechoic torn tendon stump (Figs. 3.21, 3.22, 3.23, and 3.24).[39] Cortical irregularity of the greater

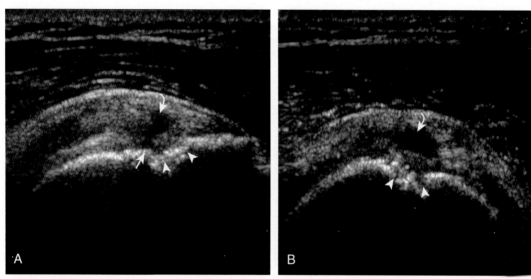

■ FIGURE 3.21 **Supraspinatus Tear: Articular, Partial Thickness.** Ultrasound Images of supraspinatus tendon in long axis (A) and short axis (B) show well-defined anechoic disruption of the tendon fibers *(curved arrow)*, which surrounds the hyperechoic tendon stump distally and creates a mixed hyperechoic-hypoechoic appearance. Note contact with the articular surface *(arrow)*, cortical irregularity of the greater tuberosity *(arrowheads)*, and lack of volume loss.

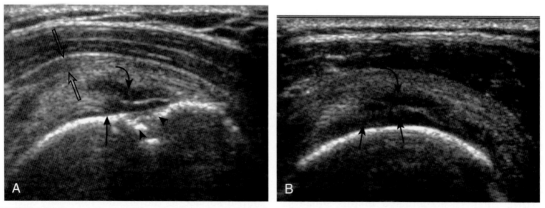

■ FIGURE 3.22 **Supraspinatus Tear: Articular, Partial Thickness.** Ultrasound images of supraspinatus tendon in long axis (A) and short axis (B) show well-defined hypoechoic disruption of the tendon fibers *(curved arrow)* with a mixed hyperechoic-hypoechoic appearance distally. Note contact with the hypoechoic hyaline cartilage at the articular surface *(arrows)*, cortical irregularity of the greater tuberosity *(arrowheads)*, and lack of volume loss. The subacromial-subdeltoid bursa is thickened and isoechoic to tendon *(open arrows)*.

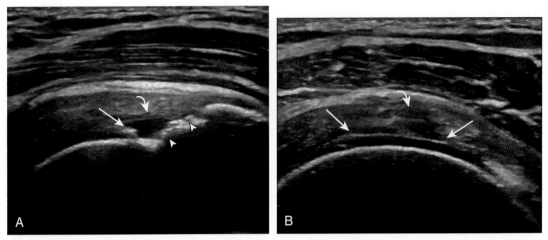

■ **FIGURE 3.23 Supraspinatus Tear: Articular, Partial Thickness.** Ultrasound images of supraspinatus tendon in long axis (A) and short axis (B) show well-defined anechoic disruption of the tendon fibers *(curved arrow)*. Note contact with the hypoechoic hyaline cartilage at the articular surface and cartilage interface sign *(arrows)* and cortical irregularity of the greater tuberosity *(arrowheads)*.

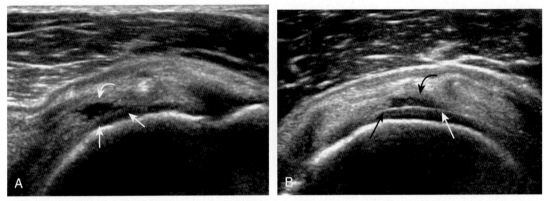

■ **FIGURE 3.24 Supraspinatus Tear: Articular, Partial Thickness.** Ultrasound images of supraspinatus tendon in long axis (A) and short axis (B) show well-defined anechoic disruption of the proximal tendon fibers *(curved arrow)* with articular extension as cartilage interface sign *(arrows)* (hypoechoic area at greater tuberosity is anisotropy).

tuberosity immediately adjacent to the tendon tear is common, related to the chronic cuff attrition at the site of the tear.[30-32] An acute tear of a previously normal cuff or a proximal tear (Fig. 3.24) will not be associated with cortical irregularity, although these tears are less common. With an articular-side partial-thickness tear, the superior surface of the tendon remains convex because global tendon volume loss is usually absent. Articular surface extension of a tear is suggested when the tear is in direct contact with the hypoechoic hyaline cartilage. The hyperechoic interface between the tendon tear and the hyaline cartilage may be accentuated in this situation (called the *cartilage interface sign*).[40] The terms *rim-rent tear* and *PASTA* (partial articular-side supraspinatus tendon avulsion) *lesion* are used specifically to describe a far-distal articular-side

partial-thickness tear, immediately adjacent to the greater tuberosity surface (Videos 3.16, 3.17. and 3.18).[17,18] Recall that the articular fibers of the distal supraspinatus tendon abruptly redirect to attach to the greater tuberosity and this tendon orientation will often create a focal hypoechoic area from anisotropy that should not be mistaken for an articular-side partial-thickness tear (see Fig. 3.69).[16,41,42]

A bursal-side partial-thickness supraspinatus tendon tear is also hypoechoic or anechoic, but it is localized to the bursal surface (Figs. 3.25, 3.26, 3.27, and 3.28).[30] Tear extension from the bursal surface to the greater tuberosity surface (or tendon footprint), without extension to the articular surface, is still considered a bursal-side partial-thickness tear. This results in focal absence of tendon or uncovering of the distal greater

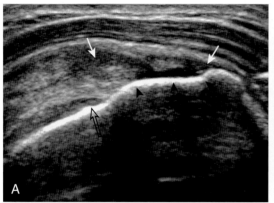
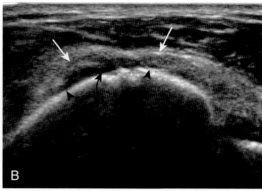

■ **FIGURE 3.25 Supraspinatus Tear: Bursal, Partial Thickness.** Ultrasound images of supraspinatus tendon in long axis (A) and short axis (B) show absence of the bursal aspect of the supraspinatus tendon and replacement with anechoic fluid *(curved arrow)*. Note the bursal extent *(between arrows)* and the greater tuberosity extent *(between arrowheads)* of tear, the absence of contact with the hyaline cartilage *(open arrow)*, and loss of the normal superior convexity. Greater tuberosity cortical irregularity is present in B.

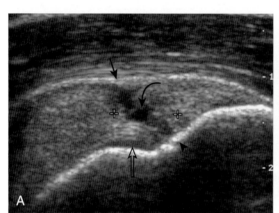
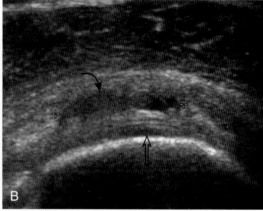

■ **FIGURE 3.26 Supraspinatus Tear: Bursal, Partial Thickness.** Ultrasound images of supraspinatus tendon in long axis (A) and short axis (B) show well-defined hypoechoic disruption of the tendon fibers *(curved arrow, between cursors)*, which extends from the bursal surface *(arrow)* to the greater tuberosity *(arrowhead)*. There is no contact with the hypoechoic hyaline cartilage at the articular surface *(open arrow)*, and this excludes a full-thickness tear.

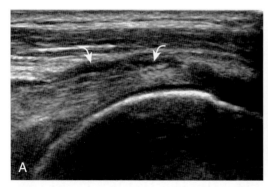
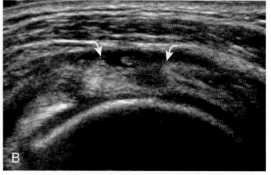

■ **FIGURE 3.27 Supraspinatus Tear: Bursal, Partial Thickness.** Ultrasound images of supraspinatus tendon in long axis (A) and short axis (B) show well-defined hypoechoic disruption of the most superficial tendon fibers *(curved arrows)*.

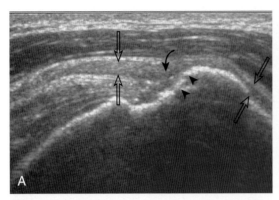
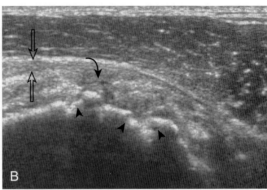

■ **FIGURE 3.28 Supraspinatus Tear: Bursal, Partial Thickness.** Ultrasound images of supraspinatus tendon in long axis (A) and short axis (B) show thinning of the tendon from loss of bursal-side fibers *(curved arrow),* torn from the greater tuberosity *(arrowheads).* Note the thickened isoechoic subacromial-subdeltoid bursa *(open arrows),* which fills the tendon tear and extends beyond the greater tuberosity. There is no extension to the articular surface.

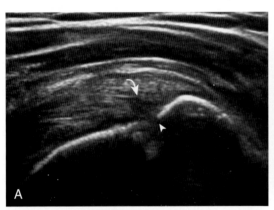
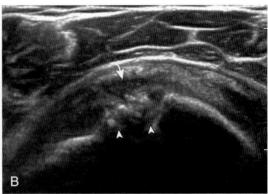

■ **FIGURE 3.29 Intra-Substance Tear.** Ultrasound images of supraspinatus in long axis (A) and short axis (B) show focal hypoechoic defect *(curved arrow)* only contacting the greater tuberosity surface with cortical irregularity *(arrowheads).*

tuberosity footprint (Video 3.19). Because of the superficial location of the tear, tendon thinning and volume loss of the cuff are usually present. This situation results in loss of the normal superior convexity of the supraspinatus tendon surface, with dipping of the deltoid muscle and subacromial-subdeltoid bursa into the torn tendon gap. Similar to other supraspinatus tendon tears, greater tuberosity cortical irregularity is typically present because the tear extends from the bursal surface to the greater tuberosity surface. If adjacent subacromial-subdeltoid bursal synovial hypertrophy is present, hypoechoic or isoechoic synovial tissue may fill the torn tendon gap, making the tear and tendon thinning less conspicuous (Fig. 3.28) (Video 3.20).

A tendon tear that does not contact the articular or bursal side of the supraspinatus is termed an *intrasubstance* or *interstitial tear.*[17,18] Such tears may be anechoic or hypoechoic, located within the

tendon substance or in contact with the greater tuberosity surface (Fig. 3.29). Cortical irregularity is often seen in the latter situation. Volume loss of the tendon is absent. Extensive intra-substance tears may either represent or be precursors of a more extensive delamination tear. The presence of a well-defined anechoic cyst within the rotator cuff is usually associated with a supraspinatus articular-side tear.[43]

FULL-THICKNESS TEAR

A full-thickness supraspinatus tendon tear is characterized by a well-defined hypoechoic or anechoic defect that disrupts the hyperechoic tendon fibers and extends from the articular to bursal surfaces of the tendon (Figs. 3.30, 3.31, 3.32, 3.33, 3.34, 3.35, 3.36, 3.37, and 3.38).[30,36] Identification of a hyperechoic interface between the hypoechoic hyaline cartilage and anechoic or

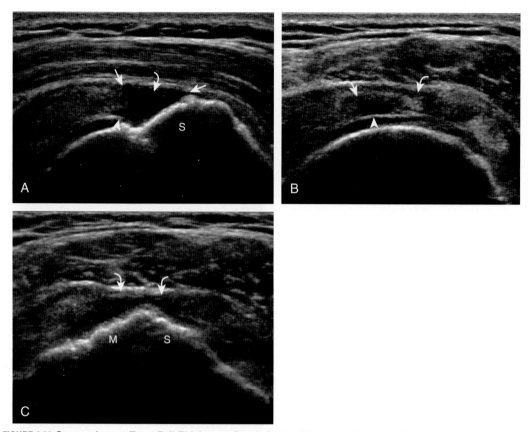

■ **FIGURE 3.30 Supraspinatus Tear: Full Thickness, Focal, Acute.** Ultrasound images of supraspinatus in long axis (A) and short axis (B and C) show anechoic focal full-thickness tear *(curved arrows)*. Note broader bursal extent *(arrows)* and more focal articular extent with cartilage interface sign *(arrowhead)* as well as cortical irregularity. *M*, Middle facet of greater tuberosity; *S*, superior facet of greater tuberosity.

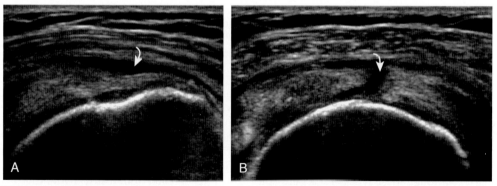

■ **FIGURE 3.31 Supraspinatus Tear: Full Thickness, Focal, Acute.** Ultrasound images of supraspinatus in long axis (A) and short axis (B) show anechoic focal full-thickness longitudinal tear *(curved arrow)* best seen in short axis. Note difficulty in visualizing the tear in long axis given longitudinal orientation and narrow width.

hypoechoic tendon tear *(cartilage interface sign)* assists in the identification of the articular extent.[40] This finding is only seen when the sound beam is perpendicular to the hyaline cartilage; the heel-toe maneuver when imaging the tendon in long axis and toggling the transducer while in short axis is helpful (see Chapter 1). Small full-thickness tears may not be associated with volume loss of the tendon, especially if filled with fluid. Narrow longitudinal tears are best visualized with the tendon in short axis (Fig. 3.31). As a tear becomes larger, flattening or concavity of the

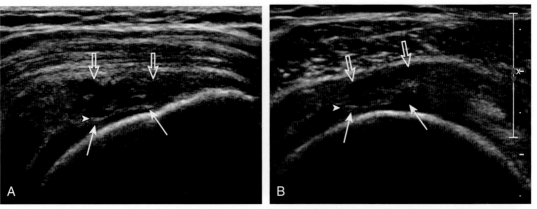

■ FIGURE 3.32 **Supraspinatus Tear: Full Thickness, Focal.** Ultrasound images of supraspinatus in long axis (A) and short axis (B) show anechoic disruption of the tendon fibers, which extends from bursal *(open arrows)* to articular *(arrows)* surfaces. Note volume loss of the tendon and a cartilage interface sign *(arrowhead)* indicating articular extension.

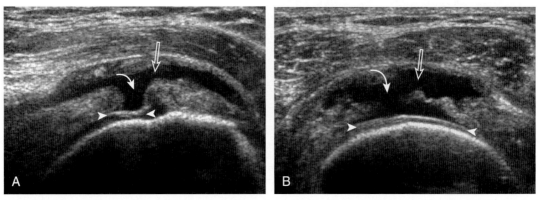

■ FIGURE 3.33 **Supraspinatus Tear: Full Thickness, Complete, Acute.** Ultrasound images of supraspinatus in long axis (A) and short axis (B) show fluid-filled anechoic disruption of the tendon fibers *(curved arrows)*, which extends from the subacromial-subdeltoid bursa *(open arrows)* to the articular surface *(arrowheads)*. Note the cartilage interface sign *(arrowheads)*, which shows the articular extent of tear.

superior supraspinatus tendon surface with volume loss is typical (Videos 3.21 and 3.22). Acute tears may occur more proximally, and more commonly are filled with anechoic fluid (Fig. 3.33).[33] An acute tear in a patient younger than 40 years or a proximal tear does not demonstrate cortical irregularity, although these types of tears are less common. When a tendon tear is identified, one should describe the location of the tendon tear, the dimensions of the tear in long axis and short axis, and extension to other adjacent tendons. A full-thickness tear that is small may be termed a *focal* or *incomplete full-thickness tear*, whereas a tear that involves the entire width of a tendon may be termed a *complete* or *full-width full-thickness tear*. Chronic tears may be associated with extensive remodeling of the greater tuberosity, and the distal torn tendon may be tapered without adjacent

fluid but possibly with isoechoic or hyperechoic synovial hypertrophy (Fig. 3.37). To determine if a supraspinatus tear involves the adjacent infraspinatus, knowledge of the greater tuberosity anatomy and tendon attachments is helpful (see Fig. 3.2). When imaging the cuff in short axis over the greater tuberosity, a tear that extends over the posterior aspect of the middle facet indicates infraspinatus involvement as well. A supraspinatus tendon tear may also extend anteriorly through the rotator interval to involve the cephalad fibers of the subscapularis tendon (see Subscapularis Tears and Tendinosis). A biceps reflection pulley tear and long head of biceps brachii tendon subluxation or dislocation may also occur in this situation (Fig. 3.39) (Videos 3.23 and 3.24).[4] The supraspinatus and infraspinatus muscles should be assessed for fatty infiltration

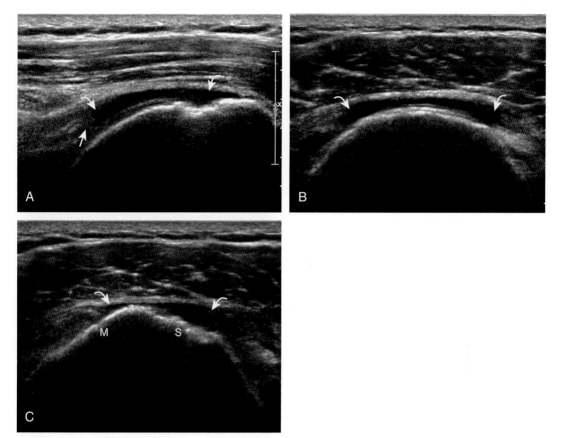

■ **FIGURE 3.34 Supraspinatus Tear: Full Thickness, Complete.** Images of supraspinatus in long axis (A) and short axis (B and C) show anechoic disruption of the tendon fibers *(between curved arrows)* with proximal tendon retraction *(arrow)*. *M,* Middle facet; *S,* superior facet of the greater tuberosity.

and atrophy in the setting of a rotator cuff tear as this finding is associated with poor surgical outcome after repair (see Rotator Cuff Atrophy).[44,45]

TENDINOSIS

The term *tendinosis* is used rather than tendinitis because active inflammatory cells are absent. Instead, a degenerative process is present with eosinophilic, fibrillar, and mucoid degeneration and possible chondroid metaplasia.[46,47] At ultrasound, focal tendinosis is characterized by a heterogeneous, somewhat ill-defined, hypoechoic area in the tendon without a defined tendon defect (Fig. 3.40).[30,48] Tendinosis must be differentiated from anisotropy as both may appear hypoechoic (see Fig. 3.11). Unlike tendon tear, tendinosis is usually less defined, it may be associated with increased tendon thickness, and it is usually not associated with adjacent cortical irregularity of the greater tuberosity.[30] Diffuse tendinosis may cause the entire tendon to appear hypoechoic, nearly equal in echogenicity to adjacent muscle

(Fig. 3.41). Unlike a massive tendon tear, a normal convex superior surface of the supraspinatus is still seen with tendinosis.

INDIRECT SIGNS OF SUPRASPINATUS TENDON TEAR

Tendon Thinning. Thinning or volume loss of the supraspinatus tendon and flattening or superior concavity of the superior supraspinatus tendon surface typically indicate tendon fiber loss. This condition can be seen with full-thickness tendon tears, especially moderate size or larger (see Figs. 3.30 and 3.38), and bursal-sided partial-thickness supraspinatus tendon tears (see Figs. 3.27 and 3.28). The presence of tendon thinning helps to exclude tendinosis because this latter condition, in contrast, shows normal or increased tendon thickness (see Figs. 3.40 and 3.41).

Cortical Irregularity. When there is cortical irregularity of the greater tuberosity immediately adjacent to a defined hypoechoic or anechoic

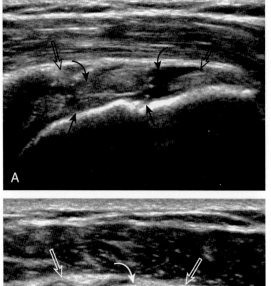

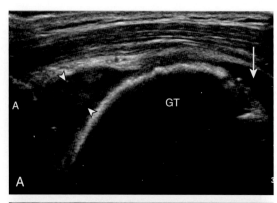

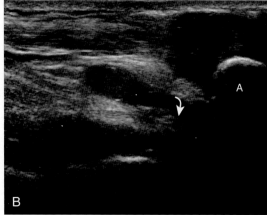

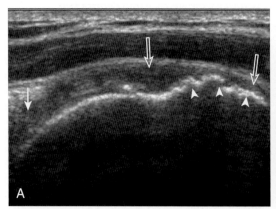

■ **FIGURE 3.35 Supraspinatus Tear: Full Thickness, Complete.** Ultrasound images of supraspinatus in long axis (A) and short axis (B) show anechoic and isoechoic heterogeneous disruption of the tendon fibers *(curved arrows)*. Note the bursal extent *(open arrows)*, articular extent with cartilage interface sign *(arrows)*, and loss of normal superior convexity.

■ **FIGURE 3.36 Supraspinatus Tear: Full Thickness, Complete.** Ultrasound image of supraspinatus in long axis (A) at greater tuberosity *(GT)* shows tendon tear filled with hypoechoic synovitis *(arrowheads)* and anechoic subacromial-subdeltoid bursal distention *(arrow)*. More proximal imaging over supraspinatus fossa (B) shows retracted supraspinatus tendon stump *(curved arrow)* and surrounding fluid medial to acromion *(A)* (left side of image is medial).

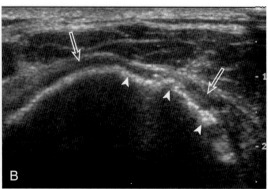

■ **FIGURE 3.37 Supraspinatus Tear: Full Thickness, Complete, Chronic.** Ultrasound images of supraspinatus in long axis (A) and short axis (B) show a torn and retracted supraspinatus tendon tear, with the tendon void filled with hypoechoic synovium, hemorrhage, and scar tissue, in continuity with the subacromial-subdeltoid bursa *(open arrows)*. There is significant volume loss of the tendon substance as the torn tendon stump is retracted *(arrow)*. Note significant irregularity and remodeling of the greater tuberosity *(arrowheads)*.

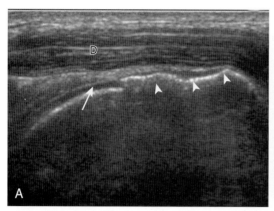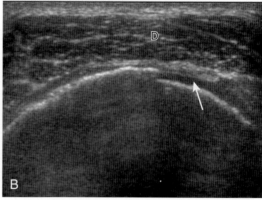

■ FIGURE 3.38 **Suprasinatus Tear: Full Thickness, Complete, Chronic.** Ultrasound images of supraspinatus in long axis (A) and short axis (B) show absence of the supraspinatus tendon because it is retracted proximally beneath the acromion. A thin hyperechoic layer represents the collapsed subacromial-subdeltoid bursa, which lies between the deltoid muscle *(D)* and the hypoechoic hyaline cartilage *(arrow)*. Note significant remodeling of the greater tuberosity *(arrowheads)*.

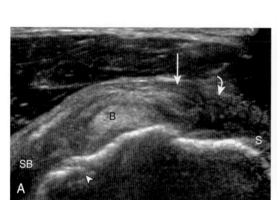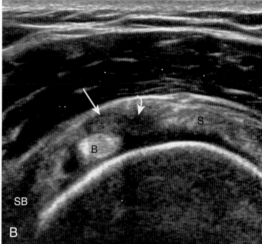

■ FIGURE 3.39 **Biceps Reflection Pulley Tear.** Ultrasound images in short axis to proximal biceps brachii tendon from two different patients (A and B) show tear of the anterior supraspinatus *(curved arrow)* and coracohumeral ligament *(arrow)*. Note (A) subchondral cortical irregularity representing the chondral print sign *(arrowhead)*. *B,* Biceps brachii long head tendon; *S,* supraspinatus; *SB,* subscapularis.

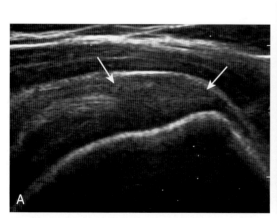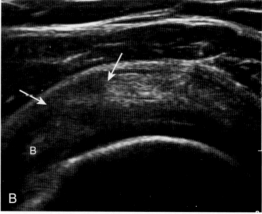

■ FIGURE 3.40 **Supraspinatus Tendinosis: Focal.** Ultrasound images of supraspinatus in long axis (A) and short axis (B) show focal, ill-defined hypoechogenicity *(arrows)* with increased tendon thickness. *B,* Biceps brachii long head tendon.

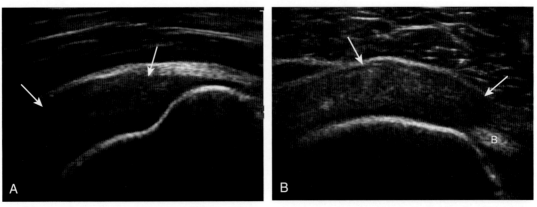

■ **FIGURE 3.41 Supraspinatus Tendinosis: Diffuse.** Ultrasound images of supraspinatus in long axis (A) and short axis (B) show diffuse hypoechogenicity throughout the tendon *(arrows)* with loss of the normal fibrillar pattern. Note smooth greater tuberosity. *B,* Biceps brachii long head tendon.

tendon abnormality of the supraspinatus, this increases the likelihood that the tendon abnormality represents a tear (see Figs. 3.21 and 3.22).[30-32] Therefore, if greater tuberosity cortical irregularity at the supraspinatus footprint is identified during scanning, special attention should be paid to this area. This finding is also helpful in the differentiation between tendon tear and tendinosis because both may appear as a hypoechoic tendon abnormality. With tendinosis, the hyperechoic greater tuberosity surface is typically smooth, as in the normal state (see Fig. 3.41). In fact, cortical irregularity of the supraspinatus footprint on radiography is associated with a rotator cuff tear in 75% of cases, while lack of cortical irregularity is associated with normal rotator cuff in 96%.[51] Cortical irregularity is common with chronic attrition tears of the supraspinatus, but it may be absent with an acute tendon tear in a younger individual or with proximal tears (see Fig. 3.33). The significance of greater tuberosity cortical irregularity is specific to the attachment of the supraspinatus tendon. Cortical irregularity of the posterior aspect of the humerus involving the bare area (an area of intra-articular cortex without hyaline cartilage) beneath the infraspinatus tendon is a common finding, possibly a normal variant, and is usually without significance.[49] However, if cortical irregularity at this site is extensive, this too can be associated with articular surface partial-thickness infraspinatus tendon tear and posterior labral tear in the setting of posterosuperior impingement syndrome.[50] Finally, cortical irregularity of the lesser tuberosity of the subscapularis tendon insertion is also a common finding and is of little clinical significance in the absence of an adjacent tendon abnormality.

Joint Effusion and Bursal Fluid. Investigators have shown that the findings of both glenohumeral

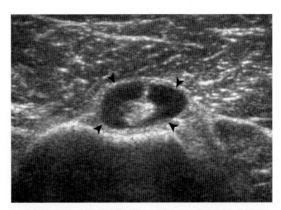

■ **FIGURE 3.42 Joint Effusion: Biceps Tendon Sheath Communication.** Ultrasound image of biceps brachii long head tendon in short axis at bicipital groove shows anechoic joint fluid *(arrowheads),* which distends the tendon sheath.

joint effusion and subacromial-subdeltoid fluid suggest rotator cuff tear with a positive predictive value of 95%.[51] To diagnose joint effusion, the long head of the biceps brachii tendon is evaluated in the bicipital groove for surrounding anechoic fluid (Fig. 3.42).[5,52] The long head of the biceps brachii tendon sheath normally communicates with the glenohumeral joint, so increased joint fluid will collect in this extension of the joint.[5,52] A tiny sliver of fluid at one side of the biceps tendon is often seen normally, but fluid greater than this is considered abnormal, especially if it is seen circumferential to the biceps tendon.[52] With regard to the posterior glenohumeral joint recess, small effusions may only be visible with the shoulder in external rotation (Video 3.25).[52] With larger joint effusions, fluid in the posterior shoulder joint recess can be seen even in neutral position deep to the infraspinatus tendon (Fig. 3.43). Subacromial-subdeltoid bursal

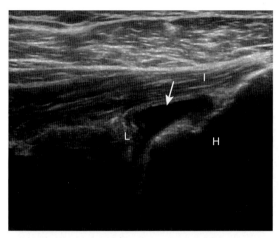

■ **FIGURE 3.43 Joint Effusion: Posterior Glenohumeral Recess.** Ultrasound image of posterior shoulder long axis to infraspinatus *(I)* shows anechoic joint fluid *(arrow)* between the posterior labrum *(L)* and the humeral head *(H)*.

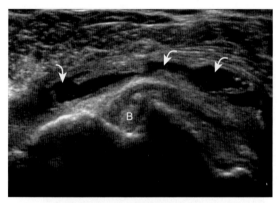

■ **FIGURE 3.44 Subacromial-Subdeltoid Fluid.** Ultrasound image over anterior shoulder short axis to the biceps brachii tendon shows a distention of the subacromial-subdeltoid bursa *(curved arrows)* filled with anechoic fluid and heterogeneous synovial hypertrophy. Note synovial hypertrophy within the tendon sheath of the biceps brachii long head tendon *(B)*.

fluid is diagnosed when the hyperechoic walls of the bursa are separated by more than 1 or 2 mm of anechoic fluid.[7] Both distention of the biceps brachii long head tendon sheath and the subacromial-subdeltoid bursa may be seen over the anterior shoulder (Fig. 3.44) (Video 3.26). Bursal fluid may also collect dependently, so the most inferior aspect of the bursa should also be evaluated to visualize small quantities of fluid (see Fig. 3.16C). Although simple joint and bursal fluid is commonly anechoic, complex fluid may appear hypoechoic or even isoechoic to adjacent muscle tissue.

Cartilage Interface Sign. Normally, the surface of the hypoechoic hyaline cartilage that covers

the humeral head is reflective and hyperechoic when the sound beam is perpendicular to the cartilage and underlying bone cortex. When an adjacent tendon is abnormally hypoechoic, or especially if there is adjacent anechoic fluid, this hyperechoic interface becomes more pronounced and is termed the *cartilage interface sign*.[40] The presence of this sign is helpful in that it indicates a tendon abnormality extends to the articular surface (see Figs. 3.24, 3.30, and 3.33) (Video 3.27).

Infraspinatus Tears and Tendinosis

Similar to the supraspinatus tendon, tears of the infraspinatus tendon may be partial-thickness tears (extending only to the articular or bursal surface, or intra-substance, and not in contact with either the articular or bursal surface) or full-thickness tears (that extend from the bursal to the articular surfaces) (Fig. 3.45). Tendon tears can appear hypoechoic or anechoic with possible tendon thinning, whereas tendinosis is typically hypoechoic with increased tendon thickness (Fig. 3.46). Partial-thickness articular-side tears of the infraspinatus have been described in the setting of internal or posterosuperior impingement syndrome.[50] This syndrome relates to impingement between the posterior aspect of the humerus and glenoid when the shoulder is externally rotated and abducted to 90 degrees, thus causing posterosuperior labral tear, marked cortical irregularity of the posterior aspect of the greater tuberosity, and partial-thickness articular infraspinatus tendon tear. Unlike the cortical irregularity of the superior aspect of the greater tuberosity associated with supraspinatus tendon tears, some degree of cortical irregularity of the posterior aspect of the humeral head in the bare area devoid of cartilage is considered a variation of normal.[49] When this irregularity is marked and associated with infraspinatus and adjacent labral disorders, posterosuperior impingement syndrome should be considered. Full-thickness tears of the infraspinatus tendon usually represent posterior extension of a supraspinatus tendon tear and are uncommonly isolated. When the entire width of the infraspinatus tendon is torn and retracted, this represents a complete or full-width full-thickness tear.

Subscapularis Tears and Tendinosis

Similar to infraspinatus tendon tears, isolated tears of the subscapularis tendon are uncommon.[53,54] Isolated full-thickness (complete or full-width) tears appear as complete tendon discontinuity, usually at the lesser tuberosity attachment (Fig. 3.47). Significant tendon retraction is common,

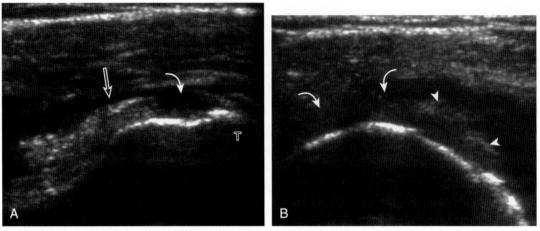

■ **FIGURE 3.45 Infraspinatus Tear: Full Thickness.** Ultrasound images long axis (A) and short axis (B) to infraspinatus show disruption of the tendon fibers *(curved arrows)* with fluid-filled subacromial-subdeltoid bursa *(open arrow)* (left side of image is proximal relative to tendon). Note the intact teres minor tendon *(arrowheads)* (left side of image is cephalad in B). *T,* Greater tuberosity.

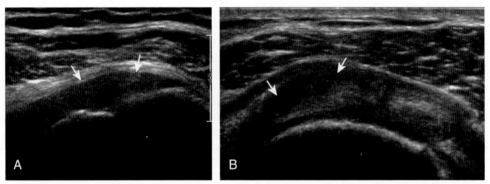

■ **FIGURE 3.46 Infraspinatus: Tendinosis.** Ultrasound images long axis (A) and short axis (B) to infraspinatus show abnormal hypoechogenicity and increased tendon thickness *(arrows)*.

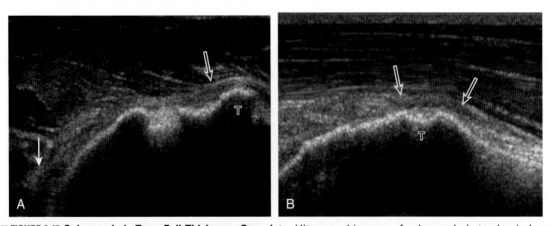

■ **FIGURE 3.47 Subscapularis Tear: Full Thickness, Complete.** Ultrasound images of subscapularis tendon in long axis (A) and short axis (B) show absence of the tendon *(open arrows)* at the lesser tuberosity *(T)* with proximal retraction *(arrow)* (left side of image is proximal in A and cephalad in B).

and this becomes more obvious with the shoulder positioned in external rotation (Video 3.28). If a fragment of bone is avulsed, this will appear as hyperechoic and shadowing, attached to the subscapularis tendon. The biceps brachii long head tendon may be dislocated into the glenohumeral joint with full-thickness subscapularis tendon tear. More commonly, subscapularis tears are isolated to the cephalad aspect in association with an anterior supraspinatus tendon (Fig. 3.48).[54] A subscapularis tear that extends from the bursal to articular surface that is isolated to the superior aspect would still be described as a focal or incomplete full-thickness tear.[55] In this setting, the long head of the biceps brachii tendon may be dislocated over the lesser tuberosity or into the substance of the subscapularis tendon at the site of the tear (see Biceps Brachii Tendon,

Subluxation and Dislocation). Partial-thickness tears may involve the articular (Fig. 3.49) or bursal surfaces or may be interstitial.[55] Tendinosis may also involve the subscapularis, which appears as heterogeneous abnormal hypoechogenicity and possible increased tendon thickness (Fig. 3.50).

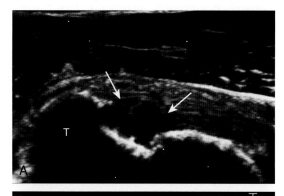

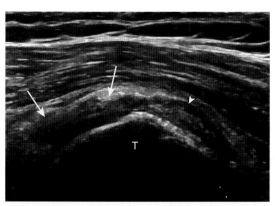

■ **FIGURE 3.48 Subscapularis Tear: Full Thickness, Incomplete or Focal.** Ultrasound image of subscapularis tendon in short axis shows the absence of the cephalad portion of the tendon *(arrows)*. Note the intact caudal fibers *(arrowhead)* at the lesser tuberosity *(T)* (left side of image is cephalad).

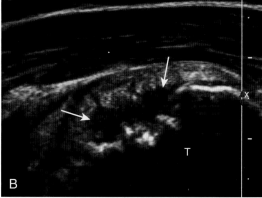

■ **FIGURE 3.49 Subscapularis Tear: Partial Thickness.** Ultrasound images of subscapularis tendon in long axis (A) and short axis (B) show focal hypoechoic articular-side tendon tear *(arrows)* (left side of image B is cephalad). *T,* Lesser tuberosity.

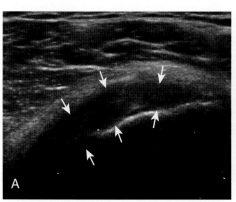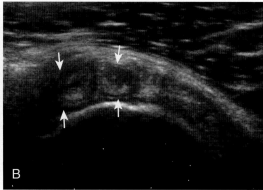

■ **FIGURE 3.50 Subscapularis: Tendinosis.** Ultrasound images of subscapularis tendon in long axis (A) and short axis (B) show increased thickness and hypoechogenicity of the cephalad portion of the subscapularis tendon *(arrows)*.

Rotator Cuff Atrophy

In the setting of a full-thickness rotator cuff tear, the supraspinatus and infraspinatus may undergo fatty degeneration or infiltration and possible atrophy.[56] This is important information because the presence of both fatty infiltration and muscle atrophy, in particular involvement of the infraspinatus, is a negative prognostic factor when considering rotator cuff repair.[44,57] The degree of rotator cuff atrophy relates to size, location, and chronicity of the rotator cuff tear.[29,57] More specifically, supraspinatus atrophy is associated with anterior cuff tears, possibly due to involvement of the rotator cable, and infraspinatus atrophy is associated with size of the full-thickness tear.[35] Isolated or more pronounced atrophy of the infraspinatus muscle is also possible, even if the rotator cuff tear is limited to the supraspinatus, possibly because of a compromised suprascapular nerve from altered biomechanics.[45] However, isolated infraspinatus atrophy may be an asymptomatic finding without associated rotator cuff tear.[58] The subscapularis and teres minor are usually unaffected. Paralabral cyst formation from a labral tear is another potential cause of both supraspinatus and infraspinatus muscle denervation when located in the suprascapular notch, or isolated to the infraspinatus when located in the spinoglenoid notch.

At ultrasound, fatty degeneration or infiltration and muscle atrophy will appear as increased echogenicity of the muscle and resultant poor differentiation between the tendon and muscle.[35,45,59] The hyperechoic tendon will demonstrate ill-defined borders in the setting of fatty infiltration, best appreciated at the musculotendinous junction

in short axis. Fatty atrophy will also result in decreased muscle bulk.[56] Imaging of the involved muscle in short axis is especially helpful in identifying decreased muscle size. One helpful landmark when imaging the infraspinatus for atrophy is the posterior scapular cortex at the level of the musculotendinous junction, where a ridge at the inferior aspect of the infraspinatus fossa of the scapula helps to define the infraspinatus and adjacent teres minor as separate muscles (Fig. 3.51). This site is useful in that the infraspinatus muscle is usually approximately twice the area compared with the adjacent teres minor. In addition, the echogenicity of the infraspinatus muscle can be compared with the teres minor, which is routinely normal even in the setting of a rotator cuff tear. Infraspinatus atrophy is diagnosed when the muscle echogenicity is greater than the teres minor, and the area of the infraspinatus is less than twice the teres minor. The supraspinatus should also be assessed for atrophy by moving the transducer superiorly from the infraspinatus between the clavicle and scapular spine.[56] Extended field of view imaging may be helpful to demonstrate both supraspinatus and infraspinatus muscle atrophy compared with the teres minor on one image (Fig. 3.52).[28] Muscle echogenicity should not be compared with the overlying deltoid because this muscle is commonly echogenic in older individuals and in diabetic patients. Ultrasound has been shown to be comparable to MRI in identification and grading of rotator cuff muscle atrophy.[56,59]

Teres minor atrophy may be seen in up to 3% of shoulders, which will appear as increased echogenicity and possible decreased muscle size compared with the infraspinatus.[60] This finding is often asymptomatic and may be due

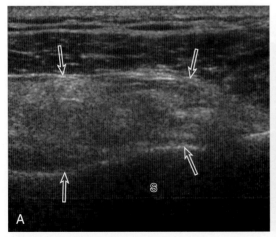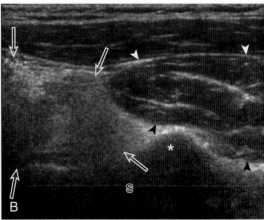

■ **FIGURE 3.51 Infraspinatus Atrophy.** Ultrasound images of infraspinatus in long axis (A) and short axis (B) show decreased size and increased echogenicity of the infraspinatus muscle *(open arrows)*, which becomes more apparent when compared with the teres minor *(arrowheads)*. S, Scapula. Note scapular ridge *(asterisk)*.

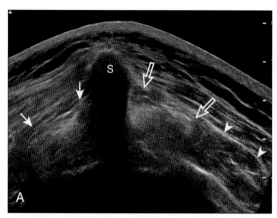
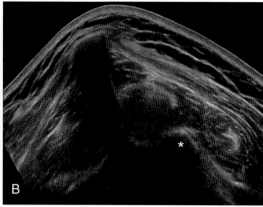

■ FIGURE 3.52 **Infraspinatus and Supraspinatus Fatty Infiltration.** Extended field of view ultrasound image (A) shows increased echogenicity of the supraspinatus *(arrows)* and infraspinatus *(open arrows)*, especially surrounding the tendons, compared with teres minor *(arrowheads)* and contralateral side (B). Note scapular ridge *(asterisk)*. *S,* Scapular spine.

to the presence of a fibrous band or variation in teres minor innervation that predisposes to nerve compression.[60-62] Uncommonly, teres minor atrophy may relate to quadrilateral space syndrome. The quadrilateral space is defined by the borders of the humerus, the long head of the triceps brachii muscle, and the teres minor and teres major. The axillary nerve and posterior circumflex humeral artery and veins traverse this space, and compression of these structures by fibrous bands, adjacent paralabral cyst, or mass may result in quadrilateral space syndrome.[63] At sonography, the teres minor or deltoid muscle, or both, may appear hyperechoic and small as a result of atrophy (Fig. 3.53).[64] To diagnose subtle abnormalities in size and echogenicity, it is helpful to make comparisons with the contralateral side or to compare the teres minor with the adjacent infraspinatus at the level of the muscle belly because normally the infraspinatus is approximately twice the size of the teres minor at this level.

Postoperative Shoulder

Evaluation of the rotator cuff after surgery can be challenging; however, ultrasound has been shown to be effective in the evaluation of the postoperative cuff with 89% accuracy.[65] One must be familiar with the types of rotator cuff repairs and aware of the appearances of the repaired and intact rotator cuff. For repair of a rotator cuff tear, a low-grade partial-thickness tear is commonly débrided, whereas a high-grade partial-thickness tear is converted to a full-thickness tear and repaired. Transosseous suture or suture anchors may be used, with the latter being single, multiple, single row, or commonly double row.[66]

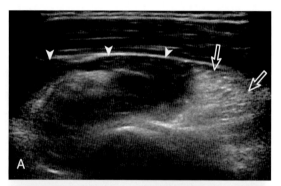
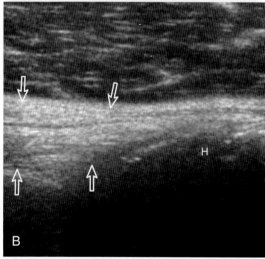

■ FIGURE 3.53 **Teres Minor Atrophy.** Ultrasound images of teres minor in short axis (A) and long axis (B) show increased echogenicity and decreased size *(open arrows)*. Note the normal appearance of the infraspinatus *(arrowheads)*. *H,* Humerus.

After rotator cuff repair, the tendon may appear thin and heterogeneous, whereas at other times, the tendon may be thickened and heterogeneously hypoechoic (Figs. 3.54, 3.55, and 3.56).[67-69] The general trend is for the repaired cuff to become more homogeneous and hyperechoic over time, with the repaired cuff beginning to appear as normal tendon by 6 months after surgery.[70] An intact tendon at 1 year tends to remain so at 2 years after surgery.[69] Hyperechoic suture material and suture anchors may be seen, as may the implantation trough, which appears as an angulated contour defect at the greater tuberosity (Fig. 3.56A). Because suture may cause shadowing of the underlying tendon that may simulate a tendon defect, imaging the cuff in short axis is helpful to show that the anechoic area is narrow and corresponds to shadowing directly under a suture, which is unlike a rotator cuff defect. If the repaired tendon is attached by suture passing through drill holes in the greater tuberosity, then suture may be seen at the lateral aspect of the greater tuberosity

as well. A hyperechoic focus attached to bone with reverberation can be seen with a metallic suture anchor. The area of the subacromial-subdeltoid bursa is commonly hypoechoic and thickened, and many times this bursa has been débrided or resected. Bone irregularity of the acromion could indicate changes related to acromioplasty.

To diagnose recurrent rotator cuff tear after repair, the most important finding is visualization of a defined tendon defect (Figs. 3.57 and 3.58).[67-69] Compressibility of the anechoic or hypoechoic tendon abnormality helps to differentiate tear from postoperative changes. Most recurrent rotator cuff tears are large or become large, with at least moderate retraction. Identification of retracted suture that is not continuous with the implantation site is additional evidence for a recurrent tear. Another feature of a recurrent cuff tear is visible suture without surrounding rotator cuff tendon (Fig. 3.58C and D). Most recurrent tendon tears occur within 3 months after surgery.[68] However, diagnosis of a recurrent tear in this

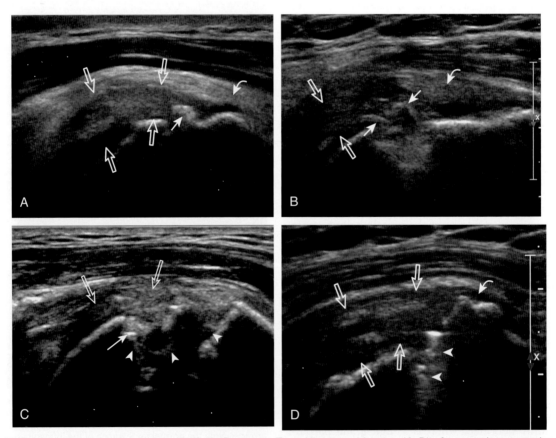

■ FIGURE 3.54 **Postoperative Rotator Cuff: No Recurrent Tear.** Ultrasound images (A–D) of supraspinatus tendon in long axis from four patients show variable appearance of repaired and intact supraspinatus tendon *(open arrows)*. Note suture material *(arrows)*, implantation trough *(arrowheads)*, and soft tissue thickening at the site of subacromial-subdeltoid bursa resection *(curved arrow)*. Echogenic metal suture anchor with reverberation artifact is seen in (D) *(arrowheads)*.

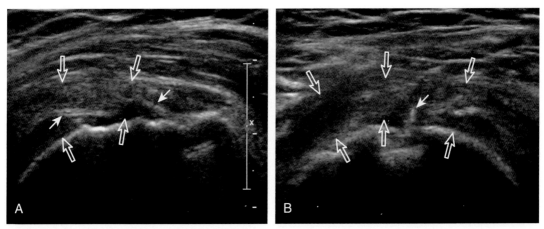

■ FIGURE 3.55 **Postoperative Rotator Cuff: No Recurrent Tear.** Ultrasound images of supraspinatus tendon in long axis (A) and short axis (B) show a heterogeneous and hypoechoic appearance *(open arrows)* with a hyperechoic suture *(arrow).*

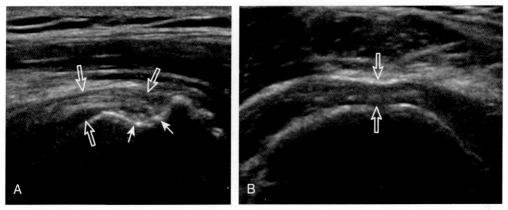

■ FIGURE 3.56 **Postoperative Rotator Cuff: No Recurrent Tear.** Ultrasound images of supraspinatus tendon in long axis (A) and short axis (B) show tendon thinning with loss of superior convexity *(open arrows)* and implantation trough *(arrows).*

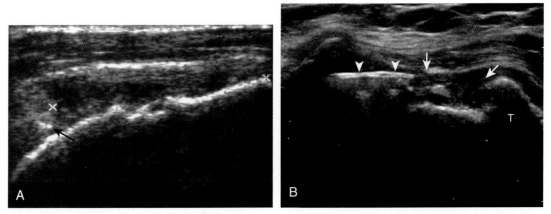

■ FIGURE 3.57 **Postoperative Rotator Cuff: Recurrent Tear.** Ultrasound image of supraspinatus tendon (long axis) (A) shows a large tendon defect *(between cursors).* Note the hyperechoic suture within the retracted proximal stump *(arrow).* Ultrasound image of supraspinatus (long axis) in a second patient (B) shows a recurrent tear *(arrows)* with displaced suture anchor *(arrowheads). T,* Greater tuberosity.

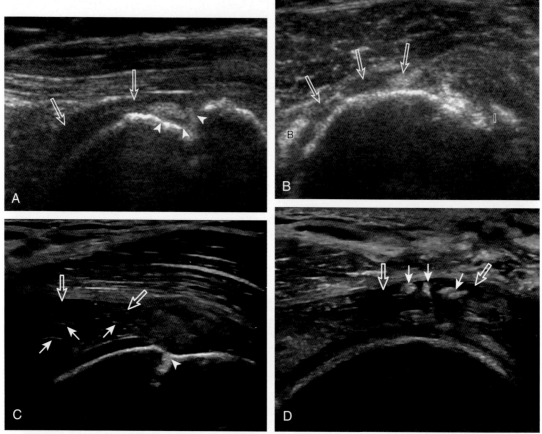

■ **FIGURE 3.58 Postoperative Rotator Cuff: Recurrent Tear.** Ultrasound images of supraspinatus in long axis (A) and short axis (B) show absence of the anterior portion of the supraspinatus *(open arrows)*. Note the tendon stump in the implantation trough *(arrowheads)*. Ultrasound images of supraspinatus in long axis (C) and short axis (D) in a second patient show a proximal tendon tear *(open arrows)* with exposed suture *(arrows)*. Note suture anchor *(arrowhead)*. *B,* Biceps; *I,* infraspinatus.

time interval should be reserved for obvious or large tears, as some tendon defects will eventually heal.[69] An equivocal ultrasound finding, especially within the first 6 to 9 months, should be reimaged after several weeks or months because such findings may improve over time, whereas a true tear often enlarges. Be aware that recurrent tendon tears may be asymptomatic, although larger defects are associated with decreased strength.[71]

Shoulder arthroplasty or joint replacement involves resection of the humeral head, placement of a metal component, and possibly resection and replacement of the glenoid surface.[66] With a conventional shoulder arthroplasty, the greater tuberosity is not resected, so the rotator cuff can be seen with ultrasound attaching normally to the humerus using routine bone landmarks. At ultrasound, the metal humeral component appears hyperechoic and smooth, with reverberation artifact, in the expected location of the humeral head (Fig. 3.59).[72,73] The normal rotator cuff

should be identified over the humeral surface attaching to the tuberosities, and therefore tendon discontinuity or non-visualization similar to the native shoulder is consistent with rotator cuff tear (Fig. 3.60). Ultrasound is ideal in evaluation of the rotator cuff after shoulder arthroplasty because artifact from the joint replacement occurs deep to the components, and the overlying rotator cuff region is easily visualized. In contrast to a conventional shoulder arthroplasty, a reverse total shoulder arthroplasty is used when there is an underlying rotator cuff tear prior to surgery. In this situation, the humeral tuberosities are resected and therefore normal bone landmarks are absent.

Tendon Calcification

Calcific deposits within the rotator cuff may take one of two forms. One form is a degenerative calcification that appears thin and linear along the axis of tendon fibers at the enthesis (Fig. 3.61)

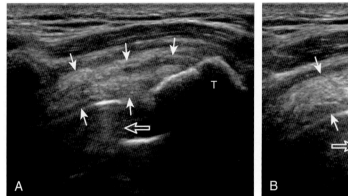
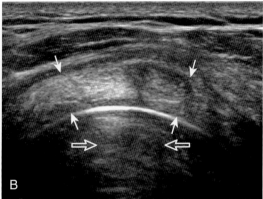

■ **FIGURE 3.59 Rotator Cuff After Shoulder Arthroplasty.** Ultrasound images of supraspinatus in long axis (A) and short axis (B) show intact rotator cuff *(arrows)* at the greater tuberosity *(T)*. Note posterior reverberation artifact *(open arrows)* deep to the arthroplasty. *(From Jacobson JA, Miller B, Bedi A, et al: Imaging of the postoperative shoulder.* Semin Musculoskelet Radiol *15:320-339, 2011.)*

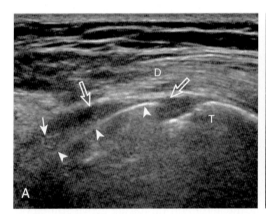
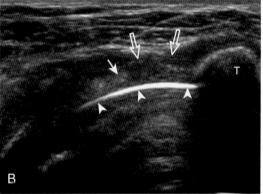

■ **FIGURE 3.60 Rotator Cuff Tear After Shoulder Arthroplasty.** Ultrasound images of the supraspinatus in long axis in two patients (A and B) show absence of the tendon *(open arrows)* over the humeral head component of the shoulder arthroplasty *(arrowheads)* and the retracted tendon stump *(arrows)*. The humeral head is high riding and in contact with the deltoid muscle *(D)*. Note posterior reverberation artifact deep to the arthroplasty. *T,* Greater tuberosity.

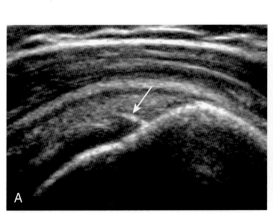
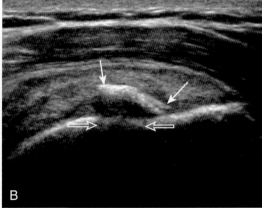

■ **FIGURE 3.61 Tendon Calcification: Degenerative.** Ultrasound images in two patients show the following: A, a well-defined linear calcific deposit *(arrow)* along the supraspinatus tendon fibers; B, a slightly larger linear calcific deposit *(arrows)* in the supraspinatus with partial shadowing *(open arrows)*.

(Video 3.29), which is commonly asymptomatic. The other form represents calcium hydroxyapatite deposition, which may be the result of decreased oxygen tension and fibrocartilaginous metaplasia although other suggested etiologies include remote trauma.[74-76] Such calcifications have three stages: pre-calcific (tendon metaplasia), calcific (including formative, resting, and resorptive phases), and post-calcific (resulting in fibrotic scar).[74] It is the resorptive phase where the calcification grows in size, becomes ill defined, and induces adjacent inflammation.[74] When symptomatic, the term *calcific tendinitis* is used given the presence of inflammatory markers, also associated with neo-vascularity and neoinnervation.[77] The underlying rotator cuff is typically intact without tendon tear. More common in women, calcific tendinosis has a reported prevalence of 24% of asymptomatic females.[78] The supraspinatus is most commonly involved, followed by the infraspinatus and sub-scapularis. Symptoms are most likely present with supraspinatus or multifocal tendon involvement.

The calcific deposits in calcific tendinosis most commonly are hyperechoic with posterior acoustic shadowing (Video 3.30), although appearances may vary (Fig. 3.62) as others have an amorphous appearance or are globular with minimal or no shadowing.[79] Cortical erosions and osseous involvement may also be present (Fig. 3.62D).[80] In approximately 7% of cases, tendon calcification shadowing is absent, and radiographs may be normal if calcifications are in the form of a thick fluid or slurry.[79] When calcific deposit echogenicity is isoechoic to tendon without shadowing, the amorphous echotexture during real-time scanning can be identified, and this replaces the normal fibrillar tendon appearance (Video 3.31). An additional method to help in this distinction is the use of anisotropy. With angulation of the transducer so that the sound beam is not perpendicular to the tendon fibers, the adjacent tendon will appear artifactually hypoechoic (Fig. 3.63). This does not significantly change the appearance of the calcifications; therefore, the hyperechoic calcific deposits become more conspicuous when they are surrounded by the hypoechoic tendon. Calcifications may be multiple in one or many tendons. In addition, large calcifications may contact the acromion during arm elevation as a form of impingement (Video 3.32).

Calcifications that are amorphous without shadowing are associated with acute symptoms, whereas well-defined calcifications with shadowing are associated with subacute or chronic symptoms.[81] In addition, larger calcifications associated with an abnormal subacromial-subdeltoid bursa are also more likely symptomatic.[82] Increased flow on color and power Doppler imaging surrounding the calcifications may be evident, a finding that correlates with patients' symptoms and a higher likelihood of the resorptive phase (Fig. 3.64).[81] Calcifications may be identified at the bursal edge of the involved tendon with possible extension into the subacromial-subdeltoid bursa (see Fig. 3.94D). Ultrasound-guided percutaneous lavage and aspiration of the calcifications have been shown to be effective and improve symptoms, although clinical outcome at 5 and 10 years may be similar regardless of treatment (see Chapter 9).[75]

Impingement Syndrome

Of the rotator cuff tendons, the supraspinatus is prone to impingement. This is because the supraspinatus passes through a confined space between the scapula and the coracoacromial arch, which consists of the acromion, the distal clavicle, the acromioclavicular joint, the coracoid process, and the coracoacromial ligament. The subacromial-subdeltoid bursa also traverses this space over the supraspinatus tendon. Any abnormality that decreases the size of this space, such as an inferior acromioclavicular osteophyte or subacromial enthesophyte, can predispose to tendon impingement. The effect on the supraspinatus tendon is that of tendinosis and possible tear, whereas the overlying subacromial-subdeltoid bursa may be distended with fluid or synovial hypertrophy. Sonography can suggest the diagnosis of early subacromial impingement when the gradual pooling of subacromial-subdeltoid bursal fluid at the acromion tip during active arm elevation is present (Fig. 3.65) (Video 3.33).[26] This sign is most important when other causes of bursal fluid are excluded, such as primary inflammatory bursitis; however, gathering of the subacromial-subdeltoid bursa during arm elevation may be an asymptomatic finding.[83] For diagnosis of subacromial impingement, the shoulder is dynamically assessed with the transducer in the coronal-oblique plane showing the bone landmarks of the acromion and the greater tuberosity (see Fig. 3.17). Sliding the transducer anterior to the acromion may show bursal thickening beneath or adjacent to the coracoacromial ligament not visible at the level of the acromion because of shadowing from the acromion (Fig. 3.65C) (Video 3.34). A subacromial enthesophyte spur may also be seen at the acromion attachment of the coracoacromial ligament, which is directed anterior and medial from the acromion toward the coracoid process (Fig. 3.66). In addition to pooling of bursal fluid, other findings of subacromial impingement include gradual distention of the subacromial-subdeltoid bursa with synovial tissue or abrupt movement of a thickened bursa (Video 3.35). Another finding

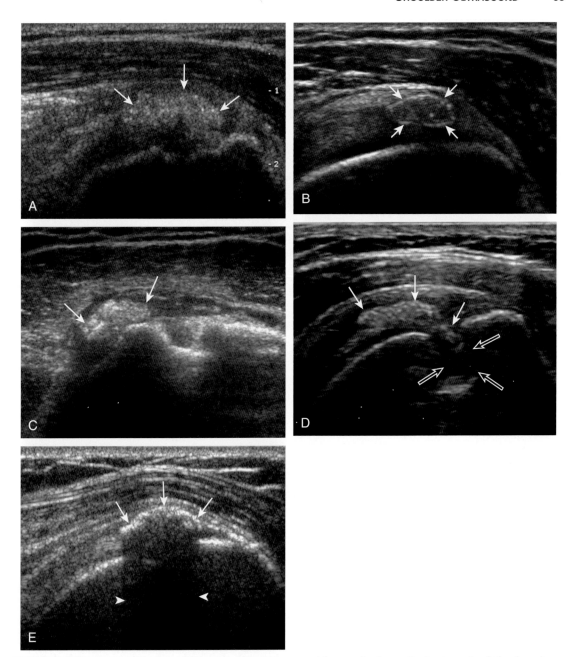

■ FIGURE 3.62 Tendon Calcification: Hydroxyapatite. Ultrasound images in five patients show the following: A, an amorphous heterogeneous nearly isoechoic calcific deposit *(arrows)* with minimal shadowing that replaces the normal fibrillar tendon architecture; B, a globular calcific deposit with internal fluid consistency *(arrows)*; C, a globular calcific deposit *(arrows)* in the subscapularis; D, a calcific deposit *(arrows)* with greater tuberosity intraosseous extension *(open arrows)*; and E, a well-defined hyperechoic supraspinatus calcific deposit *(arrows)* with posterior acoustic shadowing *(arrowheads)*.

described with subacromial impingement is superior bulging of the coracoacromial ligament when imaging the supraspinatus in short axis.[84] Later stages of subacromial impingement include abnormal upward migration of the humeral head.[25] Bone impingement may occur between the acromion and the greater tuberosity, usually in the setting of a rotator cuff tear (Video 3.36).

The presence of an os acromiale has also been associated with symptoms of cuff impingement (Fig. 3.67).

Another form of rotator cuff impingement involves the subscapularis tendon and overlying subacromial-subdeltoid bursa between the coracoid process and lesser tuberosity of the proximal humerus, termed *coracoid impingement syndrome.*

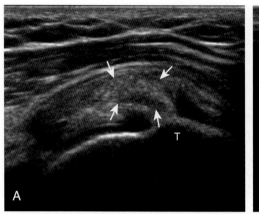
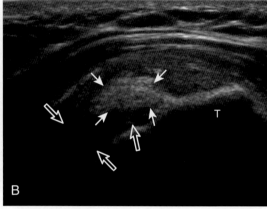

■ **FIGURE 3.63 Calcific Tendinosis: Anisotropy.** Ultrasound image of supraspinatus tendon in long axis (A) shows an ill-defined hyperechoic calcific deposit *(arrows)*. Note improved conspicuity of the calcific deposit (B) as the surrounding supraspinatus tendon is hypoechoic as a result of anisotropy *(open arrows)* after directing the ultrasound beam obliquely (heel-toe maneuver). *T,* Greater tuberosity.

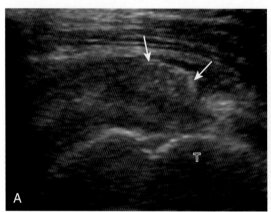
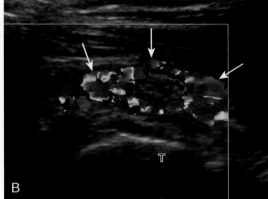

■ **FIGURE 3.64 Calcific Tendinitis: Hyperemia.** Ultrasound images of supraspinatus in long axis (gray scale in A, color Doppler in B) show amorphous hyperechoic calcific deposits within the supraspinatus tendon and the adjacent subacromial-subdeltoid bursa *(arrows)* with adjacent increased blood flow. *T,* Greater tuberosity.

Ultrasound findings in this condition include decreased distance between the coracoid process and the lesser tuberosity (range 5.9 to 9.6 mm) compared with the asymptomatic side (range 7.8 to 17.5 mm) with the ipsilateral hand placed on the opposite shoulder.[85] An additional finding is abnormal distention of the anterior aspect of the subacromial-subdeltoid bursa in the region of the subscapularis tendon and coracoid, which further distends with extension and internal rotation, correlating with anteromedial pain.[86]

Adhesive Capsulitis

Adhesive capsulitis, or frozen shoulder, is characterized by shoulder pain and limitation of motion.[87] Although often of unclear etiology, this condition is associated with diabetes mellitus, females, age greater than 40 years, trauma, and immobilization.[87] At sonography, adhesive cap-

sulitis can be initially suggested when the patient has limited external shoulder rotation while evaluating the subscapularis. Adhesive capsulitis is also suggested when there is limitation of the sliding movement of the supraspinatus tendon beneath the acromion with active arm elevation (Fig. 3.68) (Video 3.37).[27] Abnormal hypoechogenicity and hyperemia in the rotator interval, as well as thickening and increased stiffness of the coracohumeral ligament, are other described findings with adhesive capsulitis.[88-90]

■ PITFALLS IN ROTATOR CUFF ULTRASOUND

Errors in Scanning Technique

ANISOTROPY

The most common pitfall is misinterpretation of anisotropy as tendinosis or tendon tear. In

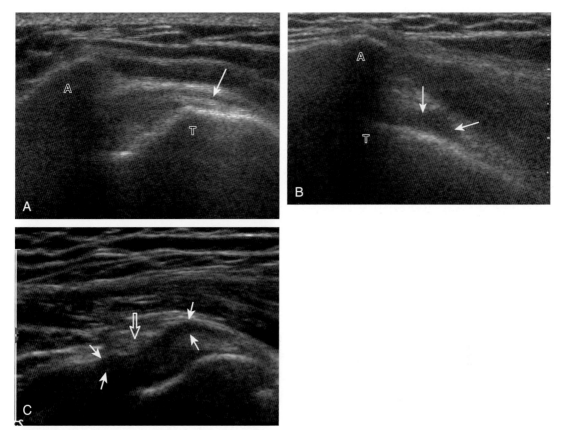

■ FIGURE 3.65 **Impingement Syndrome (Subacromial).** Ultrasound images of supraspinatus in long axis with arm in neutral position (A) and abduction (B) show gradual distention of the subacromial-subdeltoid bursa with anechoic fluid *(arrows)*. Ultrasound image of supraspinatus in long axis (C) anterior to the acromion in a different patient shows hypoechoic distention of the subacromial-subdeltoid bursa *(arrows)* with pooling on either side of the coracoacromial ligament *(open arrow)*. A, Acromion; T, greater tuberosity.

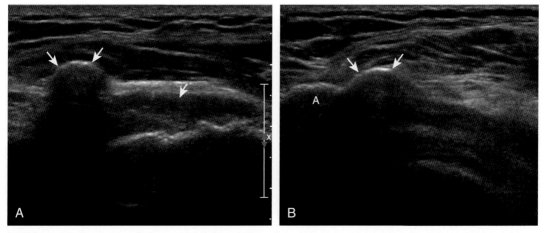

■ FIGURE 3.66 **Impingement: Subacromial Enthesophyte Spur.** Ultrasound images of supraspinatus in long axis (A) and short axis (B) show a large echogenic and shadowing subacromial enthesophyte spur *(arrows)* projecting anterior to the acromion *(A)* with adjacent supraspinatus tendinosis and tear *(curved arrow)*.

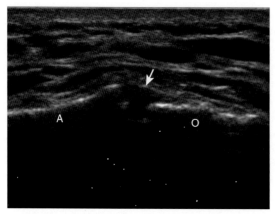

■ FIGURE 3.67 **Os Acromiale.** Ultrasound image over the acromion in the sagittal plane shows a hypoechoic cleft *(arrow)* between the acromion *(A)* and adjacent anterior acromion ossification center *(O)*.

particular, when imaging the distal supraspinatus tendon in long axis the articular fibers abruptly angulate to attach to the greater tuberosity footprint, which creates artifactual hypoechogenicity that simulates tendon tear (Fig. 3.69) (Video 3.38).[16] Redirecting the ultrasound beam perpendicular to the tendon fibers by rocking the transducer, using the heel-toe maneuver when imaging tendon in long axis or toggling the transducer when imaging the tendon in short axis, will eliminate anisotropy and show the normal hyperechoic tendon.

IMPROPER POSITIONING OF THE SHOULDER

With the shoulder in neutral position, the proximal supraspinatus is hidden beneath the acromion. Hyperextension of the shoulder (e.g., the Crass or modified Crass position) is needed to expose

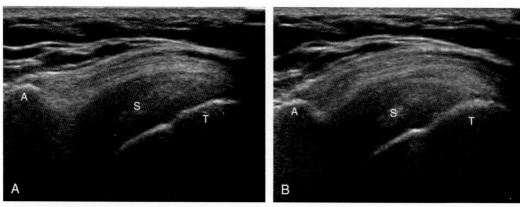

■ FIGURE 3.68 **Adhesive Capsulitis.** Ultrasound images of the supraspinatus tendon in long axis with arm in neutral position (A) and elevated to side (B) show that the supraspinatus tendon *(S)* does not slide beneath the acromion *(A)*, with arm elevation. Note the hypoechoic tendinosis of the supraspinatus tendon. *T,* Greater tuberosity.

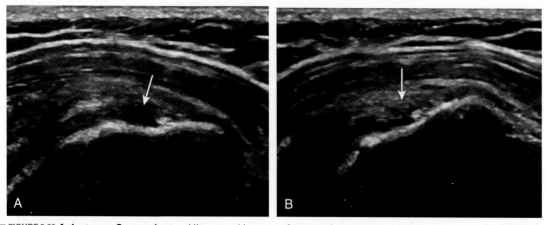

■ FIGURE 3.69 **Anisotropy: Supraspinatus.** Ultrasound images of supraspinatus tendon in long axis show (A) anisotropy *(arrow)* that simulates an anechoic tendon tear, which is no longer present (B) with repositioning of probe as sound beam becomes perpendicular to tendon fibers. Note degenerative calcifications at supraspinatus footprint.

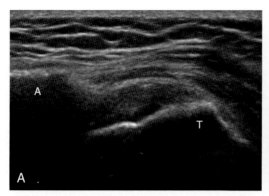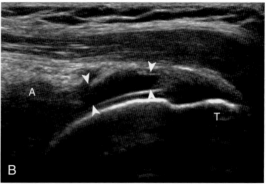

■ **FIGURE 3.70 Supraspinatus Tendon in Shoulder Neutral and Hyperextension.** Ultrasound images of supraspinatus tendon in long axis with the shoulder in neutral position (A) and hyperextension (B) show visualization of the supraspinatus tear *(arrowheads)* seen only in shoulder hyperextension. *A,* Acromion; *T,* greater tuberosity.

the entire supraspinatus tendon for evaluation (Fig. 3.70). It should be noted that distal supraspinatus pathology can adequately be seen with the shoulder in neutral position, as long as the patient's body habitus allows the arm to be vertical at the patient's side.[12] In a supine patient, the supraspinatus may also be visualized by having the patient hyperextend the arm posterior to the shoulder.[91]

INCOMPLETE EVALUATION OF THE SUPRASPINATUS TENDON

Many supraspinatus tendon tears in younger individuals occur anteriorly, often near the rotator interval.[14,17] The entire extent of the supraspinatus tendon, especially the anterior portion, must be completely evaluated. This can be ensured with visualization of the intra-articular portion of the biceps brachii tendon in the rotator interval (Fig. 3.71). When imaging the supraspinatus tendon in long axis, the transducer should be moved anteriorly on the greater tuberosity until the biceps tendon is seen. When imaging the supraspinatus tendon in short axis, the biceps tendon within the rotator interval should again be visualized to ensure that the anterior aspect of the supraspinatus tendon is evaluated.[92]

IMAGING OF THE ROTATOR CUFF TOO DISTALLY

A pitfall may occur when imaging the supraspinatus tendon in short axis. If the transducer is located too distally over the greater tuberosity beyond the rotator cuff attachment, the image of deltoid muscle lying over the proximal humerus may simulate a massive rotator cuff tear because no cuff is visible (see Fig. 3.13E). This diagnosis is easily excluded by turning the transducer 90 degrees, long axis to the supraspinatus tendon, to indicate the improper transducer location. This

is another reason evaluation of the supraspinatus ideally begins in its long axis.

Misinterpretation of Normal Structures

MISINTERPRETATION OF THE ROTATOR INTERVAL

The rotator interval is a space between the superior margin of the subscapularis tendon and the anterior margin of the supraspinatus tendon.[4] Within this interval, the intra-articular portion of the long head of the biceps brachii tendon is located, along with the biceps pulley system of capsular thickening and reflections and the superior glenohumeral and coracohumeral ligaments (see Fig. 3.13G).[4] The superior glenohumeral ligament is located at the subscapularis side of the biceps brachii tendon with fibers merging with the coracohumeral ligament, which is located superficial to the biceps tendon. The rotator interval also is the site where the glenohumeral joint communicates with the more medial subscapularis recess. The rotator interval is easily seen when the transducer is transverse to the supraspinatus tendon, although the modified Crass position may be needed to optimize visualization. The biceps tendon appears hyperechoic and is separated from the adjacent supraspinatus by a thin hypoechoic interface, which should not be misinterpreted as a tendon tear.[93] Widening of the space around the biceps brachii long head tendon in the rotator interval could indicate anterior supraspinatus or subscapularis tendon tear, biceps pulley injury, and biceps subluxation (see Fig. 3.39).[4]

MISINTERPRETATION OF THE MUSCULOTENDINOUS JUNCTION

The musculotendinous junction represents a transition from hypoechoic muscle to hyperechoic

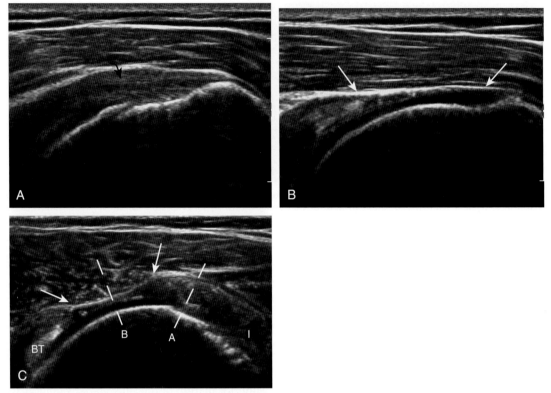

■ FIGURE 3.71 **Supraspinatus Tear.** A, Ultrasound image of supraspinatus in long axis over the middle facet posteriorly shows tendinosis. B, Ultrasound image of supraspinatus tendon in long axis anteriorly over the superior facet shows full-thickness tear *(arrows)*. C, Ultrasound image in short axis shows the supraspinatus tear *(arrows)* with the intact tendon posteriorly (A and B correspond to long axis imaging planes in A and B, respectively). *BT,* Biceps tendon; *I,* infraspinatus.

tendon. Because this transition is not uniform, a mixed hyperechoic-hypoechoic appearance may be seen. One example is the proximal aspect of the supraspinatus tendon when one visualizes the oval anterior or central tendon of the supraspinatus and the smaller and flatter posterior tendon.[16] When imaged in short axis, the intervening hypoechoic areas representing muscle tissue should not be misinterpreted as tendon tear or tendinosis (Fig. 3.72A and B). This pitfall is easily avoided by imaging the tendon in long axis, where the tapering appearance of the hypoechoic muscle tissue can be appreciated. A similar effect also involves the subscapularis, where both hypoechoic muscle and hyperechoic tendon are seen (Fig. 3.72C). This appearance is most obvious in short axis, where several hyperechoic tendon bundles can be seen with hypoechoic muscle and interfaces.

MISINTERPRETATION OF THE SUPRASPINATUS-INFRASPINATUS JUNCTION

Distally, the fibers of the supraspinatus and infraspinatus attach onto the greater tuberosity of the proximal humerus. Over the middle greater tuberosity facet, infraspinatus tendon fibers overlap superficial to the supraspinatus tendon fibers (see Fig. 3.2).[1,20] When imaging the supraspinatus in long axis over the middle facet, the overlapping and superficial infraspinatus tendon is identified given its oblique orientation relative to the supraspinatus, which also produces a series of uniform linear hypoechoic bands as a result of infraspinatus anisotropy (Fig. 3.73). This striped appearance is more conspicuous during real-time scanning because the fairly equally spaced hypoechoic oblique lines uniformly move through the tendon (Video 3.39) and should not be misinterpreted for tendon pathology. This characteristic appearance can be used to locate the supraspinatus-infraspinatus junction for accurate characterization of rotator cuff pathology. Another finding to assist in identification of the supraspinatus-infraspinatus tendon junction is identification of the characteristic bone contours of the middle facet, which appears flat relative to the humeral head when imaging in long axis (see Fig. 3.10D).[1]

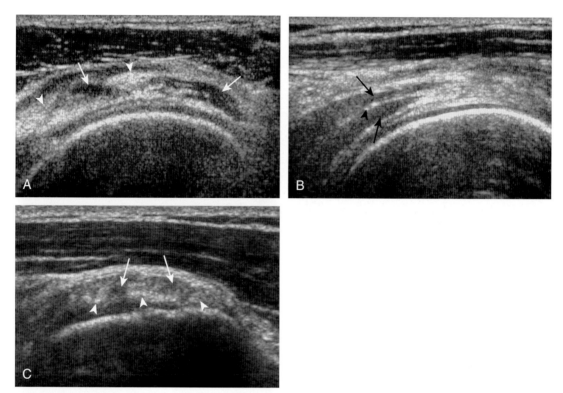

■ **FIGURE 3.72 Musculotendinous Junction.** Ultrasound images of supraspinatus in short axis (A) and long axis (B) and ultrasound image of subscapularis tendon in short axis (C) show intervening hypoechoic muscle *(arrows)* and hyperechoic tendon *(arrowheads)*.

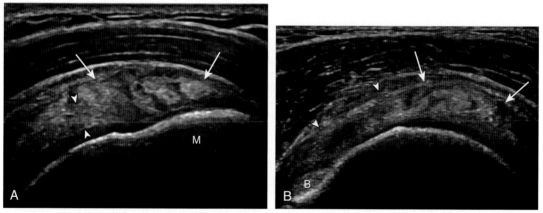

■ **FIGURE 3.73 Supraspinatus-Infraspinatus Tendon Junction.** Ultrasound images of supraspinatus tendon in long axis (A) and short axis (B) show the infraspinatus tendon (arrows) with linear, regularly spaced hypoechoic areas representing anisotropy that overlap the posterior aspect of the supraspinatus *(arrowheads)*. *M,* Middle facet of greater tuberosity; *B,* long head of biceps brachii tendon.

Misinterpretation of Pathology

SUBACROMIAL-SUBDELTOID BURSA SIMULATING TENDON

Although the abnormal subacromial-subdeltoid bursa is often distended with anechoic or hypoechoic fluid, the bursa may contain complex fluid or synovial hypertrophy. In these latter conditions, the echogenicity within the bursa may be isoechoic or even hyperechoic to adjacent muscle, and it may be nearly equal in echogenicity to tendon (Fig. 3.74). In the presence of a bursal-side partial-thickness tear (see Fig. 3.28) or a full-thickness tendon tear (see Fig. 3.37), a thickened and hyperechoic subacromial-subdeltoid bursa may lie within the torn tendon gap and

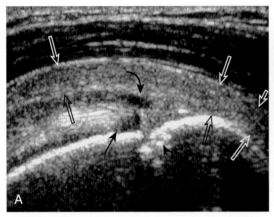

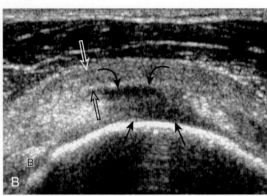

■ **FIGURE 3.74 Full-Thickness Supraspinatus Tear With Bursal Thickening.** Ultrasound images of supraspinatus in long axis (A) and short axis (B) show a well-defined hypoechoic defect, which extends from the bursal surface *(curved arrows)* to the articular surface *(arrows)*, with bone irregularity of the greater tuberosity *(arrowhead)*. Note diffuse echogenic distention of the subacromial-subdeltoid bursal *(open arrows)*, which extends beyond the greater tuberosity. *B,* Biceps tendon.

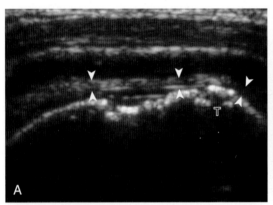

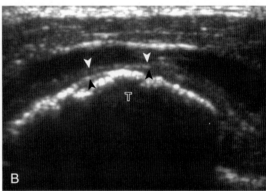

■ **FIGURE 3.75 Massive Supraspinatus Tear.** Ultrasound images of supraspinatus in long axis (A) and short axis (B) show complete absence of the supraspinatus tendon. Note the hyperechoic linear subacromial-subdeltoid bursal wall *(arrowheads)*, which extends beyond the greater tuberosity *(T)* and therefore does not represent rotator cuff tendon fibers.

simulate intact tendon fibers. The thickened bursa can be differentiated from tendon by the lack of fibrillar architecture and identification of the bursal tissue that extends beyond the greater tuberosity, unlike the rotator cuff. A similar situation may occur in the setting of a massive cuff tear, in which the thin hyperechoic wall of the subacromial-subdeltoid bursa may simulate intact fibers (Fig. 3.75). Because the bursal wall extends beyond the greater tuberosity distal to the rotator cuff tendon attachment to bone, this too excludes tendon fibers as the cause.

RIM-RENT TEAR VERSUS INTRA-SUBSTANCE TEAR

A rim-rent tear is an articular-side partial-thickness tendon tear that involves the most distal aspect of the tendon at the greater tuberosity insertion

(see Fig. 3.23).[17,18] When a well-defined hypoechoic or anechoic tendon abnormality is at this location, one must determine whether the abnormal echogenicity is in contact with the articular surface (representing a rim-rent tear) or is only in contact with the greater tuberosity surface within the supraspinatus tendon (an intra-substance tear) (see Fig. 3.29). In the latter situation, an intra-substance tear is not seen at arthroscopy or bursoscopy. Therefore, it is critical to determine whether intra-articular extension is seen, which appears as contact between the tendon tear and the hypoechoic hyaline cartilage with a possible cartilage interface sign (Fig. 3.76).

TENDINOSIS VERSUS TENDON TEAR

Because tendinosis and tendon tear may both appear hypoechoic, one must rely on other

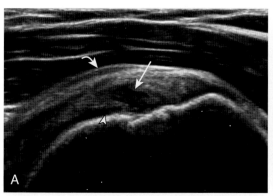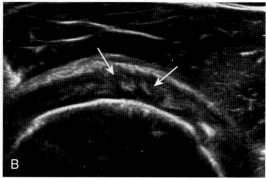

■ **FIGURE 3.76 Intra-Substance Tear: Supraspinatus.** Ultrasound images of supraspinatus in long axis (A) and short axis (B) show a well-defined hypoechoic tear *(open arrow)* with adjacent bone irregularity that does not come into contact with either the hyaline articular cartilage *(arrowhead)* or the subacromial-subdeltoid bursa *(curved arrow)*.

TABLE 3.2 Ultrasound Features of Tendon Tear and Tendinosis	
Tear	**Tendinosis**
Anechoic	Hypoechoic
Well defined	Ill defined
Homogeneous	Heterogeneous
Thin	Increased thickness
Bone irregularity[a]	Smooth cortex[a]

[a]Specific to greater tuberosity attachment of supraspinatus in patients older than 40 years.

sonographic findings to help with this distinction (Table 3.2).[30] If a tendon abnormality is hypoechoic, ill defined, and heterogeneous, then tendinosis is suggested (see Fig. 3.41). In contrast, if a tendon abnormality is more anechoic and well defined, then tendon tear is suggested (see Fig. 3.30). In addition, increased tendon thickness suggests tendinosis, whereas tendon thinning suggests either bursal-side partial-thickness tear or full-thickness tear. The most important sign that assists in the differentiation between supraspinatus tear and tendinosis in patients older than 40 years is cortical irregularity of the greater tuberosity. A supraspinatus tendon abnormality immediately adjacent to cortical irregularity of the greater tuberosity likely represents a tear.[30-32] This association is not necessarily found with other aspects of the rotator cuff. For example, cortical irregularity often is seen in the lesser tuberosity without adjacent subscapularis tendon abnormality. In addition, some degree of cortical irregularity of the posterior humerus beneath the infraspinatus (termed the *bare area* because it is devoid of cartilage) is considered a variation of normal.[49] However, extensive irregularity in this region,

coexisting with posterior labrum tear and partial-thickness infraspinatus tendon tear, indicates posterosuperior impingement syndrome.[50]

■ BICEPS BRACHII TENDON
Joint Effusion and Tenosynovitis

Because the tendon sheath of the long head of the biceps brachii tendon normally communicates with the glenohumeral joint, increased joint fluid can be found in this tendon sheath adjacent to the long head of the biceps brachii tendon at the level of the bicipital groove (Fig. 3.77).[5] In the absence of a glenohumeral joint effusion, a small sliver (<1 mm) or no fluid is visible distending the long head of biceps brachii tendon sheath.[52] A glenohumeral joint effusion of at least 5 mL will communicate with and distend the biceps brachii long head tendon sheath; an effusion of at least 8 mL will distend the tendon sheath an average of 2 mm.[5,52] Joint effusion, if simple, can be anechoic, whereas complex fluid may be hypoechoic, isoechoic, or hyperechoic relative to muscle, and it may resemble synovial hypertrophy. The findings of flow on color or power Doppler imaging and the lack of internal movement with transducer pressure suggest synovial hypertrophy rather than complex fluid.[69] Communicating glenohumeral joint effusion should be differentiated from tenosynovitis. If tendon sheath distention is focal, demonstrates hyperemia, and is symptomatic with transducer pressure, this suggests tenosynovitis, especially if out of proportion to distention of other glenohumeral joint recesses (Figs. 3.78 and 3.79). Fluid that remains focal or loculated at the level of the bicipital groove with palpation under ultrasound visualization also suggests tenosynovitis (Video 3.40). In contrast, a long segment of

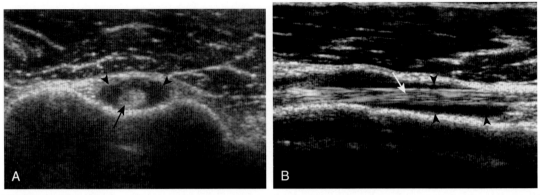

■ **FIGURE 3.77 Joint Effusion.** Ultrasound images of biceps brachii long head tendon in short axis (A) and long axis (B) show glenohumeral joint fluid *(arrowheads)*, which surrounds the biceps tendon *(arrows)* (right side of image A is medial, distal in B).

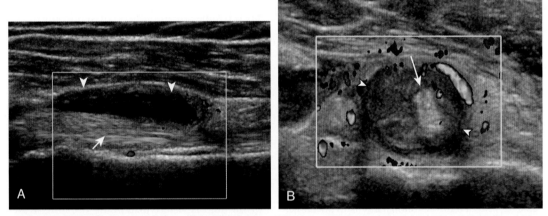

■ **FIGURE 3.78 Complex Fluid and Synovial Hypertrophy.** Ultrasound image of the biceps brachii tendon in long axis (A) shows hypoechoic complex joint fluid *(arrowheads)* that surrounds the biceps tendon *(arrow)*. Swirling of echoes was seen at real-time imaging, a finding that indicates a fluid component. B, Ultrasound image of biceps brachii long head tendon in short axis in a different patient shows synovitis *(arrowheads)* and hyperemia that surrounds the biceps tendon *(arrow)*.

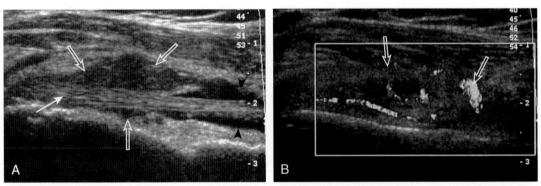

■ **FIGURE 3.79 Biceps Tenosynovitis.** Gray-scale (A) and color Doppler (B) ultrasound images long axis to the biceps brachii long head tendon show anechoic joint fluid *(arrowheads)* and hyperemic hypoechoic synovitis *(open arrows)* that surrounds the biceps tendon *(arrow)* (right side of images is distal).

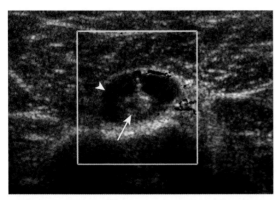

■ FIGURE 3.80 **Joint Effusion and Normal Vascularity.** Color Doppler ultrasound image of biceps brachii long head tendon in short axis shows hypoechoic glenohumeral joint fluid *(arrowhead)* that surrounds the biceps tendon *(arrow)*. Note normal vascularity (right side of image is lateral).

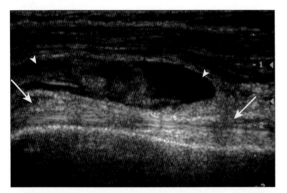

■ FIGURE 3.81 **Subacromial-Subdeltoid Fluid.** Ultrasound image of biceps brachii long head tendon in long axis shows hypoechoic fluid and isoechoic synovial hypertrophy, which distends the subacromial-subdeltoid bursa *(arrowheads)* superficial to the biceps brachii long head tendon *(arrows)* (right side of image is distal).

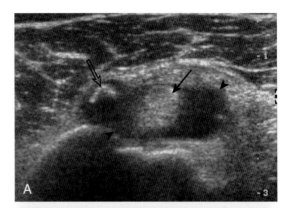

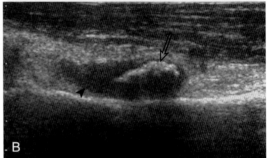

■ FIGURE 3.82 **Intra-Articular Body.** Ultrasound images of biceps brachii long head tendon in short axis (A) and long axis (B) show joint fluid *(arrowheads)* that surrounds the biceps tendon *(arrow)* with a hyperechoic and partial shadowing ossified intra-articular body *(open arrows)* (right side of image in A is medial, distal in B).

asymptomatic tendon sheath distention associated with distention of another shoulder joint recess, such as the posterior glenohumeral joint or subscapular recesses, suggests joint effusion. Normal flow seen in a branch of the anterior circumflex humeral artery should not be misinterpreted as abnormal vascularity (Fig. 3.80).[94] Distention of the subacromial-subdeltoid bursa should not be mistaken for biceps sheath abnormalities as bursal distention is often seen superficial to the biceps tendon anteriorly (Fig. 3.81). Intra-articular bodies from the glenohumeral joint are commonly seen within the biceps brachii long head tendon sheath (Fig. 3.82). The finding of joint effusion alone within the long head of the biceps brachii tendon sheath has a positive predictive value of 60% for diagnosis of rotator cuff tear; the additional finding of subacromial-subdeltoid bursal fluid increases the positive predictive value to 95%.[51]

Tendon Tear and Tendinosis

Tendinosis of the biceps brachii long head tendon appears as abnormal hypoechogenicity and possible increased thickness of the tendon but without tendon fiber disruption (Fig. 3.83). Refraction shadowing from prominent deltoid fascia superficial to the biceps tendon should not be misinterpreted as abnormality of the biceps brachii tendon (Video 3.41). Pathology of the biceps tendon most commonly occurs within 3.5 cm of the tendon origin, which may be seen proximal to and at the bicipital groove.[9] Assessment of the most proximal biceps is completed with the shoulder in the modified Crass position when the anterior aspect of the supraspinatus tendon and the rotator interval are assessed. When the biceps tendon shows anechoic clefts or an irregular superficial surface, then partial-thickness tear is present, especially when the bicipital groove is irregular from osseous spurs (Fig. 3.84).[95] As a normal variant seen in up to 50% of individuals, the aponeurotic expansion of the supraspinatus appears as a thin hyperechoic tendon immediately anterior to the biceps brachii long head tendon (Fig. 3.85) (Video 3.42).[96] This finding should

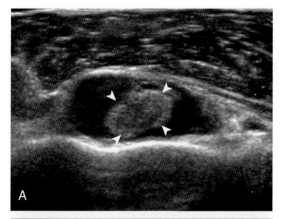

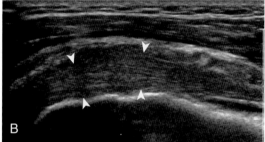

■ FIGURE 3.83 **Biceps Brachii Tendinosis.** Ultrasound images of biceps brachii long head tendon in short axis (A) and long axis (B) show increased thickness and abnormal hypoechogenicity of the tendon *(arrowheads)* with fluid distention of tendon sheath (right side of image in A is medial, distal in B).

not be misinterpreted as a longitudinal split of the biceps brachii tendon; recognition of its characteristic location and shape, as well as its attachments separate from the biceps tendon, aids in its diagnosis. Rarely, an intra-tendinous ganglion cyst may be seen within the biceps tendon.[97]

A full-thickness biceps tendon tear appears as complete fiber disruption and usually results in retraction at the torn tendon stump; therefore, the primary finding is lack of visualization of the long head of biceps tendon or an empty bicipital groove (Fig. 3.86A).[95] Visualization of echogenic synovial hypertrophy, the collapsed tendon sheath, or the adjacent subacromial-subdeltoid bursa in the bicipital groove (see Fig. 3.90C and D) should not be misinterpreted as tendon fibers; imaging distally at the pectoralis tendon and proximally in the rotator interval for the retracted stumps of the biceps tendon may be helpful. At the level of the pectoralis, the thickened and retracted distal biceps tendon stump will be located lateral to the normal short head of the biceps brachii, with or without hypoechoic or anechoic fluid, but with characteristic refraction shadowing (Fig. 3.86C and D). Often, the proximal aspect of the biceps tear is not seen in the bicipital groove or in the

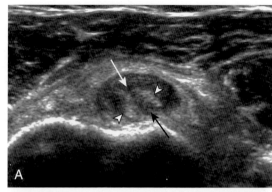

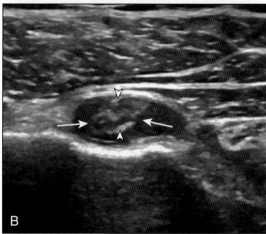

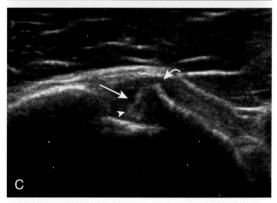

■ FIGURE 3.84 **Biceps Brachii Tendon: Partial-Thickness Tear.** Ultrasound images of biceps brachii tendon in short axis from three different patients show hypoechoic and anechoic tears *(arrows)* of the biceps tendon *(arrowheads)* with surrounding hypoechoic fluid and synovitis. Note bone spur *(curved arrow)* in C.

rotator interval because the tear has occurred more proximally at the biceps anchor at the glenoid labrum.

When the biceps brachii long head tendon is not seen in the bicipital groove, in addition to the possibility of a full-thickness tear, one must also consider the diagnosis of biceps tendon dislocation (see next paragraph for discussion).

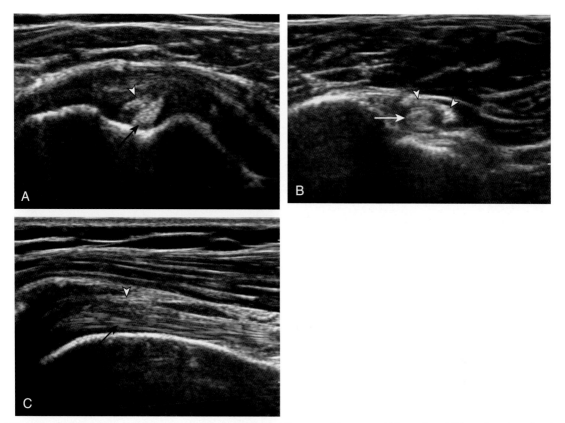

■ **FIGURE 3.85 Aponeurotic Expansion of Supraspinatus.** Ultrasound images of biceps brachii long head tendon in short axis (A, B) and long axis (C) show aponeurotic expansion *(arrowheads)* superficial to the biceps brachii long head tendon *(arrow)*.

One should inquire about prior surgery as the intra-articular portion of the biceps brachii long head tendon may be surgically transected (termed *tenotomy*) or transected and attached to the humerus (termed *tenodesis*) at the level of the bicipital groove (Fig. 3.87).

Subluxation and Dislocation

When the biceps brachii long head tendon is not normally identified in the bicipital groove, one must consider medial subluxation and dislocation.[9] With subluxation of the long head of the biceps brachii tendon, the tendon is partially out of the bicipital groove and medially displaced superficial to the lesser tuberosity (Fig. 3.88A). The biceps may also completely dislocate superficial to the lesser tuberosity (Fig. 3.89), medial to the lesser tuberosity (Fig. 3.90), into a subscapularis tendon tear (Fig. 3.91), or through a subscapularis tendon tear into the glenohumeral joint.[4] As a potential pitfall, the wall of the subacromial-subdeltoid bursa laying into the empty bicipital groove should not be mistaken for biceps tendon fibers (Fig. 3.90). In addition, with medial biceps tendon dislocation, the intra-articular location of the biceps brachii long head tendon may be difficult to identify because it may simulate the glenoid labrum or other intra-articular structure; distal imaging in short axis shows the dislocated biceps tendon coursing out of the joint and returning to a normal position lateral to the biceps brachii short head muscle. Evaluation of the proximal biceps tendon should also include external shoulder rotation to evaluate for abnormal tendon displacement (Video 3.43).[11] The contrary is also true, whereby medial dislocation of the biceps brachii long head tendon over the lesser tuberosity in neutral shoulder position may relocate into the bicipital groove with shoulder internal rotation associated with a painful snap (Video 3.44).

The long head of the biceps brachii tendon is stabilized by the bicipital reflection pulley or sling, made up of the coracohumeral and superior glenohumeral ligaments in the rotator interval (see Fig. 3.13G).[4] Tears of these structures predispose to biceps tendon instability and can be visualized with ultrasound (see Fig. 3.39 and Video 3.24).[98] Another indirect sign of biceps instability or tear is the *chondral print sign*, also visible at

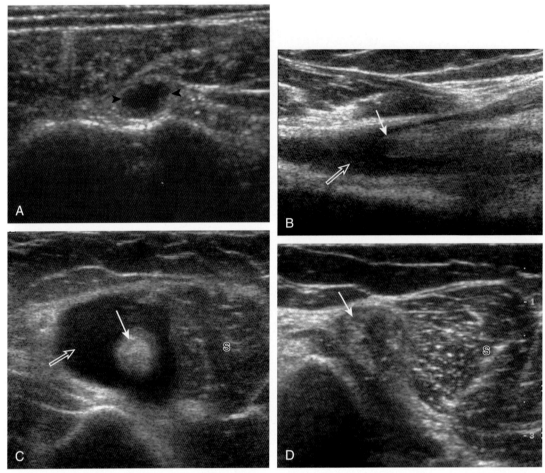

■ **FIGURE 3.86 Biceps Brachii Tendon: Full-Thickness Tear.** Ultrasound image (A) transverse over bicipital groove shows anechoic effusion or hemorrhage *(arrowheads)* and no tendon fibers. Ultrasound images of biceps brachii long head tendon more distal in long axis (B) and short axis (C) show the retracted distal stump *(arrows)* surrounded by hypoechoic fluid *(open arrows)*. Note the normal short head of the biceps brachii *(S)*. Ultrasound image (D) short axis to distal biceps in a different patient shows the heterogeneous and inferiorly retracted distal stump *(arrow)* without adjacent fluid (right side of images A, C, and D is medial, distal in B).

sonography as subchondral bone cortex irregularity adjacent to the biceps tendon in the rotator interval (see Fig. 3.39B).[99] Subluxation and dislocation of the biceps brachii tendon are often associated with partial tear of the biceps brachii long head tendon.[95]

■ SUBACROMIAL-SUBDELTOID BURSA

The subacromial-subdeltoid bursa is a synovial space, separate from the glenohumeral joint, located between the rotator cuff and the overlying acromion and deltoid muscle (see Fig. 3.1). At ultrasound it appears as a thin, uniform, 1- to 2-mm hypoechoic layer of synovial fluid surrounded by hyperechoic bursal wall and peribursal fat layers.[7,21]

Abnormal distention of the subacromial-subdeltoid bursa may be seen laterally (over supraspinatus and proximal humerus) (Video 3.45), anteriorly (over subscapularis and biceps brachii long head tendon), and posteriorly (over infraspinatus) (Fig. 3.92). A distended bursa may appear anechoic or hypoechoic from simple fluid or it may range from hypoechoic to hyperechoic as a result of complex fluid or synovial hypertrophy (Fig. 3.93). Color or power Doppler imaging may differentiate complex fluid from synovitis because blood flow suggests synovial hypertrophy. The term *bursitis* is often reserved for cases in which inflammation is truly present. Causes of subacromial-subdeltoid bursal distention include impingement (see earlier discussion in Impingement Syndrome), rotator cuff tear, hemorrhage, and amyloidosis. Inflammatory conditions should

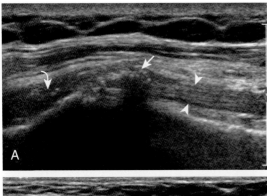

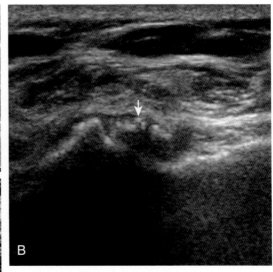

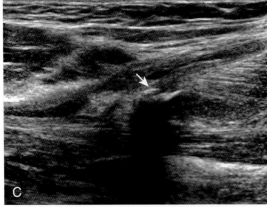

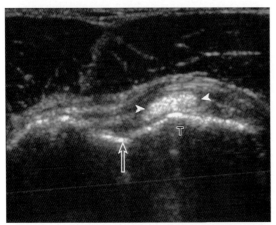

■ **FIGURE 3.87 Biceps Brachii Tenodesis.** Ultrasound images of proximal biceps brachii tendon in long axis (A) and short axis (B) show tendon *(arrowheads)* attached to the proximal humerus with echogenic suture material *(arrow)*. The biceps tendon is not seen proximally *(curved arrow)* (right side of image is distal in A). C, Ultrasound image of biceps brachii long head (long axis) in a different patient shows a failed tenodesis with echogenic suture and tendon *(arrow)* detached from the humerus and retracted distally.

■ **FIGURE 3.88 Biceps Brachii Tendon Subluxation.** Ultrasound image of biceps brachii long head tendon in short axis shows subluxation of the biceps tendon *(arrowheads)* medial to the bicipital groove *(open arrow)* and partially superficial to the lesser tuberosity *(T)* (right side of image is medial).

also be considered, such as infection (Fig. 3.94A), gout (Fig. 3.94B), and rheumatoid arthritis (Fig. 3.94C).[7] Identification of hyperechoic foci with ring-down artifact within a complex bursal fluid collection raises concern for gas-producing infection (Fig. 3.94A). Calcium hydroxyapatite deposition may be seen in the bursa (Fig. 3.94D)

(Video 3.46) or directly extending from the adjacent rotator cuff (see Fig. 3.64), both related to calcific tendinitis. With regard to rotator cuff tears, it has been shown that the presence of subacromial-subdeltoid bursal fluid has a 70% positive predictive value for rotator cuff tear; a combination of joint fluid distention of the long head of the biceps brachii tendon sheath and subacromial-subdeltoid fluid increases the positive predictive value to 95%.[51] Other causes of subacromial-subdeltoid bursal distention include synovial proliferative disorders, such as pigmented villonodular synovitis and synovial chondromatosis.

When the subacromial-subdeltoid bursa is distended, fluid often collects dependently, such as over and beyond the greater tuberosity (see Fig. 3.92B and Video 3.45).[7] In this situation, this dependent portion of the subacromial-subdeltoid bursa should be specifically evaluated as it may not be readily visualized when evaluation is focused over the rotator cuff at or proximal to the greater tuberosity. Another area of the subacromial-subdeltoid bursa that may become distended is anteriorly over the bicipital groove, often seen in evaluation of the biceps brachii long head tendon (Fig. 3.95), which should not be mistaken for a biceps tendon sheath abnormality when imaging the biceps in long axis (see Video 3.26). Imaging short axis to the biceps

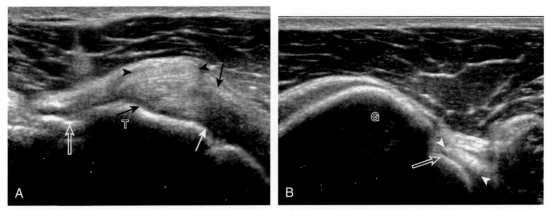

■ FIGURE 3.89 **Biceps Brachii Tendon Dislocation With Dynamic Relocation.** Ultrasound image of biceps brachii long head tendon in short axis (A) shows the biceps tendon *(arrowheads)* dislocated superficial to the lesser tuberosity *(T)* and subscapularis tendon *(arrows),* which returns to a normal location (B) at internal shoulder rotation associated with a painful snap (*open arrows,* bicipital groove). *G,* Greater tuberosity.

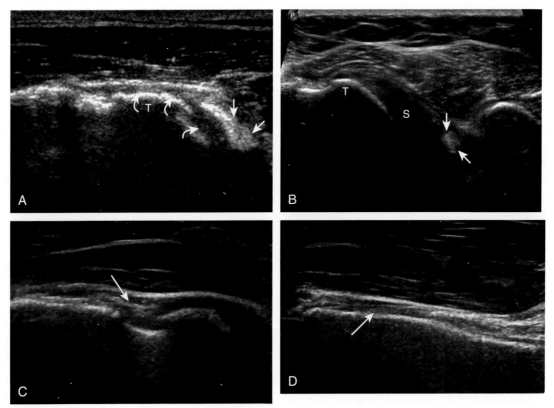

■ FIGURE 3.90 **Biceps Brachii Tendon Dislocation Medial to Lesser Tuberosity.** Ultrasound images of biceps brachii tendon in short axis in two different patients show medial dislocation of biceps *(arrows).* Note subscapularis tear *(curved arrows)* in A and normal subscapularis tendon with anisotropy *(S)* in B (right side of image is medial). *T,* Lesser tuberosity. Ultrasound images from another patient in axial (C) and (D) sagittal planes over bicipital groove show an empty bicipital groove with overlying subacromial-subdeltoid bursa wall *(arrow).*

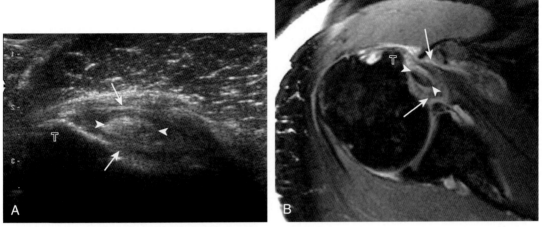

■ FIGURE 3.91 **Biceps Brachii Tendon Dislocation Into Subscapularis.** Ultrasound image (A) of biceps brachii tendon in short axis and (B) T2-weighted axial MR image show medial dislocation of the biceps tendon *(arrowheads)* within the substance of the torn subscapularis tendon *(arrows)* (right side of image A is medial). *T,* Lesser tuberosity.

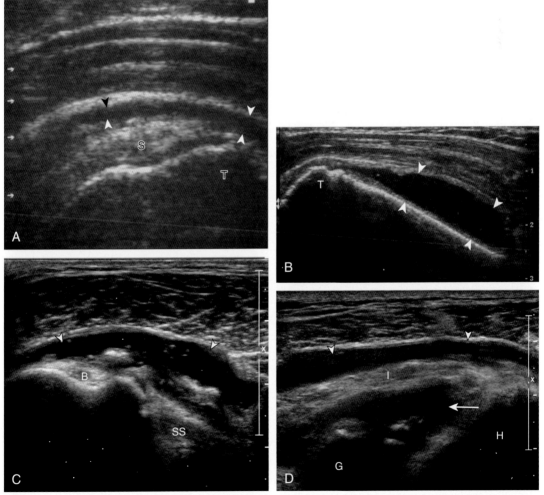

■ FIGURE 3.92 **Subacromial-Subdeltoid Bursal Distention.** Ultrasound images show anechoic distention of the subacromial-subdeltoid bursa *(arrowheads)* superficial to the (A) supraspinatus *(S)*, (B) greater tuberosity *(T)* and proximal humerus, (C) subscapularis *(SS)* and biceps brachii long head *(B)*, and (D) infraspinatus *(I)*. Note joint effusion in posterior glenohumeral recess *(arrow)* (right side of image in C is medial, and lateral in D). *G,* Glenoid; *H,* humerus.

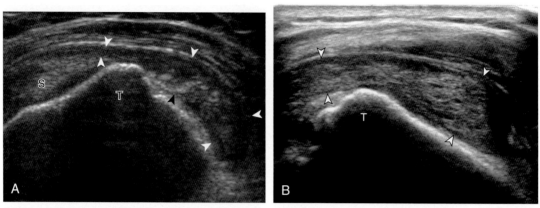

■ **FIGURE 3.93 Subacromial-Subdeltoid Bursal Distention.** Ultrasound images show heterogeneous distention from complex fluid and synovitis (A); and isoechoic/hyperechoic distention from synovial hypertrophy (B). *S,* Supraspinatus tendon; *T,* greater tuberosity.

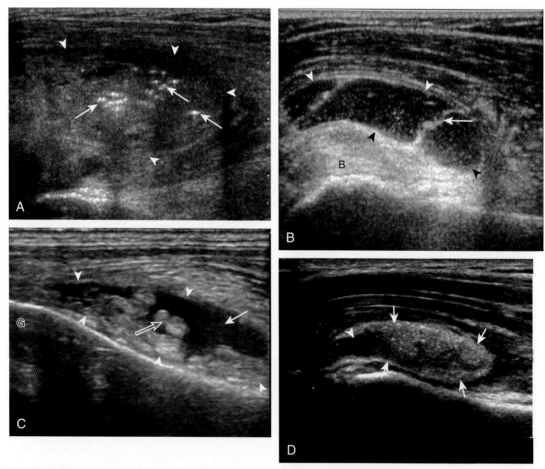

■ **FIGURE 3.94 Subacromial-Subdeltoid Bursitis.** Ultrasound images in four different patients show (A) heterogeneous distention of the bursa *(arrowheads)* with hyperechoic gas formation *(arrows)* from infection, (B) complex fluid and septations *(arrow)* from gout, (C) anechoic fluid *(arrow)* with hyperechoic synovial hypertrophy *(open arrow)* from rheumatoid arthritis, and (D) hyperechoic calcific deposit within bursa *(arrows)* with adjacent anechoic bursal fluid *(arrowhead)* from calcific tendinitis. *B,* Biceps brachii long head tendon; *G,* greater tuberosity.

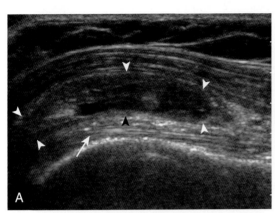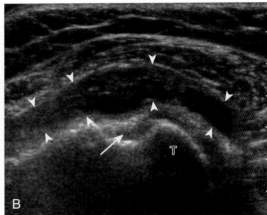

■ **FIGURE 3.95 Subacromial-Subdeltoid Bursal Distention.** Ultrasound images in long axis (A) and short axis (B) to the biceps brachii long head tendon show heterogeneous bursal distention *(arrowheads)* superficial to the biceps brachii long head tendon *(arrows)* (right side of image in A is distal, medial in B). *T,* Lesser tuberosity.

showing the distended bursa extending superficial and beyond the biceps tendon medially and laterally avoids this pitfall. Focal anterior distention of the subacromial-subdeltoid bursa with extension and internal rotation of the shoulder can be associated with symptoms related to coracoid impingement.[86]

■ GLENOHUMERAL JOINT RECESSES

The glenohumeral joint has several recesses that preferentially distend with joint fluid or other joint processes, which include the biceps brachii long head tendon sheath, the posterior glenohumeral joint recess, the subscapularis recess, and the axillary recess. These recesses should be assessed for pathology and also serve as potential sites for joint aspiration or injection. The joint recess where even small amounts of joint fluid can be seen is the biceps brachii long head tendon sheath (see Fig. 3.77).[52] As discussed earlier in the chapter, the differential diagnosis for abnormality surrounding the biceps tendon at the bicipital groove includes both localized biceps tenosynovitis (see Fig. 3.79) and a more diffuse joint process related to the glenohumeral joint. Assessing the other joint recesses assists in this differentiation. A pathologic process surrounding the biceps tendon that is out of proportion to findings in other glenohumeral joint recesses suggests a localized biceps process. Another glenohumeral joint recess includes the posterior recess, which is assessed with transducer placement over the infraspinatus tendon, where joint fluid, synovial hypertrophy, and intra-articular bodies may be identified (Fig. 3.96) (Videos 3.47 and 3.48). Small amounts of joint fluid may only

become visible at this site with the shoulder in external rotation (Video 3.49).[52] The subscapularis recess is also commonly distended and has a characteristic shape of an inverted U over the superior aspect of the subscapularis tendon near the coracoid process (Fig. 3.97). This shape distinguishes the subscapularis recess (Video 3.50) from the uncommonly distended subcoracoid bursa (Fig. 3.97 and Video 3.51); the latter is located anterior the subscapularis tendon directly inferior to the coracoid but is not located over the superior edge of the subscapularis tendon and does not communicate with the glenohumeral joint (Fig. 3.98).[6] Another feature of the subscapularis recess is its change in shape and degree of distention with shoulder movement, increasing with internal rotation and decreasing in external rotation as glenohumeral joint fluid redistributes (Video 3.50). The axillary recess is located inferior to the glenohumeral joint imaged from the axilla.

In addition to assessing for joint fluid, other joint processes such as intra-articular bodies and synovial hypertrophy can be visible in any of the abovementioned joint recesses. Cortical irregularity involving the articular surface of the humerus could represent osteophytes (see Fig. 3.96A), an osteochondral abnormality, subchondral fracture or collapse from osteonecrosis, a Hill Sachs impaction fracture (Fig. 3.99A), or possibly an erosion if adjacent synovial hypertrophy is present (Fig. 3.99B and C). The latter should be differentiated anatomically from cortical irregularity of the greater tuberosity, which is not an inflammatory erosion but related to rotator cuff tear (see Figs. 3.21 and 3.22). The adjacent hyaline cartilage and humeral head can also be assessed for layering of monosodium urate crystals (called the *double contour sign*) in gout.[100]

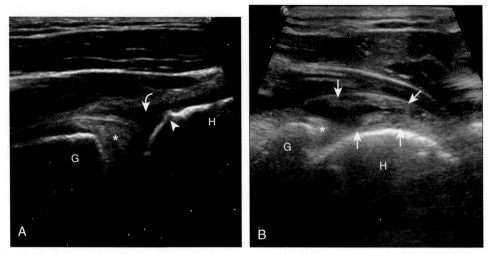

■ **FIGURE 3.96 Posterior Glenohumeral Joint Recess.** Ultrasound images in long axis to the infraspinatus tendon in two different patients show (A) anechoic fluid *(curved arrow)* with adjacent osteophyte *(arrowhead)*, and (B) anechoic fluid with isoechoic synovial hypertrophy *(arrows)* (*asterisk* indicates labrum; right side of images is lateral). *H,* Humeral head; *G,* glenoid.

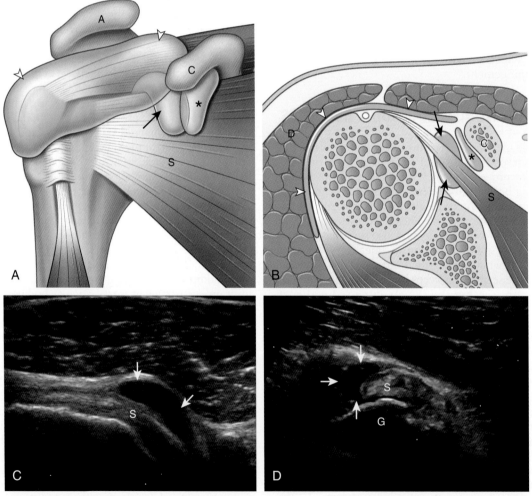

■ **FIGURE 3.97 Subscapularis Recess.** Anterior (A) and axial (B) illustrations show subscapularis recess *(arrows)*, subcoracoid bursa *(asterisk),* and subacromial-subdeltoid bursa *(arrowheads).* Ultrasound images of subscapularis in (A) long axis and (B) short axis show anechoic fluid distention of the subscapularis recess *(arrows)* (right side of image A is medial; right side of image B is inferior). Note inverted U shape. *G,* Glenoid; *S,* subscapularis tendon; *D,* deltoid: *C,* coracoid process; *A,* acromion. *(A and B from Ruangchaijatuporn T, et al: Skeletal Radiol 46:445-462, 2017.)*

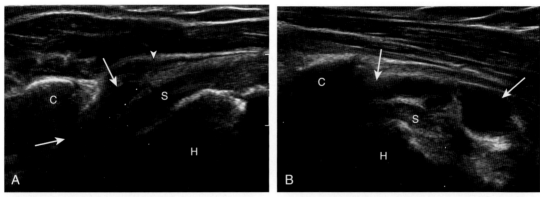

■ **FIGURE 3.98 Subcoracoid Bursa.** Ultrasound images in (A) axial and (B) sagittal planes over subscapularis (*S*) shows anechoic fluid distention of the subcoracoid bursa *(arrows)* extending from beneath the coracoid process (*C*) over the medial subscapularis. Note thickened subacromial-subdeltoid bursa *(arrowhead)* (left side of image is medial in A and cephalad in B). *H,* Humerus.

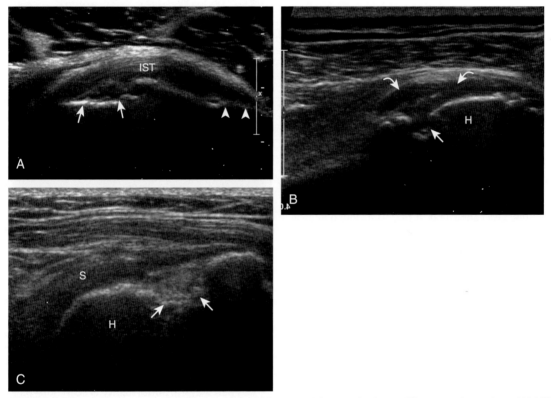

■ **FIGURE 3.99 Glenohumeral Articular Abnormalities.** Ultrasound images in three different patients show (A) Hill Sachs impaction fracture *(arrows)* from prior anterior dislocation *(arrowheads,* greater tuberosity), (B) complex fluid in posterior joint recess *(curved arrows)* with humeral head erosion *(arrow),* and (C) humeral head erosion *(arrows)* beneath supraspinatus tendon *(S). H,* Humeral head; *IST,* infraspinatus tendon.

■ GLENOID LABRUM AND PARALABRAL CYST

The glenoid labrum is a fibrocartilaginous structure located at the rim of the glenoid, which serves to help stabilize the glenohumeral joint. The normal labrum appears as a hyperechoic, triangular structure attached to the bony glenoid (see Fig. 3.18B).[101] Heterogeneous hypoechogenicity of the labrum indicates degeneration, whereas a well-defined hypoechoic or anechoic cleft indicates labral tear (Fig. 3.100) (Video 3.52). Ultrasound has a higher accuracy (98%) in differentiating posterior labral tear from other conditions (normal or degeneration) when compared to differentiating

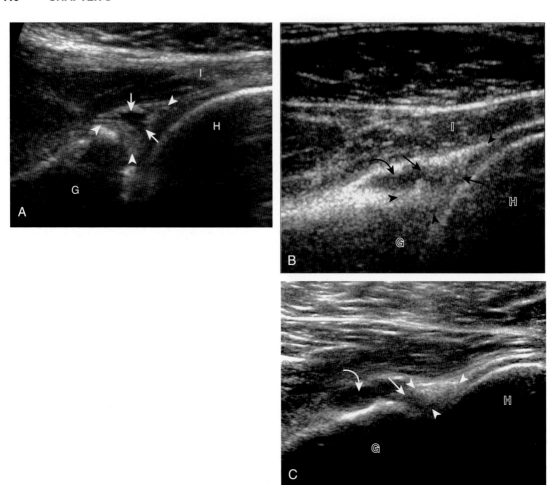

■ **FIGURE 3.100 Labral Tear.** A to C, Ultrasound images in long axis to the infraspinatus in three different patients show a hypoechoic cleft *(arrows)* within the posterior labrum *(arrowheads)*. There is an associated paralabral cyst in B and C *(curved arrows)* (right side of image is distal relative to the infraspinatus tendon). *G,* Glenoid; *H,* humeral head; *I,* infraspinatus.

abnormal posterior labrum from normal (accuracy 88%).[101] In patients with anterior shoulder instability, the sensitivity of ultrasound in depicting anterior labral pathology has ranged from 88% to 95%.[102-105] One major limitation of ultrasound in evaluation of the labrum is difficultly in visualizing the entire extent of the labrum. The anterior labrum is more difficult to demonstrate compared with the posterior labrum because of the thickness of the overlying soft tissues; evaluation with dynamic imaging may be helpful.[106] Similarly, the superior labrum is only visible in perhaps 30% of patients because of the overlying osseous structures (see Fig. 3.19F). Nonetheless, routine evaluation of the posterior labrum is easily accomplished during evaluation of the infraspinatus tendon, including the adjacent spinoglenoid notch where paralabral cyst formation may occur. Evaluating the posterior labrum with the shoulder in external rotation may improve visualization of

labral tears in the presence of a joint effusion. The transducer can also be placed long axis to the supraspinatus muscle between the clavicle and scapular spine, in an attempt to visualize the superior labrum and to evaluate the suprascapular notch for a paralabral cyst.

When a cystic abnormality is seen adjacent to the glenoid labrum, the diagnosis of paralabral cyst should be considered (Fig. 3.101) (Video 3.53).[107] In this setting, an underlying labral tear is usually present.[108] Ultrasound may show the joint fluid extension through the labral tear, which communicates with the paralabral cyst analogous to a parameniscal cyst in the knee. Paralabral cysts may extend away from the labral tear into the suprascapular notch (at the superior margin of the scapula) and at the spinoglenoid notch (between the scapula and base of the scapular spine). One must not mistake a suprascapular vein transiently distended in shoulder external

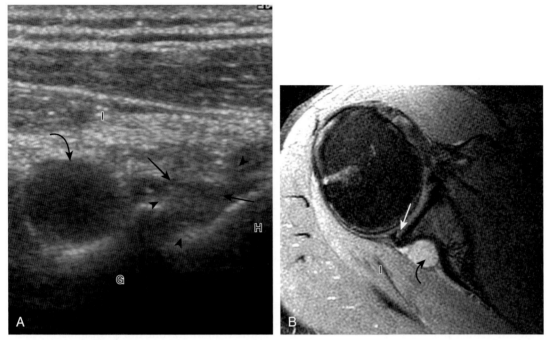

■ FIGURE 3.101 **Paralabral Cyst.** Ultrasound images in long axis to the infraspinatus (A) and T2-weighted axial MR image (B) show a hypoechoic cleft *(arrows)* within the diffusely hypoechoic posterior labrum *(arrowheads)*. There is an associated spinoglenoid notch paralabral cyst *(curved arrows)*. Note atrophy of the infraspinatus *(I)*, appearing small and hyperechoic in A and with increased signal in B. *G,* Glenoid; *H,* humeral head.

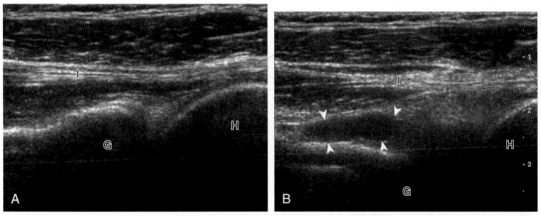

■ FIGURE 3.102 **Transient Suprascapular Vein Distention.** Ultrasound images in long axis to the infraspinatus in neutral (A) and external rotation (B) show transient distention of the suprascapular vein *(arrowheads)* (right side of image is distal relative to the infraspinatus). *G,* Glenoid; *H,* humeral head; *I,* infraspinatus. No flow was present at power Doppler imaging, which is common given slow flow. Collapse of the suprascapular vein is a differentiating feature from paralabral cyst.

rotation for a paralabral cyst in the spinoglenoid notch (Fig. 3.102) (see Video 3.15); however, fixed distention or venous varix may cause suprascapular nerve compression.[109] Because normal blood flow is not routinely identified at ultrasound in the suprascapular vein when distended during shoulder external rotation, one must rely on the collapse of the suprascapular vein with internal rotation to differentiate from a true paralabral cyst. One

potential complication of a posterior paralabral cyst is suprascapular nerve entrapment with resulting muscle denervation, which may involve the infraspinatus (when spinoglenoid) or of both supraspinatus and infraspinatus (when suprascapular in location) (see Fig. 3.52). Acute denervation causes muscle edema, and chronic denervation may cause fatty infiltration, causing the affected muscle to show increased echogenicity; decreased muscle size indicates atrophy. Although visualization of the normal suprascapular nerve may be difficult, identification of the adjacent suprascapular artery with color or power Doppler imaging assists in its localization. The suprascapular nerve courses inferiorly along the superior and posterior margin of the scapula through the suprascapular and spinoglenoid notches. The suprascapular artery is found within the spinoglenoid notch but superficial to the superior transverse scapular ligament outside of the suprascapular notch.[110] Ultrasound-guided percutaneous aspiration of a paralabral cyst can be performed (see Chapter 9), although the cyst may recur unless the underlying labral tear is repaired or treated.

■ GREATER TUBEROSITY

It is not uncommon to identify a greater tuberosity fracture during routine ultrasound evaluation of the rotator cuff after trauma. This is because a greater tuberosity fracture may be overlooked at radiography, and the patient may then present for ultrasound to evaluate for rotator cuff tear. At sonography, a greater tuberosity fracture appears as a cortical step-off and discontinuity at the junction of the humeral articular surface and greater tuberosity (Fig. 3.103) (Video 3.54).[111] The distal aspect of the fracture is often seen over the lateral aspect of the greater tuberosity or near the humeral metaphysis. The step-off deformity of a fracture should not be mistaken for cortical irregularity of the greater tuberosity related to rotator cuff tear. In the latter situation, focal pitting and cortical irregularity are present at the supraspinatus footprint, whereas fracture is characterized by a long segment cortical step-off and discontinuity at the margins of the greater tuberosity. Often, there is point tenderness directly over the fracture.

■ PECTORALIS MAJOR

Evaluation of the pectoralis major muscle tendon is typically a focused examination directed by a patient's history or symptoms. The pectoralis muscle consists of two heads—a clavicular head that originates from the medial two thirds of the clavicle and a sternal head that consists of manubrial and abdominal laminae that originate from the sternum and a portion of the costal cartilage, ribs, and abdominal fascia. As the tendons of the two pectoralis muscular heads extend toward the humerus, they twist 180 degrees so that the clavicular head moves anterior to the sternal head.[112] Approximately 15 mm medial to the humerus, the resulting anterior and posterior laminae of the distal tendons fuse and then attach to the humerus just lateral to the bicipital groove approximately 4 to 6 cm in sagittal length.[113,114]

Evaluation of the pectoralis begins with the biceps brachii long head tendon in short axis over the bicipital groove.[115] The transducer is then moved inferior from the subscapularis tendon, where the pectoralis tendon is identified as it extends over the biceps tendon to attach on the humerus (see Fig. 3.4D). Imaging should continue superiorly and inferiorly through the entire 4- to 6-cm tendon attachment to ensure complete evaluation. Evaluation of the musculotendinous junction in the sagittal plane is also helpful, as the more inferior sternal head can be seen moving superior and deep to the more superior clavicular head. This is a common site for partial-thickness tears to involve the sternal head.

Tendon tears appear as hypoechoic or anechoic tendon disruption.[114-116] Tendon retraction indicates full-thickness tear of at least one of the pectoralis heads. Most pectoralis major tears are partial-thickness tears (one head is torn while the other is intact) located at the musculotendinous

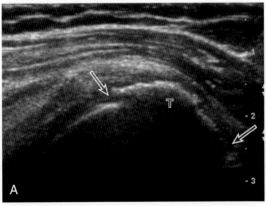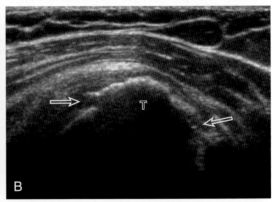

■ **FIGURE 3.103 Greater Tuberosity Fracture.** Ultrasound images in long axis (A) and short axis (B) to the supraspinatus tendon show cortical discontinuity and step-off deformity *(open arrows)*. *T,* greater tuberosity.

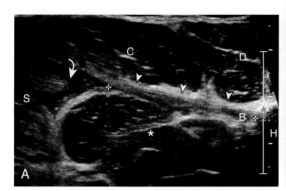
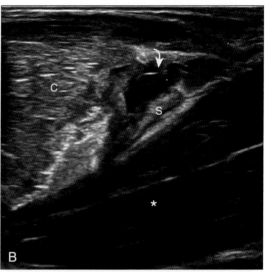

■ FIGURE 3.104 **Pectoralis Major Tear: Partial**. Ultrasound images in long axis (A) and short axis (B) to the pectoralis major show the torn and retracted *(curved arrow)* sternal head *(S)* superficial to the short head of the biceps brachii and coracobrachialis muscles *(asterisk)*, deep to intact clavicular head *(C)*. Note intact fused distal tendon *(arrowheads)* superficial to biceps brachii tendon *(B)* (left side of image A is medial and image B is cephalad). *H*, Humerus.

junction, most commonly of the sternal head. In this situation, hematoma is optimally visualized with the transducer in the sagittal plane at the musculotendinous junction where the sternal head rotates beneath the clavicular head (Fig. 3.104) (Video 3.55). In the transverse plane, the tear and hematoma are visualized at the musculotendinous junction medial to the fused tendon superficial to the short head of the biceps brachii muscle. A normal appearing fused tendon is identified superficial to the biceps brachii long head tendon.[115,116] A full-thickness full-width pectoralis major tear involves both the clavicular and sternal heads (Fig. 3.105). Distal tears at the humeral attachment may also be seen with possible hyperechoic and shadowing avulsion fracture.

■ ACROMIOCLAVICULAR JOINT

The acromioclavicular joint is routinely evaluated in shoulder sonography. If there is difficulty finding this structure, it can be palpated directly or located by following the clavicle laterally. The acromioclavicular joint can also be located by scanning superiorly from the bicipital groove region in the transverse plane. The normal acromioclavicular joint has smooth cortical margins with less than 3 mm of hypoechoic joint capsule distention.[117] The intra-articular fibrocartilage disk appears hyperechoic but may be difficult to identify. Several pathologic processes involve the acromioclavicular joint.[23] The most

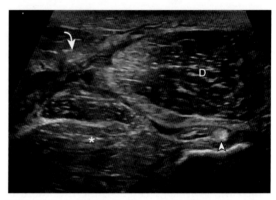

■ FIGURE 3.105 **Pectoralis Major Tear: Complete**. Ultrasound image long axis to the pectoralis major shows the torn and retracted sternal and clavicular heads *(curved arrow)* without visible distal tendon. Note long head of biceps brachii tendon *(arrowhead)* and short head of biceps brachii and coracobrachialis *(asterisk)* (left side of image is medial). *D*, Deltoid.

common pathologic condition is degenerative osteoarthritis (Fig. 3.106A), seen frequently after the age of 40 years. In this situation, the capsule may be distended, and later there will be bone irregularity, osteophyte formation, and joint space narrowing (often seen with dynamic imaging). The intra-articular fibrocartilage disk is disintegrated in most individuals after the age of 40 years from routine overuse and degenerative change.[118] Cysts may be associated with the acromioclavicular joint, which can produce a mass on physical examination (Fig. 3.106B). This may

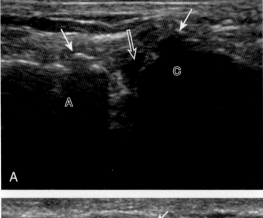

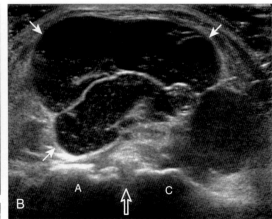

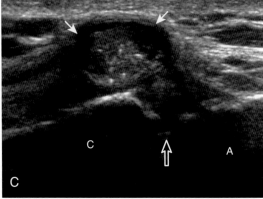

■ FIGURE 3.106 **Acromioclavicular Joint Degeneration and Cysts**. Ultrasound images long axis to the clavicle in three different patients show (A) cortical irregularity *(arrows)* from osteophytes and hypoechoic intra-articular fluid *(open arrow)* caused by degeneration, (B) a complex cyst *(arrows)* that originates from the acromioclavicular joint *(open arrow)*, and (C) synovial fluid *(arrows)* that has extended superiorly through a massive cuff tear and the acromioclavicular joint *(open arrow)* (termed the *geyser sign*). *A,* Acromion; *C,* clavicle.

be the result of glenohumeral joint fluid that tracks into the acromioclavicular joint in the setting of a chronic and massive supraspinatus tendon tear, called the *geyser sign* (Fig. 3.106C). If there is widening of the acromioclavicular joint, considerations include trauma and inflammation (Video 3.56). In the setting of the prior trauma, one may see widening of the joint, elevation of the clavicle, and hyperechoic step-off fracture; the acromioclavicular joint can also be assessed dynamically for ligament disruption (Video 3.57), as described earlier in the section on ultrasound examination techniques (Fig. 3.107).[23,24] With chronic injury, the acromioclavicular joint may be widened as a result of distal clavicular resorption, termed *distal clavicular osteolysis*, often seen with weight lifting and overhead activities (Fig. 3.108).[119] When widening and cortical irregularity of the distal clavicle and adjacent acromion are associated with fluid or synovial distention of the joint capsule and hyperemia, inflammatory conditions, such as rheumatoid arthritis and infection, should be considered. Infection is more common in intravenous drug abusers and those with septicemia,

and ultrasound-guided joint aspiration should be completed to exclude the diagnosis (see Chapter 9) (Fig. 3.109).

■ STERNOCLAVICULAR JOINT

Ultrasound may be used to evaluate the sternoclavicular joint.[23] A septic joint appears as distention of the joint capsule, with variable echogenicity fluid and synovitis (Fig. 3.110). Bone erosions, as well as joint space widening or subluxation, may occur. The findings of joint distention greater than 10 mm that extends over both the clavicle and sternum, elevated Westergren red blood cell sedimentation rate, and fever are strong indicators of infection.[120] Ultrasound-guided percutaneous aspiration is recommended if there is any concern for infection. In older women, it is not uncommon for degenerative changes of a sternoclavicular joint with capsular thickening to present as a palpable mass. Ultrasound can also diagnose subluxation or dislocation of the sternoclavicular joint (Fig. 3.111). The sternoclavicular joint should also be

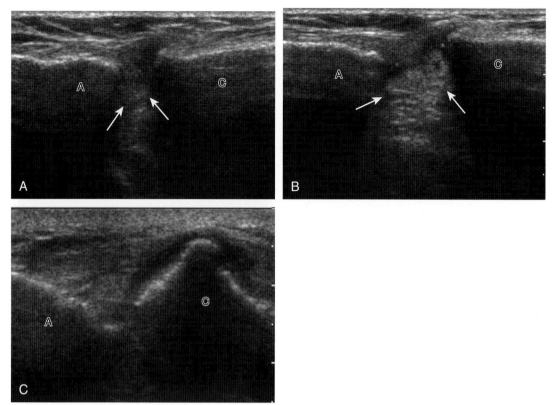

■ **FIGURE 3.107 Acromioclavicular Joint Injury.** Ultrasound images long axis to the clavicle in two different patients show (A) widening of the acromioclavicular joint *(arrows)*, which (B) increases with dynamic maneuvers. C, Longitudinal image of a different patient shows superior displacement of the clavicle relative to the acromion. *A,* Acromion; *C,* clavicle.

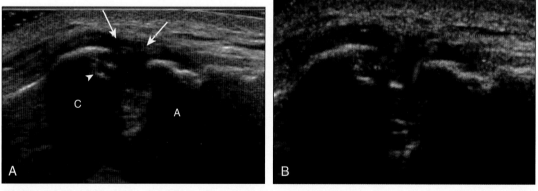

■ **FIGURE 3.108 Distal Clavicular Osteolysis.** Gray-scale (A) and color Doppler (B) ultrasound images long axis to the clavicle *(C)* show widening of the acromioclavicular joint with hypoechoic capsule distention *(arrows)*, clavicular erosions *(arrowhead)*, and hyperemia. *A,* Acromion.

assessed dynamically as subluxation may be dependent on patient arm positioning. Comparison with the contralateral side is important in diagnosing subtle subluxation. Any suspected posterior subluxation or dislocation should be evaluated with computed tomography to assess for adjacent vascular abnormalities (Fig. 3.112).

■ MISCELLANEOUS DISORDERS

Other types of shoulder diseases are often identified as examination is directed by the patient's history or symptoms. However, unlike in other peripheral joints, sonographic evaluation of the shoulder should follow a protocol similar to that

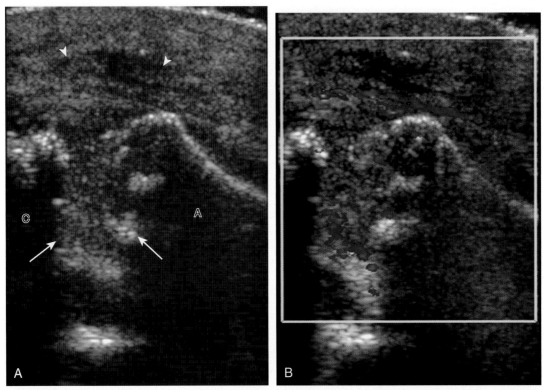

■ FIGURE 3.109 **Acromioclavicular Joint Infection.** Gray-scale (A) and color Doppler (B) ultrasound images long axis to the clavicle show a widened and irregular acromioclavicular joint from erosions *(arrows)* with soft tissue swelling *(arrowheads)* and hyperemia (B). *A,* Acromion; *C,* clavicle.

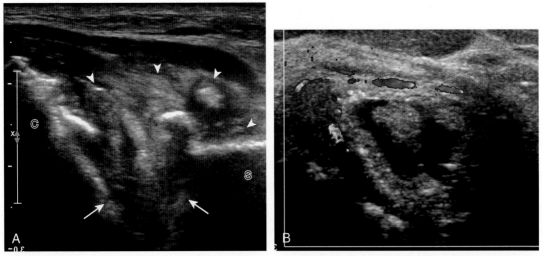

■ FIGURE 3.110 **Sternoclavicular Joint Infection.** Gray-scale (A) and color Doppler (B) ultrasound images in long axis to the clavicle show a widened and irregular sternoclavicular joint *(arrows)* with soft tissue swelling, fluid, and debris *(arrowheads)* and hyperemia (B). *C,* Clavicle; *S,* sternum.

described earlier because pain from the rotator cuff is often referred to the arm and symptoms may be misleading. At the completion of the shoulder examination, a focused examination at the site of point tenderness is recommended to identify pathology that may not otherwise be evident during the routine shoulder ultrasound examination.

Lymph node enlargement and other masses can be seen during ultrasound evaluation of the

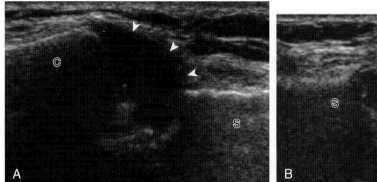
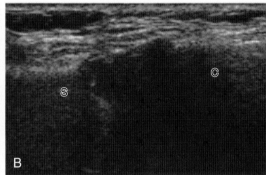

■ FIGURE 3.111 **Sternoclavicular Joint Dislocation: Anterior**. Ultrasound image in long axis to the clavicle shows (A) anterior dislocation of the clavicular head *(C)* relative to the sternum *(S),* with hypoechoic swelling at the sternoclavicular joint *(arrowheads)*. Asymptomatic contralateral sternoclavicular joint (B) shows normal alignment.

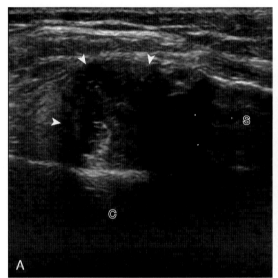
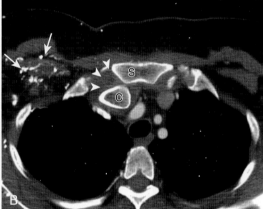

■ FIGURE 3.112 **Sternoclavicular Joint Dislocation: Posterior**. Ultrasound image (A) long axis to the clavicle and (B) contrast-enhanced axial CT image show posterior dislocation of the clavicular head *(C)* relative to the sternum *(S)* with hypoechoic swelling at the sternoclavicular joint *(arrowheads)*. Note the chest wall collateral vessels *(arrows)* resulting from right subclavian vein occlusion.

shoulder. A normal axillary lymph node appears oval, with a hypoechoic cortical rim (which decreases in thickness in older age), hyperechoic hilum, and a hilar pattern of vascularity if any. The central hyperechoic area is the result not of fat but of the reflective interfaces between the sinusoids and fat (Fig. 3.113).[121] An axillary lymph node that demonstrates eccentric thickening of the cortex, diffuse thickening of the cortex with hilar thinning, absence of the hilum, roundness, or a peripheral vascular pattern on color or power Doppler imaging suggests malignancy (Video 3.58).[122] A strict size criterion is not effective because even lymph nodes smaller than 5 mm (largest diameter) have almost 10% risk for malignancy in the setting of breast cancer.[123]

Often, ultrasound-guided percutaneous or excisional biopsy is required if malignancy is suspected (Figs. 3.114 and 3.115). Other soft tissue masses, if not originating from a synovial joint, are often not specific for one diagnosis, and ultrasound-guided percutaneous biopsy is usually required.

The identification of a soft tissue mass at ultrasound is often not specific for one diagnosis, although it limits the differential diagnosis by determining whether a mass is cystic or solid. A heterogeneous fluid collection not representing a bursal fluid collection could represent hematoma or abscess (see Chapter 2). One relatively common mass includes a soft tissue lipoma (see Chapter 2). In the setting of limb amputation, a solid soft tissue mass could represent a neuroma. These

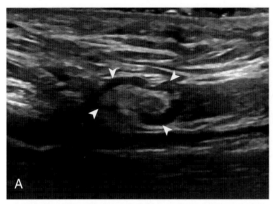

■ **FIGURE 3.113 Axillary Lymph Node: Normal.** Ultrasound image shows an asymptomatic axillary lymph node *(arrowheads)* with an echogenic hilum and a thin hypoechoic cortex.

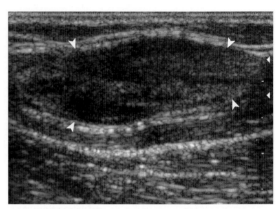

■ **FIGURE 3.115 Axillary Lymph Node: Lymphoma.** Ultrasound image shows an elongated lymph node *(arrowheads)* with cortical expansion and near obliteration of the echogenic hilum.

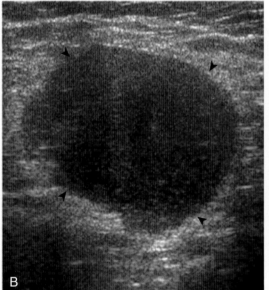

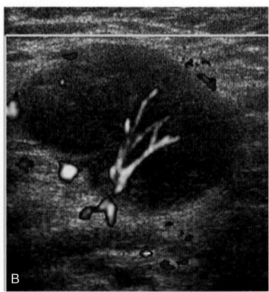

■ **FIGURE 3.114 Axillary Lymph Node: Hyperplastic.** Gray-scale (A) and power Doppler (B) ultrasound images show abnormal hypoechoic cortical expansion, obliteration of the echogenic hilum, and a round shape *(arrowheads),* although a predominant hilar pattern of vascularity is maintained.

masses are often hypoechoic but heterogeneous, and continuity between the mass and a peripheral nerve is essential to the diagnosis (Fig. 3.116). Because neuromas normally develop at a transected peripheral nerve, transducer palpation is important to determine which neuroma is symptomatic, to guide appropriate treatment.

There is one tumor-like abnormality that is specific to the shoulder, which is the elastofibroma.[124] This is not a true tumor, but a pseudotumor of fibroelastic tissue, possibly resulting from mechanical friction between the chest wall and the scapula. At ultrasound, elastofibroma appears heterogeneous and hyperechoic, with interspersed curvilinear hypoechoic strands at ultrasound (Fig. 3.117) (Video 3.59). The key to the diagnosis is the location because 99% of these lesions occur at the scapular tip, deep to the serratus anterior and latissimus dorsi muscles. This pseudotumor is most common in older women and may be bilateral in up to 66%.

Patients may also present with a palpable abnormality of the chest wall. One such etiology is a normal variant called the sternalis muscle. This variant occurs in 2% to 11% of the population and is located over the most medial aspect of the pectoralis at the sternum, just lateral to midline and elongated parallel to the rectus

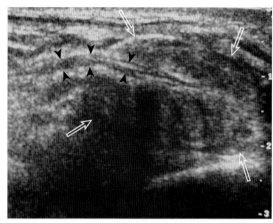

■ FIGURE 3.116 **Amputation Neuroma.** Ultrasound image shows a round, heterogeneous, but predominantly hypoechoic, mass *(open arrows),* with partial posterior shadowing, in continuity with the transected peripheral nerve *(arrowheads)* after forequarter amputation.

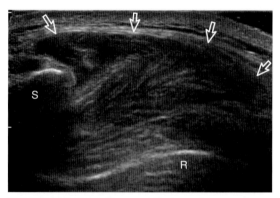

■ FIGURE 3.117 **Elastofibroma.** Ultrasound image shows a mixed echogenicity mass *(open arrows)* with internal hypoechoic strands. *R,* Rib; *S,* scapula.

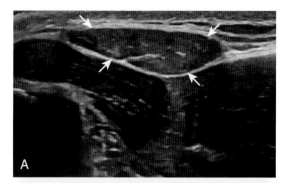

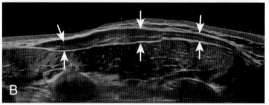

■ FIGURE 3.118 **Sternalis Muscle.** Ultrasound image shows that palpable mass corresponds to muscle tissue *(open arrows). R,* Rib; *S,* scapula.

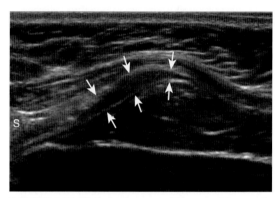

■ FIGURE 3.119 **Xiphoid Process.** Ultrasound image in the sagittal plane over lower sternum *(S)* shows a prominent and palpable unossified xiphoid process *(arrows).*

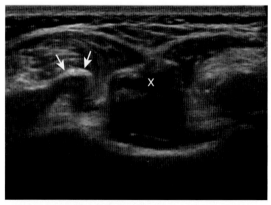

■ FIGURE 3.120 **Slipping Rib Syndrome.** Ultrasound image in the transverse plane over the lower anterior chest wall shows the cartilaginous end of a rib *(arrows),* which snapped over the xiphoid process *(X)* dynamically.

abdominis.[125] At ultrasound, the expected location of a sternalis muscle and the sonographic characteristics of normal muscle tissue allow a correct diagnosis (Fig. 3.118). A more common cause of a palpable nodule just below the sternum is the xiphoid process. The variable size, ossification, and shape of the xiphoid process can create a palpable mass. At ultrasound, the location, shape, and ultrasound appearance of either bone or cartilage is characteristic of a xiphoid process (Fig. 3.119). Some individuals present a painful snap associated with the chest wall during activities. The dynamic capabilities of ultrasound are useful to diagnose slipping rib syndrome, in which the abnormal mobility of a lower anterior rib end can cause snapping when it abruptly slips over an adjacent rib or xiphoid process (Fig. 3.120) (Video 3.60).[126]

SUGGESTED READINGS

4. Petchprapa CN, Beltran LS, Jazrawi LM, et al: The rotator interval: a review of anatomy, function, and normal and abnormal MRI appearance. *AJR Am J Roentgenol* 195(3):567–576, 2010.

8. Jacobson JA, Shoulder US: anatomy, technique, and scanning pitfalls. *Radiology* 260(1):6–16, 2011.

25. Bureau NJ, Beauchamp M, Cardinal E, et al: Dynamic sonography evaluation of shoulder impingement syndrome. *AJR Am J Roentgenol* 187(1):216–220, 2006.

30. Jacobson JA, Lancaster S, Prasad A, et al: Full-thickness and partial-thickness supraspinatus tendon tears: value of US signs in diagnosis. *Radiology* 230(1):234–242, 2004.

31. Wohlwend JR, van Holsbeeck M, Craig J, et al: The association between irregular greater tuberosities and rotator cuff tears: a sonographic study. *AJR Am J Roentgenol* 171(1):229–233, 1998.

37. de Jesus JO, Parker L, Frangos AJ, et al: Accuracy of MRI, MR arthrography, and ultrasound in the diagnosis of rotator cuff tears: a meta-analysis. *AJR Am J Roentgenol* 192(6):1701–1707, 2009.

38. Nazarian LN, Jacobson JA, Benson CB, et al: Imaging algorithms for evaluating suspected rotator cuff disease: Society of Radiologists in Ultrasound consensus conference statement. *Radiology* 267(2):589–595, 2013.

54. Morag Y, Jamadar DA, Miller B, et al: The subscapularis: anatomy, injury, and imaging. *Skeletal Radiol* 40(3):255–269, 2011.

59. Wall LB, Teefey SA, Middleton WD, et al: Diagnostic performance and reliability of ultrasonography for fatty degeneration of the rotator cuff muscles. *J Bone Joint Surg Am* 94(12):e83, 2012.

66. Jacobson JA, Miller B, Bedi A, et al: Imaging of the postoperative shoulder. *Semin Musculoskelet Radiol* 15(4):320–339, 2011.

76. Uhthoff HK, Loehr JW: Calcific tendinopathy of the rotator cuff: pathogenesis, diagnosis, and management. *J Am Acad Orthop Surg* 5(4):183–191, 1997.

115. Chiavaras MM, Jacobson JA, Smith J, et al: Pectoralis major tears: anatomy, classification, and diagnosis with ultrasound and MR imaging. *Skeletal Radiol* 44(2):157–164, 2015.

The complete references for this chapter can be found on *www.expertconsult.com.*

ELBOW ULTRASOUND

■ ELBOW ANATOMY

The elbow is a synovial joint composed of three elbow joint articulations: the trochlea and ulna, the capitellum and the radial head, and the proximal ulna and radius (Fig. 4.1). The elbow joint has prominent joint recesses located in the coronoid and radial fossae anteriorly and within the olecranon fossa posteriorly. Within each joint recess exists an intracapsular but extrasynovial fat pad, which becomes displaced with joint distention. The medial elbow joint is stabilized by the ulnar collateral ligament, of which the anterior bundle is most important, extending from the humerus anteriorly to the sublime tubercle and several centimeters distal along the ulna (Fig. 4.1C).[1] Other components of the ulnar collateral ligament include posterior and oblique bundles.[2] Laterally, the elbow joint is stabilized by the lateral collateral ligament complex, which is composed of the radial collateral ligament, the annular ligament, and a smaller accessory radial collateral ligament (Fig. 4.1D).[3] An additional component, the lateral ulnar collateral ligament, extends from the lateral epicondyle to the supinator cress of the proximal ulna; however, proximally the lateral ulnar collateral ligament is continuous with the lateral collateral ligament and typically only appears as a discrete structure extending distal from the annual ligament.[3-5]

Anterior to the elbow joint, the brachialis inserts on the ulna, and the biceps brachii tendon inserts on the radial tuberosity. With regard to the biceps brachii, a dual insertion exists where the short head is superficial and inserts more distal relative to the long head on the radial tuberosity.[6] Posteriorly, the triceps brachii inserts on the olecranon process of the proximal ulna, over which is located the olecranon bursa. The lateral and long heads of the triceps brachii represent the most superficial layer of the distal triceps, whereas the deep aspect with a relatively shorter tendon is the medial head.[7] The anconeus is located between the olecranon process and the lateral epicondyle of the humerus. Medially, the common flexor tendon, consisting of the flexor carpi radialis, palmaris longus, flexor carpi ulnaris, and flexor digitorum superficialis, originates on the medial epicondyle of the distal humerus. Laterally, the common extensor tendon, composed of the extensor carpi radialis brevis, extensor digitorum, extensor digiti minimi, and extensor carpi ulnaris, originates at the lateral epicondyle of the distal humerus. The extensor carpi radialis brevis is the most anteriorly located of the group; the extensor carpi radialis longus originates proximal to the lateral epicondyle on the lateral humeral metaphysis.

The space between the olecranon process of the ulna and the medial epicondyle is bridged by the cubital tunnel retinaculum (or Osborne fascia) and contains the ulnar nerve. Just distal to this, the ulnar nerve enters the true cubital tunnel, between the dual origins of the flexor carpi ulnaris and deep to the arcuate ligament.[8] The median nerve is located medial to the brachial artery and courses distally between the ulnar and humeral heads of the pronator teres. The radial nerve is located at the posterior aspect of the humeral shaft and then courses distally and laterally beneath the brachioradialis, where a deep branch courses between the two heads of the supinator muscle and a superficial branch courses beneath the brachioradialis and into the forearm.

■ ULTRASOUND EXAMINATION TECHNIQUE

Table 4.1 is an elbow ultrasound examination checklist. Examples of diagnostic elbow ultrasound reports are shown in Box 4.1 and Box 4.2.

General Comments

Ultrasound examination of the elbow may be completed with the patient sitting and the elbow placed on an examination table, or the patient may lie supine. A high-frequency transducer of at least 10 MHz is typically used because most of the structures are superficial. Evaluation of the elbow may be focused over the area that is clinically symptomatic or that is relevant to the

✳ TABLE 4.1 Elbow Ultrasound Examination Checklist

Location	Structures of Interest
Anterior	Brachialis
	Biceps brachii
	Median nerve
	Anterior joint recess
Medial	Ulnar collateral ligament
	Common flexor tendon and pronator teres
	Ulnar nerve
Lateral	Common extensor tendon
	Lateral collateral ligament complex
	Radial head and annular recess
	Capitellum
	Radial nerve
Posterior	Posterior joint recess
	Triceps brachii
	Olecranon bursa

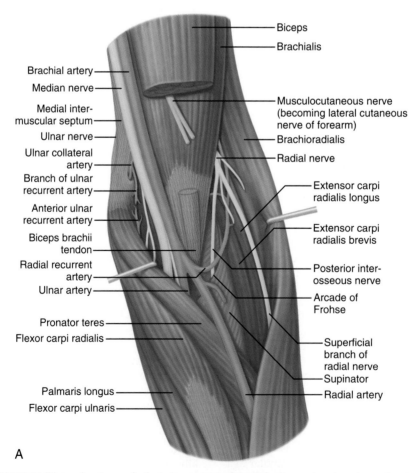

A

■ **FIGURE 4.1 Elbow Anatomy.** A, Anterior aspect of the left elbow showing deep structures.

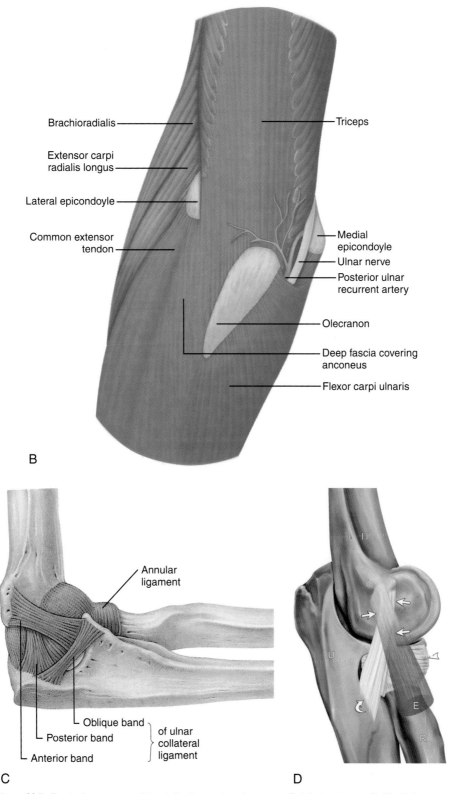

FIGURE 4.1, cont'd B, Posterior aspect of the left elbow showing superficial structures. C, Medial aspect of the left elbow joint. D, Lateral aspect of the left elbow joint shows radial collateral ligament complex. *H*, Humerus; *U*, ulna; *R*, radius; *E*, common extensor tendon; *arrows*, radial collateral ligament; *arrowhead*, annular ligament; *curved arrow*, lateral ulnar collateral ligament. *(A-C: From Standring S: Gray's anatomy: The anatomical basis of clinical practice, ed 39, Edinburgh, 2005, Churchill Livingstone.)*

BOX 4.1 Sample Diagnostic Elbow Ultrasound Report: Normal, Complete

Examination: Ultrasound of the Elbow
   Date of Study: March 11, 2011
   Patient Name: Kevin Saunderson
   Registration Number: 8675309
   History: Elbow pain, evaluate for tendon abnormality
   Findings: No evidence of joint effusion or synovial process. The biceps brachii and brachialis are normal. The common flexor and extensor tendons are also normal. No significant triceps brachii abnormality. The anterior bundle of the ulnar collateral ligament and lateral collateral ligament complex are normal. The ulnar nerve, radial nerve, and median nerve at the elbow are unremarkable. No abnormality in the cubital tunnel region with dynamic imaging. Additional focused evaluation at site of maximal symptoms was unrevealing.
   Impression: Unremarkable ultrasound examination of the elbow.

BOX 4.2 Sample Diagnostic Elbow Ultrasound Report: Abnormal, Complete

Examination: Ultrasound of the Elbow
   Date of Study: March 11, 2011
   Patient Name: Ricky Bobby
   Registration Number: 8675309
   History: Elbow pain, evaluate for tendon abnormality
   Findings: There is a partial-thickness tear of the distal biceps brachii tendon involving the superficial short head tendon with approximately 2 cm of retraction but with intact long head. Dynamic evaluation shows continuity of the long head excluding full-thickness tear. No joint effusion. The triceps brachii, common extensor, and common flexor tendons are normal. The ulnar, radial, and median nerves are unremarkable, including dynamic evaluation of the ulnar nerve. Unremarkable ulnar and lateral collateral ligaments. No bursal distention.
   Impression: Partial-thickness tear of the distal biceps brachii tendon.

patient's history. Regardless, a complete examination of all areas should always be considered for one to become familiar with normal anatomy and normal variants and to develop quick and efficient sonographic technique.[9]

Anterior Evaluation

The primary structures evaluated from the anterior approach are the brachialis, the biceps brachii, the median nerve, and the anterior elbow joint

recess. For sonographic evaluation, the elbow is comfortably extended, and the hand is supinated. Evaluation begins with the transducer short axis to the humerus. An ideal starting position is at the level of the distal humerus where the undulating contours of the humeral articular surface covered by hypoechoic hyaline cartilage appear similar to the surface of a clam shell (Fig. 4.2). The pyramid-shaped hypoechoic muscle immediately anterior to the distal humerus is the brachialis. The pulsating brachial artery is identified more superficial and medial, which is a helpful landmark in that the biceps brachii tendon is immediately lateral to the brachial artery and superficial to the brachialis. Medial to the brachial artery is the honeycomb appearance of the median nerve with the pronator teres muscle more medial. Lateral to the brachialis is the brachioradialis, and within the oblique fascia plane separating these two muscles are located the superficial and deep branches of the radial nerve, which appear hypoechoic. The lateral antebrachial cutaneous nerve is located superficial and immediately lateral to the biceps brachii tendon (Fig. 4.2B) as a continuation of the musculocutaneous nerve that courses between the brachialis and biceps brachii muscles more proximally (Fig. 4.2C).[10]

When evaluating the biceps brachii tendon in short axis, the two individual hyperechoic long and short heads may be difficult to visualize although the tendon often appears somewhat bilobed (Fig. 4.3A). However, toggling the transducer to create anisotropy will show the long head tendon lateral and the short head tendon medial, separated by a thin echogenic endotenon septum (Fig. 4.3B).[11] When moving the transducer distally, the long head tendon will rotate and move deep to the short head tendon.[6] The lacertus fibrosis or bicipital aponeurosis can be seen extending from the biceps brachii tendon to the pronator teres and flexor musculature, superficial to the brachial artery and median nerve, by placing the transducer over the anterior elbow angled from the biceps brachii tendon distal and medial (Fig. 4.3C).

The transducer is then moved proximal again to where the biceps brachii is superficial to the brachialis and is rotated 90 degrees (Fig. 4.4). At this location, the biceps tendon will be hyperechoic and fibrillar with a uniform thickness over the brachialis muscle (Fig. 4.4B). As the biceps brachii tendon courses deep along the outer contour of the brachialis, the tendon will become hypoechoic from anisotropy (Fig. 4.4C). Using the heel-toe maneuver, the sound beam is angled superiorly in order to image the tendon perpendicular to eliminate anisotropy (Fig. 4.4D). Some ultrasound machines will have beam steering, which can assist

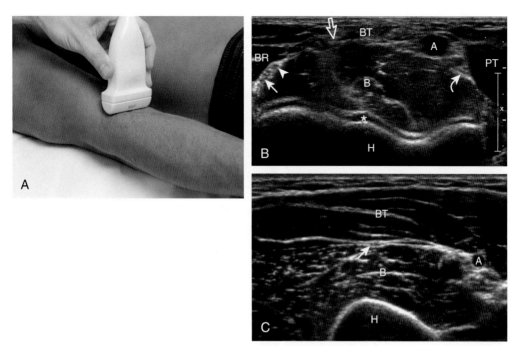

■ FIGURE 4.2 **Anterior Elbow.** A, Transverse imaging over the anterior elbow joint shows (B) brachial artery *(A)*, biceps brachii *(BT)*, brachialis *(B)*, pronator teres *(PT)*, brachioradialis *(BR)*, median nerve *(curved arrow)*, lateral antebrachial cutaneous nerve *(open arrow)*, and superficial *(arrowhead)* and deep *(arrow)* branches of radial nerve *(asterisk, hyaline articular cartilage)*. Imaging more proximal (C) shows biceps brachii muscle *(BT)*, brachialis *(B)*, and musculocutaneous nerve *(arrow)*. *H*, Humerus.

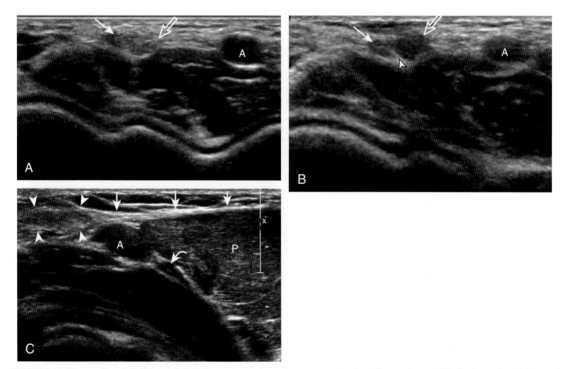

■ FIGURE 4.3 **Biceps Brachii (Short Axis).** Transverse imaging over anterior elbow shows (A) the long head *(arrow)* and short head *(open arrow)* of the biceps brachii in short axis, identified more clearly by toggling the transducer to produce anisotropy showing the intervening hyperechoic endotenon septum *(arrowhead)*. Note the lacertus fibrosus *(arrows)* in C, when the transducer is angled from the biceps tendon toward the medial epicondyle. *A*, Brachial artery; *P*, pronator teres.

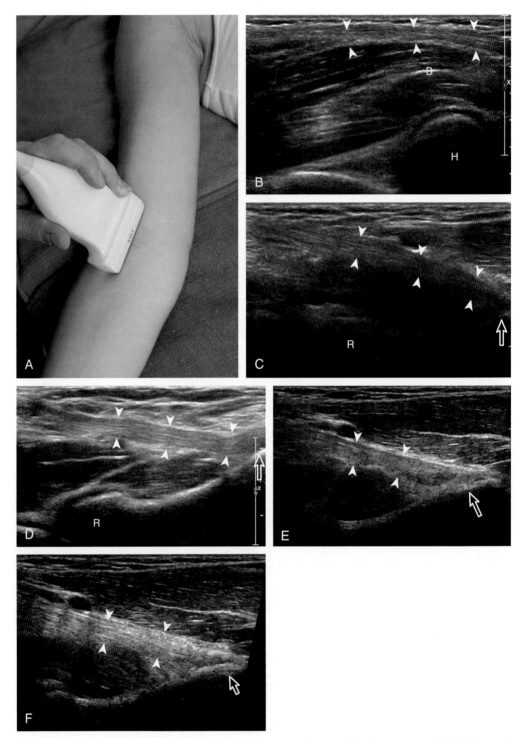

■ **FIGURE 4.4 Biceps Brachii (Long Axis).** A, Sagittal imaging over the anterior elbow shows (B) the biceps brachii tendon in long axis *(arrowheads)* superficial to the brachialis *(B)*. More distal imaging (C) shows anisotropy of the distal tendon *(arrowheads)*, which is eliminated when imaging perpendicular to the tendon (D) *(open arrow, radial tuberosity)*. In a different patient, anisotropy of the biceps brachii tendon *(arrowheads)* in E improves with beam steering in F. *H,* Humerus; *R,* radial head.

in reducing anisotropy (Fig. 4.4E and F). If the distal biceps is difficult to visualize, the elbow position may be changed with additional minimal flexion or extension.

If the distal biceps brachii tendon insertion onto the radial tuberosity in long axis is not clearly seen from an anterior approach, a medial approach should be used (Fig. 4.5), which can be accomplished in several different ways. With one method, the transducer is long axis to the biceps brachii tendon in the sagittal plane on the body, as described in the anterior approach. The transducer is then moved slightly medial until the brachial artery is identified and then the beam is angled slightly lateral toward the center of the elbow to see the biceps tendon (Fig. 4.5A). This maneuver is repeated, while adding the heel-toe maneuver until the distal tendon is visualized, where often slight elbow flexion is helpful (Fig. 4.5B). Another method is to follow the biceps brachii tendon distally in short axis, moving the transducer toward the medial elbow, and then turning long axis once the footprint is identified. A third method (the pronator window approach) is to begin with the elbow flexed and the transducer over the medial epicondyle in the coronal plane (Fig. 4.5C). The transducer is then moved toward the wrist and slightly anteriorly to visualize the radial tuberosity and the biceps brachii tendon in long axis (Fig. 4.5D).[12]

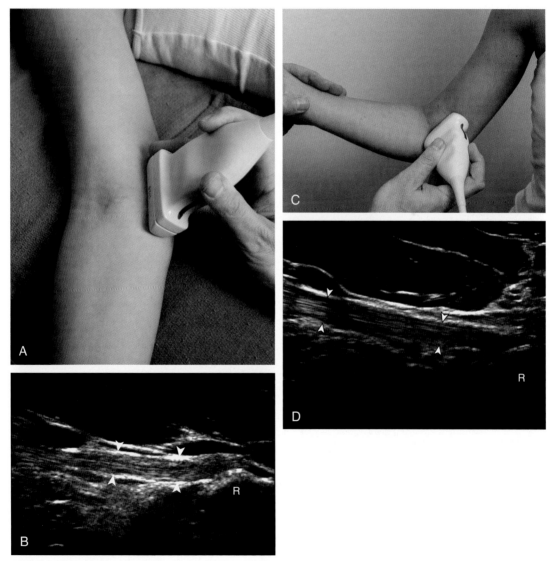

■ FIGURE 4.5 **Biceps Brachii: Medial Approach.** A, Coronal-oblique imaging over the medial elbow shows (B) the distal biceps brachii tendon *(arrowheads)*. C, imaging in the coronal plane with elbow flexion utilizes the pronator window to show (D) the biceps brachii tendon in long axis. *R*, Radial tuberosity.

Dynamic assessment of the distal biceps brachii is very helpful to distinguish partial from nonretracted full-thickness tear. While this can be effectively accomplished when evaluating the biceps tendon from a medial approach, as described (Video 4.1), an additional method to dynamically assess the biceps brachii tendon is from a lateral approach with the elbow flexed.[13] Examination with this technique begins with the transducer in short axis relative to the proximal radius (Fig. 4.6). The radial head is visualized as a curvilinear echogenic structure, and the transducer is moved toward the wrist over the radial neck, where the surrounding supinator muscle can be seen. At this level, the hand can be passively supinated and pronated to visualize movement of the biceps brachii tendon, which is perpendicular to the sound beam (Video 4.2). When the hand is fully pronated, the transducer can be moved dorsally toward the ulna to visualize the distal biceps brachii tendon (Fig. 4.7). While this dorsal evaluation with elbow flexion and pronation has limited diagnostic value in that only the distal-most segment of biceps tendon is visible between the radius and ulna, this view is

ideal when guiding a needle for biceps tendon fenestration or injection.[14]

To complete the anterior evaluation of the elbow, the transducer is returned to the sagittal plane directly in long axis to the brachialis to visualize the anterior recess of the elbow joint (Fig. 4.8A and B). Here, the coronoid fossa and smaller radial fossa are visible as concavities in the distal humerus. Within these fossae, a triangular hyperechoic intracapsular fat pad is normally seen. The hypoechoic hyaline cartilage of the trochlea and capitellum can also be identified. Returning to the original short axis view of the brachial artery, the normal median nerve is again identified in short axis and can be followed distally as it courses between the humeral and ulnar heads of the pronator teres, a potential site of nerve entrapment (Fig. 4.8C and D). The ulnar head of the pronator teres is located between the median nerve and the ulnar artery.

Medial Evaluation

For medial evaluation, the elbow is slightly flexed to bring the anterior bundle of the ulnar collateral

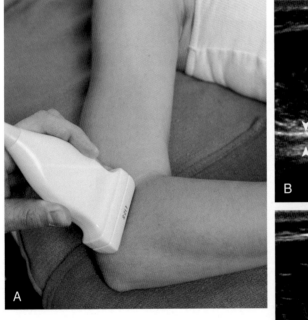

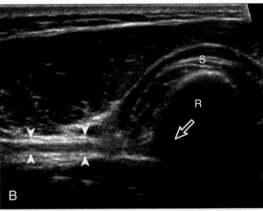

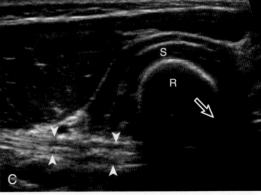

■ **FIGURE 4.6 Biceps Brachii: Lateral Approach.** A, Coronal images over the lateral elbow with elbow flexion in supination (B) and pronation (C) show biceps brachii tendon *(arrowheads)*. Note radial tuberosity rotation *(open arrows)* between pronation and supination. *R, Radius; S,* supinator muscle.

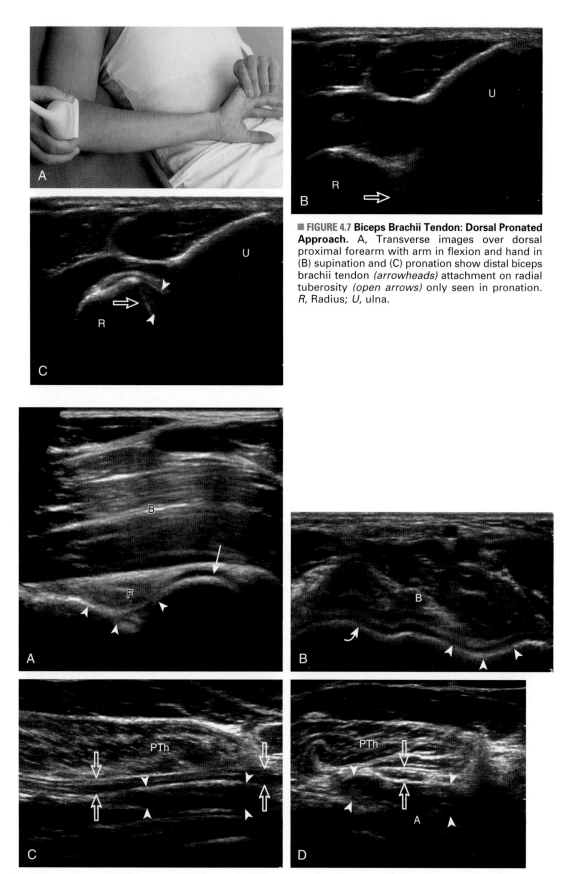

■ FIGURE 4.7 **Biceps Brachii Tendon: Dorsal Pronated Approach.** A, Transverse images over dorsal proximal forearm with arm in flexion and hand in (B) supination and (C) pronation show distal biceps brachii tendon *(arrowheads)* attachment on radial tuberosity *(open arrows)* only seen in pronation. *R*, Radius; *U*, ulna.

■ FIGURE 4.8 **Anterior Elbow Joint Recesses and Median Nerve.** A, Ultrasound image in long axis to brachialis *(B)* shows coronoid fossa *(arrowheads)*, anterior elbow fat pad *(F)*, and trochlea hyaline cartilage *(arrow)*. B, Ultrasound image short axis to brachialis *(B)* shows coronoid *(arrowheads)* and radial *(curved arrow)* fossae and hypoechoic hyaline cartilage. Ultrasound images show the median nerve *(open arrows)* in (C) long and (D) short axis and relationship to the humeral head of the pronator teres *(PTh)*, the ulnar head of pronator teres *(arrowheads)*, and the ulnar artery *(A)*.

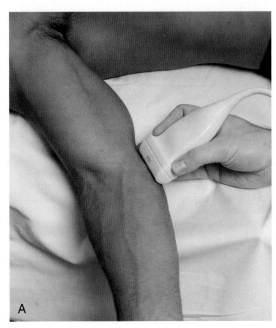

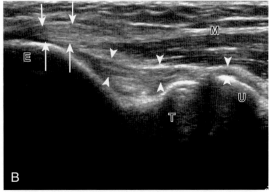

■ FIGURE 4.9 **Ulnar Collateral Ligament and Common Flexor Tendon Evaluation.** A, Coronal imaging over the medial elbow shows (B) the anterior bundle of the ulnar collateral ligament *(arrowheads)*, the common flexor tendon *(arrows)* and musculature *(M)*, the medial epicondyle *(E)*, trochlea *(T)*, and ulna *(U)*.

ligament into the coronal plane.[15] Sonographic evaluation of the medial elbow structures begins by visually identifying or palpating the medial epicondyle of the humerus. The transducer is then placed in long axis to the forearm with the proximal aspect over the medial epicondyle (Fig. 4.9). The characteristic hyperechoic bony contour of the medial epicondyle and the sloped surface of the humerus distally to its articulation with the ulna should be identified. In this imaging plane long axis to the forearm, as indicated by the characteristic bone contours, both the common flexor tendon and the anterior bundle of the ulnar collateral ligament can be identified (Fig. 4.9B). The origin of the common flexor tendon should be seen at the superficial aspect of the medial epicondyle as hyperechoic and fibrillar, with transition to hypoechoic musculature more distally. In addition, the anterior bundle of the ulnar collateral ligament is seen attached to the medial epicondyle as hyperechoic and fibrillar, but somewhat more compact than that of tendon. If not perpendicular to the ligament, the anterior bundle of the ulnar collateral ligament will be hypoechoic from anisotropy, but still fairly uniform in thickness where it extends distally over the joint space to insert on the proximal ulna.[16] The anterior bundle of the ulnar collateral ligament has a somewhat variable appearance at its proximal attachment to the humerus; it may appear as a uniform bundle, or it may fan out more proximally,

interspersed with hyperechoic fatty tissue.[17] The distal aspect of the ulnar collateral ligament anterior bundle attaches to the sublime tubercle and the ulna more distally.[1] The normal joint recess of the elbow extends proximally between the anterior bundle of the ulnar collateral ligament and adjacent humerus, but it should not extend medially from this point at the humeral attachment of the ligament or distal over the ulna. The long axis view is the key plane in the imaging of both the common flexor tendon and anterior bundle of the ulnar collateral ligament, although if a pathologic process is identified, further characterization is completed by imaging in short axis to these structures. In addition, the ulnar collateral ligament and medial joint space can be evaluated with dynamic valgus stress with the elbow in slight flexion (at least 30 degrees) to assess for ligamentous injury.[18-20]

After evaluation of the common flexor tendon and anterior bundle of the ulnar collateral ligament is completed, attention is turned to the cubital tunnel region. For this evaluation, the elbow is turned outward so that the bony protuberances of the olecranon process and the medial epicondyle can be visualized and are palpable. Evaluation should begin with the elbow extended; if the elbow is flexed at this point, it is possible that the ulnar nerve may dislocate and be difficult to locate, and identification of an anconeus epitrochlearis becomes difficult as well (see discussion later in

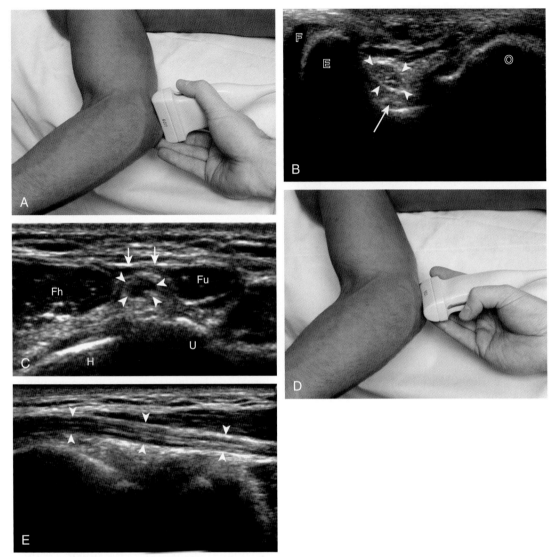

■ **FIGURE 4.10 Ulnar Nerve and Cubital Tunnel Evaluation.** A, Transverse imaging over the medial elbow between the medial epicondyle and olecranon process shows (B) the ulnar nerve *(arrowheads)* posterior to the medial epicondyle *(E)*. Note the common flexor tendon *(F)*, olecranon process *(O)*, and posterior bundle of the ulnar collateral ligament *(arrow)*. C, Transverse imaging distal to B shows the ulnar nerve *(arrowheads)* in the cubital tunnel *(arrows,* arcuate ligament). D, Longitudinal imaging shows (E) the ulnar nerve *(arrowheads)*. *Fh,* Humeral head of flexor carpi ulnaris; *Fu,* ulnar head of flexor carpi ulnaris; *H,* humerus; *U,* ulna.

this chapter). The ultrasound transducer is placed in the transverse plane between the olecranon process and the medial epicondyle, and the characteristic hyperechoic and shadowing bone contours of these structures are seen (Fig. 4.10A and B). The ulnar nerve is visible as speckled or honeycomb in appearance from hypoechoic nerve fascicles and hyperechoic connective tissue; however, the ulnar nerve posterior to the medial epicondyle often appears hypoechoic from physiologic edema but should not be enlarged.[21] The ulnar nerve may also be bilobed or bifid. Superficial to the ulnar nerve, the cubital tunnel retinaculum (or Osborne

fascia) is located and, when present, appears as a thin structure between the olecranon and medial epicondyle. The posterior bundle of the ulnar collateral ligament is deep to the ulnar nerve. Distally, the ulnar nerve can be followed into the true cubital tunnel between the humeral and ulnar heads of the flexor carpi ulnaris and under the arcuate ligament (Fig. 4.10C). With rotation of the transducer 90 degrees, the ulnar nerve can be evaluated in long axis (Fig. 4.10D and E).

The cubital tunnel region should also be assessed dynamically for pathology.[22] With the transducer again placed in the transverse plane

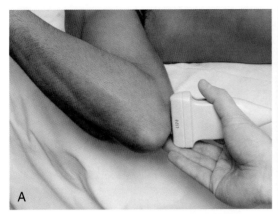
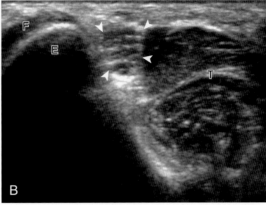

■ **FIGURE 4.11 Ulnar Nerve Dynamic Evaluation.** A, Imaging transverse to the humeral shaft at the level of the medial epicondyle in elbow flexion shows (B) the ulnar nerve *(arrowheads)* and the triceps *(T)* posterior to the medial epicondyle *(E)*. F, Common flexor tendon.

between the medial epicondyle and olecranon process and fixed over the medial epicondyle, the elbow is passively flexed (Fig. 4.11). During this maneuver, the olecranon process moves out of the imaging plane and is replaced by the hypoechoic triceps brachii muscle. Initially performing this maneuver passively is helpful to control the speed of flexion. In addition, the movement can be momentarily stopped and the transducer repositioned if the bone contour of the medial epicondyle apex is not visualized. Normally during elbow flexion, the ulnar nerve moves toward the apex of the medial epicondyle but should not translate over the epicondyle anteriorly. Abnormal ulnar nerve translation over the medial epicondyle may be felt as a palpable snap through the transducer, and typically it returns back into normal position as the elbow is extended. One should avoid too much pressure with the transducer during this dynamic evaluation because this may inhibit the abnormal ulnar nerve translation; intermittent reduction in transducer pressure during the maneuver avoids this pitfall. Ulnar nerve dislocation has been described in up to 20% of asymptomatic individuals, although abnormal movement predisposes to nerve irritation and injury.[23] Isolated ulnar nerve dislocation should also be differentiated from snapping triceps syndrome. In this latter situation, in addition to ulnar nerve dislocation, there is subluxation of the triceps muscle medial head over the medial epicondyle of the humerus in elbow flexion.[22]

Lateral Evaluation

For evaluation of the lateral elbow structures, the arm is rotated inward and slightly flexed. Structures of interest laterally include the common extensor tendon, the lateral collateral ligament complex, the radial head and annular recess, and the capitellum. Unlike the medial aspect of the elbow, the lateral epicondyle is not clearly visible to the eye and is more difficult to palpate; therefore, bone landmarks as seen at sonography are used for orientation. To begin, the transducer is placed in long axis relative to the forearm over the lateral elbow (Fig. 4.12A), and the characteristic hyperechoic shadowing contour of the radial head is readily identified (Fig. 4.12B). More proximal scanning in this plane reveals the radius articulation with the capitellum, and, more proximally, the relatively flattened contour of the lateral epicondyle. At this site, the hyperechoic and fibrillar common extensor tendon and the deeper radial collateral ligament can be seen attaching to the lateral epicondyle (Fig. 4.12C).[3] Although the long axis view is optimum in identification of the common extensor tendon given the characteristic bone landmarks for orientation, any abnormality should also be characterized in short axis as well. Care should be taken to include evaluation of the most anterior aspect of the common extensor tendon, where tendon abnormalities most commonly occur. Distinguishing the common extensor tendon from the underlying radial collateral ligament in long axis may be difficult as both are hyperechoic and fibrillar; however, knowledge of their footprint anatomy on the lateral epicondyle is helpful as the superficial common extensor tendon originates from the proximal 46% of the bone surface and a bony ridge separating the footprints may also be seen.[24] In addition, during real-time scanning the common extensor tendon and radial collateral ligament can be differentiated as they are slightly oblique to each other and an echogenic interface

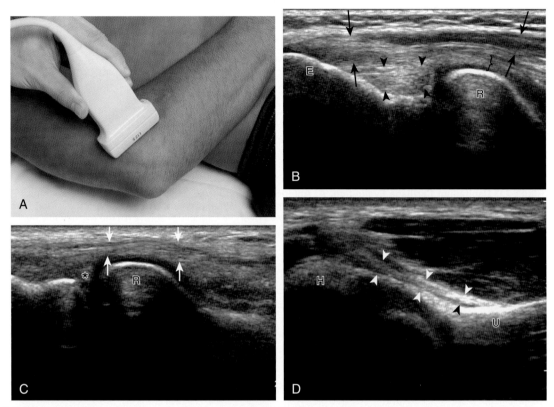

■ **FIGURE 4.12 Common Extensor Tendon and Lateral Collateral Ligament Evaluation.** A, Lateral imaging in long axis to the forearm over the radial head shows (B and C) the radial head *(R)*, common extensor tendon *(arrows)*, radial collateral ligament *(arrowheads)*, and annular ligament *(bracket)*. Note triangular synovial fold *(asterisk)* in B. Transducer placement angled from the annular ligament to the ulna shows (D) the lateral ulnar collateral ligament *(arrowheads)* from the humerus *(H)* and annular ligament to the crista supinator of the ulna *(U)*. F, Lateral epicondyle.

may be seen.[3] Lastly, the radial collateral ligament extends distal to the annular ligament superficial to the radial head, whereas the more superficial common extensor tendon courses distal and becomes muscle. At the radiocapitellar joint, a hyperechoic, triangular, meniscus-like synovial reflection or fold, also termed the *posterolateral plica*, extends from the radial collateral ligament and joint capsule into the joint.[25-27] To visualize the lateral ulnar collateral ligament, the transducer is centered over the annual ligament long axis to the radial collateral ligament and then angled dorsally to visualize its attachment to the crista supinator of the ulna; this ligament often appears hypoechoic from anisotropy but should be uniform in thickness (Fig. 4.12D).[3-5] The annual ligament is also evaluated in long axis (in the transverse plane over the radial head). At the level of the radial neck, the collapsed annular recess is difficult to discern unless it is abnormally distended (see Fig. 4.20B).

With elbow extension and the transducer anterolateral in the sagittal plane, the thin uniform hypoechoic layer of hyaline cartilage can be seen over the anterior aspect of the capitellum (Fig. 4.13A). With movement of the transducer posteriorly over the capitellum, the irregular cortex represents a normal appearance void of cartilage and should not be misinterpreted as an osteochondral abnormality.[26] With the elbow in flexion and the transducer posterior in the sagittal plane, the central and posterior aspect of the capitellum hyaline cartilage can also be visualized (Fig. 4.13B).

For evaluation of the radial nerve, one approach is to first find the oblique fascial plane between the brachioradialis and the brachialis anteriorly in the transverse plane, where the deep and superficial branches of the radial nerve are seen as round and hypoechoic (Fig. 4.14A; see Fig. 4.2B). These individual branches can be followed proximally in short axis where they join to form the radial nerve (Fig. 4.14B). Evaluation can

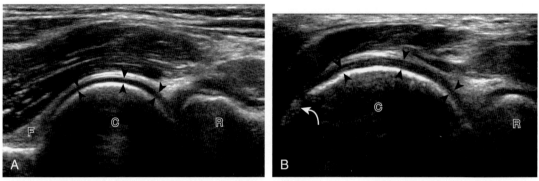

■ FIGURE 4.13 **Capitellum Cartilage Evaluation.** A, Anterior imaging in the sagittal plane over the capitellum *(C)* shows the hyaline articular cartilage *(arrowheads)*, radial head *(R)*, and anterior fat pad *(F)* in the radial fossa. Posterior imaging in the sagittal plane with the elbow flexed over the capitellum shows (B) the hypoechoic hyaline cartilage *(arrowheads)*. Note the normal bone irregularity *(curved arrow)*.

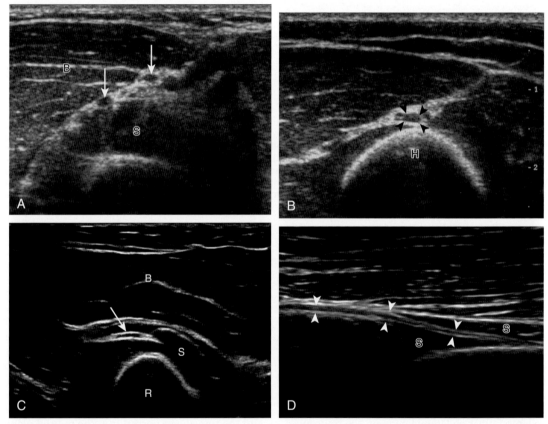

■ FIGURE 4.14 **Radial Nerve Evaluation.** Transverse imaging over anterior elbow (see Fig. 4.2A) shows (A) the superficial and deep branches of the radial nerve *(arrows)* deep to the brachioradialis *(B)*. Proximal imaging (B) shows that the radial nerve branches have joined to form radial nerve *(arrowheads)* adjacent to the posterior humerus *(H)*. Distal imaging shows deep branch of radial nerve *(arrow)* in short axis (C) and long axis *(arrowheads)* (D) within two heads of the supinator muscle *(S)*. R, Radius.

continue more proximal to follow the radial nerve as it traverses the intermuscular fascia and follows the posterior cortex of the humerus. Following the radial nerve branches distally, the deep branch is seen entering into the supinator muscle becom- ing the posterior interosseous nerve (Fig. 4.14C). The transducer is turned 90 degrees to evaluate the radial nerve and its branches in long axis as well (Fig. 4.14D). The deep branch of the radial nerve often changes shape as it passes beneath

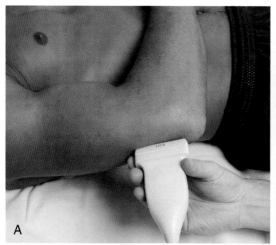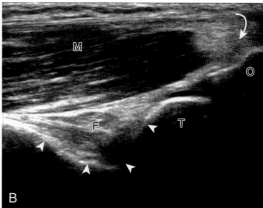

■ **FIGURE 4.15 Posterior Joint Recess and Triceps Evaluation (Long Axis).** A, Imaging in the sagittal plane over the elbow flexed shows (B) the triceps brachii muscle *(M)* and tendon *(curved arrow)*, olecranon fossa *(arrowheads)*, and hyperechoic fat pad *(F)*. Note the trochlea *(T)* with hypoechoic hyaline cartilage and the olecranon *(O)*.

the *arcade of Fröhse* and should not be interpreted as nerve swelling.[27] The superficial branch of the radial nerve may also be followed distally into the forearm.

Posterior Evaluation

To evaluate the posterior structures of the elbow, the patient's elbow is flexed to 90 degrees. If the patient is supine, this can be accomplished by asking the patient to place his or her hand across the abdomen. Structures of interest include the posterior joint recess, the triceps brachii, and the soft tissues over the olecranon. By placing the transducer posteriorly in the sagittal plane over the proximal elbow, the characteristic hyperechoic shadowing bone contours of the humerus are identified (Fig. 4.15). As the humeral diaphysis approaches the elbow joint, there is a pronounced concavity, which represents the olecranon fossa. This is also demonstrated in the transverse plane relative to the humerus (Fig. 4.16). This fossa is normally filled with the hyperechoic posterior elbow fat pad and is the site of evaluation for joint fluid, intra-articular bodies, and other joint processes. The hypoechoic trochlear and capitellum hyaline cartilage can also be identified. Superficial to the olecranon recess, the hypoechoic triceps brachii muscle and more distal hyperechoic tendon can be seen inserting onto the olecranon process. The superficial layer of the triceps brachii represents the confluence of the lateral and long heads, whereas the deeper layer with a very short tendon represents the medial head of the triceps brachii.[28] With elbow extension, the soft tissues superficial to the olecranon process can be evaluated for olecranon

bursal fluid. A thick layer of gel should be used to float the transducer so as to avoid compression and displacement of olecranon bursal fluid away from view. Although the sagittal plane is most important in evaluation of the described posterior anatomy, pathology should also be characterized in the orthogonal transverse.

■ JOINT AND BURSAL ABNORMALITIES

Although a joint effusion may distend the anterior and less commonly the annular joint recesses, the posterior olecranon recess in elbow flexion is the most sensitive location for identification of joint fluid (Fig. 4.17).[29] Imaging in the sagittal plane over the posterior joint recess demonstrates superior and posterior displacement of the hyperechoic fat pad when the joint is distended, similar to findings at radiography. Fat pad displacement, both in the anterior and posterior joint fossae, may result from anechoic simple fluid, although complex fluid may vary from hypoechoic to hyperechoic (Fig. 4.18). Heterogeneous joint fluid may be caused by hemorrhage or infection (Fig. 4.19). Synovial hypertrophy, commonly diffuse, may also distend the joint recesses and may appear hypoechoic (or, less commonly, isoechoic or hyperechoic) relative to the subcutaneous fat. The findings of joint recess compressibility, redistribution or motion of joint recess contents with transducer pressure or joint movement, and lack of internal flow on color Doppler imaging suggest complex fluid rather than synovial hypertrophy when their gray-scale appearances

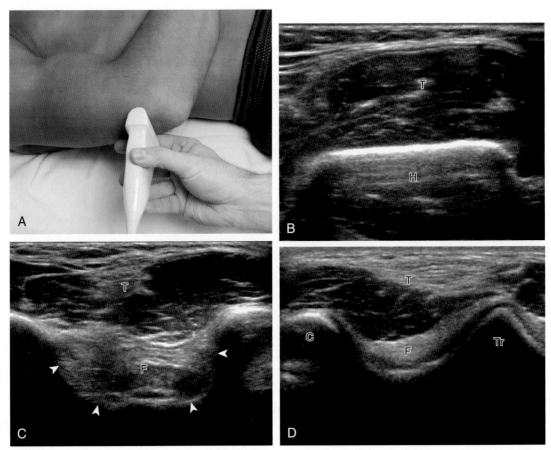

■ **FIGURE 4.16 Posterior Joint Recess and Triceps Evaluation (Short Axis).** A, Imaging transverse to the distal humerus shows (B to D) the triceps muscle *(T)* and gradual flattening of the humerus surface *(H)* to form the olecranon fossa *(arrowheads)*. Note the posterior fat pad *(F)* and the hypoechoic hyaline cartilage of the trochlea *(Tr)* and capitellum *(C)*.

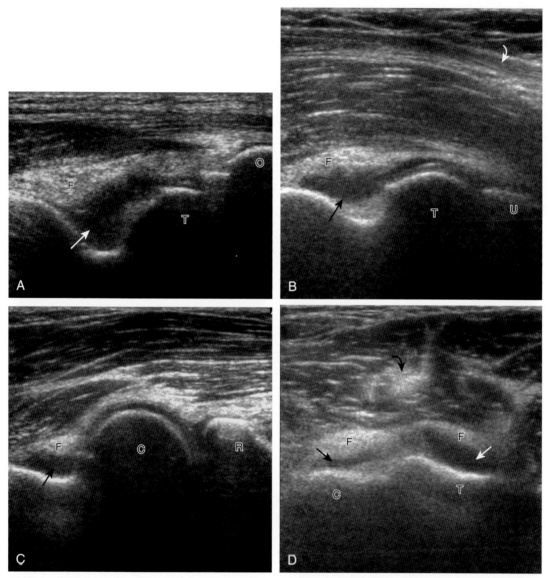

■ **FIGURE 4.17 Elbow Joint Effusion.** (A) Posterior sagittal, (B) anterior sagittal, (C) anterolateral sagittal, and (D) anterior transverse ultrasound images show anechoic joint fluid *(arrows)* with displacement of the hyperechoic fat pads *(F)* within (A) the olecranon fossa, (B and D) the coronoid fossa, and (C and D) the radial fossa (*curved arrow*, biceps brachii tendon). *C*, Capitellum; *R*, radial head; *O*, olecranon; *T*, trochlea; *U*, coronoid process of ulna.

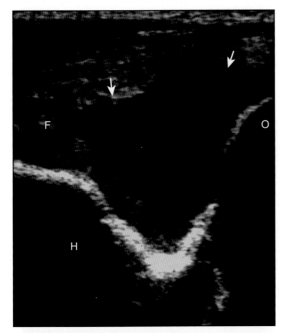

■ **FIGURE 4.18 Septic Elbow Joint.** Sagittal ultrasound image over the posterior elbow shows heterogeneous hypoechoic distention of the posterior joint recess *(arrows)* with displacement of the hyperechoic fat pad *(F)*. *H,* Humerus; *O,* olecranon.

are similar. Synovial hypertrophy may be the result of infection (Fig. 4.20), rheumatoid arthritis (Fig. 4.21), and other inflammatory arthritides (Fig. 4.22) or less likely an adjacent bone process, such as intra-articular osteoid osteoma (Fig. 4.23).[30] Chronic synovial hypertrophy can result in significant distention of the joint recesses, potentially compressing the ulnar nerve (Fig. 4.24) and radial nerve (Fig. 4.25). In the setting of synovitis, cortical discontinuity and irregularity could represent bone erosions (see Fig. 4.21). Other synovial proliferative disorders, such as pigmented villonodular synovitis and synovial chondromatosis (Fig. 4.26), should be considered, with possible calcified hyperechoic foci identified within the synovium in the latter condition.

In addition to evaluation for fluid or synovial hypertrophy, joint recesses should also be evaluated for intra-articular bodies, which if calcified or ossified will be hyperechoic, with possible shadowing. Common sites for intra-articular bodies include the olecranon, coronoid, and annular recesses (Fig. 4.27). The articular hyaline cartilage should be evaluated for an osteochondral abnormality, particularly over the capitellum, in this setting because the donor site for the intra-articular

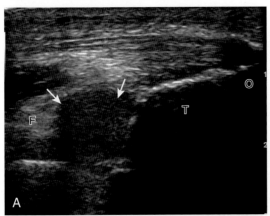

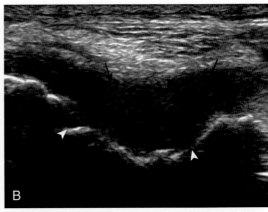

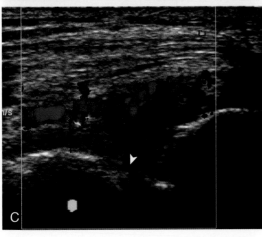

■ **FIGURE 4.19 Septic Elbow Joint.** Sagittal (A) and transverse (B) ultrasound images of the posterior elbow show heterogeneous and hypoechoic joint fluid with internal echoes *(arrows)* that displaces the hyperechoic fat pad *(F)* within the olecranon fossa. C, Note hyperemia of the joint capsule and synovium on color Doppler imaging and cortical irregularity *(arrowhead)*. *O,* Olecranon; *T,* trochlea.

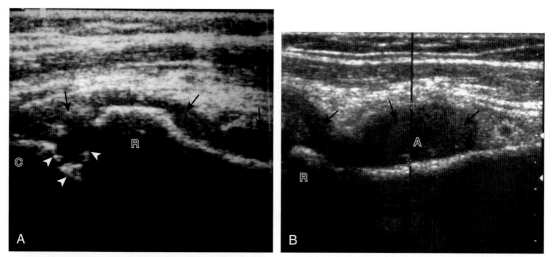

■ **FIGURE 4.20 Elbow Joint Infection: Coccidioidomycosis.** Coronal ultrasound images (A) over and (B) distal to the radial head *(R)* show hypoechoic synovial hypertrophy *(arrows)* that extends into the annular recess (A). Note subchondral bone erosions *(arrowheads). C,* Capitellum.

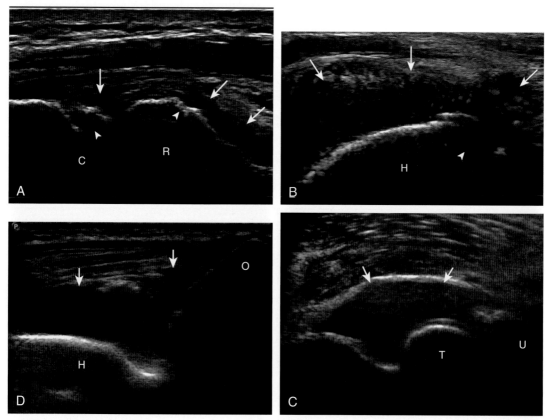

■ **FIGURE 4.21 Rheumatoid Arthritis.** Ultrasound images of the lateral (A) and medial (B) elbow show hypoechoic synovial hypertrophy *(arrows)* and erosions *(arrowheads)* with hyperemia. Ultrasound images of the anterior (C) and posterior (D) elbow from a different patient show hypoechoic synovial hypertrophy distending the joint recesses *(arrows). R,* Radius; *C,* capitellum; *H,* humerus; *O,* olecranon; *T,* trochlea; *U,* ulna.

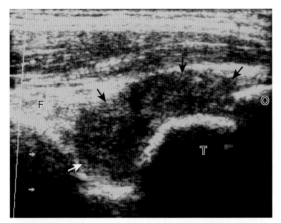

■ FIGURE 4.22 **Seronegative Spondyloarthropathy.** Sagittal ultrasound image over the posterior elbow shows synovial hypertrophy as hypoechoic to isoechoic *(arrows)*, which distends the posterior elbow recess with fat pad displacement *(F)*. *O*, Olecranon; *T*, trochlea.

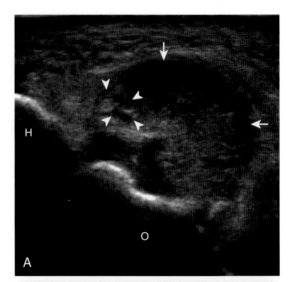

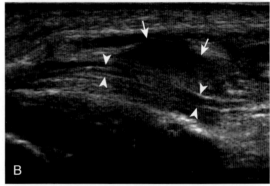

■ FIGURE 4.24 **Ulnar Nerve Compression: Rheumatoid Arthritis.** Ultrasound images in short axis (A) and long axis (B) to the ulnar nerve *(arrowheads)* show compression by adjacent hypoechoic to isoechoic synovial hypertrophy *(arrows)*. *H*, Humerus; *O*, olecranon.

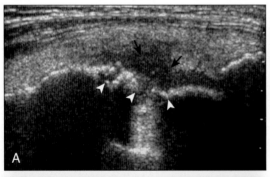

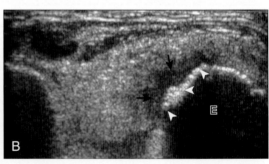

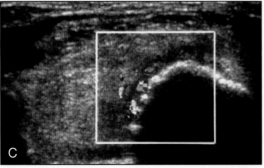

■ FIGURE 4.23 **Intra-Articular Osteoid Osteoma.** Sagittal (A) and transverse (B) ultrasound images at the posterior aspect of the medial epicondyle (E) show focal hypoechoic synovial hypertrophy *(arrows)*, cortical irregularity, and bone proliferation *(arrowheads)* at the site of an osteoid osteoma nidus. C, Note hyperemia on color Doppler images. *(From Ebrahim FS, Jacobson JA, Lin J, et al: Intraarticular osteoid osteoma: sonographic findings in three patients with radiographic, CT, and MR imaging correlation. AJR Am J Roentgenol 177:1391-1395, 2001.)*

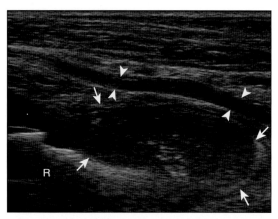

■ FIGURE 4.25 **Radial Nerve, Deep Branch Compression: Rheumatoid Arthritis.** Ultrasound image in long axis to deep branch of radial nerve *(arrowheads)* shows compression by annular recess distended with synovial hypertrophy *(arrows)*. R, Radius. *(Courtesy V. Flores, MD, Fort Worth, Texas. From Jacobson JA, Fessell DP, Lobo Lda G, et al: Entrapment neuropathies I: upper limb (carpal tunnel excluded). Semin Musculoskelet Radiol 14:473-486, 2010.)*

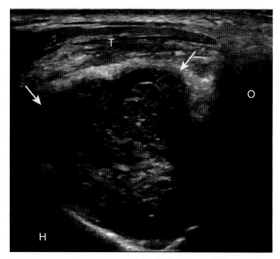

■ FIGURE 4.26 **Synovial Chondromatosis.** Sagittal image over the posterior elbow shows heterogeneous but predominantly hypoechoic synovial hypertrophy distending the posterior joint recess in the olecranon fossa *(arrows)*. H, Humerus; O, olecranon; T, triceps brachii.

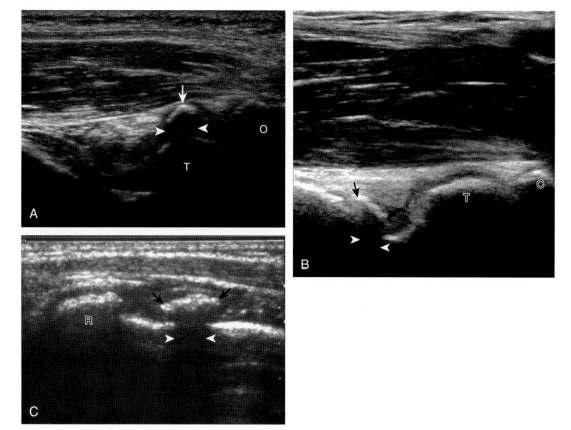

■ FIGURE 4.27 **Intra-Articular Bodies.** A, Sagittal ultrasound images over the olecranon recess posteriorly, (B) the coronoid recess anteriorly, and (C) the annular recess show hyperechoic *(arrows)* and shadowing *(arrowheads)* ossified intra-articular bodies. C, Coronoid process; O, olecranon; R, radial head; T, trochlea.

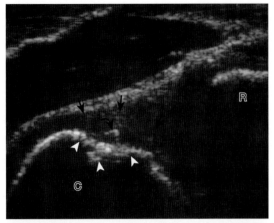

■ **FIGURE 4.28 Osteochondral Abnormality of Capitellum.** Sagittal ultrasound image shows bone irregularity of the capitellum *(arrowheads)*, with thickening and increased echogenicity of the overlying hyaline cartilage *(arrows)*. Note bone fragment *(curved arrow)*. *C*, Capitellum; *R*, radius.

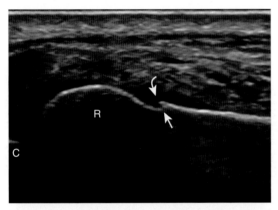

■ **FIGURE 4.29 Radius Neck Fracture.** Sagittal ultrasound image over the radial neck shows step-off deformity *(arrow)*, which represents a radius fracture with adjacent hypoechoic soft tissue hemorrhage *(curved arrow)*. *C*, Capitellum; *R*, radial head.

body may be identified (Fig. 4.28). In patients with trauma, joint effusion may be hemorrhagic, and the finding of step-off deformity of the radial head or neck indicates fracture (Fig. 4.29). Lastly, the synovial fold or plica adjacent to the radial head should be evaluated, as a heterogeneous, thickened (>3 mm), or elongated appearance with possible adjacent synovitis can indicate *synovial fold syndrome* (Fig. 4.30) (Video 4.3).

The olecranon bursa is located superficial to the olecranon process of the ulna and is a common site of pathology. Although the normal and collapsed olecranon bursa is difficult to identify, anechoic or hypoechoic distention makes this structure quite conspicuous. When evaluating the olecranon bursa the transducer should be floated

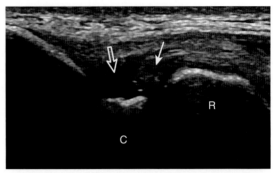

■ **FIGURE 4.30 Synovial Fold Syndrome.** Coronal ultrasound image over the radial head *(H)* and capitellum *(C)* shows heterogeneous and irregular synovial fold *(arrow)* with adjacent hypoechoic synovial hypertrophy.

on a thick layer of gel to eliminate any transducer pressure, which may displace bursal fluid from view (Video 4.4). If the bursal distention is hypoechoic, isoechoic, or hyperechoic, considerations include complex fluid and synovial hypertrophy. Similar to joint recess distention, the findings of joint recess compressibility, redistribution or motion of bursal contents with transducer pressure, and lack of internal flow on color Doppler imaging suggest complex fluid over synovial hypertrophy when their gray-scale appearances are similar. The appearance of hyperechoic synovial hypertrophy with internal hyperechoic foci is characteristic for gout (Video 4.5) (Fig. 4.31).[31] Other causes of bursal distention include trauma (Fig. 4.32), rheumatoid arthritis (Fig. 4.33), and infection. The characteristic location and well-defined borders distinguish the olecranon bursa from a nonspecific fluid collection or abscess. If there is concern for infection, ultrasound-guided percutaneous aspiration may be considered (Fig. 4.32A). The presence of cortical irregularity could indicate adjacent erosions related to inflammation. Another bursa in the elbow, the bicipitoradial bursa, is described later in the discussion of the biceps brachii tendon.

■ TENDON AND MUSCLE ABNORMALITIES

Biceps Brachii

Distal biceps brachii tendon tears most commonly occur near the tendon's insertion 1 to 2 cm proximal to the radial tuberosity.[32] Usually secondary to forced extension against active elbow flexion, this injury increases in prevalence with increasing age, typically seen after the age of 40 years. Full-thickness tears are commonly associated with significant retraction of the torn tendon stump, visualized several centimeters proximal to the

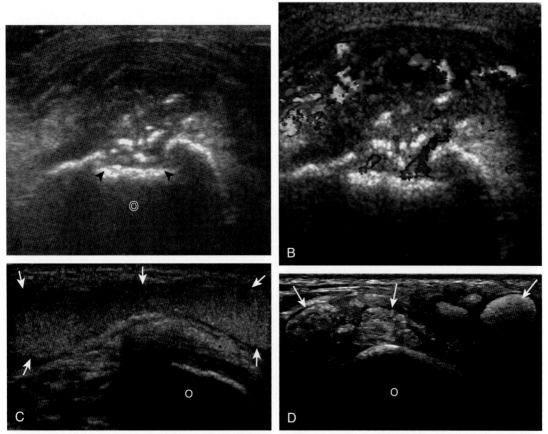

■ FIGURE 4.31 **Olecranon Bursitis: Gout**. Transverse ultrasound image over the olecranon process *(O)* shows (A) heterogeneous bursal distention *(arrows)* with cortical erosions *(arrowheads)* and adjacent hyperechoic tophi. B, Note hyperemia with color Doppler imaging. Sagittal ultrasound images in two different patients show (C) hyperechoic distention of the olecranon bursa, and (D) hyperechoic tophi *(arrows)*.

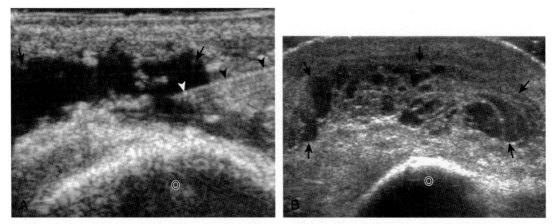

■ FIGURE 4.32 **Olecranon Bursitis: Trauma**. Transverse ultrasound images over the olecranon process *(O)* from two different patients show (A) hypoechoic *(arrows)* and (B) heterogeneous distention *(arrows)* of the olecranon bursa from trauma. Note the needle *(arrowheads)* directed into the bursa in A under ultrasound guidance.

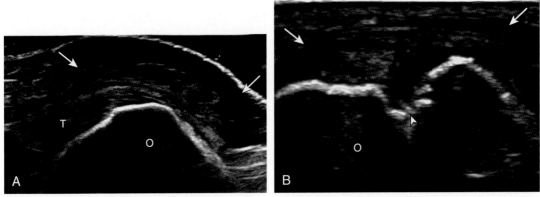

■ **FIGURE 4.33 Olecranon Bursitis: Rheumatoid Arthritis.** Sagittal (A) and transverse (B) ultrasound images over the olecranon process *(O)* shows heterogeneous but predominantly hypoechoic synovial hypertrophy *(arrows)* with an erosion *(arrowhead)*. *T,* Triceps brachii.

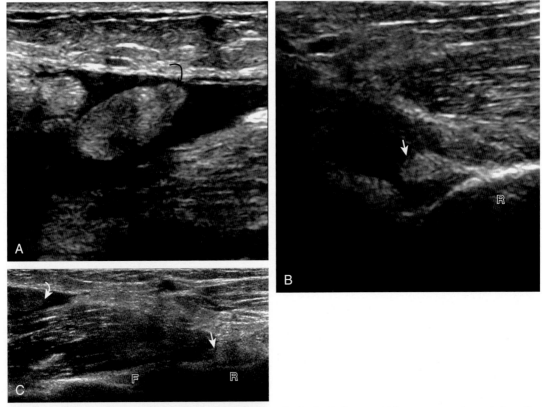

■ **FIGURE 4.34 Biceps Brachii: Full-Thickness Tear (Retracted).** Sagittal ultrasound images over the anterior elbow show (A) a proximal retracted and lax torn biceps tendon stump *(curved arrow)* with adjacent anechoic hemorrhage and (B) a distal tendon stump *(arrow)* with adjacent anechoic hemorrhage at the radial tuberosity *(R)*. C, An extended field of view image shows the full extent of retraction *(between curved arrow and arrow)*. *F,* Anterior fat pad.

radius directly superficial to the brachialis muscle and at the level of the elbow joint (Fig. 4.34). However, retraction may be minimal or absent when the bicipital aponeurosis (or lacertus fibrosus) is intact, which extends from the biceps medially

(Fig. 4.35).[32,33] Like other tendon tears, a full-thickness tear is characterized by anechoic or hypoechoic tendon fiber disruption. The presence of tendon retraction at the tendon tear, often with associated refraction shadowing, is a useful

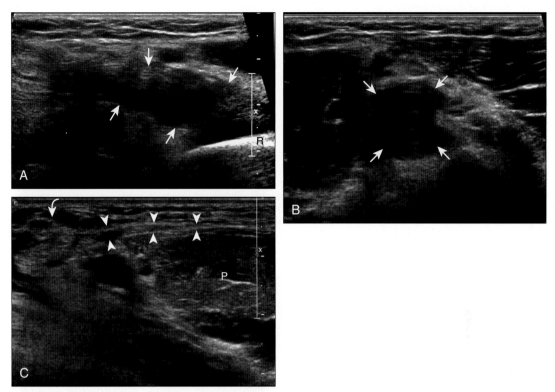

■ **FIGURE 4.35 Biceps Brachii: Full-Thickness Tear (Nonretracted).** Sagittal ultrasound images over anterior elbow show (A) complete disruption of distal biceps tendon *(arrows)*. Short axis ultrasound images at level of tear (B) and more proximal (C) show hypoechoic tendon tear *(arrows)* and more proximal tendon *(curved arrow)*. Note intact lacertus fibrosis in C *(arrowheads)*. *R*, Radius; *P*, pronator teres.

finding to indicate a full-thickness tear.[34] Uncommonly, injury may be isolated to the lacertus fibrosis (Video 4.6).

The diagnosis of nonretracted full-thickness tear, partial-thickness tear, and tendinosis of the distal biceps brachii tendon becomes more problematic because of the oblique course of the distal tendon and resulting anisotropy.[33] Tendinosis will appear as abnormal hypoechogenicity with possible increased thickness of the tendon (Video 4.7) (Fig. 4.36), whereas partial-thickness tears have superimposed hypoechoic or anechoic tendon fiber disruption or clefts and tendon thinning. In contrast, the distal biceps brachii tendon should be uniform in thickness even when hypoechoic from anisotropy. Distal tendon tears may only involve one of the two heads and therefore would be considered partial thickness.[6] Isolated tear of the superficial short head may be seen, where distal shadowing from the torn and retracted tendon stump may create difficulty in evaluation of the deeper long head (Figs. 4.37 and 4.38). To differentiate a partial-thickness tendon tear from a nonretracted full-thickness tear, evaluation with dynamic imaging is very helpful (see Fig. 4.6).[13] In the setting of a full-thickness tear, the

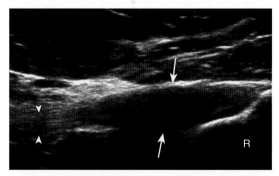

■ **FIGURE 4.36 Biceps Brachii: Tendinosis.** Coronal-oblique ultrasound image in long axis to distal biceps tendon from a medial approach shows a hypoechoic distal biceps tendon with increased thickness *(arrows)* that was painful with transducer pressure. Note normal biceps brachii tendon more proximal *(arrowheads)*. *R*, Radial tuberosity.

visualized proximal tendon segment will show little or no movement when the hand is moved from pronation to neutral (Video 4.8). In contrast, a partial-thickness tear will show movement or translation of the tendon equal to the amount of rotation of the radial tuberosity, indicating that

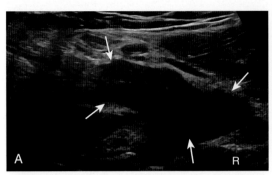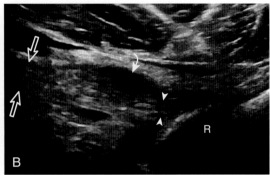

■ **FIGURE 4.37 Biceps Brachii: Partial-Thickness Tear.** A, Sagittal ultrasound image in long axis to the distal biceps tendon from an anterior approach shows hypoechoic thickening of the distal tendon *(arrows)*. B, coronal ultrasound image in long axis to the biceps brachii tendon from a medial approach shows the retracted tear of the short head *(curved arrow)* and intact long head *(arrowheads)*. Note combined short and long heads proximal to tear *(open arrows)*. R, Radial tuberosity.

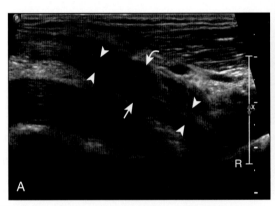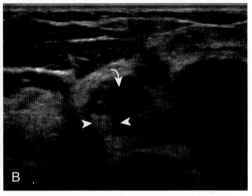

■ **FIGURE 4.38 Biceps Brachii: Partial-Thickness Tear.** Long axis (A) and short axis (B) ultrasound images relative to the biceps tendon show torn and retracted superficial short head *(curved arrow)* and intact deep long head tendon *(arrowheads)* with adjacent hypoechoic hemorrhage. Note refraction shadowing deep to the short head tendon stump *(arrow)*. R, Radial tuberosity.

fibers remain attached to the radial tuberosity (Videos 4.9 and 4.10). Dynamic evaluation can be performed when imaging from a medial or lateral approach in elbow flexion.[12] It has been reported that ultrasound can differentiate full-thickness from partial-thickness tear with 95% sensitivity and 91% accuracy.[34] After surgical repair of a torn biceps brachii tendon, ultrasound can be used to assess for re-tear; increased tendon thickness of an intact repair correlates with improved outcome (Video 4.11).[35]

Another pathologic process associated with the distal biceps brachii tendon that can cause interpretation difficulties is the bicipitoradial bursa. This normal bursa surrounds the distal biceps brachii tendon as it approaches the radial tuberosity.[36] When the bursa is distended, it may contain anechoic simple fluid, or it may appear as heterogeneous hypoechoic, isoechoic, and hyperechoic complex fluid and synovial hypertrophy with possible flow on color or power Doppler imaging (Fig. 4.39).[37] When symptomatic, this condition has also been called cubital bursitis and may compress the superficial branch of the radial nerve (Fig. 4.40).[36] Because of the potential heterogeneous appearance, this bursa may be confused with a nonspecific heterogeneous mass at imaging. The key to an accurate diagnosis of bicipitoradial bursitis is identification of its U-shaped configuration as it surrounds the distal biceps brachii tendon (Video 4.12). Although any inflammatory or proliferative condition that involves a bursa may affect the bicipitoradial bursa, including lipoma arborescens, this condition is most commonly the result of repetitive trauma.[36,38] No tendon sheath is present at the distal biceps brachii tendon, so the diagnosis of tenosynovitis is not possible at this location.

Triceps Brachii

Injuries to the triceps brachii may take the form of direct impact injury or distal avulsion. As with any muscle, a direct impact can cause muscle tear

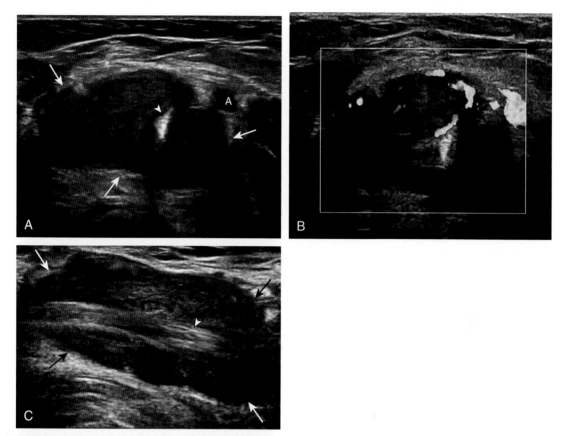

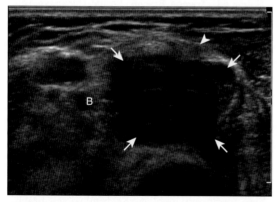

■ FIGURE 4.39 **Bicipitoradial Bursitis.** Ultrasound images in (A, B) short axis and (C) long axis to the distal biceps brachii tendon *(arrowhead)* show complex bicipitoradial bursa *(arrows)* surrounding the biceps tendon with hyperemia on color Doppler image (B). *A,* Brachial artery.

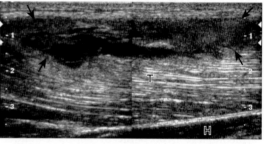

■ FIGURE 4.41 **Triceps Brachii: Direct Impact Injury.** Ultrasound image in long axis to the triceps *(T)* shows partial muscle fiber disruption with anechoic, isoechoic, and hyperechoic hemorrhage *(arrows)*. *H,* Humerus.

■ FIGURE 4.40 **Bicipitoradial Bursitis and Radial Nerve Compression.** Transverse ultrasound image over anterolateral elbow shows distended bicipitoradial bursa *(arrows)* with adjacent compression of the superficial branch of the radial nerve *(arrowhead)*. *B,* Biceps brachii.

and hemorrhage, most typically at the muscle belly with a heterogeneous but predominantly hypoechoic appearance (Fig. 4.41). Overuse of a muscle in the setting of *delayed onset muscle soreness* (DOMS) can produce a focal or diffuse hyperechoic

area of the involved muscle with possible muscle enlargement but without fiber disruption (Fig. 4.42), seen in the triceps brachii as well as other upper extremity muscles such as the biceps brachii and brachioradialis.[39] Distally, triceps tendon tears and avulsions at the olecranon process are possible. A full-thickness tear appears as complete anechoic or hypoechoic tendon disruption with retraction. Tendinosis will appear as abnormal hypoechogenicity and tendon enlargement with intact fibers,

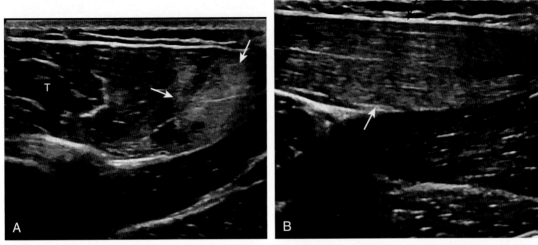

■ **FIGURE 4.42 Delayed Onset Muscle Soreness.** Ultrasound images short axis (A) and long axis (B) to the triceps brachii *(T)* show abnormal hyperechoic area with enlargement.

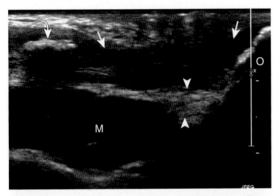

■ **FIGURE 4.43 Triceps Brachii: Partial-Thickness Tear.** Ultrasound image in long axis to the triceps shows tear of the combined lateral and long head attachment *(between arrows)* with retracted enthesophyte bone fragment *(curved arrow).* Note intact deep medial head tendon *(arrowheads).* M, Medial triceps brachii head muscle; *O,* olecranon.

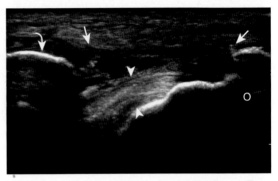

■ **FIGURE 4.44 Triceps Brachii: Partial-Thickness Tear.** Ultrasound image in long axis to the triceps shows tear of the combined lateral and long head attachment *(between arrows)* with retracted enthesophyte bone fragment *(curved arrow).* Note intact deep medial head tendon *(arrowheads). O,* Olecranon. *(From Downie R, Jacobson JA, Fessell, DP, et al: Sonography of partial-thickness tears of the distal triceps brachii tendon. J Ultrasound Med 30:1351–1356, 2011. Reproduced with permission from the American Institute of Ultrasound in Medicine.)*

whereas a partial-thickness tendon tear appears as incomplete hypoechoic or anechoic tendon fiber disruption. Partial-thickness tears most commonly involve the superficial layer of the tendon, which is the combined lateral and long head attachments, characteristically associated with a fractured and displaced enthesophyte (Figs. 4.43 and 4.44) (Videos 4.13 and 4.14).[40] The avulsed bone fragment may measure up to 2 cm with retraction up to 4 cm. No donor site is usually identified at the olecranon process as the ossific fragment represents an avulsed enthesophyte spur. The deeper medial head, which is predominantly muscle with a very short tendon attachment, remains intact to exclude full-thickness tear. Another abnormality of the triceps muscle, called *snapping triceps syndrome,* is described later, under the discussion of the ulnar nerve and cubital tunnel. Lastly, although a well-defined enthesophyte commonly involves the distal triceps brachii tendon from degeneration, the presence of an ill-defined enthesophyte with adjacent abnormal tendon and hyperemia could indicate an inflammatory enthesopathy, as seen with seronegative spondyloarthropathies such as psoriatic arthritis (Fig. 4.45).

Common Flexor and Extensor Tendons

Abnormalities of the common flexor tendon origin at the medial epicondyle (Fig. 4.46) and

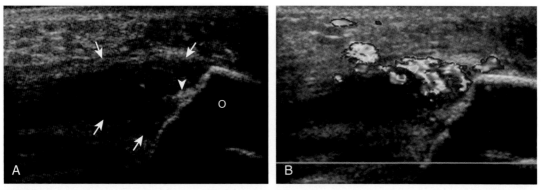

■ **FIGURE 4.45 Inflammatory Enthesopathy: Psoriatic Arthritis.** A and B, Ultrasound images in long axis to distal triceps brachii tendon show hypoechoic swelling of the distal tendon with hyperemia *(arrows)* and cortical irregularity of the olecranon from bone proliferation *(arrowhead). O,* Olecranon.

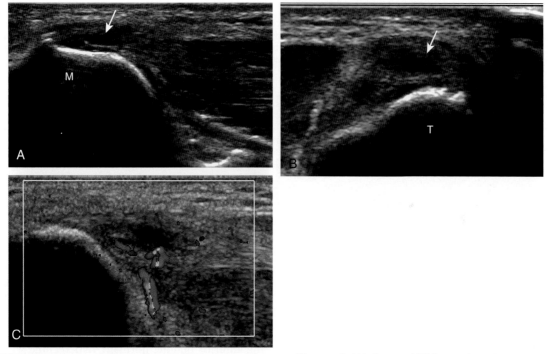

■ **FIGURE 4.46 Common Flexor Tendon Abnormality.** Ultrasound images in (A) short and (B) long axis to the common flexor tendon at the medial epicondyle *(M)* show hypoechoic tendinosis and anechoic interstitial tear with neovascularity on color Doppler image (C).

the common extensor tendon origin at the lateral epicondyle (Figs. 4.47 and 4.48) are commonly referred to as epicondylitis, or golfer's and tennis elbow, respectively.[41] The term *epicondylitis* is a misnomer in that the tendon is primarily involved and not the epicondyle, and the abnormality consists of degeneration, tendinosis, and possible tendon tear rather than true active inflammation.[42] This process is most often from trauma or overuse conditions, and with regard to lateral epicondylitis, the extensor carpi radialis brevis component of the common

extensor tendon (seen most anterior) is most commonly affected.[43] At sonography, tendinosis appears as abnormal hypoechogenicity and possible tendon enlargement (>4.2 mm if common extensor tendon), with possible hyperechoic calcification and adjacent bone irregularity.[42,44,45] Hyperemia on color or power Doppler imaging from neovascularity is variable and correlates with patient symptoms. A superimposed partial-thickness tear appears as anechoic clefts and incomplete fiber discontinuity.[42,46] Uncommonly, a full-thickness

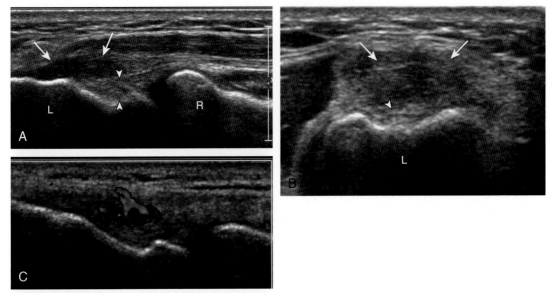

■ **FIGURE 4.47 Common Extensor Tendinosis.** Ultrasound images in (A) short and (B) long axis to the common extensor tendon at the lateral epicondyle *(L)* show hypoechoic tendinosis and with neovascularity on color Doppler image (C). Note normal radial collateral ligament *(arrowheads). R,* Radial head.

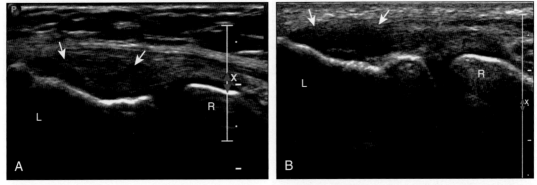

■ **FIGURE 4.48 Common Extensor Tendon Abnormality.** Ultrasound images from two different patients (A and B) in long axis to the common extensor tendon show abnormal hypoechoic tendinosis *(arrows),* with superimposed anechoic interstitial tear in B. *L,* Lateral epicondyle; *R,* radial head.

tear of the common extensor tendon can be seen with complete discontinuity and retraction (Fig. 4.49). In the setting of common extensor tendon abnormalities, the adjacent radial collateral ligament should also be evaluated.[3,47] The size of an intrasubstance common extensor tendon tear and the presence of a radial collateral ligament tear indicate poor outcome after non-operative treatment (Fig. 4.50).[46]

■ LIGAMENT ABNORMALITIES

The medial elbow joint is stabilized by the ulnar collateral ligament, which consists of a strong anterior bundle, a posterior bundle, and a weaker oblique bundle. Evaluation primarily focuses on the anterior bundle, normally hyperechoic with compact fibers that extend from the undersurface of the medial epicondyle to the sublime tubercle and more distally along the proximal ulna, although its appearance may be hypoechoic from anisotropy.[16,17,48] A partial tear or sprain of the ulnar collateral ligament appears as hypoechoic thickening and heterogeneity of the ligament, but without complete ligament fiber disruption (Fig. 4.51). A remote or chronic injury may result in an intact but lax ligament (Fig. 4.52). A full-thickness tear appears as complete fiber discontinuity, with variable anechoic, hypoechoic, and isoechoic fluid and hemorrhage (Fig. 4.53).[49] Distinguishing between a partial-thickness and full-thickness tear may be difficult, especially if the tear is subacute and hemorrhage is present.

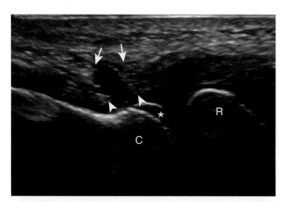

FIGURE 4.49 Common Extensor Tendon and Radial Collateral Ligament: Full-Thickness Tear. Ultrasound image in long axis to the common extensor tendon shows full-thickness anechoic disruption of the tendon *(between arrows)*. Note adjacent tear of the deeper radial collateral ligament *(between arrowheads)* *(asterisk, capitellum hyaline cartilage)*. *C*, Capitellum; *R*, radial head.

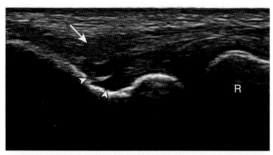

FIGURE 4.50 Common Extensor Tendon Abnormality and Radial Collateral Ligament Tear. Ultrasound image in long axis to the common extensor tendon shows mild hypoechoic tendinosis *(arrow)* and radial collateral ligament tear *(arrowheads)*. *R*, Radial head.

To assist with the differentiation, dynamic imaging is employed (Videos 4.15, 4.16, and 4.17). Under sonographic observation, the flexed elbow (at least 30 degrees) is placed into valgus stress with the hand supinated. This stress maneuver can be accomplished with the assistance of another person or with the patient holding the upper arm if the patient is seated or by using gravity if the patient is lying down with the arm extending off of the bed; the latter method produces results similar to a stress device.[18,50] In addition to visible separation of the torn ligament ends, abnormal joint space widening immediately beneath the ligament indicates ligament tear.[19,51] During valgus stress, joint gapping greater than 1 mm difference compared with the contralateral asymptomatic

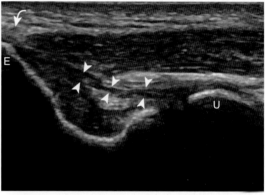

FIGURE 4.52 Ulnar Collateral Ligament: Remote Injury. Ultrasound image in long axis to the anterior bundle of the ulnar collateral ligament shows attenuated ligament *(arrowheads)*. During valgus stress, the ligament was intact, although there was asymmetrical joint space widening *(curved arrow, common flexor tendon)*. *E*, Medial epicondyle; *U*, ulna.

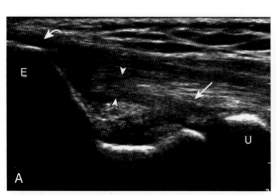

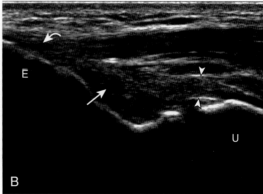

FIGURE 4.51 Ulnar Collateral Ligament: Partial-Thickness Tear. Ultrasound images from two different patients in long axis to the anterior bundle of the ulnar collateral ligament *(arrowheads)* show abnormal distal hypoechoic thinning in A *(arrow)* and hypoechoic proximal defect in B *(arrow)*. With valgus stress, the joint space did not widen, and intact ligament fibers were seen *(curved arrow, common flexor tendon)*. *E*, Medial epicondyle; *U*, ulna.

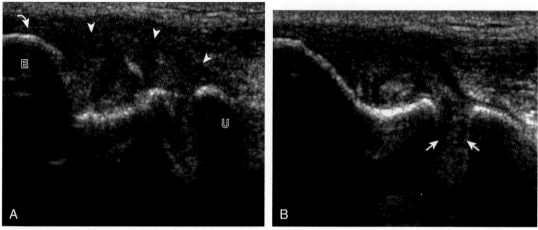

■ **FIGURE 4.53 Ulnar Collateral Ligament: Full-Thickness Tear.** Ultrasound image in long axis to the anterior bundle of the ulnar collateral ligament shows (A) abnormal hypoechoic swelling with no discernible fibers *(arrowheads)*. Note the widened medial joint space *(arrows)*, which increased with valgus stress in B *(curved arrow,* common flexor tendon). *E,* Medial epicondyle; *U,* ulna.

elbow resulted in an accuracy of 87% in the diagnosis of ulnar collateral ligament tear requiring surgery; a threshold of 2.5 mm can be used for diagnosis of full-thickness tear.[52] The use of stress ultrasound complements MR arthrography in evaluation of the ulnar collateral ligament to increase accuracy to 98% compared with the use of only one imaging method alone.[52] Abnormal hypoechoic areas and calcifications of the ulnar collateral ligament are often seen in asymptomatic professional baseball pitchers.[20]

At the lateral aspect of the elbow, the radial collateral ligament, the annular ligament, and the lateral ulnar collateral ligament can be identified.[3,4] As in the ulnar collateral ligament, partial tears appear as partial hypoechoic fiber disruption, whereas full-thickness tears appear as complete ligament fiber discontinuity (Fig. 4.54). Joint instability may also be demonstrated with varus stress in the setting of a full-thickness tear (Video 4.18). The proximal aspect of the radial collateral ligament is in close proximity to the common extensor tendon, and both may be abnormal (see Fig. 4.49). The lateral elbow can also be evaluated during hand supination and pronation for abnormal radial head movement or abnormal snapping of the annular ligament.

■ PERIPHERAL NERVE ABNORMALITIES

Ulnar Nerve

The elbow has several sites where the ulnar nerve is prone to injury or entrapment.[53] Between the medial epicondyle and the olecranon process, as the ulnar nerve passes beneath the cubital tunnel retinaculum (or Osborne fascia), the ulnar nerve may be affected by acute trauma, chronic repetitive injury with elbow flexion, and ulnar nerve subluxation and dislocation. More distally, the ulnar nerve may be compressed where it enters the true cubital tunnel, formed by the humeral and ulnar origins of the flexor carpi ulnaris bridged by the arcuate ligament.[8] The ultrasound diagnosis of ulnar nerve entrapment at this site or *cubital tunnel syndrome* relies on the visualization of hypoechoic enlargement of the ulnar nerve just proximal to the cubital tunnel, usually with a transition to normal size within the cubital tunnel (Video 4.19). A cross-sectional area of the ulnar nerve greater than 9 mm² at the site of maximal enlargement, or an increase in size with a ratio of greater than 2.8 compared to proximal is considered abnormal (Fig. 4.55).[54,55]

The ulnar nerve is also evaluated dynamically where transient dislocation of the ulnar nerve may occur with absence of a cubital tunnel retinaculum.[56] In this condition, the ulnar nerve dislocates medially and anteriorly over the medial epicondyle with elbow flexion, which predisposes to nerve irritation and injury (Fig. 4.56) (Videos 4.20 and 4.21).[57,58] With elbow extension, the ulnar nerve relocates to normal position. Up to 20% of individuals with ulnar nerve dislocation may be asymptomatic, so imaging findings should be correlated with clinical findings. Another related pathologic process associated with ulnar nerve dislocation is *snapping triceps syndrome* (Fig. 4.57) (Videos 4.22 and 4.23).[22] This condition is characterized by abnormal dislocation of the ulnar nerve and subluxation of the medial head of the

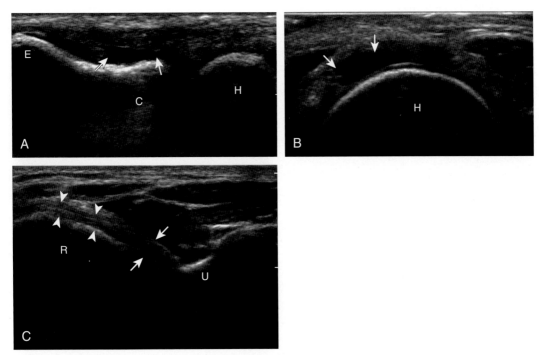

■ **FIGURE 4.54 Radial Collateral Ligament Abnormalities.** Ultrasound image (A) in long axis to the radial collateral ligament shows anechoic fluid *(arrows)* within radial collateral ligament tear. Ultrasound image (B) transverse to radial head and long axis to annular ligament shows anechoic fluid *(arrows)* within annular ligament tear. Ultrasound image (C) in long axis to lateral ulnar collateral ligament *(arrowheads)* shows hypoechoic thickening *(arrows)*. *C*, Capitellum; *E*, lateral epicondyle; *H*, radial head; *R*, radius; *U*, ulna.

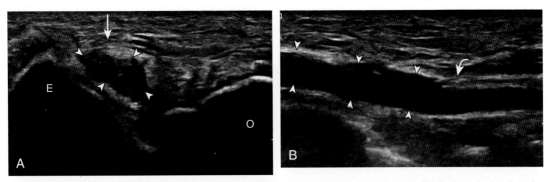

■ **FIGURE 4.55 Cubital Tunnel Syndrome.** Ultrasound images in (A) short axis and (B) long axis to the ulnar nerve show hypoechoic enlargement of the ulnar nerve *(arrowheads)* deep to the cubital tunnel retinaculum *(arrow)*, proximal to its entrance into the cubital tunnel *(curved arrow, arcuate ligament)*. *E*, Medial epicondyle; *O*, olecranon.

triceps muscle with elbow flexion and reduction in elbow extension, which may result in the palpation of two snaps rather than one with isolated ulnar nerve dislocation. One treatment for cubital tunnel syndrome and ulnar nerve dislocation is surgical transposition of the ulnar nerve, which may then be subcutaneous superficial to the pronator teres (Fig. 4.58A) or submuscular in location (Fig. 4.58B).

Another potential cause of ulnar nerve compression is an anconeus epitrochlearis muscle, which is a normal variant that occurs in up to 23% of the population (Fig. 4.59).[21] The anconeus epitrochlearis muscle has a variable size but characteristically is hypoechoic with hyperechoic fibroadipose tissue similar to other muscles and extends from the triceps brachii toward the medial epicondyle in place of Osborne fascia. The diagnosis of anconeus epitrochlearis is easiest when the elbow is in extension, where no muscle tissue should be present between the olecranon and medial epicondyle, which is in contrast to

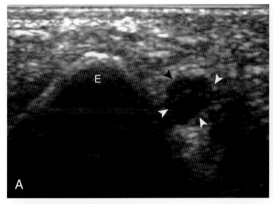

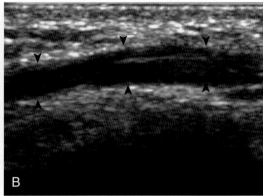

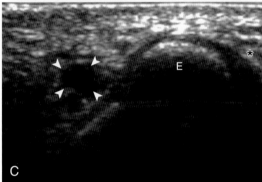

■ FIGURE 4.56 **Cubital Tunnel Syndrome From Transient Ulnar Nerve Dislocation.** Ultrasound images in (A) short axis and (B) long axis to the ulnar nerve in elbow extension show hypoechoic enlargement of the ulnar nerve *(arrowheads)*. Ultrasound image (C) in short axis to the ulnar nerve in elbow flexion shows dislocation of the ulnar nerve anteriorly over the medial epicondyle *(E)* from its normal location (*asterisk*), which reduced with elbow extension.

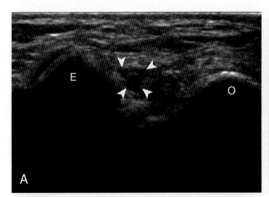

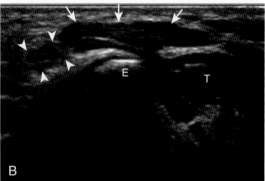

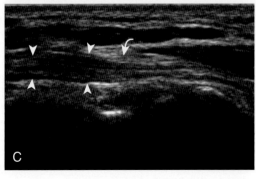

■ FIGURE 4.57 **Snapping Triceps Syndrome.** Ultrasound images in short axis to the ulnar nerve in (A) elbow extension and (B) elbow flexion show hypoechoic enlargement of the ulnar nerve *(arrowheads)*. Note the anterior dislocation of the ulnar nerve anterior to the apex of the medial epicondyle *(E)* with elbow flexion in B, accompanied by the medial head *(arrows)* of the triceps muscle *(T)*. Ultrasound image (C) in long axis to ulnar nerve shows hypoechoic swelling *(arrowheads)* (*curved arrow*, arcuate ligament). *O*, Olecranon.

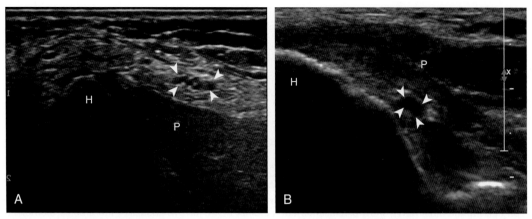

■ FIGURE 4.58 **Ulnar Nerve Transposition.** Ultrasound image (A) in short axis to the ulnar nerve shows the location of the ulnar nerve *(arrowheads)* over the pronator teres muscle *(P)*. Ultrasound image (B) of a different patient shows the ulnar nerve *(arrowheads)* deep to the pronator teres muscle *(P)*. Note normal size and appearance of the ulnar nerve. *H,* Humerus.

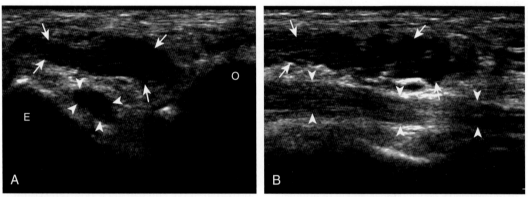

■ FIGURE 4.59 **Anconeus Epitrochlearis Muscle.** Ultrasound image in (A) short axis and (B) long axis to the ulnar nerve *(arrowheads)* shows the anconeus epitrochlearis muscle *(arrows)* between the olecranon *(O)* and medial epicondyle of the humerus (E). *(From Jacobson JA, Fessell DP, Lobo Lda G, et al: Entrapment neuropathies I: upper limb (carpal tunnel excluded). Semin Musculoskelet Radiol 14:473–486, 2010.)*

elbow flexion, where the triceps brachii is normally located adjacent to the medial epicondyle. Dynamic imaging with elbow flexion may also show crowding deep to Osborne fascia from an anconeus epitrochlearis as well as abnormal snapping (Figs. 4.59 and 4.60) (Video 4.24). Lastly, the ulnar nerve may also be compressed by adjacent elbow joint abnormalities, such as synovial hypertrophy (see Fig. 4.24), intra-articular bodies, and intra-articular hemorrhage after trauma (Fig. 4.61).

Median Nerve

The median nerve courses along the anteromedial aspect of the elbow and may be entrapped at several locations, although less commonly compared to nerve entrapment at the wrist as part of

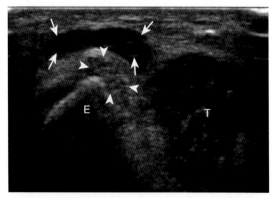

■ FIGURE 4.60 **Anconeus Epitrochlearis: Subluxation.** Ultrasound image in short axis to the ulnar nerve *(arrowheads)* with the elbow in flexion shows abnormal subluxation of the anconeus epitrochlearis muscle *(arrows)* over the medial epicondyle *(E)*. *T,* Triceps brachii muscle.

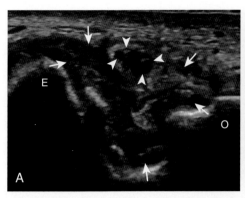

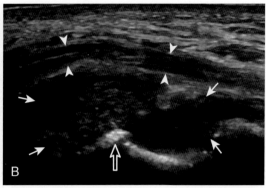

■ FIGURE 4.61 **Ulnar Nerve Compression: Intra-Articular Hemorrhage.** Ultrasound images in (A) short axis and (B) long axis to the ulnar nerve show displacement of the ulnar nerve *(arrowheads)* by intra-articular hemorrhage and synovial hypertrophy *(arrows)* from intra-articular humerus fracture *(open arrow). E,* Medial epicondyle; *O,* olecranon.

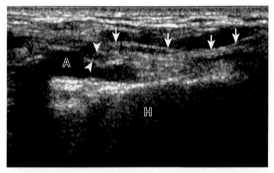

■ FIGURE 4.62 **Median Nerve Entrapment.** Ultrasound image in long axis to the ligament of Struthers over the anteromedial distal humerus shows the median nerve *(arrowheads)* beneath the ligament of Struthers *(arrows).* Note the supracondylar process *(curved arrow)* at the humeral attachment of the ligament of Struthers and the brachial artery *(A). H,* Humerus.

carpal tunnel syndrome.[53] One site of potential entrapment is at the level of the distal humerus, where the ligament of Struthers may extend from a normal variant bone excrescence of the anterior humerus (called the *supracondylar process*) to the medial epicondyle with compression of the median nerve (Fig. 4.62).[59] In the antecubital region, the median nerve may be entrapped between the humeral and ulnar heads of the pronator teres and may cause *pronator teres syndrome.* More distally, a branch of the median nerve, the anterior interosseous nerve, may also be a site of compression from fibrous bands or an anomalous muscle. Primary findings of median nerve entrapment are typically absent with ultrasound; evaluation of the distal innervated musculature should be completed because increased echogenicity from atrophy may be a clue to the nerve entrapment (Fig. 4.63).[60]

Radial Nerve

Pathologic processes of the radial nerve include nerve injury associated with the spiral groove of the humerus, termed *spiral groove syndrome,* characterized by wrist drop and sensory findings but with spared triceps brachii function.[8,53] One cause of radial nerve injury at this site is a fracture of the humeral shaft, where the injured radial nerve can range from an enlarged nerve segment (Fig. 4.64) to complete nerve transection (Fig. 4.65).[61] In this latter condition, the transected nerve ends are retracted appearing hypoechoic and enlarged. Direct transducer pressure over the proximal nerve end can elicit referred symptoms. The radial nerve may also be injured with increased thickness at the level of the spiral groove from external compression (termed *Saturday night palsy*) (Video 4.25). A hypoechoic and swollen radial nerve may also show constriction by the intermuscular septum and fibrous bands (Fig. 4.66).

Another site of radial nerve entrapment involves the deep branch of the radial nerve as it courses distally and posteriorly between the two heads of the supinator within the radial tunnel. Two distinct clinical entities may result. One entity is *radial tunnel syndrome,* which is controversial in that proximal lateral forearm pain is present without motor function or electrodiagnostic test abnormalities.[62] At imaging, denervation changes have been described with radial tunnel syndrome, especially in the supinator muscle, without nerve enlargement. In contrast, *posterior interosseous nerve syndrome* presents with painless lack of finger and thumb extension with abnormal electrodiagnostic tests without wrist drop. Imaging of posterior interosseous nerve syndrome shows abnormal enlargement of the radial nerve deep branch just proximal to its entrance between the two heads

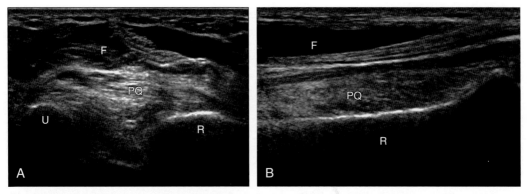

■ FIGURE 4.63 **Anterior Interosseous Nerve Syndrome.** Ultrasound images in (A) long axis and (B) short axis to the pronator quadratus *(PQ)* show abnormal increased echogenicity of the pronator quadratus relative to the more superficial flexor muscles *(F)* from denervation. *R*, Radius; *U*, ulna.

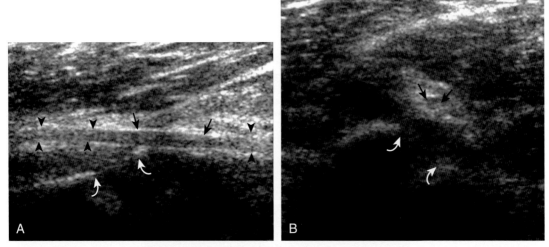

■ FIGURE 4.64 **Radial Nerve Injury After Humeral Fracture.** Ultrasound images in (A) long axis and (B) short axis to the radial nerve *(arrowheads)* at the radial groove show minimal hypoechoic swelling of the intact radial nerve *(arrows)* at the site of the humerus fracture *(curved arrows)*.

of the supinator muscle and distal compression (Fig. 4.67).[63] Causes of such compression may relate to the arcade of Frohse, fibrous bands at the leading edge of the supinator, prior trauma, or less commonly abnormal recurrent blood vessels (termed the *leash of Henry*).[53] The deep branch of the radial nerve normally flattens as it enters the supinator, which should not be misinterpreted as nerve compression when imaging in long axis.[27] This pitfall can be avoided by noting lack of nerve enlargement proximally and imaging the radial nerve in short axis to show no change in nerve area. A mass, ganglion cyst (Fig. 4.68), bicipito-radial bursa (see Fig. 4.40), or adjacent elbow joint process (see Fig. 4.25) may cause secondary nerve compression. The extensor musculature and supinator should also be assessed for echogenic denervation changes and possible atrophy.

Peripheral Nerve Sheath Tumors

Other possible peripheral nerve conditions that are not specific to the peripheral nerves around the elbow include peripheral nerve sheath tumors (see Chapter 2). Benign forms include schwannoma and neurofibroma and appear as a defined hypoechoic mass with low-level internal echoes.[64] Plexiform neurofibromas involve peripheral nerves more extensively (Fig. 4.69) (Video 4.26). Peripheral nerve sheath tumors may be associated with increased through-transmission and can simulate a complex cyst; however, the presence of increased flow on color Doppler imaging indicates a solid mass. The presence of peripheral nerve continuity with the mass indicates a peripheral nerve sheath tumor. Malignant counterparts may also contain anechoic cystic or necrotic areas.

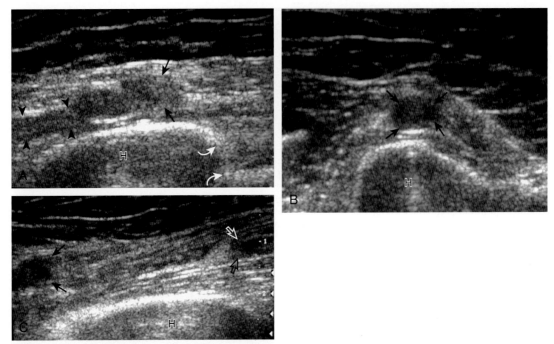

■ **FIGURE 4.65 Radial Nerve Transection After Humeral Fracture.** Ultrasound images in (A) long axis and (B) short axis to the radial nerve show the retracted nerve stump *(arrows)* in continuity with the hypoechoic and enlarged radial nerve *(arrowheads)* *(curved arrows,* humerus fracture). C, Ultrasound image in long axis more distally shows the retraction between the proximal stump *(arrows)* and the distal nerve stump *(open arrows). H,* Humerus.

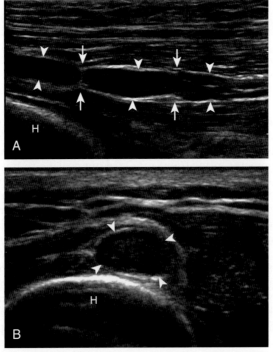

■ **FIGURE 4.66 Radial Groove Syndrome.** Ultrasound images in (A) long axis and (B) short axis to the radial nerve show diffuse nerve swelling *(arrowheads)* and two focal constrictions *(arrows). H,* Humerus.

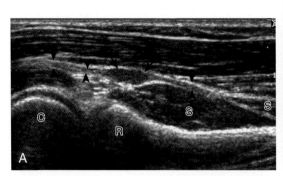

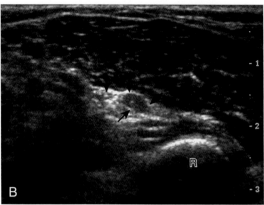

■ **FIGURE 4.67 Posterior Interosseous Nerve Syndrome.** Ultrasound images in (A) long axis and (B) short axis to the deep branch of the radial nerve *(arrowheads)* show hypoechoic enlargement *(arrows)* as the deep branch of the radial nerve enters between the two heads of the supinator muscle *(S)*. Note the normal superficial branch of the radial nerve *(curved arrow). C,* Capitellum; *R,* radial head.

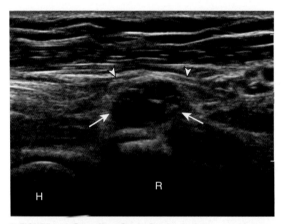

■ **FIGURE 4.68 Ganglion Cyst.** Sagittal ultrasound image of the anterolateral elbow shows a hypoechoic and multilobular ganglion cyst *(arrows)* and radial nerve superficial branch compression *(arrowheads). H,* Humerus; *R,* radial head.

■ EPITROCHLEAR LYMPH NODE

Most solid masses around the elbow that are not related to the joint are not specific for a single diagnosis; however, one must be aware of an enlarged epitrochlear lymph node, which, if correctly identified, can suggest a specific diagnosis. An epitrochlear lymph node is located at the medial aspect of the elbow just proximal to the medial epicondyle of the distal humerus between muscle and the subcutaneous tissues. A normal lymph node is oval, with an echogenic central hilum and a hypoechoic rim. The echogenic center results from interfaces between the fatty tissue and sinusoids, rather than from the fat itself, because pure fat is hypoechoic or

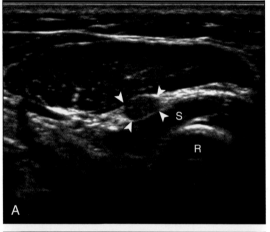

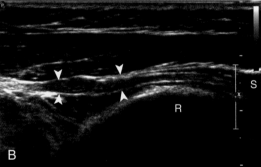

■ **FIGURE 4.69 Neurofibroma.** Ultrasound images in (A) short axis and (B) long axis to the deep branch of the radial nerve *(arrowheads)* show diffuse involvement and enlargement. *R,* Radius; *S,* supinator.

anechoic at ultrasound. When a lymph node is enlarged but maintains an oval shape, normal echogenic hilum, and hilar vascular pattern, then hyperplasia from inflammation is suggested. One such example is *cat-scratch disease* (Fig. 4.70), in

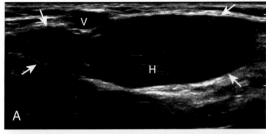

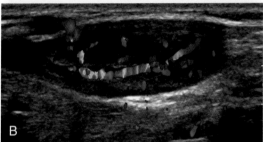

■ FIGURE 4.70 **Epitrochlear Lymph Node: Cat-Scratch Disease.** Ultrasound image over the distal medial humeral metaphysis shows hypoechoic enlargement of the epitrochlear lymph node *(arrows)* with narrowing of the echogenic hilum *(H)*. Note the hilar pattern of vascularity. *V,* Vein.

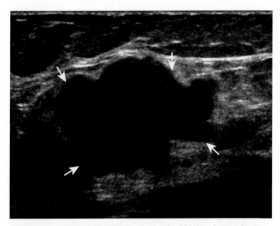

■ FIGURE 4.71 **Epitrochlear Lymph Node: Lymphoma.** Ultrasound image over medial elbow shows hypoechoic enlargement of an epitrochlear lymph node *(arrows)* with lobular margins and absence of the echogenic hilum.

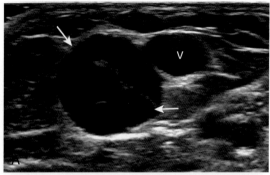

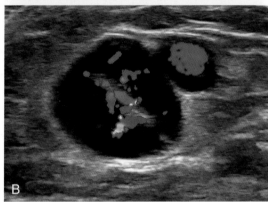

■ FIGURE 4.72 **Epitrochlear Lymph Node: Leukemia.** Ultrasound image over medial elbow shows hypoechoic enlargement of an epitrochlear lymph node *(arrows)* with lobular margins. Note narrowed echogenic hilum and hilar vascular pattern. *V,* Vein.

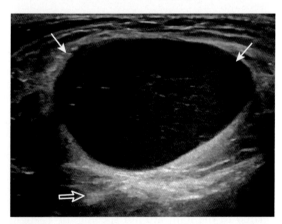

■ FIGURE 4.73 **Epitrochlear Lymph Node: Sarcoidosis.** Ultrasound image over the distal medial humeral metaphysis shows hypoechoic enlargement of an epitrochlear lymph node *(arrows)* with nearly complete obliteration of the echogenic hilum and increased posterior through transmission *(open arrow)*. Minimal blood flow was present at color Doppler imaging.

which the scratch of an animal such as a cat around the hand characteristically produces epitrochlear lymph node enlargement.[65] Inflammation adjacent to the enlarged epitrochlear lymph node can create a heterogeneous appearance to the soft tissues, which can make identification of the involved lymph node difficult. If an enlarged lymph node is round with absence of the echogenic hilum, thickening of the hypoechoic cortex, and a peripheral or mixed pattern of vascularity on color and power Doppler imaging, then malignancy is suspected, although biopsy is required to provide a diagnosis. Other examples of epitrochlear lymph node enlargement include lymphoma (Fig. 4.71), leukemia (Fig. 4.72), metastasis, and sarcoidosis (Fig. 4.73).

SELECT REFERENCES

6. Tagliafico A, Michaud J, Capaccio E, et al: Ultrasound demonstration of distal biceps tendon bifurcation: normal and abnormal findings. *Eur Radiol* 20(1):202–208, 2010.

9. Tagliafico AS, Bignotti B, Martinoli C, et al: Anatomy, variants, and scanning technique. *Radiology* 275(3):636–650, 2015.

21. Husarik DB, Saupe N, Pfirrmann CW, et al: Elbow nerves: MR findings in 60 asymptomatic subjects—normal anatomy, variants, and pitfalls. *Radiology* 252(1):148–156, 2009.

22. Jacobson JA, Jebson PJ, Jeffers AW, et al: Ulnar nerve dislocation and snapping triceps syndrome: diagnosis with dynamic sonography—report of three cases. *Radiology* 220(3):601–605, 2001.

24. Jacobson JA, Chiavaras MM, Lawton JM, et al: Radial collateral ligament of the elbow: sonographic characterization with cadaveric dissection correlation and magnetic resonance arthrography. *J Ultrasound Med* 33(6):1041–1048, 2014.

32. Chew ML, Giuffre BM: Disorders of the distal biceps brachii tendon. *Radiographics* 25(5):1227–1237, 2005.

40. Downey R, Jacobson JA, Fessell DP, et al: Sonography of partial-thickness tears of the distal triceps brachii tendon. *J Ultrasound Med* 30(10):1351–1356, 2011.

41. Jacobson JA, Miller BS, Morag Y: Golf and racquet sports injuries. *Semin Musculoskelet Radiol* 9(4):346–359, 2005.

43. Walz DM, Newman JS, Konin GP, et al: Epicondylitis: pathogenesis, imaging, and treatment. *Radiographics* 30(1):167–184, 2010.

52. Roedl JB, Gonzalez FM, Zoga AC, et al: Potential utility of a combined approach with US and MR arthrography to image medial elbow pain in baseball players. *Radiology* 279(3):827–837, 2016.

53. Jacobson JA, Fessell DP, Lobo Lda G, et al: Entrapment neuropathies I: upper limb (carpal tunnel excluded). *Semin Musculoskelet Radiol* 14(5):473–486, 2010.

The complete references for this chapter can be found on *www.expertconsult.com.*

WRIST AND HAND ULTRASOUND

■ WRIST AND HAND ANATOMY

The wrist consists of several synovial articulations among the distal radius, the distal ulna, the proximal carpal row (scaphoid, lunate, triquetrum, pisiform), and the distal carpal row (trapezium, trapezoid, capitate, and hamate). The radiocarpal joint between the distal radius and the proximal carpal row and the distal radioulnar joint between the radius and the ulna are separated by fibrocartilage, called the *triangular fibrocartilage*, which extends from the ulnar aspect of the distal radius to the base of the ulnar styloid. The midcarpal

joint is located between the carpal bones and is separated from the radiocarpal joint by two interosseous ligaments, the scapholunate and lunotriquetral ligaments. The scapholunate ligament is "U" shaped in the sagittal plane, with the open end of the U distal, and it consists of a volar portion, a thin proximal or central portion, and a thick and mechanically important dorsal portion.[1] Additional dorsal and palmar wrist ligaments are also present, named for their osseous attachments, categorized as intrinsic (intercarpal) or extrinsic (radiocarpal or ulnocarpal).[2-4]

Structures enter the wrist through several fibro-osseous tunnels. In the volar wrist, the carpal tunnel contains the median nerve and the flexor digitorum profundus, flexor digitorum superficialis, and flexor pollicis longus tendons (Fig. 5.1A–E). The fibrous flexor retinaculum extends from the pisiform and hamate to the scaphoid and trapezium, to form the roof of the carpal tunnel. The Guyon or ulnar canal is also volar adjacent to the pisiform, which contains the ulnar nerve and ulnar artery and veins. Other tendons, the flexor carpi radialis and the palmaris longus tendons, are located outside the carpal tunnel, although the flexor carpi radialis is within its own fibro-osseous canal and distally is associated with the trapezium.

The tendons of the dorsal wrist are also separated into six fibro-osseous compartments (see Fig. 5.1C). From radial to ulnar, they include the (1) abductor pollicis longus and extensor pollicis brevis, (2) extensor carpi radialis longus and brevis, (3) extensor pollicis longus, (4) extensor digitorum and extensor indicis, (5) extensor digiti minimi, and (6) extensor carpi ulnaris. A helpful bone landmark for orientation is the dorsal tubercle of the radius or Lister tubercle, which is located between the extensor carpi radialis tendons in the second compartment and the extensor pollicis longus tendon in the third compartment. The extensor carpi ulnaris is also found within a characteristic groove in the ulna.

The anatomy of the volar aspect of the fingers includes the flexor digitorum superficialis and profundus tendons. Each flexor superficialis tendon splits at the proximal interphalangeal joint, with each limb coursing to each side of the flexor digitorum profundus tendon to insert on the middle phalanx (see Fig. 5.1F–H). The flexor digitorum profundus terminates at the distal phalanx. The flexor tendons are tethered or secured to the adjacent phalanges through a series of fibrous pulleys to prevent bowstringing of the tendons with flexion (see Fig. 5.1F). The annular pulleys consist of the A1 pulley located at the metacarpophalangeal joint, the longer A2 pulley at the level of the proximal phalanx, the A3 pulley at the proximal interphalangeal joint, the A4 pulley at the level of the middle phalanx, and the A5 pulley at the distal interphalangeal joint.[5] Smaller cruciform pulleys are located between these pulleys

along the course of the flexor tendons. At the volar aspect of each metacarpophalangeal and interphalangeal joint is a fibrous structure called the *volar* or *palmar plate*. The metacarpophalangeal joints are stabilized by proper and accessory radial and ulnar collateral ligaments, with the latter extending to the volar plate.[6] The interphalangeal joints are also stabilized by radial and ulnar collateral ligaments. The soft tissue distally at the volar aspect of distal phalanx is called the *pulp*.

At the dorsal aspect of each finger, the extensor digitorum tendon attaches to the middle phalanx as a central band, whereas slips of the extensor tendon that contribute to the lateral bands attach

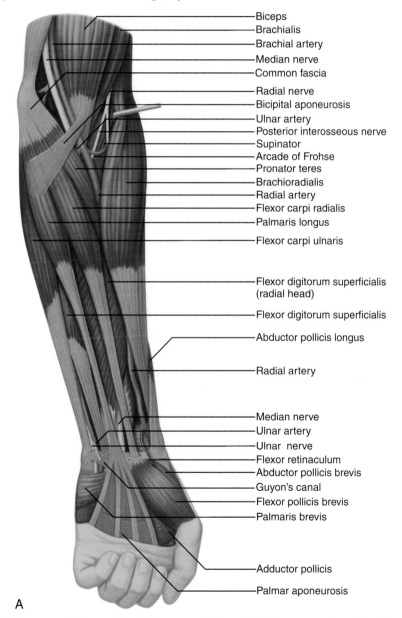

A

■ **FIGURE 5.1 Forearm, Wrist, and Hand Anatomy.** A, Superficial flexor muscles of the left forearm.

Continued

to the distal phalanx. The metacarpophalangeal joints have an overlying aponeurotic sheet or extensor hood, which consists of transverse-oriented sagittal bands that stabilize the extensor tendons.[7] The metacarpophalangeal and inter-phalangeal joints are synovial articulations with prominent dorsal joint recesses.[8]

■ ULTRASOUND EXAMINATION TECHNIQUE

Tables 5.1 and 5.2 are ultrasound examination checklists. Examples of diagnostic wrist and hand ultrasound reports are shown in Box 5.1 and Box 5.2.

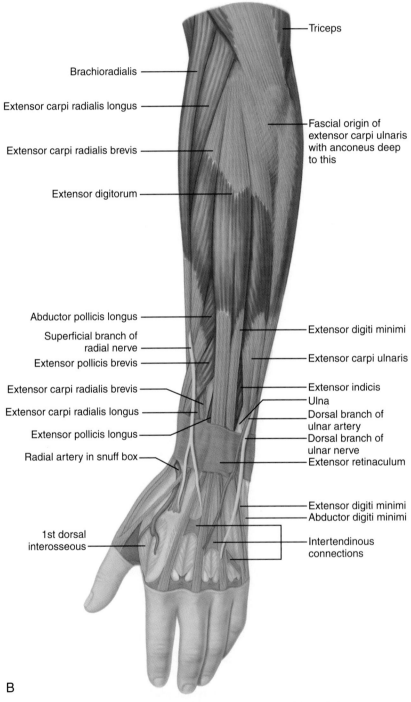

Triceps

Brachioradialis

Extensor carpi radialis longus

Extensor carpi radialis brevis

Extensor digitorum

Fascial origin of extensor carpi ulnaris with anconeus deep to this

Abductor pollicis longus

Superficial branch of radial nerve

Extensor pollicis brevis

Extensor carpi radialis brevis

Extensor carpi radialis longus

Extensor pollicis longus

Radial artery in snuff box

Extensor digiti minimi

Extensor carpi ulnaris

Extensor indicis

Ulna

Dorsal branch of ulnar artery

Dorsal branch of ulnar nerve

Extensor retinaculum

Extensor digiti minimi

Abductor digiti minimi

1st dorsal interosseous

Intertendinous connections

B

■ **FIGURE 5.1 , cont'd** B, Superficial extensor muscles of the left forearm.

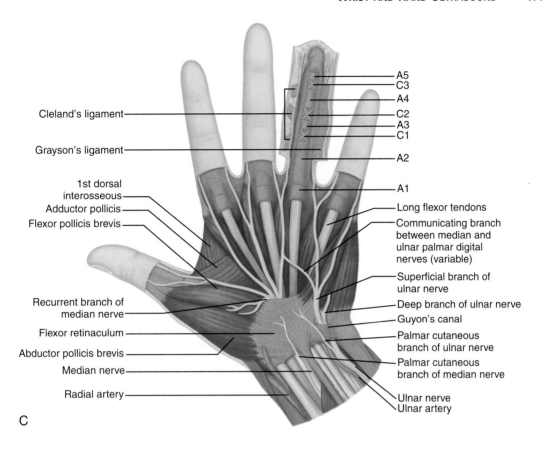

C, Palmar aspect of hand including annular *(A)* and cruciate *(C)* pulleys of the digit.

Labels: A5, C3, A4, C2, A3, C1, A2, A1

Cleland's ligament
Grayson's ligament
1st dorsal interosseous
Adductor pollicis
Flexor pollicis brevis
Recurrent branch of median nerve
Flexor retinaculum
Abductor pollicis brevis
Median nerve
Radial artery

Long flexor tendons
Communicating branch between median and ulnar palmar digital nerves (variable)
Superficial branch of ulnar nerve
Deep branch of ulnar nerve
Guyon's canal
Palmar cutaneous branch of ulnar nerve
Palmar cutaneous branch of median nerve
Ulnar nerve
Ulnar artery

C

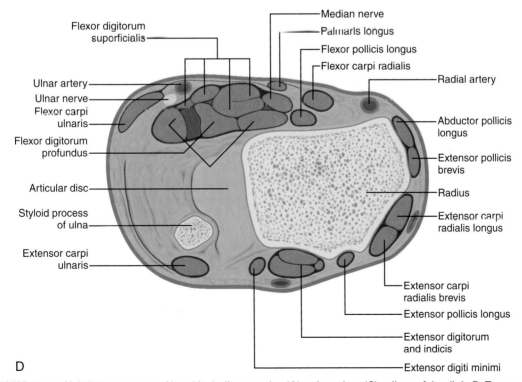

D, Transverse section through the distal left forearm at the level of the ulnar styloid.

Flexor digitorum superficialis
Ulnar artery
Ulnar nerve
Flexor carpi ulnaris
Flexor digitorum profundus
Articular disc
Styloid process of ulna
Extensor carpi ulnaris

Median nerve
Palmaris longus
Flexor pollicis longus
Flexor carpi radialis
Radial artery
Abductor pollicis longus
Extensor pollicis brevis
Radius
Extensor carpi radialis longus
Extensor carpi radialis brevis
Extensor pollicis longus
Extensor digitorum and indicis
Extensor digiti minimi

D

■ **FIGURE 5.1, cont'd** C, Palmar aspect of hand including annular *(A)* and cruciate *(C)* pulleys of the digit. D, Transverse section through the distal left forearm at the level of the ulnar styloid.

Continued

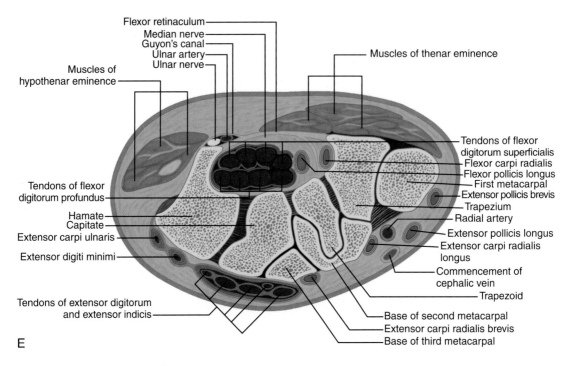

Flexor retinaculum
Median nerve
Guyon's canal
Ulnar artery
Ulnar nerve

Muscles of thenar eminence

Muscles of
hypothenar eminence

Tendons of flexor
digitorum profundus

Hamate
Capitate
Extensor carpi ulnaris

Extensor digiti minimi

Tendons of extensor digitorum
and extensor indicis

Tendons of flexor
digitorum superficialis
Flexor carpi radialis
Flexor pollicis longus
First metacarpal
Extensor pollicis brevis
Trapezium
Radial artery
Extensor pollicis longus
Extensor carpi radialis
longus
Commencement of
cephalic vein
Trapezoid
Base of second metacarpal
Extensor carpi radialis brevis
Base of third metacarpal

E

■ FIGURE 5.1, cont'd E, Transverse section through the left wrist at the level of the hamate bone. F, Palmar and lateral views showing the annular *(A)* and cruciform *(C)* pulleys of the flexor tendon sheath.

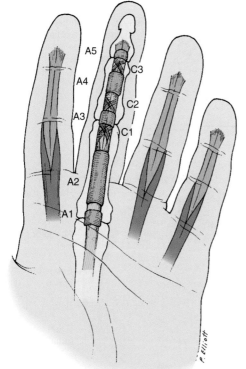

A5
A4
A3
A2
A1
C3
C2
C1

P. Elliott

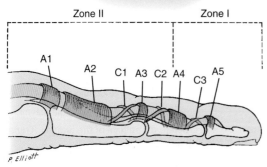

Zone II   Zone I

A1   A2   C1   A3   C2   A4   C3   A5

P. Elliott

F

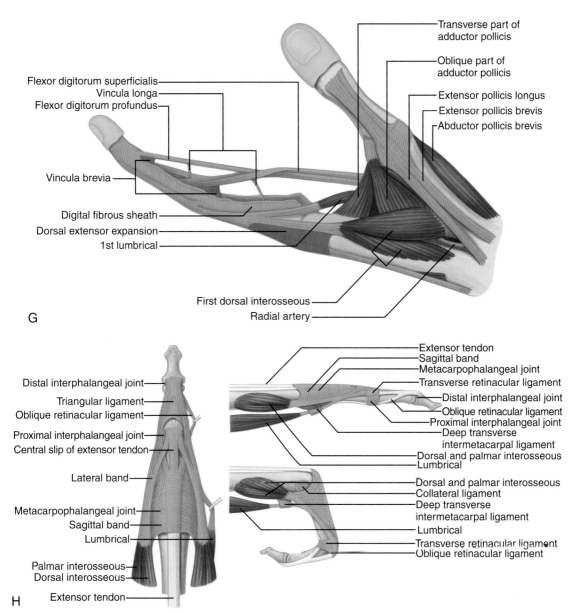

Transverse part of adductor pollicis

Oblique part of adductor pollicis

Extensor pollicis longus
Extensor pollicis brevis
Abductor pollicis brevis

Flexor digitorum superficialis
Vincula longa
Flexor digitorum profundus

Vincula brevia

Digital fibrous sheath
Dorsal extensor expansion
1st lumbrical

First dorsal interosseous
Radial artery

G

Extensor tendon
Sagittal band
Metacarpophalangeal joint
Transverse retinacular ligament
Distal interphalangeal joint
Oblique retinacular ligament
Proximal interphalangeal joint
Deep transverse intermetacarpal ligament
Dorsal and palmar interosseous
Lumbrical

Distal interphalangeal joint
Triangular ligament
Oblique retinacular ligament

Proximal interphalangeal joint
Central slip of extensor tendon

Lateral band

Dorsal and palmar interosseous
Collateral ligament
Deep transverse intermetacarpal ligament
Lumbrical
Transverse retinacular ligament
Oblique retinacular ligament

Metacarpophalangeal joint
Sagittal band
Lumbrical

Palmar interosseous
Dorsal interosseous

H   Extensor tendon

■ FIGURE 5.1, cont'd G, Lateral view of the hand showing the flexor tendons of the finger. H, Dorsal view, lateral view, and lateral view in flexion show the extensor mechanism of the finger. *(From Standring S:* Gray's anatomy: the anatomical basis of clinical practice, *ed 39, Edinburgh, 2005, Churchill Livingstone.)*

General Comments

Ultrasound examination of the wrist and hand is typically completed with the patient sitting and the hand resting on the examination table. This position allows easy comparison between each side if needed. A high-frequency transducer of at least 10 MHz is typically used because most of the structures are superficial, and a transducer with a small footprint is often helpful to maintain contact with the soft tissues under examination. I favor thick transmission gel over a stand-off pad. Evaluation of the wrist and hand may be focused over the area that is clinically symptomatic or relevant to the patient's history. Regardless, a complete examination of all areas should always be considered for one to become familiar with normal anatomy and normal variants and to develop an efficient and comprehensive sonographic technique.

Wrist: Volar Evaluation

MEDIAN NERVE, FLEXOR DIGITORUM TENDONS, AND VOLAR JOINT RECESSES

The primary structures evaluated from the volar aspect at midline are the median nerve, the flexor

TABLE 5.1 Wrist and Hand Ultrasound Examination Checklist

Location	Structures of Interest/ Pathologic Features
Volar (1)	Median nerve
	Flexor tendons
	Volar joint recesses
Volar (2)	Scaphoid
	Flexor carpi radialis
	Radial artery
	Volar ganglion cyst
Volar (3)	Ulnar nerve and artery
Dorsal (1)	Extensor tendons
	Dorsal joint recesses
Dorsal (2)	Scapholunate ligament
	Dorsal ganglion cyst
Dorsal (3)	Triangular fibrocartilage complex

TABLE 5.2 Finger Ultrasound Examination Checklist

Location	Structures of Interest
Volar	Flexor tendons
	Pulleys
	Volar plate
	Joint recesses
Dorsal	Extensor tendon
	Joint recesses
Other	Collateral ligaments

BOX 5.1 Sample Diagnostic Wrist Ultrasound Report: Normal, Complete

Examination: Ultrasound of the Wrist
  Date of Study: March 11, 2011
  Patient Name: Derrick May
  Registration Number: 8675309
  History: Numbness, evaluate for carpal tunnel syndrome
  Findings: The median nerve is unremarkable in appearance, measuring 8 mm^2 at the wrist crease and 7 mm^2 at the pronator quadratus. No evidence of tenosynovitis. The radiocarpal, midcarpal, and distal radioulnar joints are normal without effusion or synovial hypertrophy. The wrist tendons are normal without tear or tenosynovitis. Normal dorsal component of the scapholunate ligament. No dorsal or volar ganglion cyst. Unremarkable Guyon canal. Additional focused evaluation at site of maximal symptoms was unrevealing.
  Impression: Unremarkable ultrasound examination of the wrist.

BOX 5.2 Sample Diagnostic Wrist Ultrasound Report: Abnormal, Complete

Examination: Ultrasound of the Wrist
  Date of Study: March 11, 2011
  Patient Name: Jacobim Mugatu
  Registration Number: 8675309
  History: Numbness, evaluate for carpal tunnel syndrome
  Findings: The median nerve is hypoechoic and enlarged, measuring 15 mm^2 at the wrist crease and 7 mm^2 at the pronator quadratus. No evidence for tenosynovitis. The radiocarpal, midcarpal, and distal radioulnar joints are normal without effusion or synovial hypertrophy. The wrist tendons are normal without tear or tenosynovitis. Normal dorsal component of the scapholunate ligament. No dorsal ganglion cyst. A 7-mm volar ganglion cyst is noted between the radial artery and flexor carpi radialis tendon. Unremarkable Guyon canal. Additional focused evaluation at site of maximal symptoms was unrevealing.
  Impression:
1. Ultrasound findings compatible with carpal tunnel syndrome.
2. A 7-mm volar ganglion cyst.

tendons, and the volar aspects of the wrist joints. Examination begins short axis to the tendons and median nerve in the center of the wrist. For evaluation of the median nerve, the transducer is placed in the transverse plane at the level of the wrist crease, which is at the proximal aspect of the carpal tunnel (Fig. 5.2). Normal peripheral nerves have a honeycomb appearance when they are imaged in short axis from hypoechoic nerve fascicles and surrounding hyperechoic connective tissue (Fig. 5.2B).[4] Toggling the transducer to angle the sound beam along the long axis of the median nerve will help to show the characteristic appearance of the nerve when the sound beam is perpendicular (Video 5.1). Because peripheral nerve trunks are composed of both hypoechoic and hyperechoic elements, the median nerve appears relatively hypoechoic when surrounded by hyperechoic tissue in the carpal tunnel and relatively hyperechoic when surrounded by hypoechoic muscle in the forearm. At the wrist crease, the median nerve is identified by its hypoechoic nerve fascicles, which are most conspicuous surrounded by the adjacent hyperechoic tendons. If differentiation between the median nerve and adjacent tendons is difficult, median nerve identification is easily accomplished with movement of the transducer proximally in the transverse plane. During this maneuver, the normal median nerve courses radial to the flexor

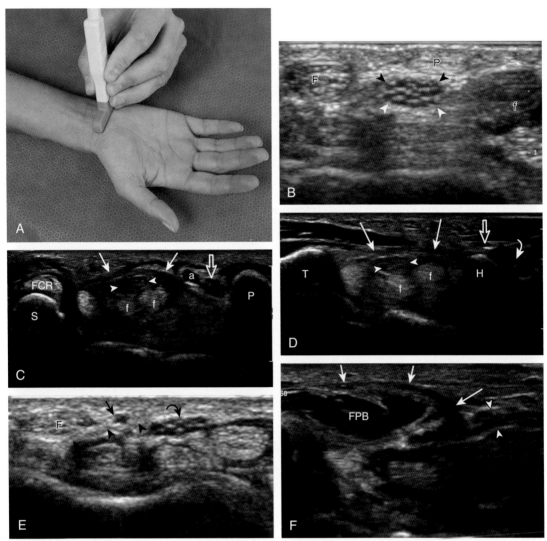

■ **FIGURE 5.2 Carpal Tunnel and Volar Wrist Evaluation (Transverse).** A, Transverse imaging over the volar wrist crease shows (B) the median nerve *(arrowheads)*, flexor carpi radialis *(F)*, palmaris longus *(P)*, flexor digitorum tendons *(f)*. Transverse imaging (C) at proximal carpal tunnel shows flexor retinaculum *(arrows)* and bone landmarks of scaphoid *(S)* and pisiform *(P)*. Transverse imaging at distal carpal tunnel shows flexor retinaculum *(arrows)* and bone landmarks of trapezium *(T)* and hamate hook *(H)*. Note in (C and D) median nerve *(arrowheads)*, flexor tendons *(f)*, flexor carpi radialis *(FCR)*, and ulnar artery *(a)*. Also note ulnar nerve *(open arrow)* in (C) and distal (D) superficial branch *(open arrow)* and deep branch *(curved arrow)*. Transverse imaging proximal at wrist crease (E) shows the palmar cutaneous branch *(arrow)* of the median nerve *(curved arrow)* superficial to the flexor retinaculum *(arrowheads)*. Sagittal-oblique imaging a distal carpal tunnel (F) shows thenar motor branch *(arrows)* of median nerve *(arrowheads)* coursing proximal into thenar musculature. *FPB*, Flexor pollicis brevis.

tendons and then moves ulnar and deep between the flexor digitorum superficialis and profundus (Fig. 5.3) (Video 5.2).[9] In addition, the median nerve now appears relatively hyperechoic as a result of the connective tissue and fat because it is surrounded by hypoechoic muscle. The characteristic course, location, and echogenicity assist in identification of the median nerve. An additional method to differentiate the median nerve from the adjacent flexor tendons at the wrist crease in the transverse plane is angulation of or toggling

the transducer along the long axis of the tendons. This maneuver causes the hyperechoic tendons to become hypoechoic as a result of anisotropy, whereas the hypoechoic median nerve fascicles remain unchanged (Video 5.1). Evaluation of the median nerve is then continued distally into the carpal tunnel, where the thin and hyperechoic flexor retinaculum can be visualized, which attaches to the pisiform and trapezium proximally (Fig. 5.2C) and the hamate and scaphoid distally (Fig. 5.2D). A small branch of the median nerve,

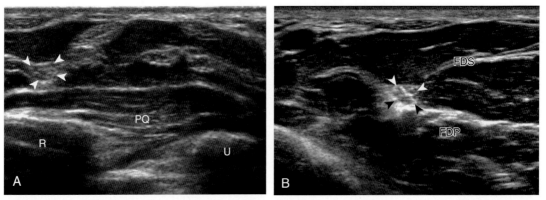

■ **FIGURE 5.3 Volar Forearm Evaluation (Distal, Transverse).** Sequential transverse ultrasound images (A and B) moving proximal to the volar wrist crease show that the median nerve *(arrowheads)* moves deep between the flexor digitorum profundus *(FDP)* and flexor digitorum superficialis *(FDS)*. *PQ,* Pronator quadratus; *R,* radius, *U,* ulna.

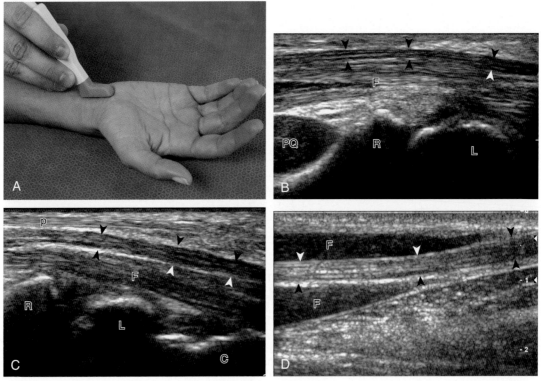

■ **FIGURE 5.4 Carpal Tunnel and Volar Wrist Evaluation (Longitudinal).** A, Sagittal imaging over the volar wrist crease shows (B to D) the median nerve *(arrowheads)*, flexor digitorum *(F)*, palmaris longus *(p)*, pronator quadratus *(PQ)*, radius *(R)*, lunate *(L)*, and capitate *(C)*. Note the median nerve proximal to the wrist crease in D, which appears relatively hyperechoic proximally and hypoechoic distally (left side of image is proximal).

the palmar cutaneous branch, originates proximal to the carpal tunnel and courses superficial to the flexor retinaculum and ulnar to the flexor carpi radialis tendon (Fig. 5.2E).[10] The thenar motor branch can also be visualized at the carpal tunnel outlet originating from the palmar ulnar aspect of the radial division of the median nerve, coursing vertically in a palmar direction and extending proximal between the abductor pollicis brevis and

flexor pollicis brevis (Fig. 5.2F).[11] The transducer is turned 90 degrees to visualize the median nerve in long axis (Fig. 5.4) (Video 5.3). The variable appearance of peripheral nerve echogenicity relative to the surrounding tissue echogenicity is well demonstrated when imaging the median nerve in long axis in the distal forearm (Fig. 5.4D). Proximal to the wrist joint in the transverse plane, the pronator quadratus can be identified extending between the distal radius and ulna, a soft tissue landmark that is used for proximal measurement of the median nerve (Fig. 5.3A).

Attention is then turned back to the flexor tendons, with each tendon evaluated in both short axis and long axis. The flexor digitorum superficialis and profundus are identified about the median nerve as described earlier, proximally as hypoechoic muscle and distally as fibrillar and hyperechoic tendons (see Figs. 5.2 and 5.3). Just beyond the wrist crease, the thin hyperechoic flexor retinaculum is seen as it extends from the proximal scaphoid pole to the pisiform and from the trapezium to the hook of the hamate, which represents the roof the carpal tunnel (see Fig. 5.2D). If the retinaculum is not imaged perpendicular to the ultrasound beam, it will appear hypoechoic as a result of anisotropy. The flexor digitorum tendons travel through the carpal tunnel to the digits, whereas the palmaris longus tendon, typically directly superficial to the median nerve, remains outside of the carpal tunnel. In the sagittal plane and long axis to the flexor tendons, the volar radiocarpal and midcarpal joint recesses are identified by the adjacent bone contours; the volar lip of the distal radius, the lunate bone, and the capitate bone have characteristic shapes (see Fig. 5.4B and C). Between the distal radius and the lunate is the volar recess of the radiocarpal joint,

and between the lunate and capitate bones is the volar recess of the midcarpal joint. The distal radioulnar joint is identified with placement of the transducer in the transverse plane between the distal radius and ulna.

SCAPHOID, FLEXOR CARPI RADIALIS TENDON, RADIAL ARTERY, AND VOLAR GANGLION CYSTS

Evaluation of the radial aspect of the volar wrist begins in the transverse plane at the wrist crease. In this position, the various tendons of the volar wrist are identified. Just radial to the median nerve and somewhat similar in size is the flexor carpi radialis tendon, located outside the carpal tunnel in its own fibro-osseous canal (see Fig. 5.2B). Ultrasound evaluation is completed in both long and short axis from proximal to the distal insertion of the flexor carpi radialis tendon on the second and third metacarpals, although some fibers insert onto the trapezium tuberosity.[12] With placement of the transducer over the distal aspect of the flexor carpi radialis tendon in long axis (Fig. 5.5), the characteristic bilobed or peanut-shaped bone contours of the scaphoid bone are identified deep to this tendon (Fig. 5.5C). The normal smooth and hyperechoic bone surface of the scaphoid bone is evaluated for cortical step-off fracture. Returning to the wrist crease in the transverse

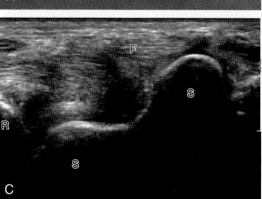
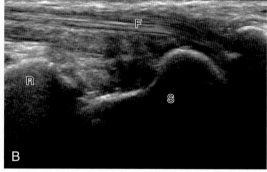
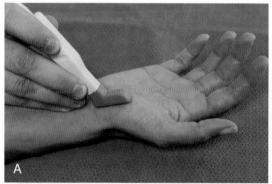

■ **FIGURE 5.5 Volar Radial Wrist Evaluation (Longitudinal).** A, Sagittal-oblique imaging over the thumb base shows (B and C) the flexor carpi radialis tendon *(F)* and scaphoid *(S)*. R, Radius.

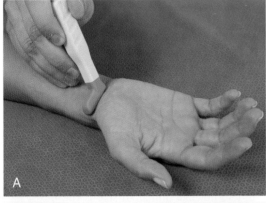

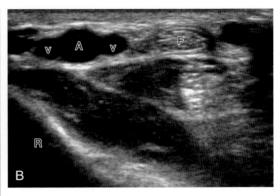

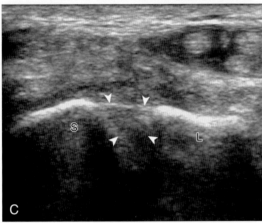

■ **FIGURE 5.6 Volar Radial Wrist Evaluation (Transverse).** A, Transverse imaging shows (B) the flexor carpi radialis tendon *(F)*, radial artery *(A)*, and veins *(v)*. Transverse imaging between scaphoid *(S)* and lunate *(L)* shows *(C)* volar portion of the scapholunate ligament *(arrowheads)*. R, Radius.

plane (Fig. 5.6A), the radial artery and veins are identified immediately radial to the flexor carpi radialis tendon (Fig. 5.6B). With the flexor carpi radialis tendon and radial artery in view, the transducer is moved both proximally and distally from the radiocarpal joint to evaluate for ganglion cysts. Placement of the transducer in the transverse plane between the scaphoid and lunate will show the normal hyperechoic and fibrillar volar component of the scapholunate ligament (Fig. 5.6C).

ULNAR ARTERY, VEIN, AND NERVE (GUYON CANAL)

Evaluation of the ulnar aspect of the volar wrist begins in the transverse plane at the wrist crease. Moving the transducer ulnar to the carpal tunnel (Fig. 5.7A), the bone landmark of the pisiform is identified (Fig. 5.7B). Between the pisiform and the ulnar artery, the ulnar nerve is identified as hypoechoic nerve fascicles and surrounding hyperechoic connective tissue. The ulnar veins are usually not visible because they are easily compressed by pressure of the ultrasound trans-

ducer. As the transducer is moved distally, the hyperechoic and shadowing surface of the hook of the hamate is seen deep to the ulnar nerve and artery. The ulnar nerve branches, with a deep motor branch coursing along the ulnar side of the hamate hook and one to two predominantly sensory branches superficial to the hamate hook (Fig. 5.7C). This area should be evaluated as trauma can cause ulnar nerve and artery abnormalities as a result of compression by the hook of the hamate. Proximal to the pisiform, the flexor carpi ulnaris is identified as well as the dorsal cutaneous branch of the ulnar nerve coursing from volar to dorsal beneath the flexor carpi ulnaris (Fig. 5.7D).[13] Evaluation of the ulnar artery and nerve is also completed in long axis (Fig. 5.8).

Wrist: Dorsal Evaluation

DORSAL WRIST TENDONS AND DORSAL JOINT RECESSES

The primary structures of the dorsal wrist are the various extensor and abductor tendons of the six wrist compartments, and the dorsal radiocarpal,

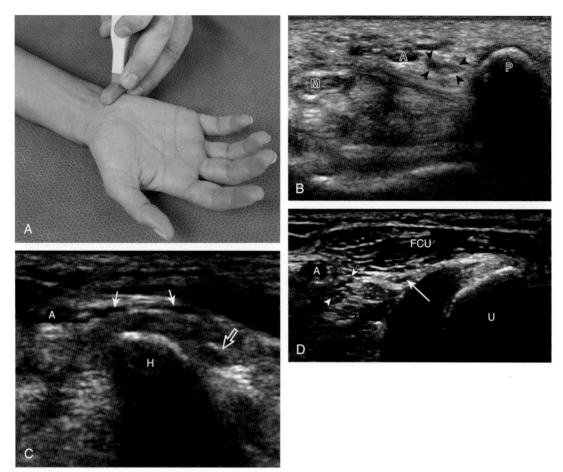

■ FIGURE 5.7 **Guyon Canal Evaluation (Transverse).** A, Transverse imaging over Guyon canal shows (B) the ulnar nerve *(arrowheads)* radial to the pisiform *(P)*. Imaging distal to B over the hook of the hamate *(H)* shows (C) the superficial *(arrows)* and deep *(open arrow)* branches of the ulnar nerve. *A*, Ulnar artery; *M*, median nerve. Imaging proximally at distal third of forearm shows (D) dorsal cutaneous branch of the ulnar nerve *(arrow)* deep to flexor carpi ulnaris *(FCU)* and adjacent ulnar nerve *(arrowheads)*. *U*, Ulna.

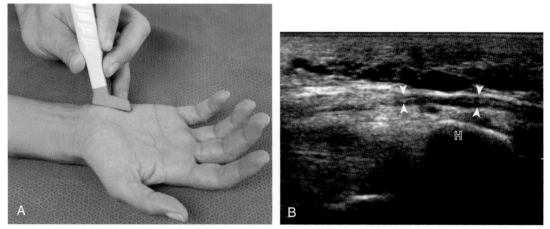

■ FIGURE 5.8 **Guyon Canal Evaluation (Longitudinal).** A, Sagittal imaging shows (B) the ulnar nerve *(arrowheads)* and hook of the hamate *(H)* (left side of image is proximal).

midcarpal, and distal radioulnar joint recesses. Evaluation of the dorsal tendons begins in the transverse plane over the Lister tubercle of the dorsal radius (Fig. 5.9A and B). This structure serves as an important starting point for dorsal wrist evaluation and assists in orientation and accurate identification of the wrist tendons. The Lister tubercle is seen as a pronounced bony prominence. Once the Lister tubercle is identified, the tendon immediately ulnar to it is the extensor pollicis longus of the third extensor compartment (Fig. 5.9B). Often there is an additional smaller dorsal radial protuberance at the ulnar aspect of the extensor pollicis longus as well. With movement of the transducer in the radial direction (Fig. 5.9C), the extensor carpi radialis brevis and then the extensor carpi radialis longus tendons are seen in the second extensor compartment (Fig. 5.9D). On further radial movement of the transducer, the extensor pollicis brevis and abductor pollicis longus tendons are seen in the first extensor compartment (Fig. 5.9D). It may be helpful to remember that the names of the tendons alternate from longus to brevis, beginning at the extensor pollicis longus and moving in a radial direction. The extensor pollicis longus tendon courses toward the thumb superficial to the extensor carpi radialis and ulnaris tendons in an oblique fashion proximally to distally. Therefore when short axis to the extensor carpi radialis brevis and longus tendons are moving distally, the extensor pollicis longus is seen moving in an ulnar to radial direction over the extensor carpi radialis brevis and longus tendons, a potential site of intersection syndrome (Fig. 5.9E) (Video 5.4). In the region of the first extensor wrist compartment, the superficial branch of the radial nerve can be seen as it courses from the volar to the dorsal aspect of the distal forearm superficial to the first extensor wrist compartment tendons and extensor retinaculum, near branches of the cephalic vein (Fig. 5.9F).

Beginning again in the transverse plane at the Lister tubercle, transducer movement ulnar from the extensor pollicis longus tendon (Fig. 5.10A) shows the extensor indicis and multiple tendons of the extensor digitorum in the fourth wrist compartment, and the extensor digiti minimi in the fifth wrist compartment near the distal radioulnar joint (Fig. 5.10B). The posterior interosseous nerve is identified deep within the radial aspect of the fourth dorsal extensor compartment (Fig. 5.9B).[14] Over the most ulnar aspect of the ulna, the extensor carpi ulnaris tendon is identified in a concave groove of the ulna in the sixth extensor compartment (Fig. 5.10C). The extensor carpi ulnaris tendon often has a normal thin hypoechoic longitudinal cleft that should not

be interpreted as a tendon tear.[15,16] The dorsal retinaculum and the deeper subsheath stabilize the extensor carpi ulnaris, with the latter attaching to the ulna.[17] Up to 50% of the extensor carpi ulnar tendon can be located outside of the groove and still be considered normal.[18]

Each of the extensor tendons is also imaged in long axis throughout the wrist (Fig. 5.11). The extensor retinaculum courses transversely but slightly oblique over the extensor tendons and appears hyperechoic, measuring up to 1.7 mm thick and 23 mm wide in cross section (Fig. 5.11B).[19] If imaged oblique to the ultrasound beam, the extensor retinaculum can appear artifactually hypoechoic as a result of anisotropy, which should not be misinterpreted as tenosynovitis.[16] Similar to the volar wrist, the dorsal recesses of the radiocarpal joint (between the radius and proximal carpal row), the midcarpal joint, and the distal radioulnar joint are identified with recognition of the characteristic bone contours for orientation. The radiocarpal and midcarpal joint recesses are optimally evaluated in the sagittal plane, whereas the distal radioulnar joint is evaluated in the transverse plane (Fig. 5.10B).

SCAPHOLUNATE LIGAMENT (DORSAL COMPONENT) AND DORSAL GANGLION CYSTS

Similar to the dorsal tendons, evaluation of the scapholunate ligament begins in the transverse plane over the Lister tubercle (Fig. 5.9A). As the transducer is then moved distally, the bone contours of the radius are interrupted by the radiocarpal joint, and the next osseous structure visualized is the scaphoid. With movement of the transducer in the ulnar direction, the adjacent lunate bone is brought into view. Between the dorsal aspects of the scaphoid and the lunate is a triangular area where one sees the dorsal aspect of the scapholunate ligament, which has a compact hyperechoic fibrillar echotexture (Fig. 5.12).[20] Directly superficial to the dorsal aspect of the scapholunate ligament, the dorsal radiocarpal ligament (or dorsal radiotriquetral ligament) is identified.[3,4] This area is a common site for dorsal wrist ganglion cysts.

TRIANGULAR FIBROCARTILAGE COMPLEX

The triangular fibrocartilage complex consists of the triangular fibrocartilage, the meniscus homologue, the extensor carpi ulnaris tendon sheath, and the volar and dorsal radiocarpal ligaments. For evaluation of the triangular fibrocartilage, the transducer is placed in the sagittal plane over the dorsal lateral wrist to identify the bone contours of the distal ulna and then moved toward

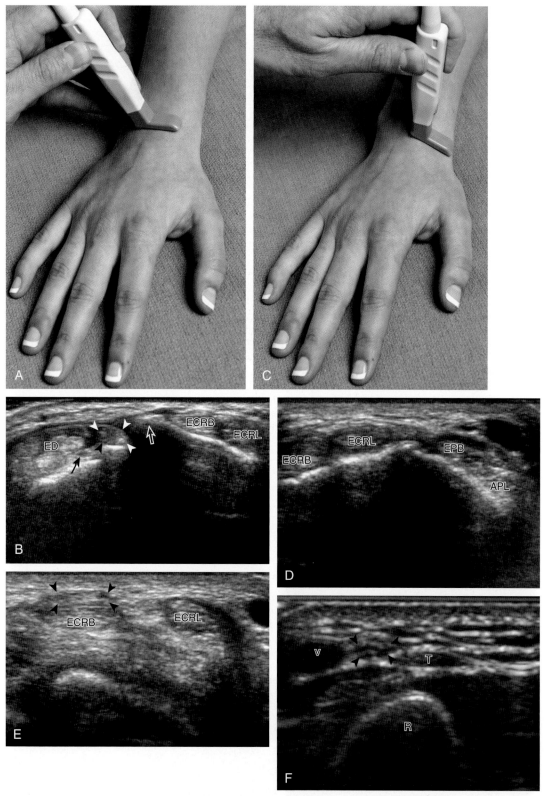

■ FIGURE 5.9 **Dorsal Wrist Evaluation (Extensor Compartments 1 to 3).** A, Transverse imaging over the Lister tubercle of the radius shows (B) the extensor pollicis longus tendon *(arrowheads)* ulnar to the Lister tubercle *(open arrow)*. Note posterior interosseous nerve *(arrow)* and extensor digitorum *(ED)* in the fourth extensor compartment. C, Transverse imaging radial to A shows (D) the second and first extensor compartments. Distal imaging over the second wrist compartment shows (E) the extensor pollicis longus *(arrowheads)* moving superficial to the extensor carpi radialis tendons. F, The superficial branch of the radial nerve *(arrowheads)* can be identified superficial to the first extensor wrist compartment (T) and near a branch of the cephalic vein *(v)*. *APL,* Abductor pollicis longus; *ECRB/L,* extensor carpi radialis brevis and longus; *EPB,* extensor pollicis brevis; *R,* radius.

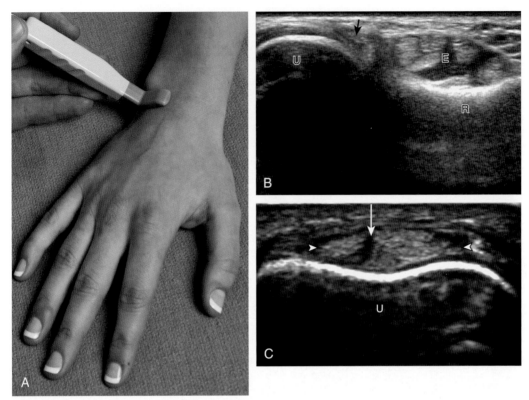

■ **FIGURE 5.10 Dorsal Wrist Evaluation (Extensor Compartments 4 to 6).** A, Transverse imaging ulnar to that shown in Fig. 5.9A shows (B) the extensor digitorum and extensor indicis *(E)*, the extensor digiti minimi *(arrow)*, and the distal radioulnar joint between the radius *(R)* and ulna *(U)*. Transverse imaging over the lateral ulna shows (C) the extensor carpi ulnaris *(arrowheads)*. Note normal hypoechoic cleft *(arrow)*.

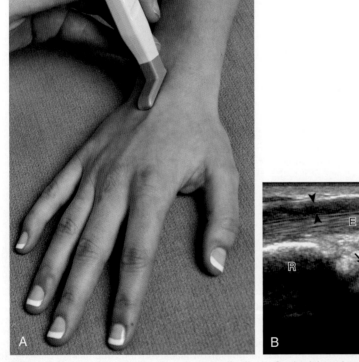

■ **FIGURE 5.11 Dorsal Wrist Evaluation (Longitudinal).** A, Sagittal imaging shows (B) the extensor retinaculum *(arrowheads)*, extensor tendons *(E)*, and dorsal recesses of radiocarpal *(arrows)* and midcarpal *(curved arrow)* joints. *C*, Capitate; *L*, lunate; *R*, radius.

the coronal plane with the wrist in slight radial deviation (Fig. 5.13A). A hyperechoic slab of tissue is identified as it extends from the ulnar styloid base to the radius, which represents the triangular fibrocartilage (Fig. 5.13B).[3] The radial attachment of the triangular fibrocartilage must be identified to ensure complete evaluation as this may be a site of traumatic tears. Evaluation of the triangular fibrocartilage can be difficult given its orientation

in the transverse plane extending away from the transducer, and often a lower frequency transducer is helpful. The meniscus homologue is seen as a hyperechoic triangular structure with its base adjacent to the extensor carpi ulnar tendon and in contact with the triquetrum, and this should not be mistaken for the triangular fibrocartilage, which is thinner, more proximal, and directly over the ulnar head.

Finger Evaluation

VOLAR

At the volar aspect of the finger in long axis (Fig. 5.14A), both the hyperechoic and fibrillar flexor digitorum superficialis and profundus tendons can be seen at the level of the metacarpophalangeal joint with the overlying A1 pulley (Fig. 5.14B).[5] The pulleys often have a trilaminar appearance at ultrasound, consisting of the superficial reflective surface of the pulley, the relatively hypoechoic pulley, and the deeper hyper-reflective surface of the adjacent flexor tendon sheath. With regard to imaging the flexor tendons in long axis, the individual tendons can be distinguished from each other with isolated passive movement of the distal phalanx because this will cause movement of the

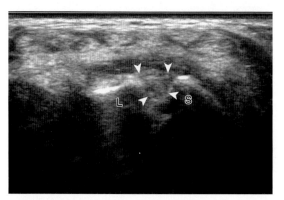

■ FIGURE 5.12 **Scapholunate Ligament Evaluation (Dorsal Component).** Transverse imaging over the proximal carpal row shows the dorsal aspect of the scapholunate ligament *(arrowheads)*. *L*, Lunate; *S*, scaphoid.

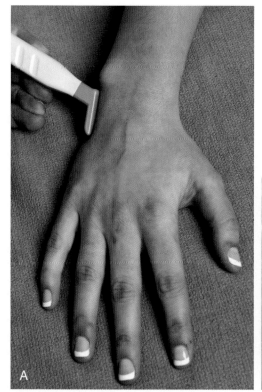

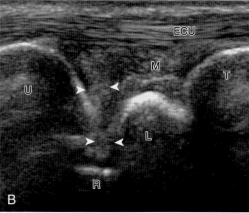

■ FIGURE 5.13 **Triangular Fibrocartilage Evaluation.** A, Coronal-oblique imaging dorsal to the ulnar styloid shows (B) the triangular fibrocartilage *(arrowheads)* and the meniscus homologue *(M)*. *ECU,* Extensor carpi ulnaris; *L,* lunate; *R,* radius; *T,* triquetrum; *U,* ulna. *(Courtesy Tracy Boon, Ann Arbor, Michigan.)*

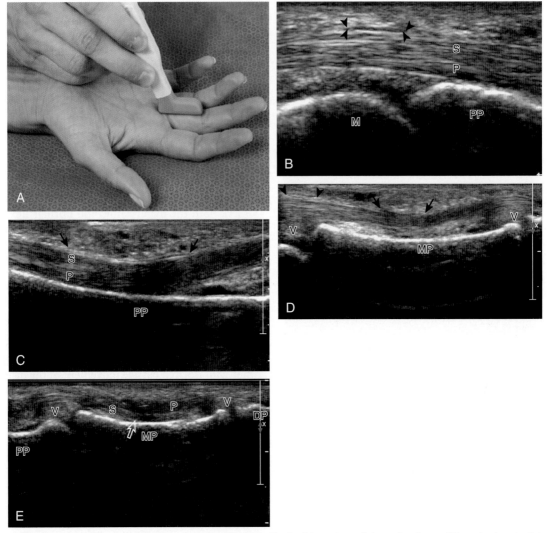

■ **FIGURE 5.14 Volar Finger Evaluation (Longitudinal).** A, Sagittal imaging of the volar finger (B) at the level of the metacarpophalangeal joint, (C) the proximal phalanx, and (D and E) the middle phalanx shows the flexor digitorum profundus *(P)* and superficialis *(S)* tendons and volar plates *(V)*. Note (B) the A1 pulley *(arrowheads)*, (C) A2 pulley *(arrows)*, (D) A3 pulley *(arrowheads)*, and A4 pulley *(arrows)*. The attachment of the flexor digitorum superficialis *(open arrow)* is seen in the parasagittal plane. *DP*, Distal phalanx; *M*, metacarpal; *MP*, middle phalanx; *PP*, proximal phalanx.

flexor digitorum profundus. At the level of the proximal phalanx, the A2 pulley can be identified; slight obliquity of the transducer may make the pulley appear hypoechoic from anisotropy and can aid in its identification (Fig. 5.14C). The A2 pulley normally is thicker distally, which assists in its identification. At the level of the proximal interphalangeal joint, the hyperechoic volar (or palmar) plate is identified (Fig. 5.14D and E). The A3 and A4 pulleys are also identified superficial to the flexor tendons, at the level of the proximal interphalangeal joint and middle phalanx, respectively (Fig. 5.14D).[5] Just distal to the proximal interphalangeal joint, the flexor digitorum superficialis inserts on the middle phalanx in the parasagittal plane, whereas the

flexor digitorum profundus extends distally over the volar plate of the distal interphalangeal joint in the sagittal plane to insert on the distal phalanx (Fig. 5.14E). The flexor digitorum superficialis inserts on the middle phalanx by dividing into two bundles, with each segment moving around the flexor digitorum profundus tendon. This is best appreciated by imaging in short axis (Fig. 5.15A and B). More proximally over the palm of the hand (Fig. 5.16), the lumbrical and interosseous muscles can be identified, as can the common and proper palmar digital arteries and nerves. The metacarpophalangeal and interphalangeal joints are also evaluated in the sagittal plane for volar plate abnormality and joint recess distention from fluid or synovial disorders.

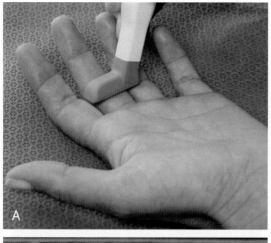

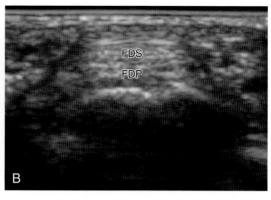

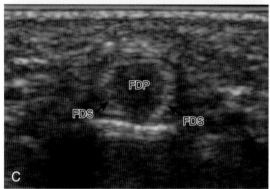

■ **FIGURE 5.15 Volar Finger Evaluation (Transverse).** A, Transverse imaging over the proximal phalanx (B) and middle phalanx (C) shows the flexor digitorum profundus *(FDP)* and superficialis *(FDS)* tendons. Note anisotropy of the FDP.

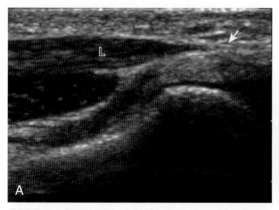

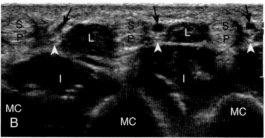

■ **FIGURE 5.16 Palmar Hand Evaluation.** Parasagittal imaging (A) shows the distal aspect *(arrow)* of a lumbrical muscle *(L)*. Transverse imaging (B) shows the flexor digitorum superficialis *(S)* and profundus *(P)* tendons, the common digital arteries *(arrows)* and nerves *(arrowheads)*, and interosseous muscles *(I)*. *MC*, Metacarpal.

DORSAL

At the dorsal aspect of each digit, the thin, hyperechoic, and fibrillar extensor digitorum tendon extends over the metacarpophalangeal joint in the sagittal plane (Fig. 5.17A and B). At the level of the proximal interphalangeal joint, the central band of the extensor tendon inserts on the middle phalanx (Fig. 5.17C and D). With movement of the transducer just off midline of the phalanx, the slips of the extensor tendon to the lateral bands can be seen (Fig. 5.17E), which insert distally on the distal phalanx (Fig. 5.17F). The ultrasound beam penetrates through the nail and allows visualization of the underlying hypoechoic nail bed, subungual space, and the surface of the distal phalanx (Fig. 5.17F). At the level of the metacarpophalangeal joint, the transducer is positioned short axis to the extensor tendon, and the finger is flexed to evaluate for subluxation of the tendon, which would indicate sagittal band injury. The joints of each digit are also evaluated for distention from fluid or synovial hypertrophy, where the dorsal joint recess extends proximally beneath the extensor tendon. In addition, the hypoechoic hyaline articular cartilage of each joint can be visualized, which is accessible with flexion of the digits (Fig. 5.17G–I). A triangular region of connective tissue is normally found superficial to the metacarpophalangeal joint articulation (Fig. 5.17H).[8] The dorsal

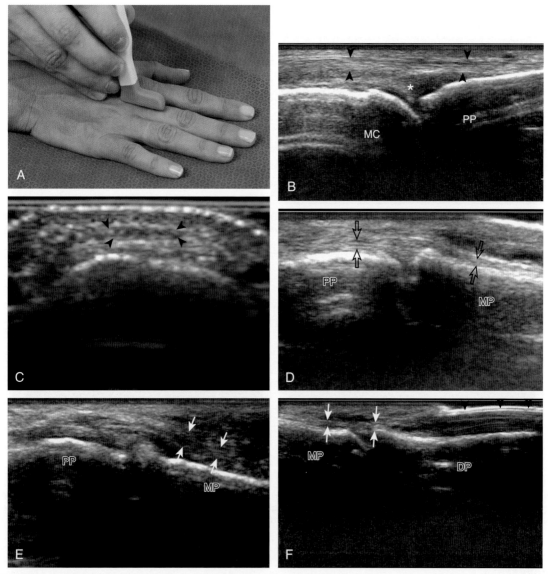

■ **FIGURE 5.17 Dorsal Finger Evaluation.** A, Sagittal imaging of the dorsal finger shows (B) the extensor tendon *(arrowheads)*, also seen in transverse imaging (C). Note the hypoechoic hyaline cartilage covering the metacarpal head and triangle-shaped area of connective tissue *(asterisk)*. Imaging over the proximal interphalangeal joint shows (D) the attachment of the central band *(open arrows)*. Parasagittal imaging (E) shows a lateral band *(arrows)*, attaching distally (F) on the distal phalanx *(DP)*. Note the nail *(arrowheads)*.

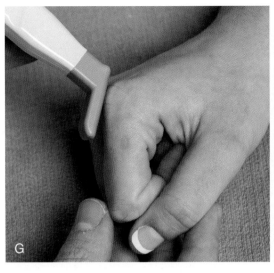
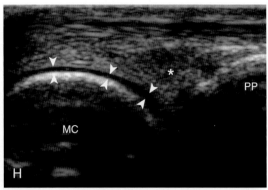
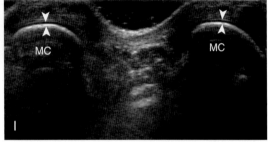

■ **FIGURE 5.17, cont'd** With finger flexion (G), ultrasound images show metacarpal articular cartilage *(arrowheads)* in the (H) sagittal and (I) transverse planes. Note overlying triangle-shaped connective tissue *(asterisk)* and extensor tendon. *MC*, Metacarpal head; *MP*, middle phalanx; *PP*, proximal phalanx.

metacarpophalangeal joints are imaged in both the sagittal and transverse planes to evaluate for synovial hypertrophy and erosions.

LIGAMENTS

The collateral ligaments of the digits can also be assessed with ultrasound in the coronal plane around each individual joint. To specifically evaluate the ulnar collateral ligament of the first metacarpophalangeal joint, the hand is placed around a rolled-up towel, and the transducer is placed in the coronal plane relative to the first metacarpophalangeal joint (Fig. 5.18A). The (proper) ulnar collateral ligament proper will appear in long axis as hyperechoic with a compact fibrillar echotexture, extending from a broad concavity in the metacarpal to the proximal phalanx (Fig. 5.18B).[21] Because the subcutaneous fat directly overlying the ulnar collateral ligament is hyperechoic, the ligament may appear relatively hypoechoic but should be fibrillar and of relatively uniform thickness. Additionally, the ligament may appear artifactually hypoechoic where it is oblique to the sound beam from anisotropy. The overlying adductor pollicis aponeurosis, which is specific to the ulnar collateral ligament of the first metacarpophalangeal joint, is seen as a thin hypoechoic structure over the ulnar collateral ligament. Flexion

of the interphalangeal joint will produce isolated movement of the adductor pollicis aponeurosis, which assists in its identification (Video 5.5). An additional dynamic maneuver in assessment of any collateral ligament is stressing the joint (valgus for ulnar ligaments, varus for radial ligaments). This is accomplished with minimal stress and is helpful because joint fluid will often move into the ligament tear under ultrasound visualization to improve detection. Other ulnar and radial collateral ligaments of the digits similarly appear as compact and hyperechoic fibrillar structures, which extend across each joint.

■ JOINT ABNORMALITIES

There are multiple synovial articulations of the hand and wrist and each individual site should be evaluated for joint abnormalities. In the sagittal plane, the volar and dorsal recesses of the radiocarpal and midcarpal joints are assessed for abnormal distention (Fig. 5.19A and B). The distal radioulnar joint is also assessed from both dorsal and volar aspects in the transverse plane (Fig. 5.19C). The digits are assessed in the sagittal plane over each joint, including the dorsal and volar joint recesses (Fig. 5.19D and E). Anechoic distention of a joint recess typically represents simple fluid,

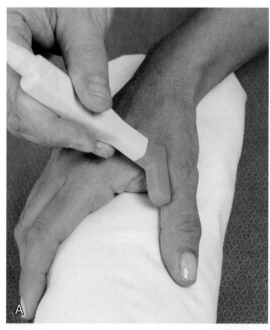

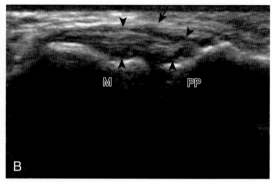

■ FIGURE 5.18 **Ulnar Collateral Ligament of First Metacaropophalangeal Joint.** A, Coronal imaging over the ulnar collateral ligament of the first metacarpophalangeal joint shows (B) the fibrillar appearance of the proper ulnar collateral ligament *(arrowheads)*. Note the characteristic contours of the metacarpal at the ulnar collateral ligament attachment. *M,* Metacarpal; *PP,* proximal phalanx. The adductor pollicis aponeurosis is partially seen *(arrow)* superficial to the ulnar collateral ligament.

although possible etiologies include degenerative, reactive, traumatic, and inflammatory causes; if there is concern for infection, ultrasound-guided aspiration should be considered. In the setting of trauma, one must evaluate the osseous structures at any focal area of symptoms for cortical step-off deformity, which would indicate fracture.

If a joint recess distention is not anechoic, considerations include complex fluid (Fig. 5.20) versus synovial hypertrophy (Fig. 5.21). Differentiation between these two etiologies may be difficult as both may appear hypoechoic or isoechoic compared with the overlying subcutaneous tissues. If joint recess distention collapses with transducer pressure or joint movement (Video 5.6), or if swirling of echoes within the recess are identified, and if there is no internal flow on color Doppler imaging, then complex fluid is suspected. In contrast, if there is no displacement, little compressibility of the joint recess, and internal flow on color Doppler imaging, then synovial hypertrophy is likely (Fig. 5.21) (Video 5.7).[22] Ultrasound-guided aspiration may be needed to make this determination. Because dorsal wrist ganglion cysts occur at the site of the dorsal radiocarpal joint recess and may appear similar, dynamic imaging with compression and joint movement also helps in their differentiation; a ganglion cyst is typically multilocular and noncompressible (see Fig. 5.89),

whereas a fluid-filled joint recess is compressible and unilocular (Video 5.6).[23] Possible etiologies for both complex fluid and synovial hypertrophy include hemorrhage and inflammation, which includes infection (Fig. 5.22), rheumatoid arthritis (Fig. 5.23) (Video 5.7), psoriatic arthritis (Fig. 5.24), systemic lupus erythematosus (Fig. 5.25), and gout (Fig. 5.26) (Video 5.8), among other inflammatory arthritides.

Synovial hypertrophy appears as nondisplaceable and poorly or noncompressible distention of a joint recess that is hypoechoic (Fig. 5.27) or less frequently isoechoic or hyperechoic compared with the adjacent subdermal fat (Fig. 5.27C).[24] Active inflammatory synovitis is usually hypoechoic with hyperemia on color Doppler imaging. When evaluating superficial structures, the transducer should be "floated" on a thick layer of gel with minimal transducer pressure so as to not compress the vascularity. The ultrasound finding of synovial thickening without hyperemia is not specific for one diagnosis and may be seen with osteoarthritis as well as asymptomatic subjects; therefore, assessing multiple joints and review of history, laboratory values, distribution, and radiographic findings are important for the synthesis of a concise diagnosis of inflammatory arthritis.[25] While uncommon with osteoarthritis, inflammatory changes as shown by ultrasound are more prevalent with erosive

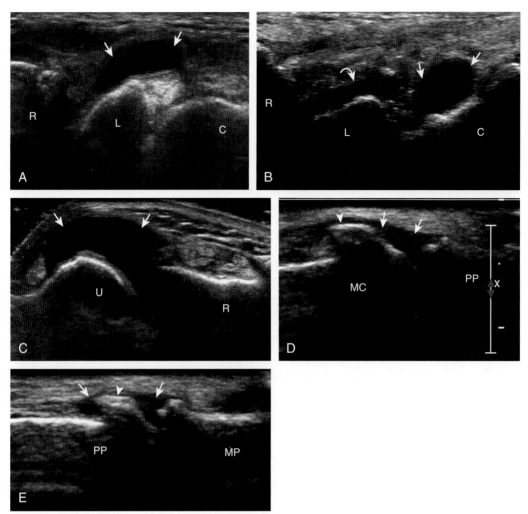

■ **FIGURE 5.19 Joint Effusion.** Sagittal ultrasound images over the dorsal wrist in two different patients show (A) anechoic distention *(arrows)* of the radiocarpal joint dorsal recess and (B) anechoic distention *(arrows)* of the midcarpal joint dorsal recess. Note collapsed radiocarpal joint recess *(curved arrow)* in B. Ultrasound image in the transverse plane shows (C) anechoic distention *(arrows)* of the distal radioulnar joint dorsal recess. Sagittal ultrasound images of the (D) metacarpophalangeal and (E) proximal interphalangeal joints show dorsal recess distention *(arrows)*. Note dorsal osteophytes from osteoarthritis *(arrowheads)*. *C,* Capitate; *L,* lunate; *MC,* metacarpal; *MP,* middle phalanx; *PP,* proximal phalanx; *R,* radius; *U,* ulna.

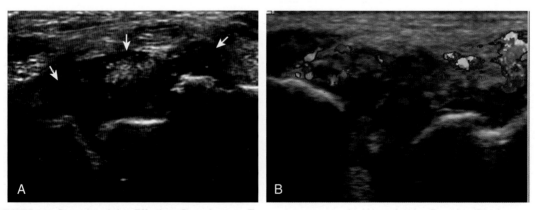

■ **FIGURE 5.20 Complex Joint Effusion: Pseudogout.** Transverse gray-scale (A) and color Doppler (B) ultrasound images over dorsal radiocarpal joint recess show mixed echogenicity but predominantly hypoechoic distention *(arrows)* and hyperemia.

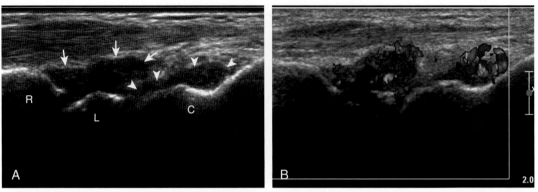

■ **FIGURE 5.21 Synovial Hypertrophy: Rheumatoid Arthritis.** Sagittal gray-scale (A) and color Doppler (B) ultrasound images over the dorsal wrist show hypoechoic distention of the radiocarpal *(arrows)* and midcarpal *(arrowheads)* dorsal joint recesses with hyperemia. *C*, Capitate; *L*, lunate; *R*, radius.

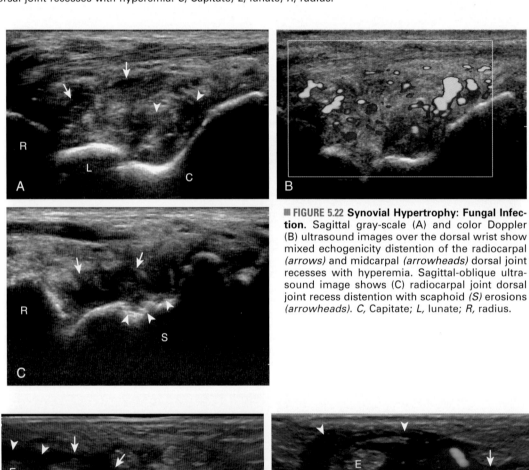

■ **FIGURE 5.22 Synovial Hypertrophy: Fungal Infection.** Sagittal gray-scale (A) and color Doppler (B) ultrasound images over the dorsal wrist show mixed echogenicity distention of the radiocarpal *(arrows)* and midcarpal *(arrowheads)* dorsal joint recesses with hyperemia. Sagittal-oblique ultrasound image shows (C) radiocarpal joint dorsal joint recess distention with scaphoid *(S)* erosions *(arrowheads)*. *C*, Capitate; *L*, lunate; *R*, radius.

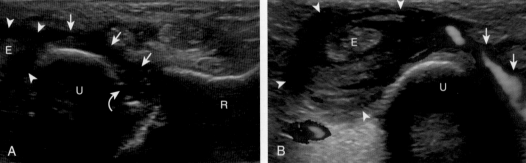

■ **FIGURE 5.23 Synovial Hypertrophy: Rheumatoid Arthritis.** A, Transverse ultrasound images show hypoechoic synovial hypertrophy distending the dorsal recess of the distal radioulnar joint *(arrows)* with hyperemia (B) and erosion *(curved arrow)*. Note adjacent tenosynovitis *(arrowheads)* of extensor carpi ulnaris (E). *R*, Radius; *U*, ulna.

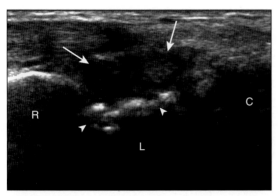

■ FIGURE 5.24 **Synovial Hypertrophy: Psoriatic Arthritis.** Ultrasound image of dorsal wrist in sagittal plane shows hypoechoic synovial hypertrophy *(arrows)* and erosions *(arrowheads). R,* Radius; *L,* lunate; *C,* capitate.

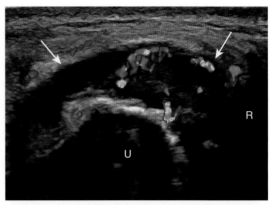

■ FIGURE 5.25 **Synovial Hypertrophy and Effusion: Systemic Lupus Erythematosus.** Transverse ultrasound image shows anechoic fluid and hypoechoic synovial hypertrophy with hyperemia of the distal radioulnar joint dorsal recess *(arrows). U,* Ulna; *R,* radius.

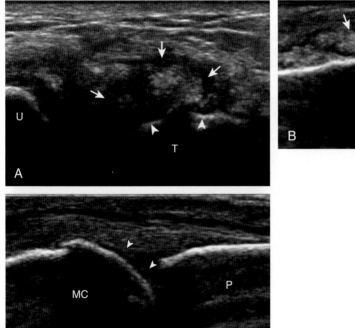

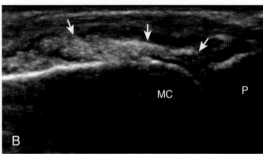

■ FIGURE 5.26 **Complex Joint Fluid and Tophus: Gout.** A, Coronal ultrasound image shows echogenic tophus with hypoechoic halo *(arrows)* with adjacent carpal erosions *(arrowheads).* B and C, Sagittal ultrasound images of the metacarpophalangeal joint shows echogenic effusion *(arrows)* and hyaline cartilage icing *(arrowheads)* from urate crystals (the double contour sign). *MC,* Metacarpal head; *P,* proximal phalanx; *T,* triquetrum; *U,* ulna.

osteoarthritis.[26,27] Synovial proliferative disorders such as pigmented villonodular synovitis and synovial chondromatosis are other considerations when synovial hypertrophy is identified. In the latter condition, superimposed hyperechoic calcifications may be seen in the synovial tissue.

If inflammatory synovitis is suspected, the hypoechoic hyaline articular cartilage and the subjacent bone cortex should be evaluated for erosions where thinning or defects of the hyaline cartilage may be identified (Figs. 5.28, 5.29, 5.30, and 5.31). An osseous erosion appears as discontinuity or irregularity of the normally smooth and hyperechoic bone cortex visible in two planes.[24,28] While the cause for an erosion can be from many inflammatory conditions, a large erosion at the

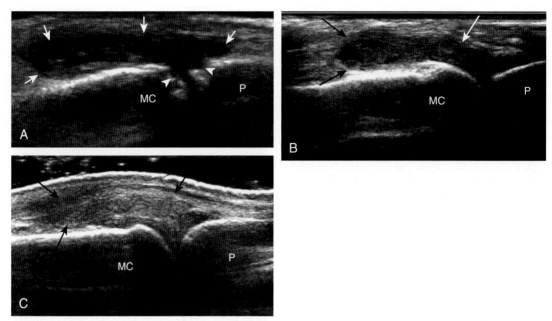

■ **FIGURE 5.27 Synovial Hypertrophy: Rheumatoid Arthritis.** Sagittal ultrasound images of the metacarpophalangeal dorsal joint recesses in three patients show predominantly (A) hypoechoic synovial hypertrophy *(arrows)* and erosions *(arrowheads)*, (B) predominantly hypoechoic, and (C) isoechoic synovial hypertrophy. *MC*, Metacarpal head; *P*, proximal phalanx.

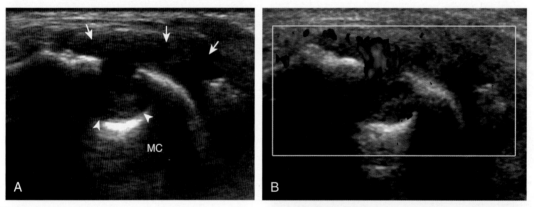

■ **FIGURE 5.28 Erosions: Rheumatoid Arthritis.** Ultrasound images show (A, B) hypoechoic synovial hypertrophy *(arrows)* that extends into a metacarpal *(MC)* erosion *(arrowheads)* with hyperemia.

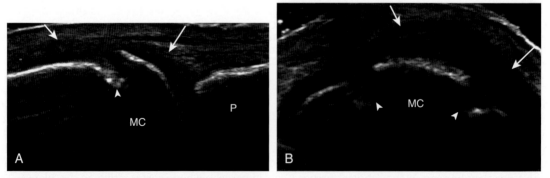

■ **FIGURE 5.29 Erosions: Rheumatoid Arthritis.** Ultrasound images of the dorsal second metacarpophalangeal joint in the sagittal (A) and transverse (B) planes show hypoechoic synovial hypertrophy *(arrows)* and metacarpal head *(MC)* erosions *(arrowheads)*. *P*, Proximal phalanx.

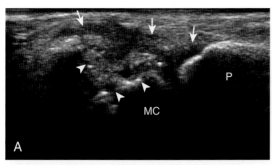
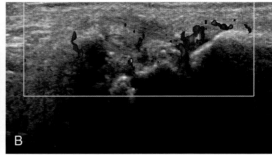

■ **FIGURE 5.30 Erosions: Rheumatoid Arthritis.** Sagittal ultrasound image (A) of the second metacarpal head shows synovial hypertrophy that ranges from hypoechoic to hyperechoic *(arrows)* that extends into the metacarpal *(MC)* erosion *(arrowheads)* with hyperemia in B. *P,* Proximal phalanx.

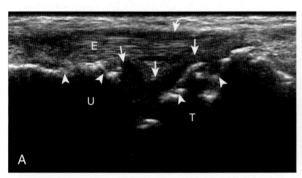
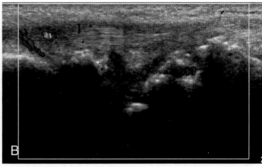

■ **FIGURE 5.31 Erosions: Rheumatoid Arthritis.** Coronal ultrasound image over lateral wrist shows predominantly hypoechoic synovial hypertrophy *(arrows)* with erosions *(arrowheads)* of the ulna *(U)* and triquetrum *(T)* with hyperemia in B. Note tenosynovitis *(curved arrow)* of the extensor carpi ulnaris *(E)*.

second or fifth metacarpal head, or distal ulna, suggests rheumatoid arthritis as the etiology.[29] Compared with radiography, ultrasound is more sensitive in detection of hand and wrist erosions and has the benefit of evaluating synovial thickness and hyperemia; however, the sensitivity of ultrasound in diagnosis of wrist erosions is only 40%.[30] When a bone erosion is suspected, the presence of adjacent synovitis increases the likelihood of a true erosion as there are many other causes for bone irregularity.[16] Correlation with history, radiography, and other joints is essential because a false-positive rate of 29% has also been reported; prominent concavities of the distal metacarpals and irregular osteophytes may simulate erosions.[31] A small depression in the dorsal metacarpal at the edge of the hyaline cartilage can be a normal variation, especially at the second metacarpal (Fig. 5.32).[8] Unlike a true erosion, this cortical depression is usually smooth and shallow (less than 2 mm) without cortical disruption; however, the absence of synovial hypertrophy is a critical finding to suggest a normal variation.[8] In addition to the metacarpal heads, cortical irregularity is normally seen at the lunate and triquetrum related to vascular channels and can simulate erosions (Fig. 5.33).

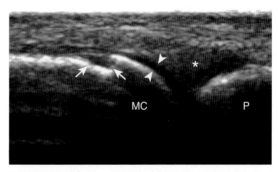

■ **FIGURE 5.32 Metacarpal Head Pseudoerosion.** Sagittal ultrasound image over the dorsum of the second metacarpal shows shallow pseudoerosion *(arrows)*. Note hyaline cartilage *(arrowheads)* of metacarpal head *(MC)*, proximal phalanx *(P)*, and triangle-shaped connective tissue *(asterisk)*.

Because ultrasound is very sensitive in the identification of bone cortex surface abnormalities and irregularity, the various causes of such findings should be considered. In addition to an erosion, bone proliferation from a seronegative spondyloarthropathy or an osteophyte from osteoarthritis may also appear as cortical irregularity, and correlation with history, distribution of findings, and radiographs are essential. Bone irregularity

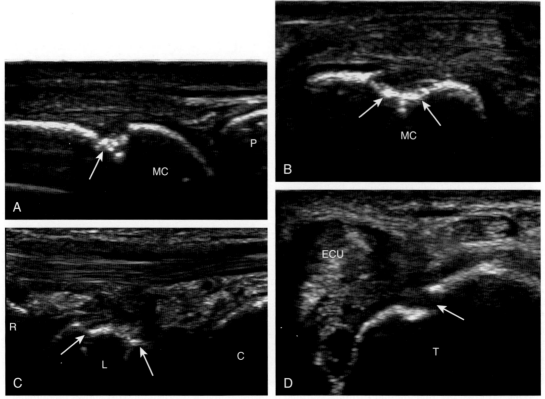

■ **FIGURE 5.33 Pseudoerosions.** Ultrasound images of (A, B) third metacarpal head (sagittal and transverse planes), (C) lunate, and (D) distal ulna show cortical irregularity *(arrows)* without adjacent synovitis. *MC,* Metacarpal; *P,* proximal phalanx; *R,* radius; *L,* lunate; *C,* capitate; *T,* triquetrum; *ECU,* extensor carpi ulnaris.

from degenerative change can be differentiated from seronegative spondyloarthropathy in several ways. With degenerative change, bone proliferation is at the margins of a synovial articulation (osteophytes) (Fig. 5.34; see Fig. 5.19D and E), whereas bone proliferation from a spondyloarthritis can occur anywhere along the surface of a bone and particularly occurs at tendon or ligament attachments related to enthesitis (Fig. 5.35), characterized by abnormal hypoechoic tendon or ligament, hyperemia, and bone proliferation or erosion at the tendon or ligament footprint.[32]

There are various protocols for inflammatory arthritis screening of the wrist and hand. In suspected rheumatoid arthritis, ultrasound can provide information for diagnosis and prognosis.[33] The second metacarpal is an important target to assess with suspected rheumatoid arthritis because it is a frequent site of involvement; assessment in the coronal plane at the radial aspect should complement dorsal assessment in the sagittal and transverse planes (see Fig. 5.29).[34] Evaluation of the dorsal recesses of the three wrist joints (radioulnar, radiocarpal, midcarpal), as well as the third metacarpophalangeal, is also essential.[22,34,35] Focused assessment at any symptomatic site should

also be completed, with consideration for the fifth metatarsophalangeal joint of the foot, another common site of rheumatoid arthritis involvement.[36] A limited bilateral examination of the hand and wrist for assessment of rheumatoid arthritis has been proposed, which includes the three joints of each wrist, and the metacarpophalangeal joints of each index and long fingers, although other protocols additionally include the proximal interphalangeal joints of the index and long fingers.[35,37] However, a global or comprehensive examination of all key and symptomatic joint recesses of the wrist and hand for synovial hypertrophy can be completed efficiently with ultrasound. The presence of synovial hypertrophy with hyperemia and erosions increases the likelihood of an inflammatory arthritis.[38,39] Joint abnormalities may also be seen with systemic lupus erythematosus in a similar distribution to rheumatoid arthritis but is less common (see Fig. 5.25).[40] With regard to other inflammatory arthritis conditions, ultrasound assessment may be directed by symptoms or radiographic findings. For example, bone proliferation of psoriatic arthritis may occur at various sites, including the carpus or a single digit at ligament attachments (see Fig. 5.35).[41,42] A gouty

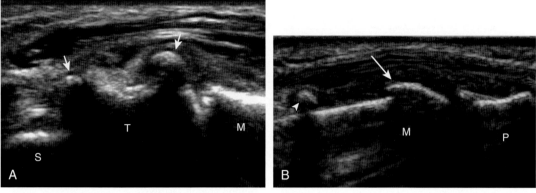

■ **FIGURE 5.34 Osteophytes: Osteoarthritis.** Ultrasound images of the thumb from two different patients (A and B) show osteophytes *(arrows)* and intra-articular body *(arrowhead)*. *S*, Scaphoid; *T*, trapezium; *M*, first metacarpal; *P*, proximal phalanx.

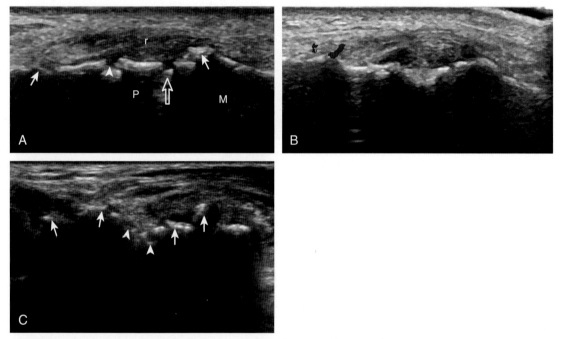

■ **FIGURE 5.35 Enthesopathy: Psoriatic Arthritis.** A and B, Ultrasound images of the long axis to the radial collateral ligament *(r)* of a proximal interphalangeal joint *(open arrow)* show areas of bone proliferation at the ligament attachments *(arrows)* and an erosion *(arrowhead)* with adjacent hypoechoic soft tissue swelling and (B) hyperemia. C, Transverse ultrasound image over the dorsal wrist shows diffuse areas of bone proliferation *(arrows)* and erosions *(arrowheads)* with overlying hypoechoic soft tissue swelling. *M*, Middle phalanx; *P,* proximal phalanx.

tophus may also occur at variable sites, and monosodium urate crystals may be seen as complex fluid or layering over the hyaline cartilage (the double contour sign) (see Fig. 5.26).[43]

■ TENDON AND MUSCLE ABNORMALITIES

Possible tendon abnormalities of the wrist and hand include tenosynovitis (and paratendinitis if

inflammation surrounds a tendon that has no tendon sheath), tendinosis, and tendon tear. Tenosynovitis is characterized by distention of the synovial sheath around the tendon. Similar to a joint recess, distention of a tendon sheath may be predominantly anechoic (Figs. 5.36 and 5.37). If tendon sheath distention is not anechoic, possibilities include complex fluid versus synovial hypertrophy (Fig. 5.38). Compressibility, movement of internal echoes with transducer pressure, and lack of flow on color Doppler imaging suggest

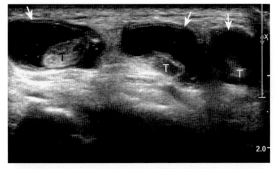

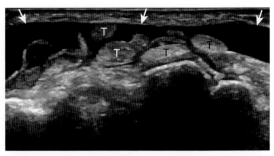

■ FIGURE 5.36 Tenosynovitis: Rheumatoid Arthritis. Ultrasound over the dorsal wrist in short axis to the extensor tendons *(T)* shows predominantly anechoic fluid distention of the tendon sheaths *(arrows)*.

■ FIGURE 5.37 Tenosynovitis: Pseudogout. Ultrasound over the dorsal wrist in short axis to the extensor tendons *(T)* shows anechoic fluid distention of the tendon sheath *(arrows)*.

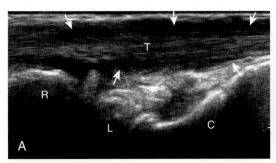

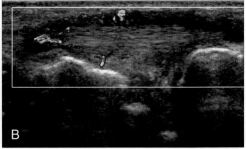

■ FIGURE 5.38 Tenosynovitis: Rheumatoid Arthritis. A, Gray-scale and (B) color Doppler ultrasound images in long axis to the extensor tendons of the wrist *(T)* show hypoechoic synovial hypertrophy *(arrows)* with increased flow. *C,* Capitate; *L,* lunate; *R,* radius.

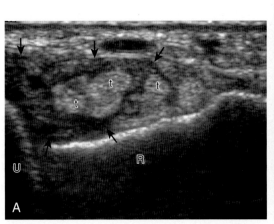

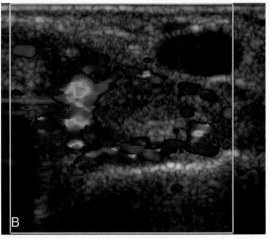

■ FIGURE 5.39 Tenosynovitis: Systemic Lupus Erythematosus. A, Gray-scale and (B) color Doppler ultrasound images in short axis to the extensor tendons of the wrist *(t)* show hypoechoic to isoechoic synovial hypertrophy *(arrows)* with increased flow. *R,* Radius; *U,* ulna.

complex fluid rather than synovial hypertrophy, whereas non-compressibility and flow on color Doppler imaging suggest synovial hypertrophy (Video 5.9).[44] Synovial hypertrophy is most commonly hypoechoic, or less commonly isoechoic or hyperechoic compared with subdermal fat (Fig. 5.39).[24] Tenosynovitis may cause erosion of an adjacent bone, such as the ulnar styloid with rheumatoid arthritis (Fig. 5.40). Evaluation of tendon sheaths in rheumatoid arthritis, especially the extensor carpi ulnaris and second flexor tendon, can indicate early disease and further progression.[45] Less commonly, tendon sheath involvement may also occur in systemic lupus erythematosus (Fig. 5.39) (Video 5.10) as well as systemic sclerosis.[40,46,47] Regardless of ultrasound appearance, possible etiologies of tenosynovitis include degenerative, traumatic, proliferative, and inflammatory, including crystal deposition (Figs. 5.41 and 5.42) (Videos 5.11 and 5.12) and infection (Fig. 5.43).[48] When evaluating for tenosynovitis, the extensor retinaculum at the level of the radiocarpal joint dorsally should not be mistaken for tenosynovitis as the normal hyperechoic retinaculum may appear artifactually hypoechoic due to anisotropy (see Fig. 5.11B).[9] With spondyloarthritis, such as psoriatic arthritis, ultrasound may show peritendon inflammation (see Fig. 5.46), as well as inflammatory enthesitis at tendon attachments, characterized by abnormal hypoechogenicity, hyperemia, erosions, and enthesophytes; correlation with radiography is helpful in differentiation between a degenerative and inflammatory enthesophyte as the latter is ill defined.[41,42,49]

A specific stenosing tenosynovitis involves the extensor pollicis brevis and abductor pollicis longus tendons in the first extensor wrist compartment, which is called *de Quervain disease.*[50] This condition is characterized by thickening of the

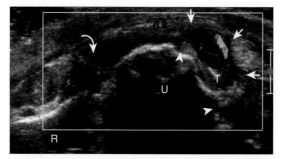

■ FIGURE 5.40 **Tenosynovitis: Rheumatoid Arthritis.** Color Doppler ultrasound image in short axis to the extensor carpi ulnaris tendon *(T)* shows hypoechoic tenosynovitis with increased blood flow *(arrows)* and ulna *(U)* erosions *(arrowheads)*. Note synovial hypertrophy from the distal radioulnar joint *(curved arrow)* as well as increased blood flow and abnormal hypoechogenicity of the extensor carpi ulnaris. *R,* Radius.

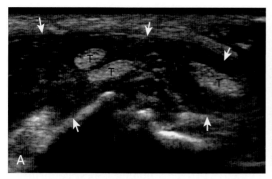
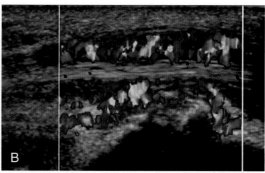

■ FIGURE 5.41 **Tenosynovitis: Gout.** A, Gray-scale short axis and (B) color Doppler long axis ultrasound images of the wrist extensor tendons *(T)* at the level of the radiocarpal joint show hypoechoic synovial hypertrophy with increased flow on color Doppler imaging *(arrows)*.

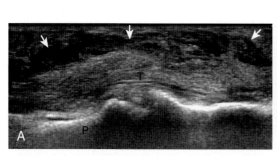
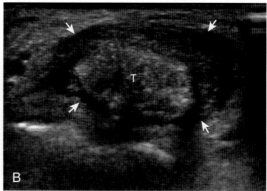

■ FIGURE 5.42 **Tenosynovitis: Gout.** Ultrasound images in (A) long axis and (B) short axis to the flexor tendons of the finger *(T)* show hypoechoic to isoechoic synovial hypertrophy *(arrows)*. *M,* Middle phalanx; *P,* proximal phalanx.

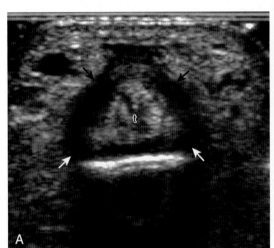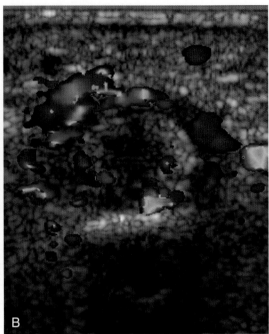

■ **FIGURE 5.43 Tenosynovitis: Infection.** Ultrasound image (A) in short axis to the flexor tendons of the finger shows hypoechoic synovial hypertrophy *(arrows)* with (B) hyperemia. *t,* Tendon.

extensor retinaculum over the involved tendons, with possible hyperemia, tendinosis, and cortical irregularity of the radius (Fig. 5.44) (Video 5.13).[27] The extensor retinaculum is thickened at the level of the radius, typically dorsally adjacent to the extensor pollicis brevis tendon, although associated tenosynovial fluid may only be seen proximal or distal to the retinaculum. A hypoechoic septum-like structure is often present that causes subcompartmentalization of the first extensor compartment, associated with an osseous ridge (more common in females), which is important when injection of the tendon sheath is considered.[50-53] The abductor pollicis longus tendon or less commonly the extensor pollicis brevis tendon may also have multiple tendon slips, termed the "lotus root sign," which should not be mistaken for longitudinal tendon tears.[52,53]

Other tendon abnormalities include tendinosis and tendon tear. Tendinosis represents tendon degeneration, typically from overuse, and is characterized by hypoechoic tendon enlargement without disruption of tendon fibers (Fig. 5.45). In the setting of inflammatory arthritis, abnormal tendon hypoechogenicity and increased flow on color Doppler imaging can indicate true tendinitis (Fig. 5.46; see Fig. 5.40). Calcium hydroxyapatite deposition appears hyperechoic with variable shadowing representing calcific tendinosis or tendinitis if in the inflammatory phase (Fig. 5.47).

The finding of incomplete hypoechoic or anechoic tendon fiber disruption indicates partial-thickness tendon tear (Fig. 5.48). Involvement of the flexor carpi radialis tendon from tendinosis or tear near the trapezium may be associated with triscaphe osteoarthritis.[12] The finding of complete fiber disruption indicates a full-thickness tendon tear (Figs. 5.49 and 5.50).[54] Tendon injuries in the digits may also include bone avulsions, which will appear as a hyperechoic fragment (Fig. 5.51) (Video 5.14). This finding is best confirmed on radiography. In this setting, tendon retraction typically occurs, which is a helpful finding that indicates a full-thickness tear. If there is a question of partial- versus full-thickness tendon tear, dynamic imaging with passive and active tendon movement can show either continuous fiber movement excluding a full-thickness tear (Videos 5.14 and 5.15) or lack of tendon translation across the abnormal site, which would indicate a full-thickness tear. Dynamic evaluation should also be used to assess for tendon subluxation. The extensor carpi ulnaris subluxation or dislocation is considered abnormal if greater than 50% of the tendon moves beyond the osseous groove in the ulna, due to extensor carpi ulnaris subsheath tear (Fig. 5.52) (Video 5.16).[17,18] An injury to the sagittal band of the extensor hood can occur and when torn, extensor tendon subluxation can be seen during finger flexion, termed *boxer knuckle* (Fig. 5.53) (Video 5.17).[55] If the patient has symptoms

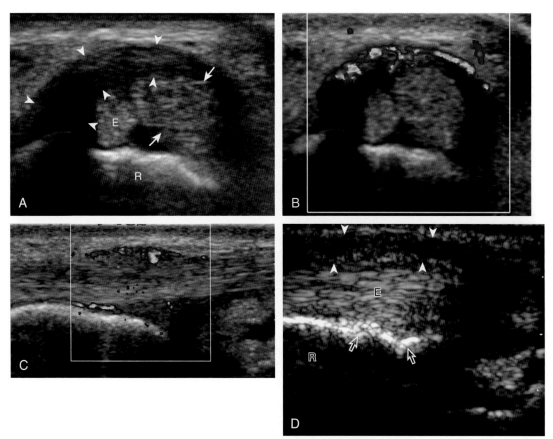

■ FIGURE 5.44 **De Quervain Disease.** Ultrasound images in (A) short axis and color Doppler (B) short axis and (C) long axis to first extensor compartment tendons show hypoechoic extensor retinaculum thickening *(arrowheads)* and increased flow on power Doppler imaging. Ultrasound image in (D) long axis in a second patient shows hypoechoic extensor retinaculum thickening *(arrowheads)* and cortical irregularity *(open arrows)* of the radius *(R). E*, extensor pollicis brevis tendon.

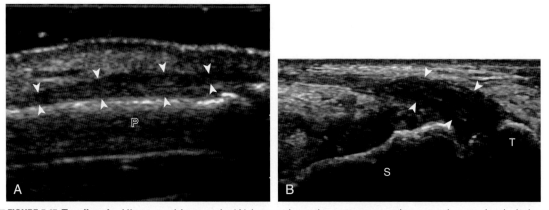

■ FIGURE 5.45 **Tendinosis.** Ultrasound images in (A) long axis to the extensor tendon over the proximal phalanx and (B) long axis to the flexor carpi radialis tendon in two different patients show hypoechoic thickening of the involved tendon *(arrowheads). P*, Phalanx; *S*, scaphoid; *T*, trapezium.

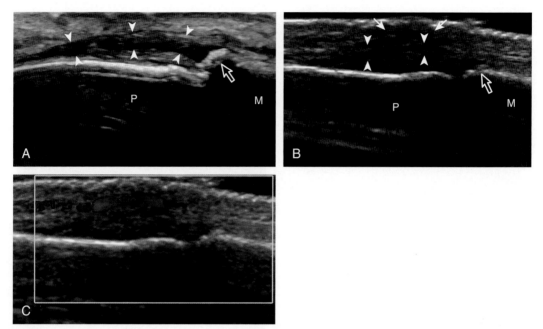

■ **FIGURE 5.46 Tendinitis: Psoriatic Arthritis.** Ultrasound images in long axis to the extensor tendon at the proximal interphalangeal joint show (A) hypoechoic tendon thickening *(arrowheads)* and enthesopathy *(open arrow)*, and in another patient (B) hypoechoic tendon thickening *(arrowheads)*, enthesopathy *(open arrow)*, and adjacent hypoechoic swelling *(arrows)* with increased blood flow in (C). *M,* Middle phalanx; *P,* proximal phalanx.

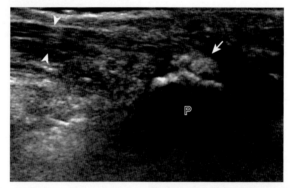

■ **FIGURE 5.47 Calcific Tendinosis: Flexor Carpi Ulnaris.** Ultrasound image in long axis to the flexor carpi ulnaris tendon *(arrowheads)* shows a calcium hydroxyapatite deposit *(arrow)* adjacent to the pisiform *(P).* Note cortical irregularity.

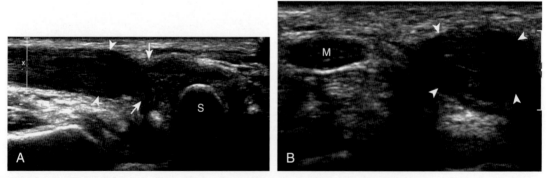

■ **FIGURE 5.48 Partial-Thickness Tear: Flexor Carpi Radialis Tendon.** Ultrasound images in (A) long axis and (B) short axis to the flexor carpi radialis show hypoechoic thickening of the flexor carpi radialis *(arrowheads)* with partial anechoic tendon fiber disruption *(arrows). M,* Median nerve; *S,* scaphoid.

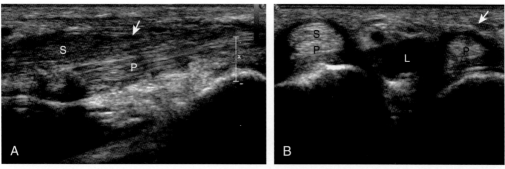

■ **FIGURE 5.49 Full-Thickness Tear: Flexor Digitorum Superficialis.** Ultrasound images in (A) long axis and (B) short axis to the flexor digitorum profundus *(P)* and superficialis *(S)* show a torn and retracted flexor digitorum superficialis *(arrow)*. *L*, Lumbrical muscle.

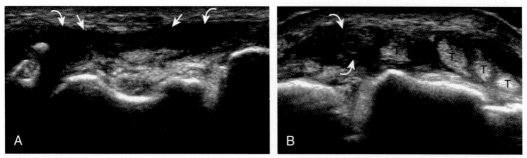

■ **FIGURE 5.50 Full-Thickness Tear: Extensor Indicis.** Ultrasound images in (A) long axis and (B) short axis to the extensor indicis show a tendon tear *(between arrows)* with retracted tendon stumps *(curved arrows)*. *T*, extensor digitorum tendons.

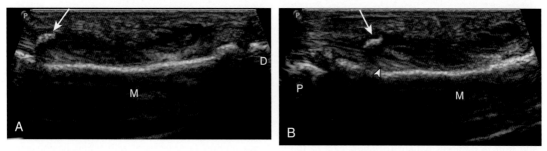

■ **FIGURE 5.51 Avulsion Fracture: Flexor Digitorum Profundus.** Sagittal ultrasound image of the volar digit shows (A) the hyperechoic retracted fracture fragment *(arrow)* avulsed from the distal phalanx (D). Parasagittal image (B) shows intact flexor digitorum superficialis tendon attaching to middle phalanx (M). *P*, Proximal phalanx. *(Courtesy S. Allred, Hamilton, Ontario.)*

of intermittent snapping, clicking, or popping, the patient is asked to reproduce the symptom while evaluating the area with ultrasound.

Ultrasound can be effective in the evaluation of pulley injuries of the digits.[5] A pulley tear will appear as abnormal hypoechogenicity or absence of the pulley (Figs. 5.54 and 5.55). An important indirect sign of a pulley tear is abnormal volar displacement of the flexor tendons, called *bow-stringing*, evaluated dynamically during active forced finger flexion (Fig. 5.56) (Video 5.18).[56-58]

Injury to the A2 pulley is common; additional involvement of the A3 pulley typically requires surgical repair.[57] Volar displacement of the flexor tendons measured from the adjacent phalanx should normally be at most 1 mm with active finger flexion against resistance.[57] Volar displacement at the distal A2 pulley greater than 3 mm indicates complete A2 pulley rupture, while a measurement greater than 5 mm indicates combined A2 and A3 complete rupture.[57] Less commonly, a pulley injury to the thumb may also be seen (Fig. 5.57). Another digit abnormality is *trigger finger*, whereby impaired flexor tendon gliding is caused by tendon constriction due to thickening of the A1 pulley (Figs. 5.57 and 5.58) (Video 5.19), with possible cyst formation, pulley

hyperemia, tendinosis, and tenosynovitis.[59,60] A1 pulley thickening is also seen in scleroderma.[61]

There are various other muscle and tendon abnormalities of the forearm, wrist, and hand, which are either uncommon or have nonspecific imaging features. However, there is a specific abnormality called *intersection syndrome*, occurring where the muscles of the first wrist compartment cross over the muscles of the second wrist compartment in the distal forearm approximately 4 to 8 cm proximal to the Lister tubercle.[62,63] At imaging, pain is produced with transducer pressure and hypoechoic swelling or adjacent fluid may be seen (Fig. 5.59). A less common distal intersection syndrome may occur where the extensor pollicis longus tendon crosses over the extensor carpi radialis longus and brevis tendons distal to the Lister tubercle.[62]

There exist a number of normal variations in the hand and wrist, including multiple tendon slips and the presence of accessory tendons and muscles, such as the extensor digitorum brevis manus, which may simulate a soft tissue mass at

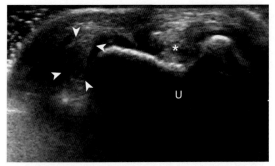

■ **FIGURE 5.52 Dislocation: Extensor Carpi Ulnaris Tendon.** Ultrasound image in short axis to the extensor carpi ulnaris tendon *(arrowheads)* shows dislocation of the tendon from its normal position *(asterisk)*. *U,* Ulna.

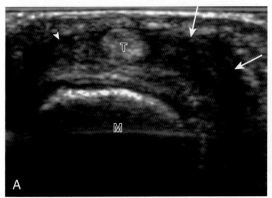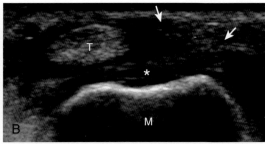

■ **FIGURE 5.53 Sagittal Band Injury.** Ultrasound image (A) short axis to the central band of the extensor tendon *(T)* shows hypoechoic thickening of the sagittal band *(arrows)* compared to normal appearance *(arrowhead)*. Ultrasound image from a different patient (B) short axis to the extensor tendon *(arrowheads)* with finger flexion shows subluxation of the tendon *(T)* from its normal position *(asterisk)* and discontinuity of the sagittal band of the extensor hood or boxer knuckle *(arrows)*. *M,* Metacarpal.

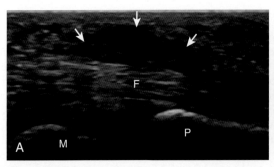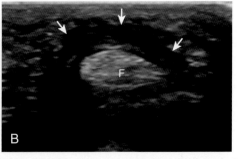

■ **FIGURE 5.54 Pulley Injury: A1.** Ultrasound images in (A) long axis and (B) short axis to the flexor tendons *(F)* of the finger show marked hypoechoic thickening of the A1 pulley *(arrows)*. *M,* Metacarpal head; *P,* proximal phalanx.

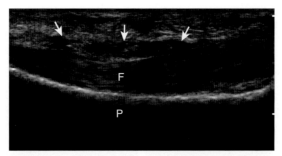

■ FIGURE 5.55 **Pulley Injury: A2.** Ultrasound image in long axis to the flexor tendons *(F)* of the finger show marked hypoechoic thickening of the A2 pulley *(arrows)*. P, Proximal phalanx.

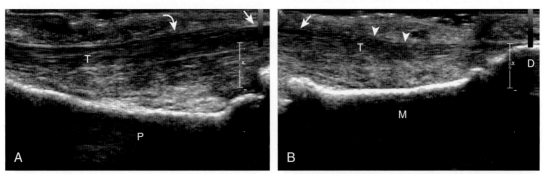

■ FIGURE 5.56 **Pulley Injury: A2 to A4.** Ultrasound images in (A and B) long axis to the flexor tendons *(T)* of the finger show disruption of the distal A2 pulley *(curved arrow)* and absence of the A3 *(arrows)* and A4 *(arrowheads)* pulleys with volar displacement of the flexor tendons (termed *bowstringing*). *D,* Distal phalanx; *M,* middle phalanx; *P,* proximal phalanx.

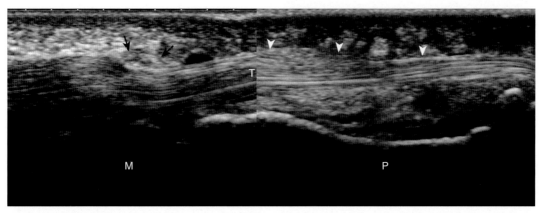

■ FIGURE 5.57 **Pulley Injury: Thumb.** Ultrasound image in long axis to the flexor tendons *(T)* of the thumb show disruption of the pulleys (A2 and oblique) *(arrowheads)* with volar displacement of the flexor tendons (termed *bowstringing*). Note deviation of flexor tendon beneath a thickened A1 pulley *(arrows)*. *M,* Metacarpal head; *P,* proximal phalanx.

physical examination (Fig. 5.60) (Video 5.20).[64,65] Variations that also involve the palmaris longus may occur and present as a palpable abnormality (Fig. 5.61).[65] Another common variant, the accessory abductor digiti minimi is discussed with ulnar nerve entrapment (see Fig. 5.73). Masses of the tendons are discussed later with other hand and wrist masses.

■ PERIPHERAL NERVE ABNORMALITIES

Carpal Tunnel Syndrome

The most common upper extremity entrapment neuropathy is carpal tunnel syndrome, which involves the median nerve at the level of the wrist.[66,67] Because the median nerve traverses the

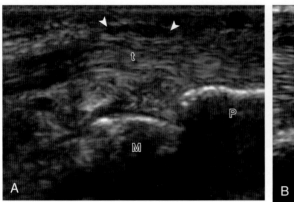 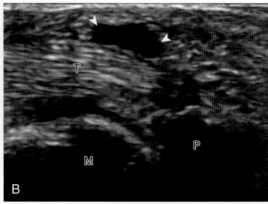

■ **FIGURE 5.58 Trigger Finger.** Ultrasound images in long axis to the second digit flexor tendons at the level of the metacarpophalangeal joint in two different patients show (A) hypoechoic thickening of the A1 pulley *(arrowheads)* and (B) cyst formation *(arrowheads)* with deviation of the flexor tendons *(t)* as they course beneath the A1 pulley, and (B). *M,* Metacarpal head; *P,* proximal phalanx.

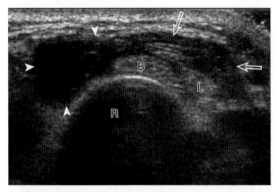

■ **FIGURE 5.59 Intersection Syndrome.** Ultrasound image in the axial plane at the distal forearm shows an abnormally hypoechoic extensor pollicis brevis muscle *(arrowheads)* where it crosses over the extensor carpi radialis brevis *(B)* and longus *(L)* with the abductor pollicis longus *(open arrows)*. *R,* Radius.

fibro-osseous carpal tunnel, a decrease in the size of the carpal tunnel or increase in the volume of its contents can cause median nerve compression, such as trauma, mass, or tenosynovitis. At sonography, carpal tunnel syndrome is characterized by hypoechoic enlargement of the median nerve as it enters into the carpal tunnel (Fig. 5.62) (Video 5.21), although distal nerve swelling is also possible (Fig. 5.63). With regard to quantitative assessment for carpal tunnel syndrome, there have been many studies that recommend different size criteria and depend on how one balances sensitivity and specificity. A median nerve area of less than 6 mm^2 usually excludes and an area greater than 12 mm^2 indicates carpal tunnel syndrome.[66] A more accurate assessment of carpal tunnel syndrome assesses a change in median nerve cross-sectional area; an increase in size greater than 2 mm^2 comparing proximal (at proximal pronator quadratus) with distal (maximal nerve enlargement at the wrist crease) can diagnose carpal tunnel syndrome with 99% accuracy (Fig. 5.64).[68] In addition, a change in median nerve area of 6 mm^2 indicates moderate and 9 mm^2 severe carpal tunnel syndrome.[69] Of note, the circumferential trace method of measuring area is preferred, given variations in the shape of the median nerve, and measurement is made inside the echogenic epineurium. Other findings of carpal tunnel syndrome include volar bowing of the retinaculum in the transverse plane and flattening of the median nerve within the carpal tunnel best seen in long axis, where the abrupt transition in size has been termed the *notch sign*.[66] Also, imaging of the carpal tunnel during movement of the digits has shown decreased transverse sliding of the median nerve in carpal tunnel syndrome.[70] Demonstration of blood flow on color Doppler imaging has also been shown to be an accurate indicator of carpal tunnel syndrome (see Fig. 5.66).[71-73] Median nerve enlargement has also been described in diabetic patients with symmetrical polyneuropathy.[74]

A bifid or high division of the median nerve, usually associated with a persistent median artery between the two nerve trunks, is a normal variant seen in 15% of the asymptomatic population that is often incomplete but not typically bilateral (Fig. 5.65).[75,76] Although not a risk factor, carpal tunnel syndrome may exist in this situation as well, where the hypoechoic and enlarged two median nerve trunk areas combined show a difference of 4 mm^2 or more comparing proximal (at pronator quadratus) and distal (at carpal tunnel) (Fig. 5.66) (Video 5.22).[77] Less commonly, a persistent median artery may be present in the

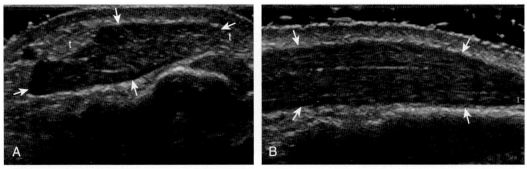

■ FIGURE 5.60 **Extensor Digitorum Brevis Manus.** Ultrasound images (A) transverse and (B) sagittal over the dorsal wrist shows a hypoechoic accessory muscle *(arrows)*, which often is seen between the extensor tendons *(t)* of the second and third digits.

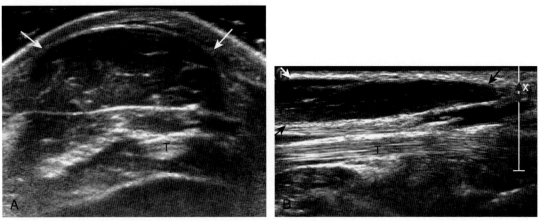

■ FIGURE 5.61 **Palmaris Longus: Inversus Variant.** Ultrasound images in (A) short axis and (B) long axis show inverted palmaris longus *(arrows)* adjacent to extensor tendons *(T).*

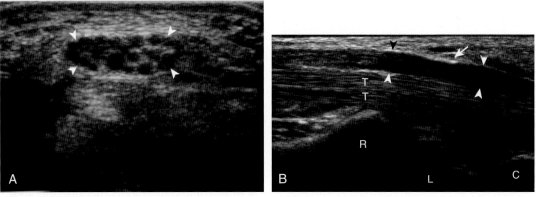

■ FIGURE 5.62 **Carpal Tunnel Syndrome.** Ultrasound images in (A) short axis and (B) long axis to the median nerve show hypoechoic nerve enlargement *(arrowheads).* Note hyperechoic flexor retinaculum immediately superficial to the median nerve in (A), and mild deviation of the median nerve *(arrow)* as it courses beneath the flexor retinaculum in (B). *C,* Capitate; *L,* lunate; *R,* radius; *T,* flexor tendons.

absence of a bifid median nerve, usually unilateral, which may simulate a prominent nerve fascicle.[78] In addition, one of the bifid median nerve trunks may take an aberrant course through the flexor digitorum superficialis musculature (Video 5.23).

After surgical carpal tunnel release for treatment of carpal tunnel syndrome, the retinaculum may be thickened or disrupted with volar displacement of the median nerve; the median nerve may return to normal size or remain enlarged regardless

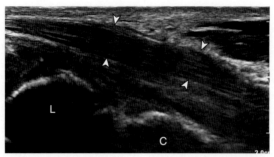

■ **FIGURE 5.63 Carpal Tunnel Syndrome.** Ultrasound image long axis to the median nerve shows hypoechoic nerve enlargement *(arrowheads)* within distal carpal tunnel. *L,* Lunate; *C,* capitate.

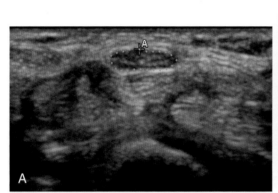
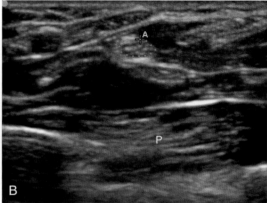

■ **FIGURE 5.64 Carpal Tunnel Syndrome: Measurement Technique.** Ultrasound images in short axis to the median nerve at the level of (A) carpal tunnel and (B) pronator quadratus *(P)* show the circumferential trace method of calculating median nerve area *(see caliper markings),* which was greater than 2 mm² difference comparing proximal to distal.

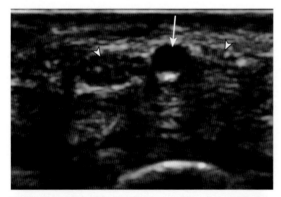

■ **FIGURE 5.65 Bifid Median Nerve and Persistent Median Artery.** Ultrasound image in short axis shows bifid median nerve *(arrowheads)* and a large persistent median artery *(arrow).*

of clinical outcome (Fig. 5.67).[79,80] After steroid injection into the carpal tunnel, the median nerve may show a decrease in size as early as 7 days after injection.[81] Uncommonly, median nerve compression in the carpal tunnel may be secondary

to extrinsic compression by a mass, ganglion cyst (Fig. 5.68), or tenosynovitis (Fig. 5.69). A rare cause of enlargement of the median nerve is *fibrolipomatous hamartoma,* in which there is diffuse fatty infiltration of the nerve separating the normal-appearing nerve fascicles (Fig. 5.70).[82]

Ulnar Tunnel Syndrome

Another less common entrapment syndrome involves the ulnar nerve in Guyon canal, called *ulnar tunnel syndrome.*[83] The cause of this syndrome is most commonly trauma. Because the hook of the hamate bone is directly deep to the ulnar nerve and artery, direct impact on the ulnar aspect of the hand can cause peripheral nerve or vascular injury, or chronic repetitive injury related to compression from the handlebar while cycling. Ulnar nerve compression may also be from an adjacent ulnar artery aneurysm (Fig. 5.71), potentially associated with ulnar artery thrombosis. At sonography, an abnormal ulnar nerve will appear hypoechoic with symptoms reproduced

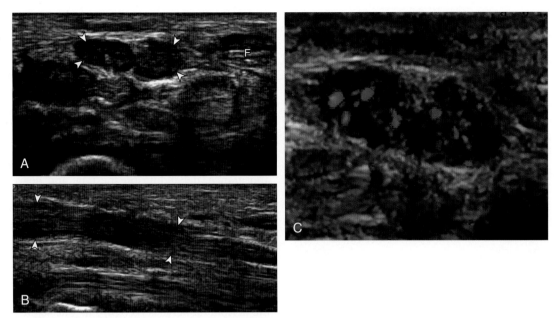

■ FIGURE 5.66 **Bifid Median Nerve and Carpal Tunnel Syndrome**. Ultrasound images in (A) short and (B) long axis show hypoechoic enlargement of each nerve trunk *(arrowheads)* with increased flow on color Doppler image (C). Note flexor carpi radialis tendon *(F)*.

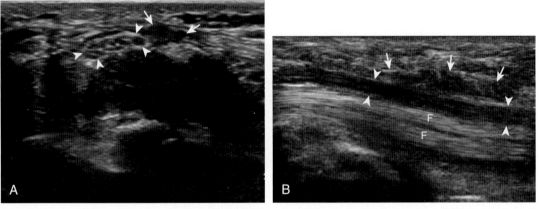

■ FIGURE 5.67 **Carpal Tunnel Syndrome: Post-Release**. Ultrasound images in (A) short axis and (B) long axis to the median nerve *(arrowheads)* in two different patients after surgical carpal tunnel release show hypoechoic thickening of the flexor retinaculum *(arrows)*. *F,* Flexor tendons.

with transducer pressure when the ulnar nerve is compressed between the transducer and the hook of the hamate bone. Ulnar artery aneurysm will appear as a heterogeneous mass in continuity with the ulnar artery, which demonstrates to-and-fro (yin-yang) flow on color Doppler imaging. No flow may be present with thrombosis. There exists a related entity called *hypothenar hammer syndrome*, in which direct trauma results in ulnar artery thrombosis or aneurysm and distal emboli to the digits, causing vascular insufficiency (Fig. 5.72).[84,85] Other causes of ulnar tunnel syndrome include

vascular abnormalities, mass, and ganglion cyst. The ulnar nerve may also be compressed by an accessory abductor digiti minimi muscle, a normal variant seen in up to 24% of the population, which is typically located superficial to the ulnar nerve and vessels although variability exists (Fig. 5.73).[65]

Radial Nerve Compression

The superficial branch of the radial nerve is located in the superficial and radial aspect of the mid-forearm. As the nerve continues distally, it crosses over the radial aspect of the forearm and the extensor pollicis brevis and abductor pollicis longus muscles. More distally, the superficial branch of the radial nerve continues into the dorsal wrist superficial to the extensor retinaculum.

Compression of the superficial branch of the radial nerve may occur in the distal forearm, called *Wartenberg syndrome*, and can be caused by hematoma or nerve injury at an intravenous catheter site given close proximity to the cephalic vein. Involvement from a mass or scar tissue is also possible (Fig. 5.74) (Video 5.24).[63,83]

Transection Neuromas

Injury to a peripheral nerve may have a variable appearance, depending on the type and degree of injury.[86] After complete nerve transection, a neuroma may develop as the normal response of a transected nerve attempting to regenerate, which results in a tangled area of nerve fibers and scar tissue.[87] At sonography, a neuroma will appear as a heterogeneous but predominantly hypoechoic mass (Fig. 5.75). Its appearance is not specific until continuity between the mass and the peripheral nerve is recognized. The segment of peripheral nerve that enters into the neuroma is often abnormally hypoechoic, which aids in its

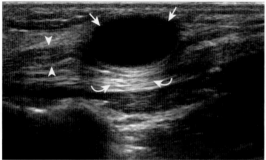

■ **FIGURE 5.68 Carpal Tunnel Syndrome: Ganglion Cyst.** Ultrasound image in long axis to the median nerve *(arrowheads)* shows an anechoic ganglion cyst *(arrows)* with increased through-transmission *(curved arrows)*.

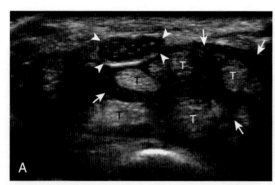
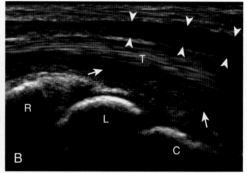

■ **FIGURE 5.69 Carpal Tunnel Syndrome: Tenosynovitis.** Ultrasound images in (A) short axis and (B) long axis to the median nerve show hypoechoic nerve enlargement *(arrowheads)*. Note hypoechoic synovial hypertrophy *(arrows)* surrounding the flexor tendons *(T)*. *C*, Capitate; *L*, lunate; *R*, radius.

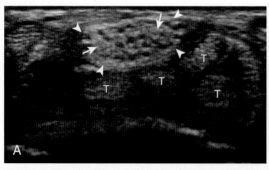
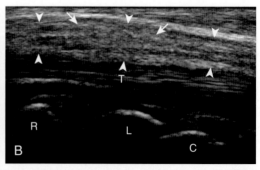

■ **FIGURE 5.70 Fibrolipomatous Hamartoma of the Median Nerve.** Ultrasound images in (A) short axis and (B) long axis to the median nerve *(arrowheads)* show hyperechoic fibrofatty tissue *(arrows)* interspersed between the hypoechoic nerve fascicles. *C*, Capitate; *L*, lunate; *R*, radius; *T*, flexor tendons.

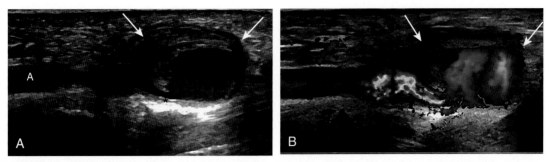

■ **FIGURE 5.71 Aneurysm: Ulnar Artery**. Ultrasound image (A) in long axis to the ulnar artery shows heterogeneous aneurysmal enlargement *(arrows)* continuous with the ulnar artery *(A)*. Note to-and-fro flow pattern on (B) color Doppler image.

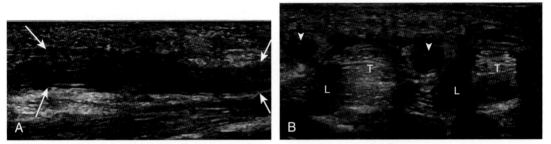

■ **FIGURE 5.72 Hypothenar Hammer Syndrome**. Ultrasound images in long axis (A) to ulnar artery shows non-compressible hypoechoic thrombus. Note distal thrombosis of common digital arteries *(arrowheads)* in (B). *T*, Flexor digitorum tendons; *L*, lumbricals.

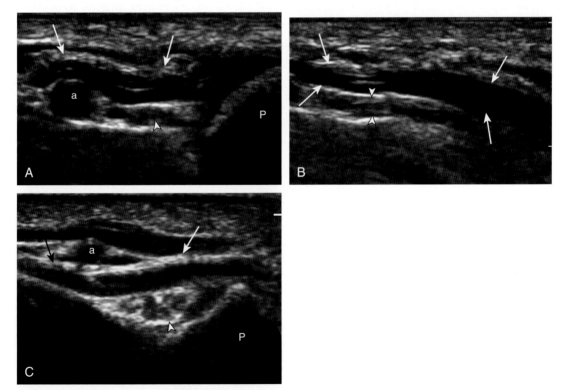

■ **FIGURE 5.73 Accessory Abductor Digiti Minimi**. Ultrasound images in (A) short axis and (B) long axis to the ulnar nerve *(arrowheads)* show the hypoechoic muscle *(arrows)* of the accessory abductor digiti minimi. Ultrasound image from a different patient (C) shows accessory abductor digiti minimi interposed between ulnar artery *(a)* and ulnar nerve *(arrowheads)*. *P*, Pisiform.

identification, in addition to referable symptoms with transducer pressure.

■ LIGAMENT AND OSSEOUS ABNORMALITIES

Scapholunate Ligament Injury

Acute trauma and repetitive overuse conditions may cause abnormalities to the wrist ligaments, cartilage, and adjacent osseous structures. With regard to the interosseous wrist ligaments, the scapholunate ligament is one of many important stabilizing structures. Normally, a ligament has a hyperechoic and fibrillar echotexture, more compact than that of tendon, which connects bone to bone. An abnormal ligament may appear hypoechoic and thickened if partially torn, or it may not be visible, possibly replaced with anechoic

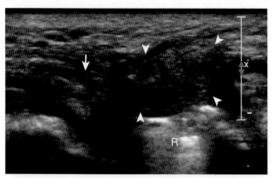

■ **FIGURE 5.74 Radial Nerve, Superficial Branch: Scar Tissue.** Ultrasound image shows the superficial branch of the radial nerve in long axis *(arrow)* entering into hypoechoic scar tissue and hematoma *(arrowheads)* after surgical repair of distal radius *(R)* fracture.

fluid or hypoechoic synovitis when completely torn (Fig. 5.76).[20,88] The space between the lunate and scaphoid bones may also be increased, which may further increase with clenched-fist maneuver or ulnar and radial deviation. The volar aspect of the scapholunate ligament, as well as the volar and dorsal aspects of the lunotriquetral ligaments, may also be evaluated.[2] In addition to the interosseous ligaments of the wrist, other intrinsic and extrinsic capsular ligaments may also be evaluated for injury or abnormality, such as the dorsal radiocarpal (or dorsal radiotriquetral) ligament, which lies dorsal and superficial to the scapholunate ligament (Fig. 5.77).

Ulnar Collateral Ligament Injury (Thumb)

In addition to the wrist ligaments, the collateral ligaments of the digits may also be evaluated for tear. One specific ligament, the ulnar collateral ligament of the first metacarpophalangeal joint, deserves emphasis because of important surgical implications.[21,89] This injury has been historically termed *gamekeeper's thumb* because the injury occurred in hunters when breaking the neck of a rabbit. More currently, this injury is called *skier's thumb*, but can occur with any abduction injury. Similar to other ligament injuries, an abnormal ulnar collateral ligament may appear hypoechoic with increased thickness (Fig. 5.78A) and possible partial (Fig. 5.78B) or complete (Fig. 5.79) ligament discontinuity with the adjacent phalanx.[90] Differentiation between a partial tear and non-displaced full-thickness tear is extremely difficult; however, the primary goal is to identify a displaced full-thickness ulnar collateral ligament tear (or Stener lesion).[21] Visualization of an echogenic

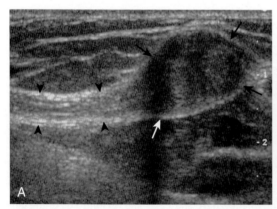
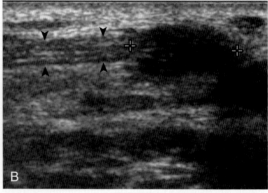

■ **FIGURE 5.75 Transection Neuromas.** Ultrasound images of the long axis to the (A) ulnar nerve and the (B) median nerve in two patients show heterogeneous but predominantly hypoechoic neuroma formation *(arrows in A; between cursors in B)*. Note continuity with the respective nerve *(arrowheads)*.

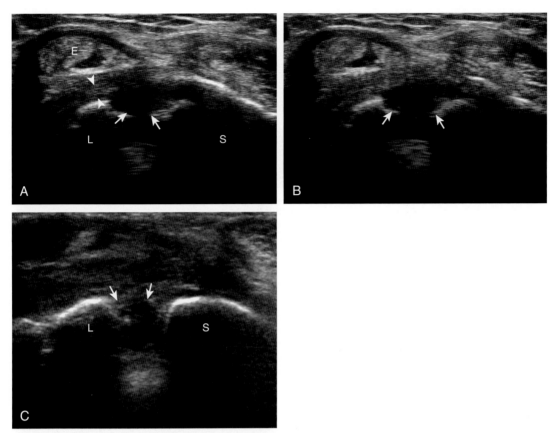

■ FIGURE 5.76 **Scapholunate Ligament Tear.** Ultrasound images transverse over the dorsal wrist at the level of the proximal carpal row (A) without and (B) with the clench fist maneuver show abnormal hypoechogenicity *(arrows)* at the expected site of the scapholunate ligament *(arrowheads,* dorsal radiocarpal ligament). Note widening of the scapholunate distance between A and B. An ultrasound image over the volar wrist (C) shows partial hypoechoic scapholunate ligament disruption. *E,* Extensor digitorum; *L,* lunate; *S,* scaphoid.

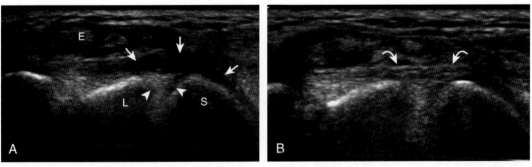

■ FIGURE 5.77 **Dorsal Radiocarpal Ligament: Tear.** Transverse ultrasound image (A) over the dorsal wrist shows hypoechoic disruption of the dorsal radiocarpal (or radiotriquetral) ligament *(arrows)* seen in long axis. Note the normal scapholunate ligament *(arrowheads)* and (B) normal contralateral side *(curved arrows)*. *E,* Extensor digitorum; *L,* lunate; *S,* scaphoid.

avulsion fracture fragment may be a clue to full-thickness tear. Gentle valgus stress of the first metacarpophalangeal joint under ultrasound observation may help demonstrate a full-thickness ligament tear and retraction if fluid is identified entering into the torn ligament gap (Video 5.25).

A Stener lesion represents a distal full-thickness ulnar collateral ligament tear of the first metacarpophalangeal joint, which is displaced proximal to the adductor pollicis aponeurosis (Fig. 5.80).[21,89] In this situation, the ligament will not heal spontaneously, and therefore surgery is indicated

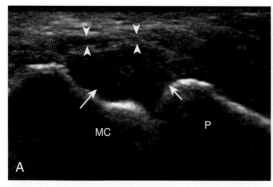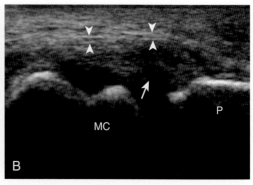

■ **FIGURE 5.78 Ulnar Collateral Ligament of the First Metacarpophalangeal Joint: Sprain and Partial Tear.** Ultrasound images in long axis to the ulnar collateral ligament in two different patients show (A) diffuse hypoechoic swelling with intact fibers *(arrows)* and (B) a focal anechoic partial-thickness tear *(arrow)*. Note the intact adductor pollicis aponeurosis *(arrowheads)*. *MC,* Metacarpal; *P,* proximal phalanx.

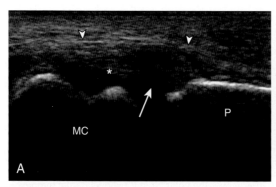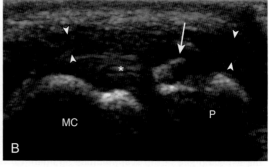

■ **FIGURE 5.79 Ulnar Collateral Ligament of the First Metacarpophalangeal Joint: Full-Thickness Tear and Avulsion.** Ultrasound images from two different patients in long axis to the ulnar collateral ligament *(asterisk)* show (A) nondisplaced full-thickness tear *(arrow)*, and (B) retraction of distal avulsion fracture fragment *(arrow)*. Note adductor aponeurosis *(arrowheads),* normal in (A) and injured in (B) appearing hypoechoic and thickened. *MC,* Metacarpal; *P,* proximal phalanx.

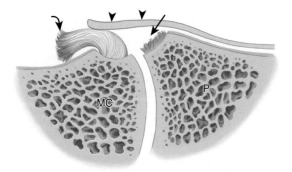

■ **FIGURE 5.80 Stener Lesion.** Illustration shows a distal full-thickness tear of the ulnar collateral ligament *(arrow)* with displacement *(curved arrow)* proximal to the metacarpophalangeal joint and adductor pollicis aponeurosis *(arrowheads)*. *MC,* Metacarpal; *P,* proximal phalanx. *(Modified from an illustration by Carolyn Nowak, Ann Arbor, Michigan; http://www.carolync-nowak.com/MedTech.html.)*

to avoid chronic instability. At ultrasound, the Stener lesion will appear as a hypoechoic but heterogeneous, round, mass-like structure located proximal to the metacarpophalangeal joint in the plane of the normal (proper) ulnar collateral ligament (Fig. 5.81) (Videos 5.25 and 5.26).[21] Shadowing is often present deep to the Stener lesion related to sound beam refraction at the torn ligament end. In addition, normal ligament fibers are absent in their expected location crossing the first metacarpophalangeal joint. A hyperechoic and possibly shadowing focus attached to the retracted ligament distally is characteristic of a bone avulsion (Fig. 5.81C). The ultrasound appearance of a Stener lesion has been likened to a yo-yo on a string, similar to findings on magnetic resonance imaging.[91] The string of the yo-yo represents the adductor pollicis aponeurosis, and the yo-yo represents the balled-up and displaced proximal portion of the ulnar collateral ligament. Although the shape of the Stener lesion can be round, oval, or elongated (Fig. 5.81B), the position of the displaced ligament is proximal to the leading edge of or possibly superficial to the adductor pollicis aponeurosis (Fig. 5.81A).[21] Flexion of the interphalangeal joint will cause the adductor pollicis aponeurosis to slide over the ulnar collateral ligament, which assists in its identification and differentiation from the adjacent Stener lesion (Videos 5.25 and 5.26). The adductor pollicis aponeurosis may be hypoechoic and thickened from injury as well (Fig. 5.82) (Video 5.27).

Other Ligament Injuries

Other collateral ligaments may be evaluated for tear, such as the radial collateral ligament of the thumb (Fig. 5.83). A hyperechoic bone fragment at a joint but not at the attachment of a ligament could relate to capsular (Fig. 5.84A) or volar plate (Fig. 5.84B) avulsion fracture. Cortical irregularity at a ligament attachment is not always due to trauma, and in the correct clinical setting, a

seronegative spondyloarthropathy should be considered. Ultrasound findings in this scenario, such as psoriatic arthritis, include cortical irregularity or erosions and bone proliferation at a ligament attachment site (termed *enthesitis*) with flow on color Doppler imaging and hypoechoic enlargement of the adjacent ligament (Fig. 5.85)

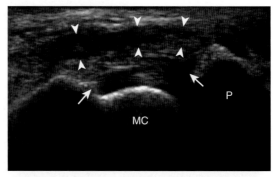

■ FIGURE 5.82 **Adductor Aponeurosis: Tear.** Ultrasound image in long axis to the ulnar collateral ligament of the first metacarpophalangeal joint shows markedly hypoechoic and thickened adductor aponeurosis *(arrowheads)* with normal ulnar collateral ligament *(arrows)*. *MC*, Metacarpal; *P*, proximal phalanx.

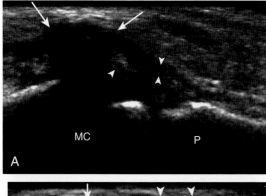

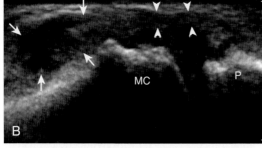

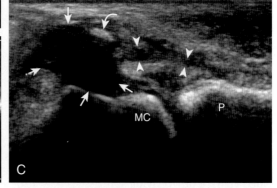

■ FIGURE 5.81 **Stener Lesion.** Ultrasound images in long axis to the ulnar collateral ligament of the first metacarpophalangeal joint in three different patients (A to C) show full-thickness tear of the ulnar collateral ligament with proximal displacement (Stener lesion) *(arrows)*. Note the adductor pollicis aponeurosis *(arrowheads)* (abnormally hypoechoic from injury) creating a yo-yo on a string appearance. Also note (C) hyperechoic avulsion fracture fragment *(curved arrow)*. *MC*, Metacarpal; *P*, proximal phalanx.

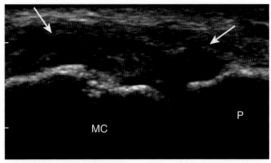

■ **FIGURE 5.83 Radial Collateral Ligament: Tear.** Ultrasound image in long axis to the radial collateral ligament of the first metacarpophalangeal joint shows abnormal hypoechogenicity *(arrows)* without visible ligament fibers. *MC*, Metacarpal; *P*, proximal phalanx.

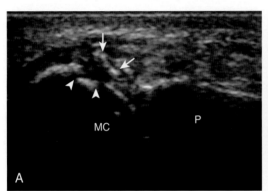
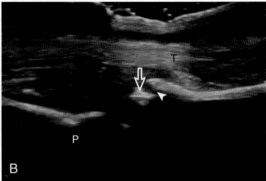

■ **FIGURE 5.84 Cortical Avulsion Fractures.** Ultrasound images from two different patients show (A) fracture fragment *(arrows)* at volar capsule attachment with donor site *(arrowheads)* from metacarpal *(MC)*, and (B) fracture fragment *(open arrow)* at volar plate attachment from base of middle phalanx *(arrowhead)*. *P*, Proximal phalanx; *T*, flexor tendons.

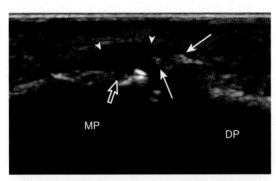

■ **FIGURE 5.85 Enthesopathy: Psoriatic Arthritis.** Ultrasound image in coronal plane at distal interphalangeal joint shows abnormal hypoechoic ulnar collateral ligament *(arrowheads)* with erosion *(open arrow)* and bone proliferation *(arrows)*. *MP*, Middle phalanx; *DP*, distal phalanx.

(Video 5.28). The overlying soft tissues may also be thickened and hypoechoic.

Ligament abnormalities of the wrist may be associated with triangular fibrocartilage abnormalities, often associated with ulnar-sided wrist pain.

Although often difficult to evaluate comprehensively with ultrasound, abnormalities of the triangular fibrocartilage will appear as abnormal hypoechogenicity, thinning, or absence (Fig. 5.86).[3,92] The radial attachment of the triangular fibrocartilage is often difficult to evaluate but must be identified to ensure complete evaluation.

An additional ligamentous-like abnormality involves the interosseous membrane between the radius and ulna of the forearm. This complex structure is comprised of a large main fiber bundle, a proximal dorsal oblique bundle, several accessory bundles, and a distal membranous portion.[93] Sonographic evaluation of the interosseous membrane begins in the transverse plane of the dorsal midforearm, and the transducer is angled slightly distally toward the ulna to elongate the interosseous membrane fibers. With injury of the interosseous membrane, the normally thin and hyperechoic appearance is replaced with hypoechoic thickening or disruption and nonvisualization (Fig. 5.87).[94] Interosseous membrane injury is an important component of the *Essex-Lopresti injury*, in which a comminuted radial head fracture at the elbow

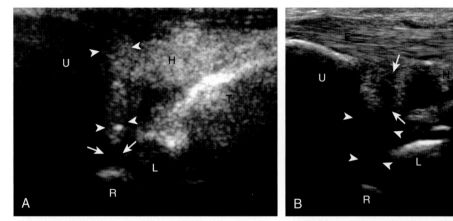

■ FIGURE 5.86 **Triangular Fibrocartilage Tears.** Ultrasound images in coronal plane at the ulnar aspect of the wrist from two different patients show abnormal hypoechogenicity *(arrows)* of the triangular fibrocartilage *(arrowheads)*. Note meniscus homologue *(H)*. *E*, Extensor carpi ulnaris tendon; *L*, lunate; *R*, radius; *T*, triquetrum; *U*, ulna.

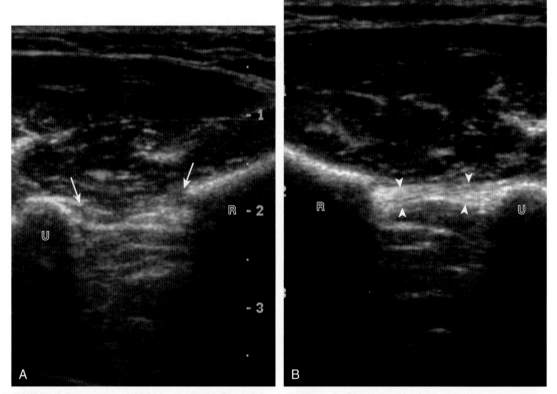

■ FIGURE 5.87 **Interosseous Membrane Tear: Essex-Lopresti Injury.** A, Oblique-transverse ultrasound image over the dorsal midforearm shows no identifiable interosseous membrane *(between arrows)*. B, Note the normal appearance in the contralateral asymptomatic forearm *(arrowheads)*. *R*, Radius; *U*, ulna.

is associated with interosseous membrane injury and distal radioulnar joint disruption.[95]

Osseous Injury

Injury to bone can be visible at sonography if a fracture extends to the visible portion of the bone cortex, commonly creating cortical disruption and

a step-off deformity or an avulsion fracture fragment (see Fig. 5.84). The finding of the focal cortical step-off deformity is fairly specific for fracture, which is unlike the cortical irregularity at the margin of a joint with osteoarthritis from an osteophyte, although correlation with radiography is essential. Hyperemia, adjacent hypoechoic soft tissue swelling, and point tenderness with transducer pressure are other important associated findings of fracture. Although fractures may occur anywhere in the hand and wrist, it is the scaphoid fracture that receives much attention because a nontreated scaphoid fracture may result in nonunion and osteonecrosis of the proximal scaphoid pole. If history of trauma and snuffbox tenderness, the scaphoid bone should be evaluated

for a cortical step-off deformity and adjacent soft tissue hematoma, which could indicate fracture (Fig. 5.88).[96] Small avulsion fractures of the hand and wrist are seen at tendon and ligament insertions and appear as focal hyperechoic, possibly shadowing foci.

GANGLION CYST

Most wrist masses are benign and are most commonly ganglion cysts. Although the cause of ganglion cysts is uncertain, they may be degenerative, related to prior injury, or idiopathic. At sonography, a ganglion cyst most commonly appears multilocular, hypoechoic or anechoic, and non-compressible (Figs. 5.89 and 5.90).[23,97-99] Increased through-transmission may be absent when the fluid locules are small.[99] Less commonly, a ganglion cyst may appear as a unilocular anechoic simple cyst and increased through-transmission.[23,97,99] Given this somewhat variable appearance of wrist ganglion cysts, it is the location of the presumed ganglion that becomes very important in consideration of the correct diagnosis. Many ganglion cysts are located dorsal, adjacent to the scapholunate ligament (Fig. 5.89).[23] A dorsal ganglion cyst should be differentiated from a distended dorsal wrist joint recess as both have similar anatomic locations; with wrist

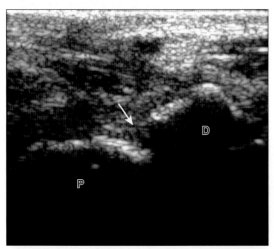

■ **FIGURE 5.88 Scaphoid Fracture.** Ultrasound image over the volar wrist in long axis to the scaphoid shows a cortical step-off deformity *(arrow)* and discontinuity. *D,* Distal pole of scaphoid; *P,* proximal pole of scaphoid.

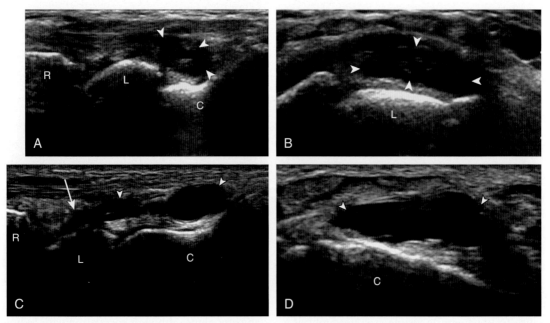

■ **FIGURE 5.89 Ganglion Cysts: Dorsal.** Dorsal ultrasound images in sagittal and transverse over the lunate *(L)* in two different patients show hypoechoic (A, B) and anechoic (C, D) multilocular ganglion cysts *(arrowheads)*. Note communication to radiocarpal joint *(arrow)* and increased through-transmission. *C,* Capitate; *R,* radius.

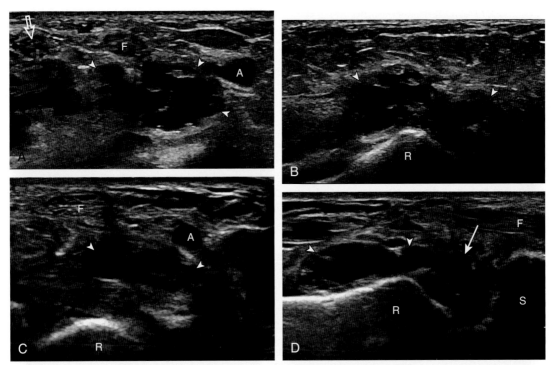

■ **FIGURE 5.90 Ganglion Cysts: Volar.** Ultrasound images transverse between the radial artery *(A)* and flexor carpi radialis tendon *(F)* and sagittal over the distal radius *(R)* in two different patients (A, B) and (C, D) show an anechoic multilocular ganglion cysts *(arrowheads)* with increased through-transmission. Note median nerve *(arrowhead)* in (A) and communication to radiocarpal joint *(arrow)* in (B).

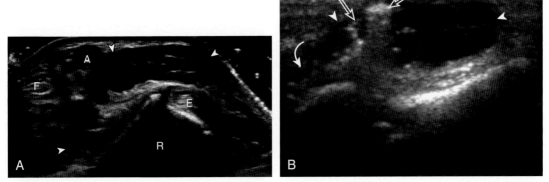

■ **FIGURE 5.91 Ganglion Cysts: Volar.** Ultrasound images transverse between the radial artery *(A)* and flexor carpi radialis tendon *(F)* in two different patients show multilocular ganglion cysts (A) extending over first extensor wrist compartment *(arrowheads)*, and (B) containing hyperechoic gas *(open arrows)*. E, First extensor wrist compartment.

movement or transducer pressure, a joint recess typically collapses, whereas a ganglion cyst is non-compressible (see Fig. 5.19) (Videos 5.29 and 5.30).[23] Another very common and often underreported site for ganglion cysts is volar, between the radial artery and the flexor carpi radialis tendon, originating from the radiocarpal joint between the radius and scaphoid and extending proximally (Fig. 5.90) (Video 5.31). A volar ganglion cyst may extend volar toward the median nerve or dorsal over the first extensor wrist compartment (Fig. 5.91A) and uncommonly contain echogenic gas from radiocarpal vacuum joint gas (Fig. 5.91B). A volar ganglion cyst may also displace (Fig. 5.92A)

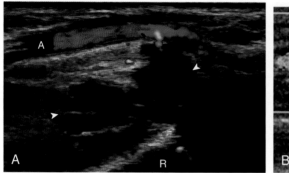
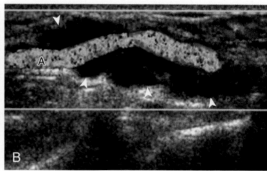

■ FIGURE 5.92 **Ganglion Cysts: Volar.** Ultrasound color Doppler images in long axis to the radial artery *(A)* in two different patients show multilocular anechoic septated ganglion cysts *(arrowheads)* that (A) displace and (B) encompass the radial artery. *R,* Radius.

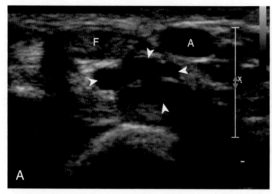
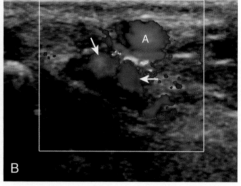

■ FIGURE 5.93 **Ganglion Cyst: Artifactual Flow.** Ultrasound (A) gray-scale and (B) color Doppler images in short axis to the radial artery show an anechoic septated ganglion cyst *(arrowheads).* Note the artifactual flow in the ganglion cyst *(arrows)* in (B) from pulsation of the adjacent radial artery *(A). F,* Flexor carpi radialis tendon.

or encompass (Fig. 5.92B) the adjacent radial artery. Pulsation from the adjacent radial artery may cause artifactual flow within the ganglion cyst and simulate internal flow on color Doppler imaging (Fig. 5.93). Volar ganglion cysts may be small and nonpalpable, but symptomatic regardless; therefore, imaging between the radial artery and flexor carpi radialis tendons in addition to over the scapholunate ligament should be part of a scanning routine for wrist pain. A ganglion cyst may occur elsewhere in the wrist and hand and may cause carpal tunnel syndrome (see Fig. 5.68) and trigger finger (see Fig. 5.58B). Any visible connection between a ganglion cyst and joint or tendon sheath should be described as this information is relevant when a ganglion cyst is treated. Percutaneous ultrasound-guided aspiration and steroid injection have been shown to be effective in the treatment of wrist ganglion cysts.[100, 101] An additional cyst that may be confused with a ganglion cyst is a *mucous cyst,* which originates from a degenerative distal interphalangeal joint and commonly extends toward the nail bed (Fig. 5.94).[102]

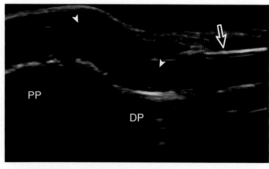

■ FIGURE 5.94 **Mucous Cyst.** Ultrasound image sagittal over the dorsal thumb shows anechoic multilocular mucous cyst *(arrowheads)* extending distally from the distal interphalangeal joint. Note nail *(open arrow). PP,* Proximal phalanx; *DP,* distal phalanx.

■ OTHER MASSES
Giant Cell Tumor of the Tendon Sheath and Similar Masses

If a solid mass is in contact with a tendon, a giant cell tumor of the tendon sheath (also called

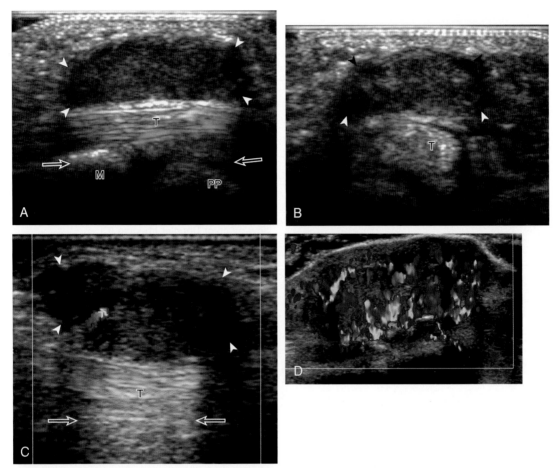

■ **FIGURE 5.95 Giant Cell Tumor of the Tendon Sheath.** Long axis (A) and short axis (B) ultrasound images show uniformly heterogeneous but predominantly hypoechoic soft tissue mass *(arrowheads)* with increased through-transmission *(open arrows)*. Long axis color Doppler images from two different patients (C and D) show similar findings with variable flow. *M*, Metacarpal; *PP*, proximal phalanx; *T*, flexor tendon.

pigmented villonodular tenosynovitis) should be strongly considered (Video 5.32).[103-105] This hypoechoic solid mass is in contact with the tendon sheath, most commonly the flexor tendons of the first through third digits but does not move with tendon translation (Fig. 5.95). Increased through-transmission may be present, as with other solid masses, and may initially be misinterpreted as a hypoechoic complex cyst; however, internal flow on color or power Doppler imaging indicates a solid mass. Another solid mass of the digit that may appear similar is a fibroma of the tendon sheath (Fig. 5.96).[106] Because solid masses are not specific for one diagnosis, pathologic confirmation is necessary.

Dupuytren Contracture

Patients with this fibrosing condition present with a palpable mass or nodularity superficial to the flexor tendons of the hand caused by thickening of the palmar aponeurosis, which can result in contracture.[107] At ultrasound, nodular or cord-like hypoechoic masses are seen superficial and parallel to one or more of the flexor tendons (Fig. 5.97).[108] Uncommonly, other soft tissue pathology may appear similar, such as a ruptured epidermal inclusion cyst (Fig. 5.98).[109,110] A condition called *knuckle pads* is associated with Dupuytren contracture, causing hypoechoic subcutaneous soft tissue thickening dorsally superficial to the proximal interphalangeal or less commonly metacarpophalangeal joints (Fig. 5.99).[111]

Glomus Tumor

A glomus tumor arises from a neuromyoarterial glomus body, most commonly beneath the nail or about the distal aspect of the digit. Clinically, this tumor may present with pain, point tenderness, and sensitivity to cold exposure. At ultrasound, a glomus tumor will appear as a

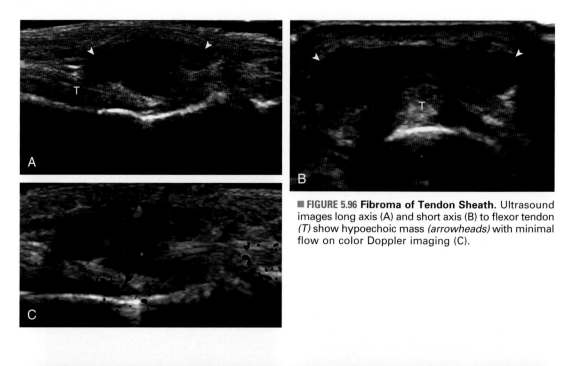

■ **FIGURE 5.96 Fibroma of Tendon Sheath.** Ultrasound images long axis (A) and short axis (B) to flexor tendon *(T)* show hypoechoic mass *(arrowheads)* with minimal flow on color Doppler imaging (C).

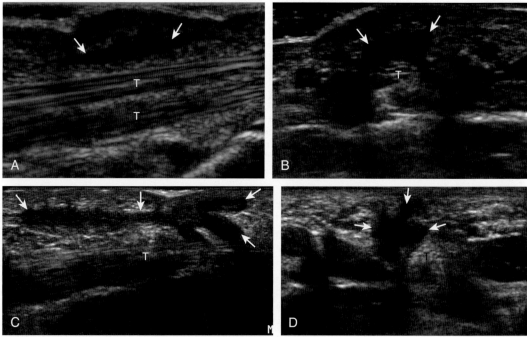

■ **FIGURE 5.97 Dupuytren Contracture (Palmar Fibromatosis).** Ultrasound images in two different patients (A and B, C and D) in long axis and short axis to the flexor tendons *(T)* show hypoechoic mass-like thickening of the palmar fascia *(arrows)*.

focal hypoechoic mass with hyperemia, increased through-transmission, and possible cortical bone remodeling (Fig. 5.100) (Video 5.33).[112] Because the imaging appearance is not specific for one diagnosis, it is the location of the abnormality that is important in suggesting the correct diagnosis.

Miscellaneous Masses

Although most solid masses are not specific for one diagnosis at ultrasound, associated imaging features may allow a precise diagnosis in some cases. For example, continuity between a mass and

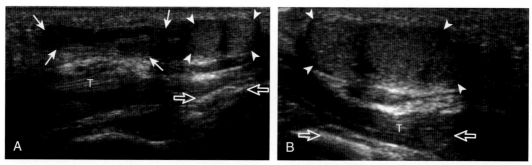

■ **FIGURE 5.98 Epidermal Inclusion Cyst: Rupture.** Ultrasound images (A and B) over the palmar aspect of the hand show an epidermal inclusion cyst *(arrowheads)* as a low-level homogeneous echo and posterior through-transmission *(open arrows)* with adjacent hypoechogenicity *(arrows)* from rupture. *T,* Flexor tendon.

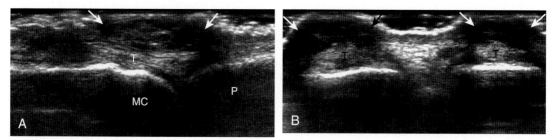

■ **FIGURE 5.99 Knuckle Pads.** Ultrasound images in long axis (A) and short axis (B) to the extensor tendons *(T)* show superficial dorsal soft tissue thickening. *MC,* Metacarpal; *P,* proximal phalanx.

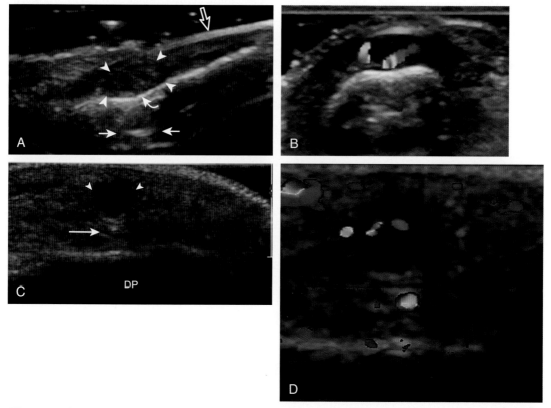

■ **FIGURE 5.100 Glomus Tumor.** Ultrasound images (A) sagittal and (B) transverse over dorsal distal finger and nail *(open arrow)* show hypoechoic glomus tumor *(arrowheads)* with increased through-transmission *(arrows)* and bone remodeling of the distal phalanx *(curved arrows).* Note increased flow in (B). Sagittal gray scale (C) and color Doppler (D) images over the volar distal phalanx *(DP)* pulp in a different patient show hypoechoic glomus tumor *(arrowheads)* with increased through-transmission *(arrows)* and hyperemia (*between cursors* in A).

peripheral nerve is consistent with a peripheral nerve sheath tumor or a nerve transection neuroma (see Chapter 2). If a heterogeneous mass shows typical to-and-fro yin-yang flow on color Doppler imaging and there is continuity with a vascular structure, then pseudoaneurysm is the likely diagnosis. Other tumors may involve the hand and the wrist, including benign tumors such as soft tissue chondromas and malignant tumors such as sarcomas. Retained soft tissue foreign bodies may produce a mass-like appearance (see Chapter 2).

SELECT REFERENCES

5. Boutry N, Titecat M, Demondion X, et al: High-frequency ultrasonographic examination of the finger pulley system. *J Ultrasound Med* 24(10):1333–1339, 2005.

8. Boutry N, Larde A, Demondion X, et al: Meta-carpophalangeal joints at US in asymptomatic volunteers and cadaveric specimens. *Radiology* 232(3):716–724, 2004.

16. Chiavaras MM, Jacobson JA, Yablon CM, et al: Pitfalls in wrist and hand ultrasound. *AJR Am J Roentgenol* 203(3):531–540, 2014.

21. Melville D, Jacobson JA, Haase S, et al: Ultrasound of displaced ulnar collateral ligament tears of the thumb: the Stener lesion revisited. *Skeletal Radiol* 42(5):667–673, 2013.

28. Lund PJ, Heikal A, Maricic MJ, et al: Ultraso-nographic imaging of the hand and wrist in rheumatoid arthritis. *Skeletal Radiol* 24(8):591–596, 1995.

41. Kaeley GS: Review of the use of ultrasound for the diagnosis and monitoring of enthesitis in psoriatic arthritis. *Curr Rheumatol Rep* 13(4):338–345, 2011.

43. Thiele RG: Role of ultrasound and other advanced imaging in the diagnosis and management of gout. *Curr Rheumatol Rep* 13(2):146–153, 2011.

50. Lee KH, Kang CN, Lee BG, et al: Ultrasono-graphic evaluation of the first extensor compartment of the wrist in de Quervain's disease. *J Orthop Sci* 19(1):49–54, 2014.

57. Klauser A, Frauscher F, Bodner G, et al: Finger pulley injuries in extreme rock climbers: depiction with dynamic US. *Radiology* 222(3):755–761, 2002.

66. Peetrons PA, Derbali W: Carpal tunnel syndrome. *Semin Musculoskelet Radiol* 17(1):28–33, 2013.

83. Jacobson JA, Fessell DP, Lobo Lda G, et al: Entrapment neuropathies I: upper limb (carpal tunnel excluded). *Semin Musculoskelet Radiol* 14(5):473–486, 2010.

99. Wang G, Jacobson JA, Feng FY, et al: Sonography of wrist ganglion cysts: variable and noncystic appearances. *J Ultrasound Med* 26(10):1323–1328, 2007. [quiz 30-1].

102. Baek HJ, Lee SJ, Cho KH, et al: Subungual tumors: clinicopathologic correlation with US and MR imaging findings. *Radiographics* 30(6):2010, 1621-1636.

108. Murphey MD, Ruble CM, Tyszko SM, et al: From the archives of the AFIP: musculoskeletal fibromatoses: radiologic-pathologic correlation. *Radiographics* 29(7):2143–2173, 2009.

The complete references for this chapter can be found on *www.expertconsult.com.*

HIP AND THIGH ULTRASOUND

■ HIP AND THIGH ANATOMY

The hip joint is a synovial articulation between the acetabulum of the pelvis and the proximal femur. The joint recess extends from the acetabulum over the femur to the level of the intertrochanteric line, just beyond the femoral neck. The joint capsule becomes thickened from the iliofemoral, ischiofemoral, and pubofemoral ligaments (Fig. 6.1), and a reflection of the joint capsule extends proximally along the femoral neck.[1] The femoral head is covered by hyaline cartilage, whereas the acetabulum is lined by hyaline cartilage in an inverted U shape with a fibrocartilage labrum attached to the acetabular rim.

Several muscles originate from the pelvis and extend across the hip joint, and others originate from the femur itself. Muscles that originate from the posterior surface of the ilium are the gluteus minimus (which inserts on the anterior facet of the greater trochanter), the gluteus medius (which inserts on the lateral and superoposterior facets of the greater trochanter), and the gluteus maximus (which inserts on the posterior femur gluteal tuberosity below the trochanters and iliotibial tract) (Figs. 6.2 and 6.3).[2] Posteriorly, the piriformis originates from the sacrum and extends inferior and lateral to insert onto the greater trochanter. Other muscles inferior to the piriformis that extend from the pelvis to the proximal femur include the superior gemellus, obturator internus, inferior gemellus, obturator externus, and quadratus femoris.[3]

At the anterior aspect of the hip joint, the iliopsoas can be seen as a continuation of the iliacus and psoas major, which inserts on the lesser trochanter, although the anatomy is complex with independent muscle bundles.[4] Other anterior muscles include the sartorius (which originates from the anterior superior iliac spine of the pelvis and inserts on the medial aspect of the proximal tibia) and the tensor fasciae latae (which originates from the posterolateral aspect of the ilium and inserts on the iliotibial tract, which, in turn, inserts on the proximal tibia) (Fig. 6.4). The rectus femoris has two origins: a direct or straight head, which originates from the anterior inferior iliac spine; and an indirect or reflected head, which originates inferior and posterior to the anterior inferior iliac spine from the superior acetabular ridge.[5] Distally in the thigh, the direct tendon forms an anterior superficial tendon with unipennate architecture, whereas the indirect tendon forms the central tendon with bipennate architecture.[6] The rectus femoris distally combines with the vastus medialis, vastus lateralis, and vastus intermedius musculature (which all originate from the femur) to form the quadriceps tendon, which

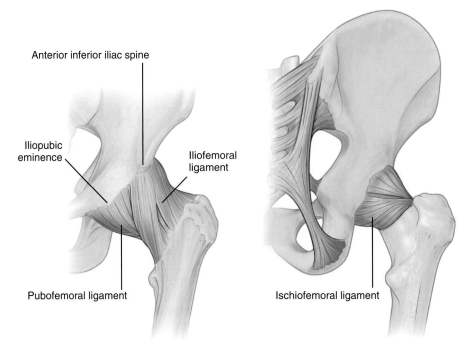

Anterior inferior iliac spine

Iliopubic
eminence

Iliofemoral
ligament

Pubofemoral ligament

Ischiofemoral ligament

■ **FIGURE 6.1 Hip Joint Anatomy**. Anterior and posterior views show the hip joint ligaments. *(From Drake R, Vogl W, Mitchell A: Gray's Anatomy for Students, Philadelphia, 2005, Churchill Livingstone.)*

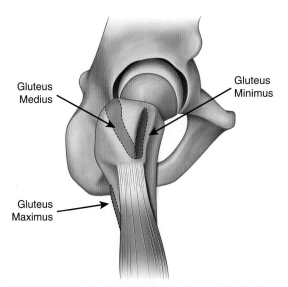

Gluteus
Medius

Gluteus
Minimus

Gluteus
Maximus

■ **FIGURE 6.2 Greater Trochanter Anatomy**. Lateral view of greater trochanter shows attachments of gluteal tendons. *(Illustration by Danielle Dobbs, Ann Arbor, Michigan.)*

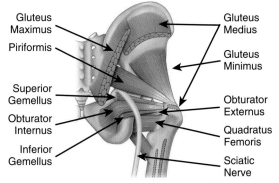

Gluteus
Maximus

Piriformis

Superior
Gemellus

Obturator
Internus

Inferior
Gemellus

Gluteus
Medius

Gluteus
Minimus

Obturator
Externus

Quadratus
Femoris

Sciatic
Nerve

■ **FIGURE 6.3 Posterior Hip Anatomy**. Posterior view shows gluteal muscles and external rotators of the hip and sciatic nerve. *(Illustration by Danielle Dobbs, Ann Arbor, Michigan.)*

inserts on the patella with superficial fibers continuing distally over the patella (termed the *prepatellar quadriceps continuation*) to the tibial tuberosity by way of the patellar tendon.[7]

Medially, the adductor musculature includes the adductor longus, the adductor brevis, and the adductor magnus, which originate from the ischium and pubis of the pelvis and insert on the femur at the linea aspera and, in the case of the adductor magnus, the adductor tubercle as well. Superficial and medial to the adductors, the gracilis muscle extends from the inferior pubic ramus to the proximal tibia as part of the pes anserinus.

The posterior thigh musculature, from medially to laterally, consists of the semimembranosus, the semitendinosus (both of which originate from the ischial tuberosity and insert on the proximal tibia, with the semitendinosus being part of the pes anserinus), and the biceps femoris (with long head

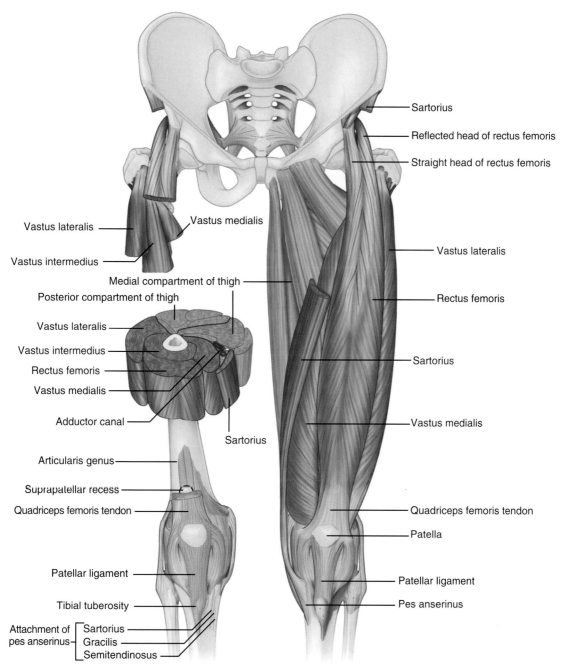

Sartorius

Reflected head of rectus femoris

Straight head of rectus femoris

Vastus medialis

Vastus lateralis

Vastus intermedius

Vastus lateralis

Rectus femoris

Medial compartment of thigh

Posterior compartment of thigh

Vastus lateralis

Vastus intermedius

Rectus femoris

Vastus medialis

Sartorius

Adductor canal

Vastus medialis

Sartorius

Articularis genus

Suprapatellar recess

Quadriceps femoris tendon

Quadriceps femoris tendon

Patella

Patellar ligament

Tibial tuberosity

Patellar ligament

Pes anserinus

Attachment of pes anserinus— Sartorius — Gracilis — Semitendinosus

■ **FIGURE 6.4** **Hip and Thigh Anatomy.** Anterior musculature. *(From Drake R, Vogl W, Mitchell A:* Gray's Anatomy for Students, *Philadelphia, 2005, Churchill Livingstone.)*

origin from the ischial tuberosity and short head origin from the femur; the biceps femoris inserts on the fibula and lateral tibial condyle) (Fig. 6.5). Proximally, the semimembranosus tendon is located anterior to the conjoined biceps femoris–semitendinosus tendon and the semitendinosus muscle belly; the semimembranosus origin on the ischium is anterolateral to the conjoint tendon origin.[8]

Other important structures of the anterior hip and thigh include (lateral to medial) the femoral nerve, artery, and vein (use the mnemonic NAVEL for *n*erve, *a*rtery, *v*ein, *e*mpty space, *l*ymphatics). A branch of the femoral nerve, the saphenous nerve, courses deep to the sartorius muscle and becomes subcutaneous inferior to the knee.[9] The sciatic nerve is seen in the posterior thigh adjacent to the biceps femoris muscle, where it bifurcates

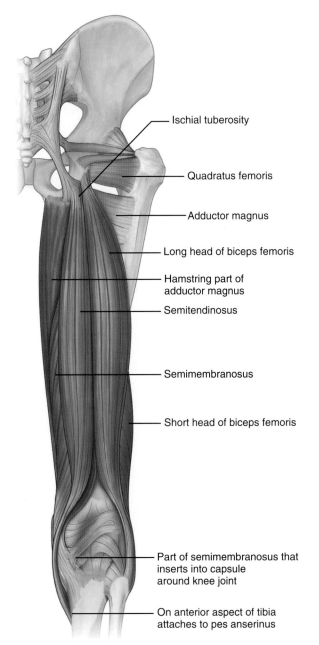

Ischial tuberosity

Quadratus femoris

Adductor magnus

Long head of biceps femoris

Hamstring part of
adductor magnus

Semitendinosus

Semimembranosus

Short head of biceps femoris

Part of semimembranosus that
inserts into capsule
around knee joint

On anterior aspect of tibia
attaches to pes anserinus

■ FIGURE 6.5 **Hip and Thigh Anatomy.** Posterior musculature. *(From Drake R, Vogl W, Mitchell A:* Gray's Anatomy *for Students,* Philadelphia, 2005, Churchill Livingstone.)

as the tibial nerve and the common peroneal nerve laterally.

Several bursae are located about the hip. The iliopsoas bursa is located anteriorly along the medial aspect of the psoas major tendon of the iliopsoas complex and normally communicates with the hip joint in up to 15% of the population.[10] The trochanteric (or subgluteus maximus) bursa is located posterolateral over the posterior and lateral facets of the greater trochanter deep to the gluteus maximus and iliotibial tract, whereas smaller subgluteus medius and subgluteus minimus bursae are located between the lateral facet and gluteus medius, and the anterior facet and gluteus minimus, respectively (see Fig. 6.16).[2] Other more variable bursae exist about the proximal femur as well.[11] Other possible bursae include the obturator externus bursa, located medially and inferior to the femoral neck, which may communicate with the posteroinferior hip joint.[12] An ischial (or ischiogluteal bursa) is found superficial to the ischial tuberosity.

In the inguinal region, the inguinal canal represents a triangular, elongated passage in the

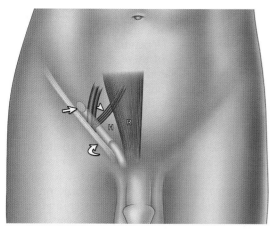

■ FIGURE 6.6 **Hip and Thigh Anatomy.** Illustration of the male right inguinal region shows the inferior epigastric artery *(arrowhead)*, deep inguinal ring *(arrow)*, inguinal ligament *(curved arrow)*, Hesselbach triangle *(H)*, and rectus abdominis *(R)*. *(From Jacobson JA, Khoury V, Brandon CJ: Ultrasound of the Groin: Techniques, Pathology, and Pitfalls. AJR Am J Roentgenol 205:1-11, 2015.)*

✳ **TABLE 6.1 Hip and Thigh Ultrasound Examination Checklist**

Location	Structures of Interest
Hip: anterior	Hip joint, iliopsoas, rectus femoris, sartorius, pubic symphysis
Hip: lateral	Greater trochanter, gluteal tendons, bursae, iliotibial tract, tensor fascia latae
Hip: posterior	Sacroiliac joints, piriformis, and other external rotators of the hip
Inguinal region	Deep inguinal ring, Hesselbach triangle, femoral artery region
Thigh: anterior	Rectus femoris, vastus medialis, vastus intermedius, vastus lateralis
Thigh: medial	Femoral artery and nerve, sartorius, gracilis, adductors
Thigh: posterior	Semimembranosus, semitendinosus, biceps femoris, sciatic nerve

lower abdominal wall located just superior to the inguinal ligament (Fig. 6.6). The inguinal canal's posterior opening, the *deep inguinal ring*, is located laterally, whereas the anterior opening, called the *superficial inguinal ring*, is located medially near the pubis. The contents of the inguinal canal include the ilioinguinal nerve, as well as the spermatic cord in males and the round ligament in females. The deep inguinal ring is located just lateral to the origin of the inferior epigastric artery from the external iliac artery. The inguinal (or Hesselbach) triangle is demarcated by the lateral margin of the rectus abdominis medially, the inguinal ligament inferiorly, and the superior epigastric artery laterally.[13] Another structure near the inguinal ligament is the lateral femoral cutaneous nerve, which exits the pelvis to extend over the lateral thigh in a somewhat variable manner. Although most common medial, it may also course superficial or lateral to the anterior superior iliac spine with variable branching.[14,15]

■ ULTRASOUND EXAMINATION TECHNIQUE

Table 6.1 is a checklist for hip and thigh ultrasound examination. Examples of diagnostic hip ultrasound reports are shown in Boxes 6.1 and 6.2.

General Comments

Ultrasound examination of the hip and anterior thigh is completed with the patient supine; the

✳ **BOX 6.1 Sample Diagnostic Hip Ultrasound Report: Normal, Complete**

Examination: Ultrasound of the Right Hip
   Date of Study: March 11, 2016
   Patient Name: Jack White
   Registration Number: 8675309
   History: Hip pain, evaluate for bursitis
   Findings: The hip joint is normal without effusion or synovial hypertrophy. Limited evaluation of the anterior labrum is unremarkable. No evidence of iliopsoas bursal distention or snapping iliopsoas tendon with dynamic imaging. The remaining anterior tendons, including the rectus femoris and sartorius, as well as the adductors, are normal.

Evaluation of the lateral hip is normal. No evidence of abnormal bursal distention around the greater trochanter. The gluteus minimus and medius tendons are normal. No abnormal snapping with dynamic evaluation.

Impression: Unremarkable ultrasound examination of the hip.

patient is prone for evaluation of the posterior thigh. For evaluation of the greater trochanteric region, the patient rolls on the contralateral side. Evaluation of the hip and thigh may be considered as two separate examinations in most circumstances. Hip or groin pain in an athlete may be caused from hip joint pathology, tendon or muscle pathology, osseous injury, or adjacent hernia, and therefore all etiologies should be considered.[16,17] The choice of transducer frequency depends on the patient's body habitus. A high-frequency linear probe is preferred to optimize resolution, although with a large body habitus a transducer of less than 10 MHz may be needed to penetrate the soft tissues adequately; a curvilinear transducer in this latter setting provides a larger field of view and is also helpful when guiding percutaneous needle procedures. A lower frequency transducer should be considered regardless of body habitus because one should examine the entire depth of the soft tissues before focusing on the more superficial structures. This approach ensures a complete and global evaluation and also serves to orient the examiner to the various muscles, an important consideration because the bone landmarks are few and deep. Evaluation of the hip and thigh may be focused over the area that is clinically symptomatic or relevant to the patient's history, keeping in mind symptoms may be multifactorial or referred. Regardless, a complete examination of all areas should always be considered for one to become familiar with normal anatomy and normal variants, and to develop a quick and efficient sonographic technique.

Hip Evaluation: Anterior

The primary structures evaluated include the hip joint and recess, iliopsoas complex and bursa,

proximal thigh musculature origin in the hip region (rectus femoris and sartorius), and pubic symphysis region. Depending on patient history and symptoms, all of these structures should be considered in the evaluation because symptoms may be referred and etiology multifactorial. Evaluation begins with the anterior hip with the transducer long axis to the femoral neck, which is in the oblique-sagittal plane (Fig. 6.7A). To find the femoral neck, one may initially image transversely over the femoral shaft to locate the curved and echogenic surface of the femur and then move the transducer proximally; once the bony protuberances of the greater and lesser trochanter are identified, the transducer is turned to the sagittal-oblique plane parallel to the femoral neck. The hip joint may also be located lateral to the femoral vasculature. The hip joint is identified long axis to the femoral neck by the characteristic bone contours of the femoral head, acetabulum, and femoral neck (Fig. 6.7B–D). It is at this location superficial to the femoral neck where the anterior joint recess is evaluated for fluid or synovial abnormalities.[1]

The anterior recess of the hip joint over the femoral neck is normally about 4–6 mm thick, and this can be explained anatomically.[1] The anterior joint capsule extends inferiorly from the acetabulum and labrum and inserts at the intertrochanteric line of the femur; however, some capsule fibers are reflected superiorly along the femoral neck to attach at the femoral head-neck junction (Fig. 6.8). Both the anterior and posterior layers of the joint capsule measure 2–3 mm each in thickness; physiologic fluid between these layers should measure less than 2 mm, and typically no fluid is identified in the normal situation.[1] The anterior layer may be slightly thicker than the posterior layer as a result of capsular thickening from ligaments and the zona orbicularis, which encircles the capsule at the femoral head-neck junction. The posterior layer may also demonstrate focal thickening at its attachment at the femoral head-neck junction. The normal anterior joint recess is usually concave or flat anteriorly but may be convex with internal hip rotation (see Fig. 6.35).[1] The true hyperechoic and fibrillar appearance of the joint capsule and its reflection is best appreciated when the femoral neck is perpendicular to the sound beam (see Fig. 6.7C); if imaged obliquely, the joint capsule may artifactually appear hypoechoic and may simulate fluid in echogenicity, especially in a patient with a large body habitus (see Fig. 6.7B). The femoral head and neck should be smooth, and the visualized portion of the hypoechoic hyaline cartilage that covers the femoral head should be uniform. The fibrocartilage labrum is hyperechoic and triangular and

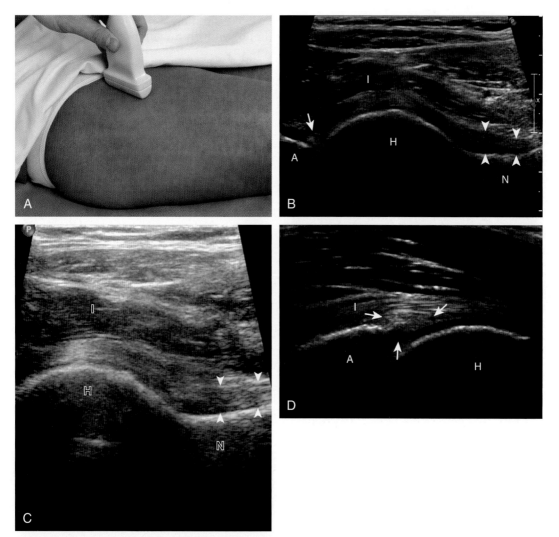

■ **FIGURE 6.7 Hip Joint Evaluation (Long Axis).** A, Sagittal-oblique imaging over the proximal femur shows (B–D) the femoral head *(H)*, femoral neck *(N)*, and collapsed anterior joint recess *(arrowheads)*. Note the acetabulum *(A)* and fibrocartilage labrum *(arrows)*. I, Iliopsoas.

extends from the margins of the acetabulum (see Fig. 6.7D). The femoral head and neck are also evaluated in short axis to the femoral neck (Fig. 6.9).

To evaluate the iliopsoas region, the transducer is first placed in the transverse plane over the femoral head because this bone landmark is easy to identify (see Fig. 6.9B). The transducer is then moved superiorly and angled parallel to the inguinal ligament (Fig. 6.10). The characteristic bone contours are seen, as well as the iliopsoas complex, the rectus femoris origin at the anterior inferior iliac spine laterally, and the femoral vessels medially. The iliopsoas complex is comprised of multiple muscular and tendon components. The muscle identified laterally represents the lateral and medial fibers of the iliacus separated by an intramuscular fascia, while the prominent tendon medially represents the psoas major tendon with its respective muscle tissue seen more medially.[4] The true iliopsoas tendon does not form until more distal. As with imaging any tendon in short axis, toggling the transducer is often helpful to visualize the tendon as hyperechoic, especially because the iliopsoas normally courses deep toward the lesser trochanter and is oblique to the sound beam. The iliopsoas should be evaluated dynamically for tendon snapping (see Snapping Hip Syndrome later in the chapter).[4] The anterior hip is also evaluated for iliopsoas bursa, which originates at the level of the femoral head and typically extends medial and possibly deep to the psoas major tendon and iliopsoas tendon. The transducer is also rotated 90 degrees to evaluate the iliopsoas tendon in long

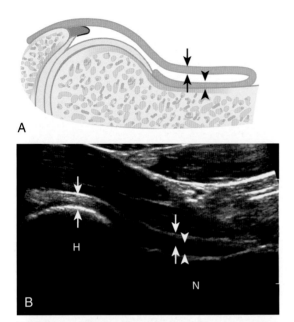

A

B

■ **FIGURE 6.8 Anterior Hip Joint Recess.** A, A sagittal-oblique illustration through the femoral head and neck and (B) an ultrasound image show the anterior layer of the joint capsule *(arrows)* and the posterior layer *(arrowheads)*. *H*, Femoral head; *N*, femoral neck. *(Modified from an illustration by Carolyn Nowak, Ann Arbor, Michigan.)*

axis; visualization of the distal iliopsoas tendon is improved with the hip in flexion abduction and external rotation (FABER) (Fig. 6.11).[18]

To evaluate the rectus femoris origin, the transducer is returned to the transverse plane over the iliopsoas complex parallel to and at the level of the inguinal ligament (see Fig. 6.10A) and then moved laterally over the anterior inferior iliac spine. The direct head is seen directly superficial to the anterior inferior iliac spine and is imaged in short and long axis (Fig. 6.12A and B) (Video 6.1). When moving the transducer laterally from the direct head in long axis, the indirect head will be seen coursing proximal and deep, appearing hypoechoic from anisotropy and producing a characteristic refraction shadow (Fig. 6.12C) (Video 6.2). One method of evaluating the indirect head of the rectus femoris is to begin anteriorly over the anterior iliac spine short axis to the direct head. The transducer is then moved over the lateral acetabulum in the transverse plane to identify the indirect head and then rotated 30 degrees to visualize the tendon in long axis (Fig. 6.12D and E).[19] To evaluate the sartorius, the transducer is returned to short axis relative to the rectus femoris direct head and moved proximally

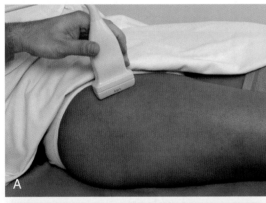

A

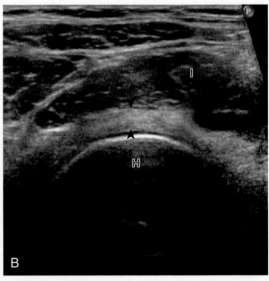

B

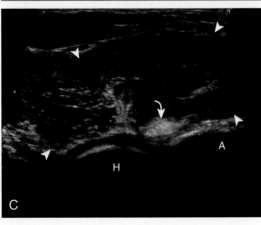

C

■ **FIGURE 6.9 Hip Joint Evaluation (Short Axis).** A, Transverse-oblique imaging shows (B) the anterior layer of the joint capsule and iliofemoral ligament *(arrowheads)* with hypoechoic hyaline cartilage over the femoral head *(H)*. C, Ultrasound image at the proximal aspect of the femoral head *(H)* shows the iliacus and psoas muscles *(arrowheads)* and psoas major tendon *(curved arrow)*. *A*, Acetabulum; *I*, iliopsoas complex.

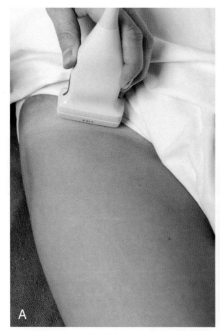

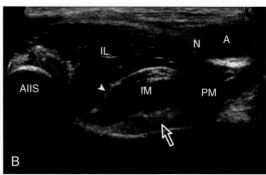

■ FIGURE 6.10 **Iliopsoas Evaluation (Short Axis).** A, Transverse-oblique imaging shows (B) the psoas major tendon *(open arrow)* and muscle *(PM)*, and the lateral *(IL)* and medial *(IM)* fibers of the iliacus with intramuscular fascia *(arrowhead)*. Note direct head of rectus femoris *(arrow)*, anterior inferior iliac spine *(AIIS)*, femoral artery *(A)*, and femoral nerve *(N)*.

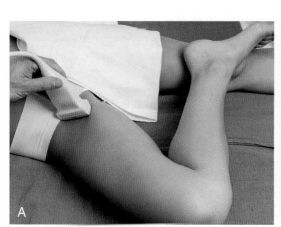

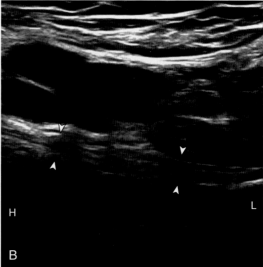

■ FIGURE 6.11 **Iliopsoas Evaluation (Long Axis).** A, Sagittal imaging with hip flexion, abduction, and external rotation shows (B) the iliopsoas tendon *(arrowheads)* and lesser trochanter *(L)*. *H,* Femoral head.

and laterally to visualize the sartorius and its origin on the anterior superior iliac spine (Fig. 6.13).

To evaluate the lateral femoral cutaneous nerve, position the transducer in the transverse plane over the proximal sartorius near the anterior superior iliac spine.[20] As the transducer is moved distally, the lateral femoral cutaneous nerve can

be seen as several nerve fascicles coursing over the sartorius from medial to lateral (Fig. 6.14A). More distally, a branch of the lateral femoral cutaneous nerve is identified in a triangular hypoechoic fatty space at the lateral aspect of the sartorius adjacent to the tensor fascia latae (Fig. 6.14B) (Video 6.3).[21] The transducer is then moved

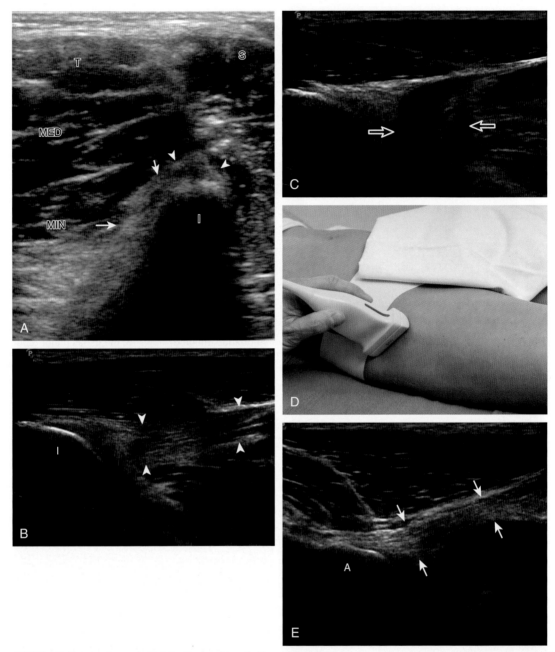

■ **FIGURE 6.12 Rectus Femoris Origin Evaluation.** A, Transverse imaging over the anterior inferior iliac spine *(I)* shows the direct head *(arrowheads)* and indirect head *(arrows)* (left side of image is lateral). B, Ultrasound image in sagittal plane shows the direct head of the rectus femoris in long axis *(arrowheads)*. C, Ultrasound image moving lateral to (B) shows refraction shadow *(open arrows)* from the indirect head of the rectus femoris and anisotropy. D, Positioning the probe lateral in 30 degrees of obliquity shows (E) the indirect head of the rectus femoris in long axis *(arrows)* and acetabulum *(A)*. *MED,* Gluteus medius; *MIN,* gluteus minimus; *S,* sartorius; *T,* tensor fasciae latae.

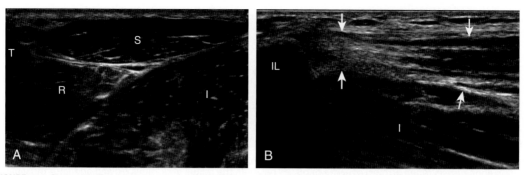

■ FIGURE 6.13 **Sartorius Evaluation.** Ultrasound images show the (A) short axis and (B) long axis of the sartorius (*S* and *arrows*). *I*, Iliopsoas complex; *IL*, anterior superior iliac spine of ilium; *R*, rectus femoris; *T*, tensor fascia latae.

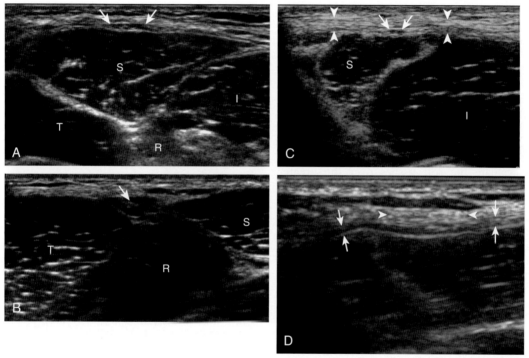

■ FIGURE 6.14 **Lateral Femoral Cutaneous Nerve Evaluation.** A, Ultrasound image in short axis to the sartorius (*S*) shows nerve fascicles *(arrows)*. B, More distally, one nerve fascicle *(arrow)* is within hypoechoic fat. C, Proximal view at the level of the inguinal ligament *(arrowheads)* shows nerve fascicles *(arrows)* in short axis and (D) long axis. *I*, Iliacus; *R*, rectus femoris; *T*, tensor fascia latae.

proximally to evaluate for potential nerve entrapment at the inguinal ligament (Fig. 6.14C and D).[22] The lateral femoral cutaneous nerve may branch proximal to the inguinal ligament and has a variable course. Although most common medial, it may also course superficial or lateral to the anterior superior iliac spine with a variable branching pattern.[14,15]

Although thigh evaluation is considered separately, patients with hip pain (especially sports-related pain or athletic pubalgia) may have abnormalities at the adductor tendon origin and

the rectus abdominis insertion, with possible abnormalities directly associated with the pubic symphysis.[23] To evaluate the pubic symphyseal region, the transducer can be placed transverse the rectus abdominis inferior to the umbilicus. The transducer is centered over one of the rectus abdominis muscles and then rotated 90 degrees in the sagittal plane. The rectus abdominis is followed distally until the echogenic surface of the pubis and overlying common aponeurosis is seen. Angling the transducer laterally at this point toward the adductor tendons can visualize the

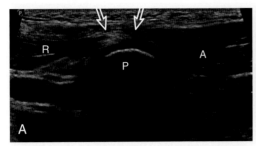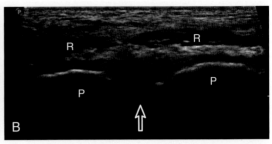

■ FIGURE 6.15 **Common Aponeurosis and Pubic Symphysis.** A, Ultrasound image in the sagittal-oblique plane shows common aponeurosis *(open arrows)* over the pubis *(P)* between the rectus abdominis *(R)* and adductor musculature *(A)*. B, Ultrasound image transverse in midline shows distal rectus abdominis muscles *(R)* and pubic symphysis *(open arrow)*.

rectus abdominis, the adductor longus, and the intervening common aponeurosis (Fig. 6.15A).[24] The symphysis pubis is then evaluated by rotating the transducer back to the transverse plane and centered over the symphysis pubis (Fig. 6.15B). Further assessment of the more distal adductor musculature is discussed with the medial thigh evaluation.

Hip Evaluation: Lateral

To evaluate the soft tissues over the greater trochanter, bone landmarks are essential (Fig. 6.16). The patient lies on the opposite side and the transducer is placed laterally over the hip of interest in the transverse plane (Fig. 6.17A). If the greater trochanter is not directly visualized, the transducer can be placed short axis to the femoral shaft more inferiorly. With movement of the transducer cephalad, the characteristic bone contours of the greater trochanter are identified laterally. The key landmark is the apex of the greater trochanter between the anterior and lateral facets, which typically is identified slightly anterior to the lateral hip (Fig. 6.17B).[2] Posterior to the lateral facet is the rounded posterior facet of the greater trochanter. The gluteus minimus tendon is identified inserting on the anterior facet, the distal gluteus medius inserting on the lateral facet, and the gluteus maximus superficial but not attaching to the posterior facet. Superficial to the gluteus minimus tendon over the anterior facet is seen the hypoechoic muscle of the gluteus medius and more superficially the iliotibial tract, with the latter appearing as a hyperechoic band of tissue as a continuation of the fascial layers that envelop the gluteus maximus posteriorly and the tensor fascia latae anteriorly (Fig. 6.16). Superficial to the gluteus medius tendon over the lateral facet is seen the iliotibial tract; if the hip is externally rotated, the gluteus maximus will also be visualized over the gluteus medius. Each

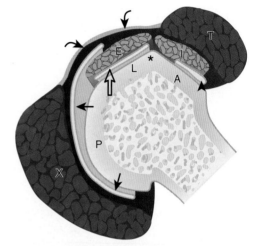

■ FIGURE 6.16 **Greater Trochanter Anatomy.** Illustration in short axis to the proximal femur (anterior is right side of image, lateral is top of image) shows gluteus minimus *(I)* attachment to the anterior facet *(A)* with interposed subgluteus minimus bursa *(arrowhead)*, gluteus medius *(E)* attachment to the lateral facet *(L)* with interposed subgluteus medius bursa *(open arrow)*, and gluteus maximus *(X)* passing over the posterior facet *(P)* with interposed trochanteric (or subgluteus maximus) bursa *(arrows)*. Note the bone apex *(asterisk)* between the anterior and lateral facets and iliotibial tract *(curved arrows)*. T, Tensor fascia latae. *(Modified from an illustration by Carolyn Nowak, Ann Arbor, Michigan.)*

greater trochanter facet should be evaluated separately in short axis and the transducer should be positioned so that the cortex of each individual facet is perpendicular to the sound beam to eliminate anisotropy of the overlying tendon and to evaluate for distended bursae (Fig. 6.17C).

The subgluteus minimus bursa, subgluteus medius bursa, and trochanteric (subgluteus maximus) bursa are located between each respective tendon and their greater trochanter facet (see Fig. 6.16).[2] Because the trochanteric bursa is

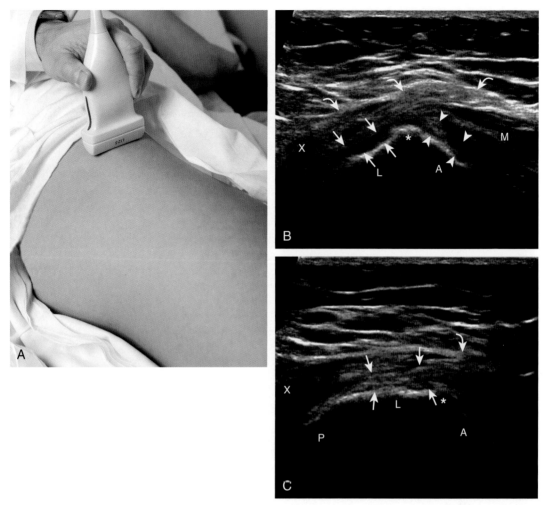

■ **FIGURE 6.17 Greater Trochanter Evaluation (Short Axis).** A, Transverse imaging over the greater trochanter with the patient in the decubitus position shows (B) bone apex *(asterisk)* between gluteus minimus *(arrowheads)* attachment on the anterior facet *(A)* and gluteus medius *(arrows)* insertion on the lateral facet *(L)*. The hypoechoic appearance of the gluteus medius in (B) from anisotropy is corrected in (C) when the transducer sound beam is directed perpendicular to the lateral facet. Note the iliotibial tract *(curved arrows)* and gluteus maximus *(X)*. *M*, Gluteus medius muscle; *P*, posterior facet of the greater trochanter.

located between the gluteus maximus and posterior facet, it is essential to position the transducer posteriorly so as not to overlook bursal distention at this site. When distended, the trochanteric bursa may also extend laterally between the gluteus medius tendon beneath the iliotibial tract.

The gluteus minimus tendon is then evaluated in long axis by moving the transducer in short axis over and perpendicular to the anterior facet, visualizing the gluteus minimus tendon, and then rotating the transducer 90 degrees but slightly anterior (Fig. 6.18A). The same technique is used over the lateral facet to evaluate the gluteus medius tendon in long axis with the transducer angled slightly posteriorly (Fig. 6.18B). Because the gluteus medius tendon is attached to two facets (lateral and superoposterior), the transducer should

be moved cephalad and posterior to visualize the full extent of the gluteus medius tendon attachment (Fig. 6.18C). In long axis, the gluteus minimus and medius tendons form a "V" moving cephalad (see Fig. 6.2).[3]

Hip Evaluation: Posterior

Evaluation of the posterior hip and pelvis is not typically considered part of a routine hip evaluation but rather is guided by patient history and symptoms. Structures of interest include the sacroiliac joints, piriformis, superior gemellus, obturator internus, inferior gemellus, obturator externus, and quadriceps femoris (see Fig. 6.3).[25] Evaluation can begin with the sacroiliac joint by first positioning the transducer in midline

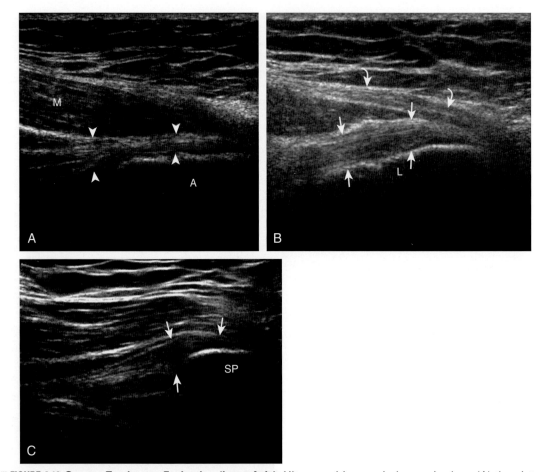

■ **FIGURE 6.18 Greater Trochanter Evaluation (Long Axis).** Ultrasound images in long axis show (A) the gluteus minimus *(arrowheads)* and (B) gluteus medius *(arrows)* tendons. Note the iliotibial tract *(curved arrows)* and gluteus medius muscle *(M).* The transducer more posterior over the superoposterior facet *(SP)* of the greater trochanter shows (C) an additional insertion site of the gluteus medius *(arrows). A,* Anterior facet; *L,* lateral facet of the greater trochanter.

over the sacrum and then moving the transducer laterally to visualize the posterior sacral foramina and more laterally to view the sacroiliac joint and adjacent posterior ilium (Fig. 6.19) (Video 6.4).[26] The posterior sacral foramina are differentiated from the sacroiliac joint by their more medial location as well as the characteristic focal disruptions in the cortex when scanning superior to inferior, which is in contrast to the more lateral and linear cortical disruption of the sacroiliac joint. The superior aspect of the sacroiliac joint is widened at the fibrocartilage or ligamentous articulation (Fig. 6.19A), whereas the more inferior true synovial articulation is narrow (Fig. 6.19B).

To identify the piriformis, a curvilinear transducer with a frequency of less than 10 MHz is essential given the required depth of penetration. The transducer is first positioned in the transverse plane over the sacroiliac joint, as described, then moved inferior into the greater sciatic notch and

angled inferiorly and laterally toward the greater trochanter (see Fig. 6.19C) to identify the piriformis in long axis (see Fig. 6.19D).[27,28] The muscle belly will be located medial to the ilium, while the tendon will be seen directly over the ilium extending to the greater trochanter. Passive hip rotation will assist in its identification because of movement of the tendon and muscle (Videos 6.5 and 6.6).

To identify the quadratus femoris, obturators, and gemelli, examination can begin in the transverse plane at the level of the ischial tuberosity and hamstring origin (Fig. 6.20A). Lateral to the ischial tuberosity and deep to the sciatic nerve is located the quadratus femoris muscle between the ischium and proximal femur. The obturator externus is located deeper and courses anteriorly. Moving cephalad, the inferior gemellus is seen (Fig. 6.20B), followed by the obturator internus (Fig. 6.20C), and then superior gemellus. The obturator

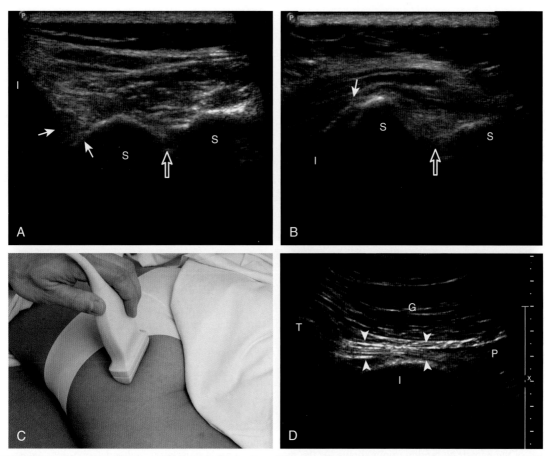

■ **FIGURE 6.19 Sacroiliac Joint and Piriformis Evaluation.** Ultrasound images in the transverse plane over (A) the upper and (B) lower sacrum *(S)* show the left sacroiliac joint *(arrows)*, posterior sacral foramen *(open arrow)*, and posterior ilium *(I)* (right side of image is at midline and left side is lateral). C, Oblique axial ultrasound image (D) shows the piriformis tendon *(arrowheads)* and muscle *(P)*. *G*, Gluteus maximus; *I*, ilium; *T*, greater trochanter.

internus is identified by its unique anatomy coursing medial over the ischial tuberosity and into the pelvis.[29] The relationship between the gemelli and the obturator internus, often considered a single functional unit, is appreciated in their short axis with the transducer in the sagittal plane (Fig. 6.20D). If the transducer is moved cephalad again and angled medial and superior toward the sacrum, the piriformis muscle will be seen (see Fig. 6.19C). In their short axis, from cephalad to caudal, the piriformis, superior gemellus, obturator internus, inferior gemellus, obturator externus, and quadratus femoris are identified deep to the sciatic nerve (Fig. 6.20D). The sciatic nerve lies deep to the piriformis but superficial to the other external hip rotators described.

Inguinal Region Evaluation

Sonography of the hip and groin region may also include evaluation for inguinal hernias as patient symptoms are often multifactorial.[30] For example, inguinal hernia and adductor tendon abnormalities often coexist in patients with femoroacetabular impingement.[16] At ultrasound an important landmark for determining the type of inguinal hernia is to identify the Hesselbach triangle, which has its base medially bordered by the lateral margin of the rectus abdominis and its apex laterally formed by the inferior epigastric artery superiorly and the inguinal ligament inferiorly (see Fig. 6.6).[17]

To begin, one sonographic technique is to scan in the transverse plane over the mid-abdomen below the umbilicus with the patient supine. At this location, the linea alba is seen as a hyperechoic fascial layer between the rectus abdominis muscles and the transducer is centered over one of the ipsilateral rectus abdominis muscles. The transducer is then moved inferior in the transverse plane, and the inferior epigastric artery will be identified beneath the rectus abdominis coursing from medial to lateral (Fig. 6.21A). The inferior

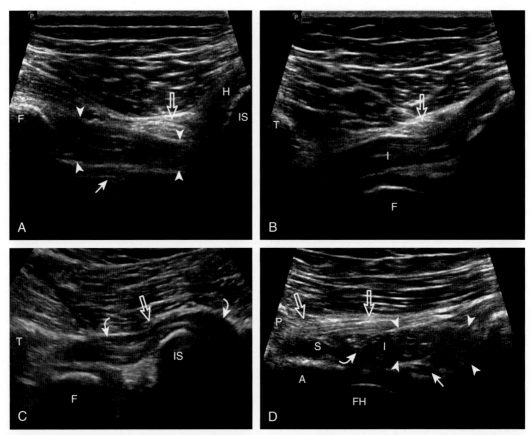

■ FIGURE 6.20 **Quadratus Femoris, Obturator, and Gemelli Evaluation.** Ultrasound image in transverse plane at the level of the hamstring tendon origin shows (A) the quadratus femoris muscle *(arrowheads)*, obturator externus *(arrow)*, and sciatic nerve *(open arrow)* deep to the gluteus maximus. The transducer is moved cephalad to show (B) the inferior gemellus *(I)*. Moving more cephalad (C) the obturator internus *(curved arrow)* is seen coursing medial over the ischium *(IS)* (using a curvilinear transducer). In short axis (D), from superior to inferior is identified the superior gemellus *(S)*, obturator internus *(curved arrow)*, inferior gemellus *(I)*, quadratus femoris *(arrowheads)*, and obturator externus *(arrow)*. Note the sciatic nerve *(open arrows)* and piriformis *(P)*. *A*, Acetabulum; *F*, femur; *FH*, femoral head; *H*, hamstring tendon origin; *IS*, ischium; *T*, greater trochanter.

epigastric artery is then followed inferiorly and laterally until it joins the external iliac artery, which is the apex of the Hesselbach triangle. This site is a very important landmark; just lateral and superior to this location is the deep inguinal ring (Fig. 6.21B). Hernias that originate lateral to the inferior epigastric artery at the deep inguinal ring and extend superficially and medially within the inguinal canal are indirect inguinal hernias. In contrast, hernias that originate in the Hesselbach triangle and move in an anterior direction are direct inguinal hernias.

At the deep inguinal ring, the transducer is then angled toward the pubis, parallel and just superior to the inguinal ligament, long axis to the inguinal canal to visualize indirect inguinal hernias if present (see Fig. 6.21C). In male patients, the serpiginous and mixed-echogenicity spermatic cord can be identified (see Fig. 6.21D and E). At this location, the patient is asked to tighten the stomach or perform the Valsalva maneuver (forced expiration against a closed airway) to evaluate for transient herniation of intra-abdominal structures or tissue; the patient can be asked to blow against the back of the hand and puff the cheeks outward. This maneuver is also repeated with the transducer directly over the Hesselbach triangle to evaluate for direct hernias. Identification of inguinal hernias must also be confirmed in the sagittal plane to avoid several diagnostic pitfalls.[17] When imaging the inguinal canal and spermatic cord (in males) in short axis, an indirect inguinal hernia will be seen moving in and out of the ultrasound plane displacing the spermatic cord. Similar to the transverse plane, a direct hernia will appear as focal abnormal anterior movement, which must be differentiated from non-focal movement of intra-abdominal fat.[17]

For evaluation of femoral hernias, the transducer is again positioned long axis to the inguinal

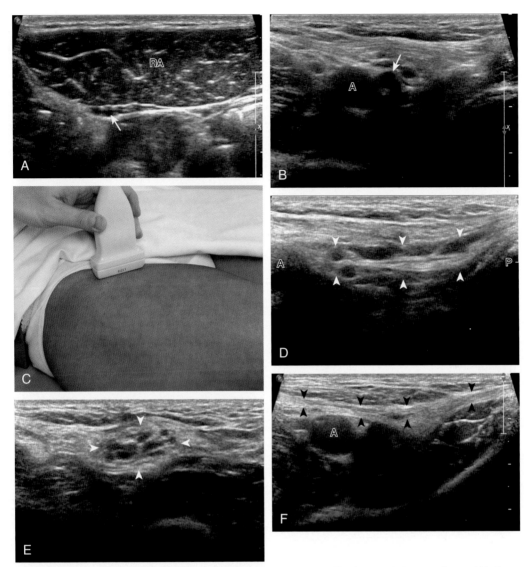

■ **FIGURE 6.21 Inguinal Region Evaluation.** Transverse imaging over the lower abdomen shows (A) the rectus abdominis muscle *(RA)* and the inferior epigastric artery *(arrow)* (right side of image is midline). Transverse imaging inferior to A shows (B) the origin of the inferior epigastric artery *(arrow)* from the external iliac artery *(A)*. C, Imaging in long axis to the inguinal canal shows (D) the spermatic cord *(arrowheads)*, also visible in short axis to the inguinal canal (E). Imaging in long axis at the inferior extent of the inguinal canal shows (F) the inguinal ligament *(arrowheads)*. *A,* External iliac artery; *P,* pubis.

ligament (see Fig. 6.21F) and moved distally over the common femoral artery just beyond the inguinal ligament during Valsalva maneuver. An adequate Valsalva maneuver is confirmed if the femoral vein distends. Ultrasound evaluation of other types of ventral abdominal hernias, such as Spigelian (located between the rectus abdominis and lateral abdominal musculature), umbilical, and incisional are usually directed by patient symptoms. Although the causes of "sports hernia" are debated, abnormality of the common aponeurosis is the predominant finding in *athletic*

pubalgia, which is described earlier in evaluation of the symphysis pubis.[31]

Thigh Evaluation: Anterior

Structures of interest anteriorly in the thigh include the four muscles that make up the quadriceps femoris (see Fig. 6.4). Examination can begin in the transverse plane over the mid-anterior thigh, where the four individual muscles can be identified (Fig. 6.22A) (Videos 6.7 and 6.8). Directly below the transducer and most superficial

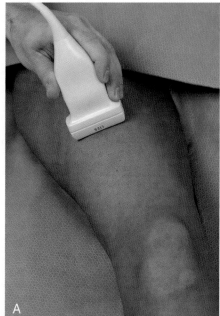

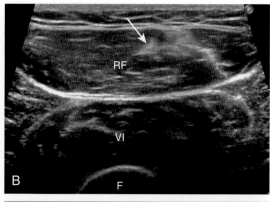

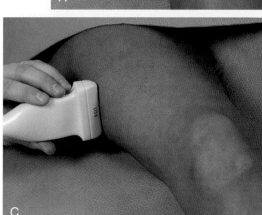

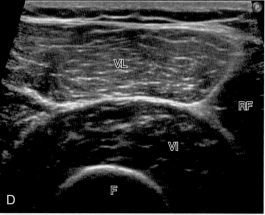

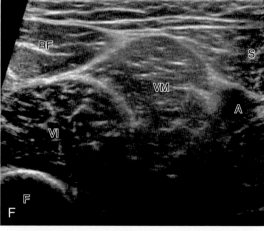

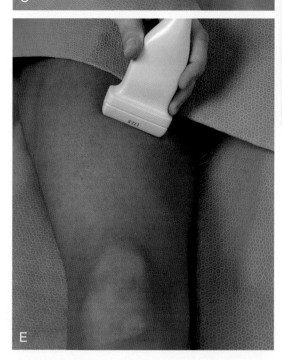

■ **FIGURE 6.22 Anterior Thigh Evaluation (Short Axis).**
A, Transverse imaging over the anterior thigh shows
(B) the rectus femoris *(RF)* with central aponeurosis
(arrow), vastus intermedius *(VI)*, and femur *(F)*.
C, Transverse imaging over the anterolateral thigh
shows (D) the vastus lateralis *(VL)*, vastus intermedius
(VI), rectus femoris *(RF)*, and femur *(F)*. E, Transverse
imaging over the anteromedial thigh shows (F) the
vastus medialis *(VM)*, rectus femoris *(RF)*, vastus
intermedius *(VI)*, femur *(F)*, femoral artery *(A)*, and
sartorius *(S)*.

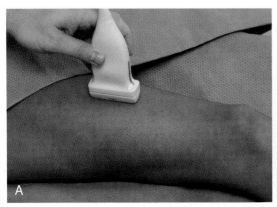
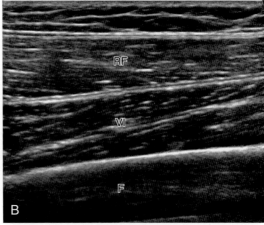
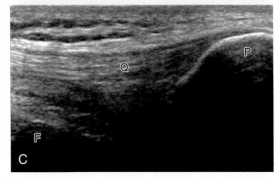

■ **FIGURE 6.23 Anterior Thigh Evaluation (Long Axis).** A, Sagittal imaging shows (B) the rectus femoris *(RF)* and vastus intermedius *(VI)* tapering distally (C) to form the quadriceps femoris tendon *(Q)*. F, Femur; P, patella.

is the rectus femoris muscle (Fig. 6.22B). Deep to this and immediately adjacent to the femur is the vastus intermedius. Lateral to these two structures is the vastus lateralis (Fig. 6.22C and D), and medial is the vastus medialis (Fig. 6.22E and F). Muscle at ultrasound is predominantly hypoechoic, although interspersed hyperechoic fibroadipose septa are identified.

The quadriceps femoris is then evaluated in long axis (Fig. 6.23). As one moves the transducer distally, the rectus femoris tapers to a tendon, followed by the vastus musculature, which forms the trilaminar quadriceps tendon that inserts on the superior pole of the patella. The superficial layer of the distal quadriceps tendon is made up of the rectus femoris, the middle layer is composed of both the vastus medialis and lateralis tendons, and the deep layer is made up of the vastus intermedius tendon. Some quadriceps tendon fibers continue over the patella (termed the *prepatellar quadriceps continuation*) to attach to the tibial tuberosity by means of the patellar tendon.[7] The distal tapering appearance of the rectus femoris is best appreciated in long axis in the sagittal plane. The individual muscles of the quadriceps can then be evaluated more proximally.

As described earlier, the rectus femoris tendon proximally originates at the ilium (see Fig. 6.12), where its direct head originates from the anterior inferior iliac spine and the indirect head originates laterally at the superior acetabular ridge. In the thigh, the direct head flattens superficially, the indirect head continues as the central aponeurosis of the rectus femoris, and more distally a posterior aponeurosis forms (see Fig. 6.22B).[6] The adjacent tensor fasciae latae is seen lateral to the rectus femoris muscle (Fig. 6.24); the fascia of the tensor fascia latae continues laterally as the iliotibial tract (see Fig. 6.16).

Thigh Evaluation: Medial

Structures of interest in the medial thigh include the femoral nerve, artery, and vein and the sartorius, gracilis, and adductor musculature. Ultrasound examination can begin with the anterior thigh as mentioned for orientation and initial identification of the rectus femoris muscle. The transducer is then moved cephalad into the medial upper thigh (see Fig. 6.22E). The femoral artery is identified at the medial aspect of the rectus femoris and vastus medialis muscles and

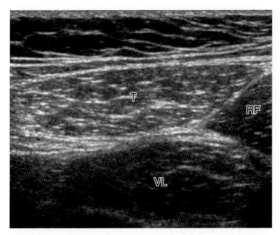

■ **FIGURE 6.24 Tensor Fasciae Latae Evaluation.** Transverse imaging over the upper thigh shows the tensor fasciae latae *(T)*, vastus lateralis *(VL)*, and rectus femoris *(RF)* (left side of image is lateral).

is a very helpful landmark (Fig. 6.25A). Directly superficial to the femoral artery is the sartorius muscle. Medial and posterior to these structures are the adductor muscles (Fig. 6.25B). The most anterior is the adductor longus, next posterior is the adductor brevis, and most posterior and largest is the adductor magnus. One mnemonic to describe the order of adductor muscles from anterior to posterior is "ALABAMa" (*a*dductor *l*ongus, *a*dductor *b*revis, *a*dductor *m*agnus). Between these respective muscles are located the anterior and posterior branches of the obturator nerve. Superficial and medial to the adductor muscles is the gracilis muscle, just below the subcutaneous tissues (Fig. 6.25C). The saphenous nerve can be identified in the distal medial thigh as it crosses from anterior to posterior deep to the sartorius and superficial to the gracilis (Fig. 6.25D), becoming subcutaneous adjacent to the great saphenous vein below the knee (Fig. 6.25E) (Video 6.9).[9] For each of these medial thigh muscles, the proximal to distal extents can be visualized in short axis. The transducer can also be turned in long axis over each muscle to visualize the proximal origins and distal attachments (Fig. 6.25F).

Thigh Evaluation: Posterior

Structures of interest in the posterior thigh include the semimembranosus, the semitendinosus, the biceps femoris, and the sciatic nerve. Ultrasound evaluation can begin in the transverse plane at three different levels: the gluteal fold, the ischial tuberosity, or the mid-posterior thigh.

GLUTEAL FOLD AND ISCHIAL TUBEROSITY

If the transducer is placed in the transverse plane at the gluteal fold (Fig. 6.26A), the characteristic appearance of the semimembranosus tendon and aponeurosis is identified deep to the semitendinosus muscle, which is a helpful landmark for orientation. In addition, the conjoined biceps femoris long head–semitendinosus tendon, the semimembranosus tendon, and the sciatic nerve are in the arrangement of a triangle. The semimembranosus is medial and the sciatic nerve lateral forming the base of the triangle, and the conjoined biceps femoris–semitendinosus tendon is the more superficial apex (Fig. 6.26B). Toggling the transducer to eliminate anisotropy is helpful to visualize the tendons as hyperechoic (Fig. 6.26C). The adductor magnus tendon can be identified medial to the semimembranosus (Fig. 6.26B).[32] As the transducer is moved cephalad toward the ischial tuberosity, the semimembranosus tendon will cross under the conjoined biceps femoris–semitendinosus tendon from medial to lateral (Fig. 6.26D).

At the ischial tuberosity in the transverse plane, the conjoined biceps femoris–semitendinosus tendon is seen in short axis and is superficial, whereas the adjacent semimembranosus tendon is lateral and deep on the ischial tuberosity (Fig. 6.26E). Lateral to the hamstring tendons is the sciatic nerve and posterior femoral cutaneous nerve, located superficial to the quadratus femoris muscle.[33] Ultrasound evaluation of the proximal hamstring tendons in short axis may be completed from the gluteal fold to ischial tuberosity as described, or one may start at the ischial tuberosity and move caudal, using palpation to assist in initially locating the ischial tuberosity. As another characteristic anatomic finding, if one moves the transducer distal from the gluteal fold, a curvilinear hyperechoic intramuscular raphe is identified within the semitendinosus (Fig. 6.26F).

To evaluate the proximal hamstring tendons in long axis, the transducer can be placed in the sagittal plane over the ischial tuberosity (Fig. 6.27A). At this site, the conjoined biceps femoris–semitendinosus tendon can be identified at the superficial aspect of the ischial tuberosity (Fig. 6.27B). To visualize the semimembranosus tendon, the transducer is moved slightly lateral to the conjoint tendon and angled toward midline (Fig. 6.27C and D). The conjoined biceps femoris–semitendinosus tendon and semimembranosus tendon can only be visualized together in long axis over a short segment where they cross just distal to the ischial tuberosity (Fig. 6.27E). The sciatic nerve is also identified in long axis laterally and should not be mistaken for tendon (Fig. 6.27F). Positioning the transducer superior to the

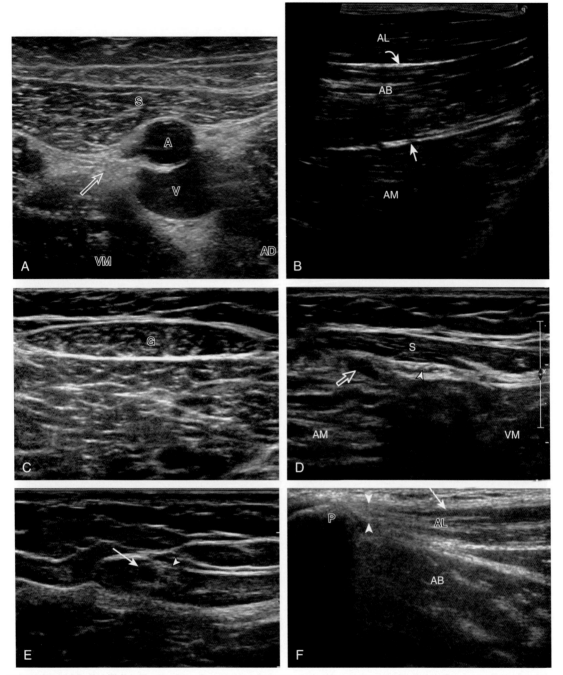

■ **FIGURE 6.25 Medial Thigh Evaluation.** Transverse imaging over the anteromedial thigh shows (A) the sartorius *(S)* immediately superficial to the femoral artery *(A)* and vein *(V)* (*open arrow*, femoral nerve). Transverse imaging over the medial thigh shows (B) the adductor longus *(AL)*, adductor brevis *(AB)*, and adductor magnus *(AM)*. Note the anterior *(curved arrow)* and posterior *(arrow)* divisions of the obturator nerve. Transverse imaging over the medial thigh shows (C) the gracilis *(G)* superficial to the adductor musculature. Transverse imaging distally (D) shows saphenous nerve *(arrowhead)* between sartorius *(S)* and gracilis *(open arrow)* (hypoechoic from anisotropy), that becomes subcutaneous inferior to the knee (E) adjacent to the great saphenous vein *(arrow)*. Coronal imaging long axis to the adductor musculature shows (F) the adductor longus *(AL)*, which originates *(arrowheads)* from the pubis *(P)* and adductor brevis *(AB)*. *AD,* Adductor musculature; *VM,* vastus medialis.

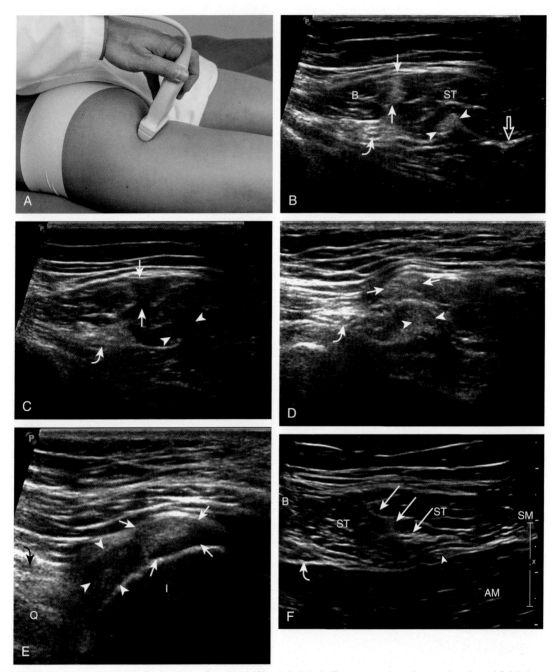

■ **FIGURE 6.26 Posterior Thigh Evaluation—Proximal (Short Axis).** A, Transverse imaging at the gluteal fold shows (B) the semimembranosus tendon *(arrowheads)*, the conjoined biceps femoris–semitendinosus tendon *(arrows)*, and semitendinosus muscle *(ST) (curved arrow,* sciatic nerve). Note biceps femoris long head muscle (B) and adductor magnus *(open arrow)*. Left side of image is lateral. Toggling the transducer (C) shows anisotropy of the tendons. More proximal imaging (D) shows the conjoined tendon *(arrows)* directly superficial to the semimembranosus tendon *(arrowheads)*. E, At the ischial tuberosity *(I),* the conjoined biceps femoris–semitendinosus tendon *(arrows)* is superficial and the semimembranosus *(arrowheads)* is deep and lateral (left side of image is lateral). Note sciatic nerve *(curved arrow)* superficial to quadratus femoris *(Q).* F, Imaging distal to gluteal fold shows characteristic raphe *(opens)* in semitendinosus muscle *(ST). AM,* Adductor magnus muscle; *SM,* semimembranosus muscle.

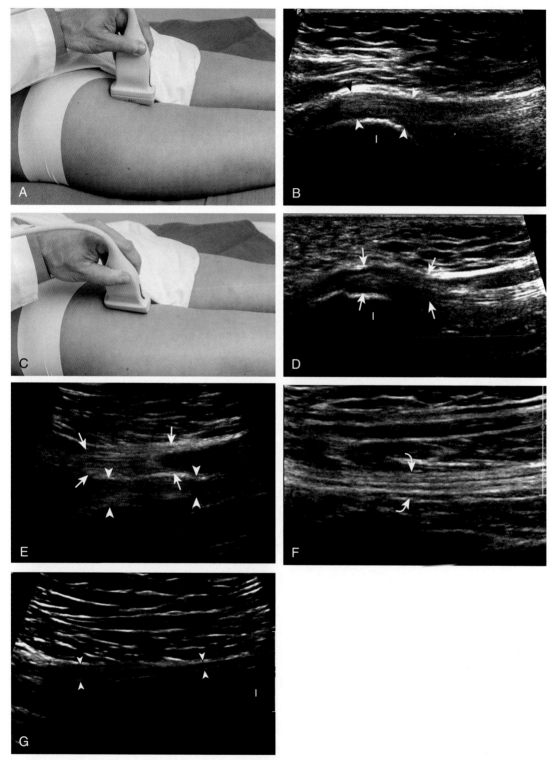

■ **FIGURE 6.27 Posterior Thigh Evaluation—Proximal (Long Axis).** A, Sagittal imaging shows (B) the conjoined biceps femoris–semitendinosus tendon *(arrows)* in long axis at superficial aspect of ischial tuberosity *(I)*. C, The transducer is moved lateral and angled toward midline to visualize (D) the semimembranosus tendon *(arrowheads)*. Just distal to the ischial tuberosity (E), both the conjoined biceps femoris–semitendinosus tendon *(arrows)* and semimembranosus tendon *(arrowheads)* are seen in long axis. More lateral (F), the sciatic nerve *(curved arrows)* is visualized. Imaging proximal to the ischial tuberosity shows (G) the sacrotuberous ligament *(open arrows)*.

ischial tuberosity and angling slightly medial can identify the sacrotuberous ligament (Fig. 6.27G), which has fibers continuous with the conjoined biceps femoris–semitendinosus tendon.[34]

MID-POSTERIOR THIGH

In the transverse plane centered over the mid-posterior thigh (Fig. 6.28A), three distinct muscles can be identified medial to lateral, which are the semimembranosus, semitendinosus, and biceps femoris muscles (Fig. 6.28B). The short head of the biceps femoris can be identified deep to the

long head at the femoral cortex at the level of the mid-femur, and the honeycomb appearance of the sciatic nerve can be identified between the biceps femoris muscle and the semitendinosus muscle. When the transducer is moved in the transverse plane distally toward the knee, the semitendinosus becomes a round tendon and moves directly superficial to the semimembranosus muscle (Fig. 6.28C–E). As the transducer is moved cephalad from the mid-thigh, the biceps femoris short head disappears from view proximal to its femoral origin, and the semimembranosus muscle forms an aponeurosis and tendon that

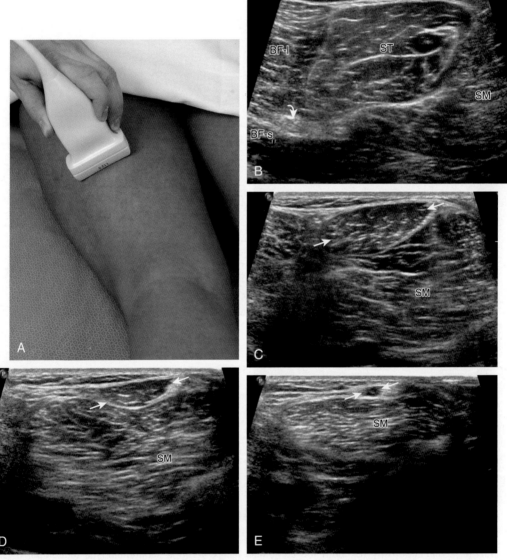

■ FIGURE 6.28 **Posterior Thigh Evaluation—Mid to Distal (Short Axis).** A, Transverse imaging at the mid posterior thigh shows (B) the semitendinosus *(ST)*, semimembranosus *(SM)*, and biceps femoris long head *(BF-l)* and short head *(BF-s)* *(curved arrow,* sciatic nerve). Note (C–E) the distal tapering of the semitendinosus *(arrows)* over the semimembranosus *(SM)* (right side of image is medial).

course beneath the semitendinosus muscle as described earlier at the gluteal fold. The individual hamstring muscle can also be imaged in long axis.

Hip Evaluation for Dysplasia in a Child

There are several opinions with regard to the ultrasound technique for hip dysplasia. Whereas one method favors the position of the femoral head and measurements, another emphasizes dynamic evaluation of position and stability using the Ortolani and Barlow maneuvers. Regardless, a minimal examination should include coronal neutral or coronal flexion positions (with optional stress and measurements) and a transverse flexion position with and without stress.[35] An ultrasound protocol for hip dysplasia may be divided into several steps. The first is a coronal view with the hip in neutral position (Fig. 6.29A). The resulting image is likened to an egg on a spoon, in which a line drawn from the flat ilium covers at least 50% of the head and an acetabular α angle is greater than 60 degrees (Fig. 6.29B and C). The α angle measures the angle between the lateral ilium (baseline) and the acetabular roof line, whereas the β angle measures the angle between the lateral ilium baseline and a line drawn through the hyperechoic labral tip from the lateral acetabulum (inclination line).[36] The ossified acetabulum and proximal femur are hyperechoic with shadowing, and the unossified femoral head and triradiate cartilage of the acetabulum appear speckled and hypoechoic. The second position is in the coronal plane with the hip flexed (Fig. 6.30A). In this position, in addition to assessment of the femoral head

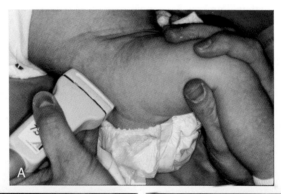

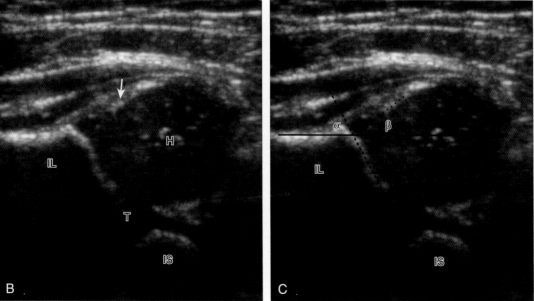

■ FIGURE 6.29 **Hip Dysplasia Evaluation (Coronal).** A, Coronal imaging over the lateral hip in neutral position shows (B) the femoral head *(H)*, ilium *(IL)*, ischium *(IS)*, triradiate cartilage *(T)*, and tip of labrum *(arrow)*. C, α and β angle measurements are indicated.

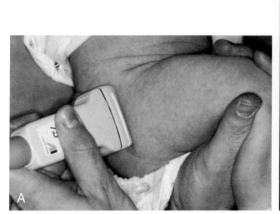

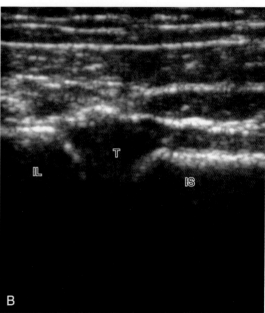

■ FIGURE 6.30 **Hip Dysplasia Evaluation (Coronal).** A, Coronal imaging with the hip in flexion and posteriorly directed stress shows (B) the normal triradiate cartilage *(T)* between the ilium *(IL)* and ischium *(IS)* without posterior displacement of the femoral head.

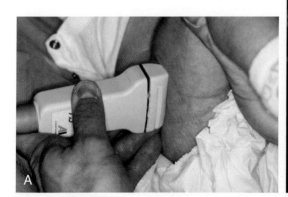

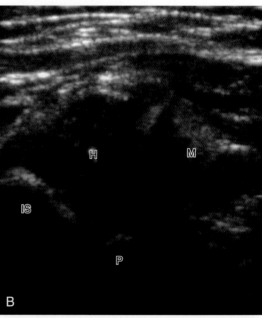

■ FIGURE 6.31 **Hip Dysplasia Evaluation (Transverse).** A, Transverse imaging with the hip in flexion and adduction with posteriorly directed stress shows (B) the normal location of the femoral head *(H)* relative to the ischium *(IS)* without subluxation or dislocation. *M,* Femoral metaphysis; *P,* pubis.

position, the transducer is moved posteriorly over the triradiate cartilage, and posteriorly directed stress is applied to evaluate for posterior subluxation of the femoral head (Fig. 6.30B). In the third position, the hip remains flexed, and the transducer is turned to the transverse plane (Fig. 6.31A). In this position, dynamic hip adduction with posteriorly directed stress (the Barlow test) (Fig. 6.31B) evaluates for hip subluxation, and hip abduction with anteriorly directed stress (the Ortolani test) evaluates for relocation if there is subluxation or dislocation of the hip.

■ JOINT AND BURSAL ABNORMALITIES

Joint Effusion and Synovial Hypertrophy

The diagnosis of a hip joint effusion in the hip relies on distention of the joint recess over the femoral neck (Fig. 6.32). In the native hip, imaging of the anterior hip recess over the femoral neck is sufficient to evaluate for joint effusion as fluid circumferentially surrounds the femoral neck; it is a misconception that joint fluid may only collect posteriorly.[37] To diagnose a joint effusion, the criterion for abnormal joint distention in a child is 2 mm of separation of the anterior and posterior

capsule layers over the anterior femoral neck (Fig. 6.33).[1] In the adult, total capsular distention of 7 mm (measured from the anterior femoral neck surface to the outer margin of the capsule, to include both anterior and posterior layers) or 1 mm of asymmetry compared with the contralateral asymptomatic hip has been shown to indicate joint distention,[38] although 5-mm of capsular separation has also been used (Fig. 6.34) (Video 6.10).[37] Imaging the femoral neck perpendicular to the sound beam reduces anisotropy of the capsule thereby improving detection of joint fluid. Leg extension and abduction may also improve visualization of a hip joint effusion. While a convex or bulging surface of the anterior joint recess suggests abnormal distention, internal

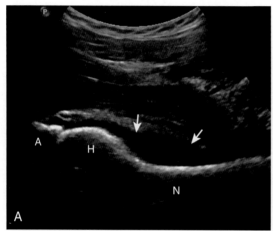
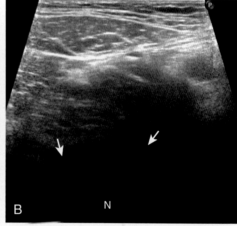

■ FIGURE 6.32 **Joint Effusion: Septic.** Ultrasound images in (A) long axis and (B) short axis to the femoral neck show anechoic anterior joint recess distention (arrows). A, Acetabulum; H, femoral head; N, femoral neck.

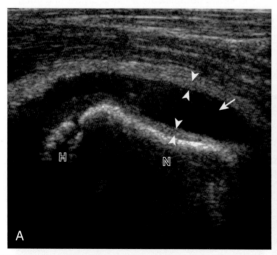
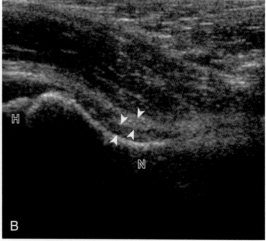

■ FIGURE 6.33 **Joint Effusion: Aseptic.** Ultrasound image in a child in (A) long axis to the proximal femur shows anechoic anterior joint recess distention (arrow). Note the joint capsule layers (arrowheads). Ultrasound image (B) of the contralateral asymptomatic hip shows normal capsular reflection (arrowheads) and no effusion. H, Femoral head epiphysis; N, femoral neck.

rotation of the leg may cause similar bulging of the normal joint capsule, which should not be misinterpreted as effusion (Fig. 6.35) (Video 6.11).[1] Uncommonly, joint effusion may extend superficially through a defect in the hip joint capsule within a pseudodiverticulum of the synovial membrane (Fig. 6.36).[1]

The normal collapsed joint recess may have a variable appearance that could potentially mimic joint effusion or synovial hypertrophy. While normally hyperechoic (if imaged perpendicular to sound beam), the capsule and its reflection may appear hypoechoic (if imaged obliquely from anisotropy or in large patient). In this latter scenario, anterior capsular measurement of less than 7 mm in thickness, owing to the normal capsule and its reflection, suggests artifact and not true joint recess distention (see Figs. 6.7 and 6.8).

The sonographic appearance of an effusion may range from anechoic (if simple fluid) to hyperechoic (if synovial hypertrophy or complex fluid from hemorrhage or infection). Neither joint recess echogenicity nor flow on color or power Doppler imaging can distinguish between aseptic and septic effusion; ultrasound-guided percutaneous aspiration should be considered if there is concern for infection.[39] In addition, it may be difficult to appreciate a small joint effusion in patients with increased soft tissues superficial to the hip and in those with a large body habitus.[40] In this situation, joint aspiration should be considered regardless of ultrasound findings if there is clinical concern for infection. A large body habitus may cause anechoic fluid to appear artifactually hypoechoic or isoechoic, even with lower-frequency transducers and tissue harmonic imaging.

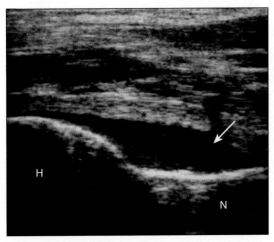

■ FIGURE 6.34 **Joint Effusion: Aseptic.** Ultrasound image in long axis to the femoral neck shows anechoic anterior joint recess distention *(arrow)* and capsule layers *(asterisks)*. *H,* Femoral head; *N,* femoral neck.

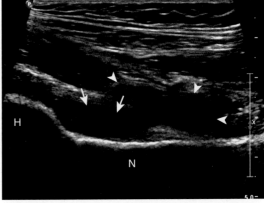

■ FIGURE 6.36 **Complex Joint Fluid.** Ultrasound image in long axis to the femoral neck shows hypoechoic anterior joint recess distention with internal echoes *(arrows)*. Note the distention of the pseudodiverticulum *(arrowheads)*. *H,* Femoral head; *N,* femoral neck.

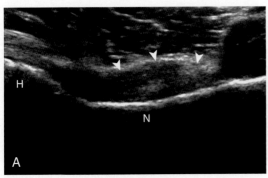
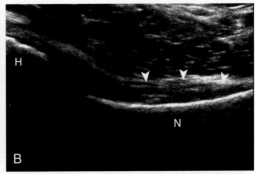

■ FIGURE 6.35 **Effects of Leg Position on Joint Capsule.** Ultrasound images in long axis to the femoral with the leg in (A) internal rotation and (B) external rotation show convex bulging of the joint capsule *(arrowheads)* with internal rotation. *H,* Femoral head; *N,* femoral neck.

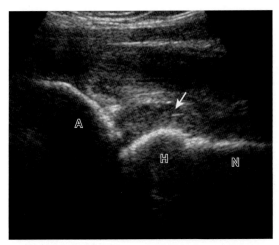

■ FIGURE 6.37 **Synovial Hypertrophy: Infection.** Ultrasound image in long axis to the femoral neck shows isoechoic anterior joint recess distention *(arrow)*. *A,* Acetabulum; *H,* femoral head; *N,* femoral neck.

Causes of hip effusion include fluid from a joint (i.e., osteoarthritis) or femoral head (i.e., osteonecrosis) abnormality, trauma, infection, and hemorrhage. Hypoechoic, isoechoic, or hyperechoic distention of the hip joint recess can be caused by either complex fluid (see Fig. 6.36) or synovial hypertrophy. In the latter condition, lack of compressibility or redistribution and absence of internal flow on color Doppler imaging suggests synovial hypertrophy. Causes of synovial hypertrophy include infection (Fig. 6.37) and inflammatory arthritis (Fig. 6.38). Other synovial proliferative disorders such as pigmented villonodular synovitis (Fig. 6.39) can appear similar, as can synovial osteochondromatosis (although the latter may show hyperechoic calcific foci). Intraarticular bodies appear as hyperechoic foci with possible posterior acoustic shadowing within the joint recess. In children, transient synovitis causes an effusion but without synovial hypertrophy visible by ultrasound.[1]

Labrum and Proximal Femur Abnormalities

Other intra-articular structures visible by ultrasound include the portions of the hypoechoic hyaline cartilage that cover the femoral head and the hyperechoic triangle-shaped fibrocartilage acetabular labrum. Labral degeneration may appear as diffuse hypoechogenicity, while a labrum tear appears as a defined hypoechoic or anechoic cleft, which is more conspicuous when there is adjacent joint fluid (Fig. 6.40). The presence of a hypoechoic or anechoic paralabral cyst is also an indicator of underlying hip labrum tear (Fig. 6.41; see 6.44).[41,42] The accuracy of

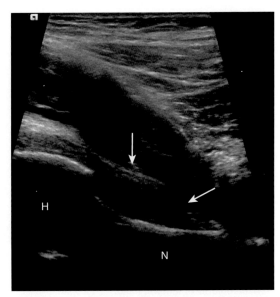

■ FIGURE 6.38 **Synovial Hypertrophy: Rheumatoid Arthritis.** Ultrasound image in long axis to the femoral neck shows hypoechoic anterior joint recess distention *(arrows)*. *A,* Acetabulum; *H,* femoral head; *N,* femoral neck.

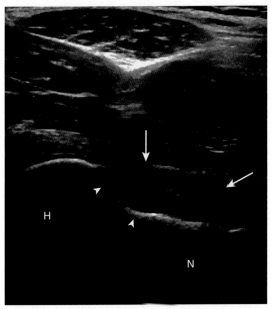

■ FIGURE 6.39 **Synovial Hypertrophy: Pigmented Villonodular Synovitis.** Ultrasound image in long axis to the femoral neck shows hypoechoic anterior joint recess distention *(arrows)* and cortical erosion *(arrowheads)*. *H,* Femoral head; *N,* femoral neck.

ultrasound in the diagnosis of hip labrum tear is variable because limitations exist given the depth of and limited access to the labrum.[43-45] However, accuracy is highest anteriorly where labral tears commonly occur. Chondrocalcinosis, which may be idiopathic or from calcium pyrophosphate

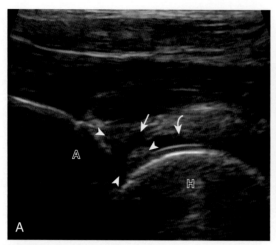

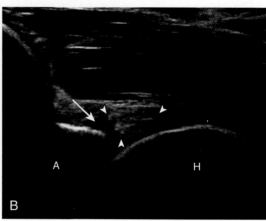

■ **FIGURE 6.40 Labral Tear.** Ultrasound images in long axis to the femoral neck from two different patients show an anechoic cleft *(arrow)* with the hyperechoic fibrocartilage labrum *(arrowheads)* in (A) and labral detachment *(arrow)* in (B). Note (A) joint effusion *(curved arrow)* adjacent to the femoral head hypoechoic hyaline cartilage. *A,* Acetabulum; *H,* femoral head.

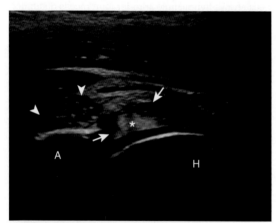

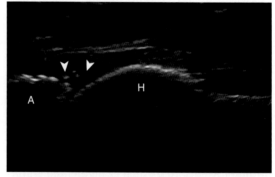

■ **FIGURE 6.42 Chondrocalcinosis.** Ultrasound image in long axis to the femoral neck shows hyperechoic foci within the labrum *(arrowheads)* representing chondrocalcinosis. *A,* Acetabulum; *H,* femoral head.

■ **FIGURE 6.41 Labral Tear and Paralabral Cyst.** Ultrasound image in long axis to the femoral neck shows an anechoic cleft *(arrows)* extending through the labrum *(asterisk)* with a hypoechoic paralabral cyst *(arrowheads)*. *A,* Acetabulum; *H,* femoral head.

dihydrate crystal deposition, will create punctate reflective echoes within the labrum (Fig. 6.42).

The cortical surfaces of the proximal femur are also assessed for abnormalities. A step-off deformity of the femoral neck can indicate a fracture.[46] An osteophyte at the femoral neck indicates osteoarthritis (Fig. 6.43). Cortical irregularity or bony protuberance of the anterosuperior femoral head-neck junction and non-spherical appearance can be seen in cam-type femoroacetabular impingement.[47-50] Dynamic imaging with hip flexion and internal rotation may show direct contact between a labral tear and femoral cortical irregularity, which supports the diagnosis (Fig. 6.44) (Videos 6.12 and 6.13). Treatment of

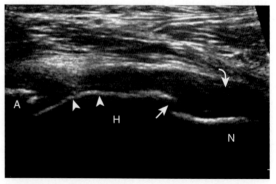

■ **FIGURE 6.43 Osteoarthritis.** Ultrasound image in long axis to the femoral neck shows a marginal osteophyte at the head-neck junction *(arrow)* and irregular contour of the femoral head *(arrowheads)*. Note the hypoechoic distention of the joint capsule *(curved arrow)*. *A,* Acetabulum; *H,* femoral head; *N,* femoral neck.

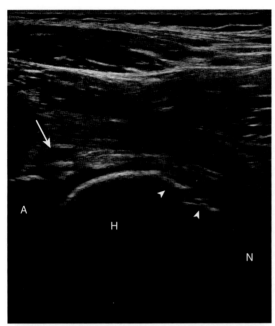

■ **FIGURE 6.44 Femoroacetabular Impingement.** Ultrasound image in long axis to the femoral neck shows cortical irregularity *(arrowheads)* of the anterior femoral head *(H)* and neck *(N)*. Note labral tear and associated anechoic paralabral cyst *(arrow)*. *A*, Acetabulum.

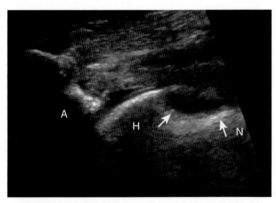

■ **FIGURE 6.45 Osteoplasty.** Ultrasound image in long axis to the femoral neck shows concavity at the femoral head-neck junction *(arrows)* from prior surgical osteoplasty. *A*, Acetabulum; *H*, femoral head; *N*, femoral neck.

femoroacetabular impingement includes osteoplasty, which will appear as a cortical defect at the femoral head-neck junction (Fig. 6.45).

Bursal Abnormalities

There are many bursae that can be found about the hip.[11] The iliopsoas bursa is located anterior to the hip joint.[51] When distended, the iliopsoas bursa is seen medial to iliopsoas complex and may extend anterior adjacent to the neurovascular structures or extend lateral and posterior to the

iliopsoas.[52] The iliopsoas bursa communicates with the hip joint in up to 15% of the population, and its distention is often related to hip joint pathology.[10] Possible communication between the iliopsoas bursa and the hip joint can be visualized in the transverse plane at the level of the femoral head immediately medial to the psoas major tendon of the iliopsoas complex (Fig. 6.46A). The iliopsoas bursa may be distended with simple fluid, complex fluid (6.46B and C), or synovial hypertrophy, which may range from anechoic to hyperechoic. Similar to joint recess distention, lack of compressibility and the presence of internal flow on color Doppler imaging suggest synovial hypertrophy. An abnormally distended bursa may extend into the abdomen and should not be confused for an intra-abdominal or psoas abscess.[53] In addition, distention of the iliopsoas bursa does not imply inflammation or true bursitis but may be due to hip pathology; the presence of pain with transducer pressure, internal flow on color Doppler imaging, and bursal distention out of proportion to hip joint recess distention suggest true inflammation and bursitis.

The greater trochanteric region is also evaluated for abnormal bursal distention.[2] The trochanteric (or subgluteus maximus) bursa originates between the gluteus maximus and posterior facet of the greater trochanter but also extends laterally between the gluteus medius tendon and overlying iliotibial tract (Fig. 6.47 and see Fig. 6.16). Evaluation with the patient lying on the contralateral side is important to access the entire posterior facet to evaluate for focal trochanteric bursal distention posteriorly. Similar to other bursae, distention of the trochanteric bursa can be from simple fluid, complex fluid, or synovial hypertrophy, related to infection (Fig. 6.48) or inflammatory arthritis (Fig. 6.49) (Video 6.14). As described earlier, the subgluteus minimus bursa (Fig. 6.50) and subgluteus medius bursa are located between the greater trochanter and their respective tendons, are smaller, and less commonly distended. In the setting of *greater trochanteric pain syndrome*, identification of a distended and inflamed bursa is rare.[54-57] Gluteus minimus and medius tendon abnormalities are typically the primary cause of symptoms and not a bursa (Fig. 6.47).[54,57-59] Uncommonly, an obturator externus bursa may be seen at the medial aspect of the lesser trochanter of the femur[12] or an ischial (ischiogluteal) bursa (Fig. 6.51) superficial to the ischial tuberosity (Video 6.15).[60]

Post-Surgical Hip

With regard to a hip replacement, the femoral head and proximal femur are typically replaced

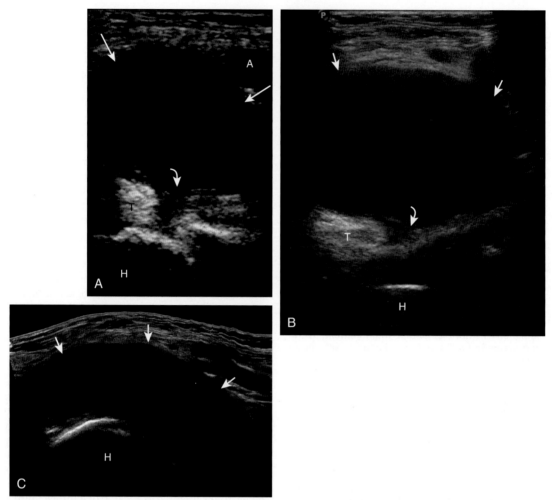

■ **FIGURE 6.46 Iliopsoas Bursal Distention.** Ultrasound image (A) transverse to the femoral head *(H)* shows anechoic distention of the iliopsoas bursa *(arrows)*. Note the communication with the hip joint *(curved arrow)* medial to the psoas major tendon *(T)* of the iliopsoas complex, adjacent to femoral artery *(A)*. Ultrasound images (B) transverse and (C) sagittal (with extended field of view) over the femoral head *(H)* in a different patient show complex fluid distention of iliopsoas bursa *(arrows)* with hip joint communication *(curved arrow)* medial to psoas major tendon *(T)* of iliopsoas complex.

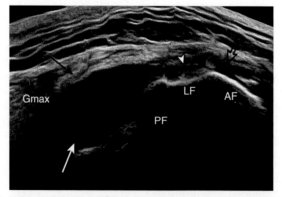

■ **FIGURE 6.47 Trochanteric (Subgluteus Maximus) Bursal Distention.** Ultrasound images in short axis to the femur show anechoic distention of the trochanteric bursa *(arrows)*. Note tear of the gluteus minimus *(open arrow)*, tendinosis of gluteus medius *(arrowhead)*, and posterior location of trochanteric bursa deep to gluteus maximus *(Gmax)*. *AF*, Anterior facet of the greater trochanter; *LF*, lateral facet; *PF*, posterior facet.

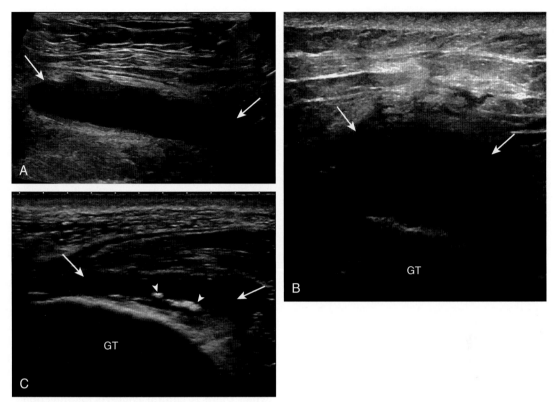

■ FIGURE 6.48 **Trochanteric (Subgluteus Maximus) Bursal Distention: Infection.** Ultrasound images from three different patients show hypoechoic bursal distention *(arrows)* adjacent to greater trochanter *(GT)*. Note echogenic gas foci *(arrowheads)* in (C).

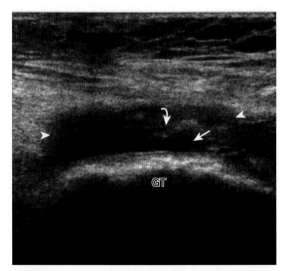

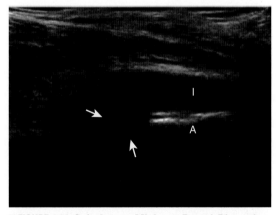

■ FIGURE 6.49 **Trochanteric (Subgluteus Maximus) Bursal Distention: Lupus.** Coronal ultrasound image, over the greater trochanter *(GT)* shows anechoic fluid *(arrow)* and hypoechoic synovial hypertrophy *(curved arrow)*, which distends the trochanteric bursa *(arrowheads)*.

■ FIGURE 6.50 **Subgluteus Minimus Bursal Distention.** Ultrasound in long axis to the gluteus minimus tendon *(I)* shows hypoechoic distention *(arrows)* of the subgluteus minimus bursa. Note severe tendinosis of the gluteus minimus tendon. *A,* Anterior facet of the greater trochanter.

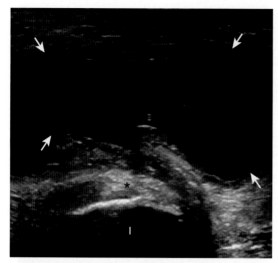

■ **FIGURE 6.51 Ischial Bursal Distention.** Ultrasound image in the transverse plane over the ischium *(I)* shows heterogeneous but predominantly hypoechoic complex bursa distention *(arrows)* *(asterisk,* conjoined biceps femoris–semitendinosus tendon of hamstring).

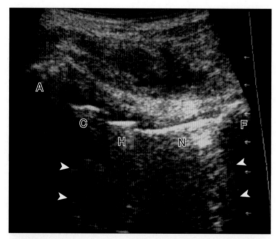

■ **FIGURE 6.52 Normal Total Hip Arthroplasty.** Ultrasound image in long axis to the femoral neck of hip arthroplasty shows the reflective surfaces of the acetabular cup *(C)*, femoral head *(H)*, and femoral neck *(N)* components with posterior reverberation artifact *(arrowheads)*. Note the native acetabulum *(A)* and femur *(F)* with posterior acoustic shadowing.

with material composed of metal or ceramic, with a plastic, metal, or ceramic acetabular cup. At sonography, these components demonstrate a hyperechoic surface and possible posterior reverberation (with a metal surface) (Fig. 6.52).[61] When imaging the proximal femur in long axis to the femoral neck, the echogenic surface contours of

the arthroplasty will show posterior reverberation artifact in contrast to the more distal native femur, which will appear hyperechoic with shadowing. The echogenic edge of the acetabular cup is also seen (if present); the adjacent native acetabulum more proximally produces posterior acoustic shadowing. Hypoechogenicity superficial to the neck of the prosthesis, and up to 6 mm superficial to the native femur at the prosthesis-bone junction has been described in asymptomatic patients after total hip arthroplasty.[62]

A hip joint effusion appears as a hypoechoic or anechoic layer over the femoral neck of the prosthesis (Fig. 6.53).[40] The margins of the effusion may be ill defined if the hip joint capsule has been resected because the fluid will then be outlined by a pseudocapsule. However, ultrasound is unreliable in the diagnosis of a small joint effusion after hip replacement due to hypoechoic post-surgical changes, which is often compounded when a patient has a large body habitus.[40] Ultrasound can be more accurate with larger joint effusions. The presence of complex fluid extending beyond the joint into the soft tissues should raise concern for infection (Fig. 6.54).[61] Regardless of sonographic findings, one should consider joint aspiration when there is clinical concern for infection. If no fluid is present at joint aspiration attempt, lavage and re-aspiration are recommended to exclude infection.[63] If percutaneous aspiration is considered using fluoroscopy, the soft tissues anterior to the femoral neck should be evaluated with cross-sectional imaging such as ultrasound to avoid the potential contamination of a sterile joint by passing a needle through overlying soft tissue infection.[64]

Other causes of joint effusion after arthroplasty include prosthesis loosening and particle disease, the latter representing inflammatory reaction to breakdown of the prosthesis components that may cause osteolysis and joint distention. An adverse periprosthetic soft tissue reaction associated with metal-on-metal hip arthroplasties has been termed *pseudotumor* and can appear as heterogeneous but predominantly hypoechoic with ultrasound (Fig. 6.55).[65,66] After hip replacement, the incision site, bursa[67] (see Fig. 6.48), and femoral shaft along the extent of the arthroplasty (Fig. 6.56), as well as any symptomatic area should also be evaluated (Video 6.16). The gluteal tendons should also be evaluated for abnormality after arthroplasty, especially if an arthroplasty is placed using a direct lateral or modified anterolateral approach.[68] Another cause of symptoms includes iliopsoas impingement from the anterior aspect of the femoral component[69] or acetabular cup[70] (Fig. 6.57) of a hip arthroplasty. Acetabular liner displacement may also be detected.[71]

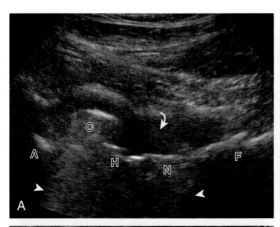

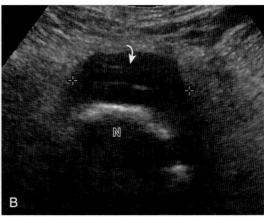

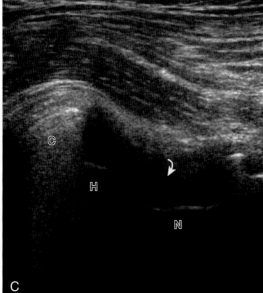

■ FIGURE 6.53 **Hip Arthroplasty and Effusion.** Ultrasound images in (A) long axis and (B) short axis to the femoral neck of a total hip arthroplasty show the reflective surfaces of the acetabular cup *(C)*, femoral head *(H)*, and femoral neck *(N)* components with posterior reverberation artifact *(arrowheads)* and overlying hypoechoic joint fluid *(curved arrows)*. Note the native acetabulum *(A)* and femur *(F)* with posterior acoustic shadowing. Ultrasound image (C) long axis to the femoral neck of a bipolar hip hemiarthroplasty shows similar findings.

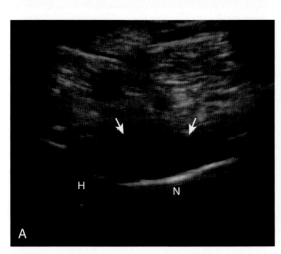

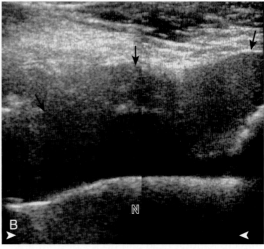

■ FIGURE 6.54 **Infected Total Hip Arthroplasty.** Ultrasound image (A) in long axis to the femoral neck of a hip arthroplasty shows hypoechoic fluid *(arrows)* over the femoral neck *(N)* and head *(H)* of the prosthesis. Ultrasound image (B) in long axis to the femoral neck of a hip arthroplasty in a different patient shows reflective surfaces of the femoral neck *(N)* component with posterior reverberation artifact *(arrowheads)*. Note the anechoic and hypoechoic complex fluid *(arrows)* extending from the joint into the adjacent soft tissues.

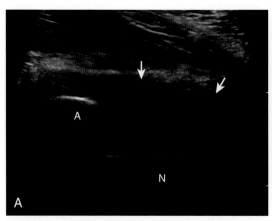
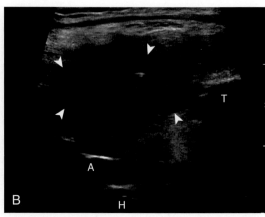

■ FIGURE 6.55 **Pseudotumor.** Ultrasound images in long axis to the femoral neck of a metal-on-metal total hip arthroplasty in the (A) sagittal and (B) coronal planes show abnormal hypoechoic distention of the pseudocapsule *(arrows)* with an adjacent lateral hypoechoic and heterogeneous mass-like area *(arrowheads)*. A, Acetabular component; H, femoral head component; N, femoral neck; T, greater trochanter.

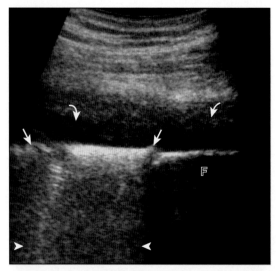

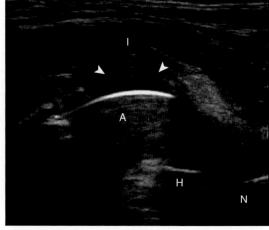

■ FIGURE 6.57 **Iliopsoas Impingement.** Ultrasound image in long axis to the femoral neck component of a total hip arthroplasty shows abnormal hypoechoic tissue *(arrowheads)* between the iliopsoas *(I)* and acetabular cup *(A)* of the arthroplasty. H, Femoral head component; N, femoral neck component.

■ FIGURE 6.56 **Infected Hip Arthroplasty Endoprosthesis.** Ultrasound image in long axis to the femoral shaft at the junction of the metal endoprosthesis *(arrows)* and native femur *(F)* shows hypoechoic complex fluid *(curved arrows)*. Note the posterior reverberation artifact from the prosthesis *(arrowheads)*.

Regardless of the type of surgery, an incision site is a common location for pathology such as infection, hematoma (Fig. 6.58A), seroma (Fig. 6.58B), and heterotopic ossification (Fig. 6.58C). Another surgical procedure of the hip involves complete femoral head and neck resection after infection *(Girdlestone procedure)*. Post-surgical changes can be seen at the femoral head-neck junction after osteoplasty for treatment of femoroacetabular impingement (see Fig. 6.45).

■ TENDON AND MUSCLE ABNORMALITIES

Tendon and Muscle Injury

Similar to other tendons in the body, a degenerative condition of tendons called *tendinosis* is characterized by abnormal tendon hypoechogenicity and possible increased thickness.[8,72,73] This term is used instead of tendinitis because there are no significant acute inflammatory cells in this situation but rather mucoid degeneration and possible interstitial tearing. Partial-thickness

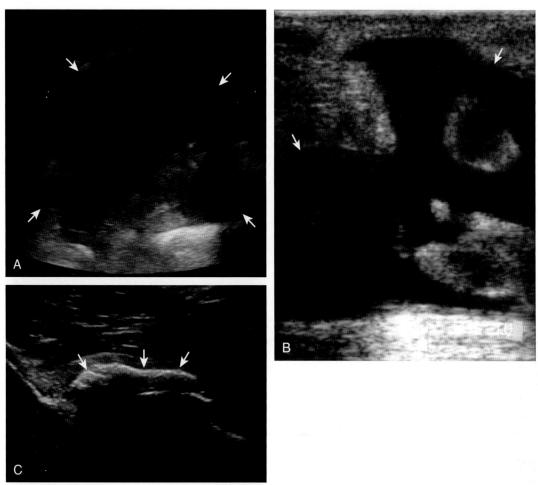

■ FIGURE 6.58 **Post Surgical Soft Tissue Abnormalities.** Ultrasound images in three different patients show (A) heterogeneous but predominantly hypoechoic hematoma *(arrows)*, (B) heterogeneous but predominantly anechoic seroma *(arrows)*, and (C) echogenic and shadowing heterotopic ossification *(arrows)*.

tendon tears are characterized by more defined hypoechoic or anechoic clefts within the involved tendon but without the complete tendon disruption and retraction that are characteristic of full-thickness tears. In this latter condition, the tendon is torn and retracted with interposed heterogeneous but predominantly hypoechoic hemorrhage. Cortical irregularity at a tendon footprint or attachment is common with chronic repetitive injury or attrition. Muscles that cross two joints are prone to tears at the musculotendinous junction; chronic injuries occur at the entheses, and direct impact injuries involve the muscle belly.

ADDUCTOR MUSCULATURE AND PUBIC SYMPHYSIS REGION

Tendinosis and partial-thickness tears commonly involve the adductor longus origin at the pubis (Fig. 6.59). This finding may be associated with

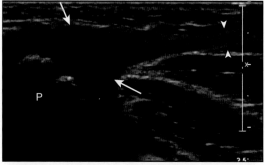

■ FIGURE 6.59 **Adductor Longus: Tendinosis and Partial Tear.** Ultrasound image in long axis to the adductor longus tendon shows hypoechoic tendinosis *(arrows)* with focal more defined interstitial tears. Note cortical irregularity of pubis *(P)* and normal distal adductor longus tendon *(arrowheads)*.

abnormality of the common aponeurosis between the rectus abdominis and the adductor longus tendons superficial to the pubis, a finding described with *athletic pubalgia* (a term preferred over "sports hernia"), appearing as hypoechoic tendon thickening with cortical irregularity (Fig. 6.60).[24,31,74] The symphysis pubis should also be evaluated for effusion, capsular thickening, and possible offset. Full-thickness adductor tears are characterized by tendon retraction and interposed hemorrhage (Fig. 6.61), with possible hyperechoic avulsed cortical fragment. Distal to the adductor origin,

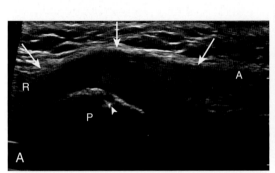
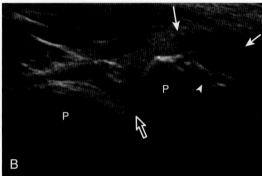

■ **FIGURE 6.60 Common Aponeurosis Injury (Chronic).** Ultrasound images in the (A) sagittal-oblique and (B) transverse planes over the pubis *(P)* show hypoechoic thickening of the common aponeurosis *(arrows)* that extends to the rectus abdominis *(R)* and adductor longus *(A)* with cortical irregularity *(arrowheads)*. Note the pubic symphysis *(open arrow)* in (B).

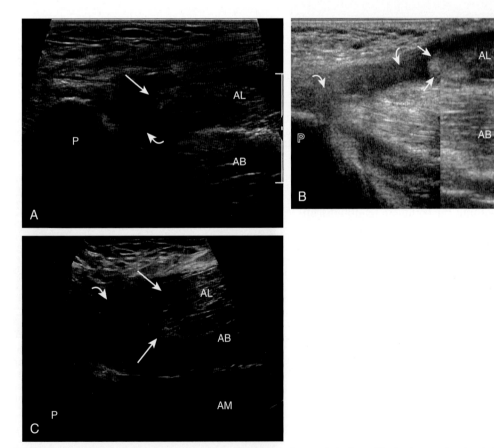

■ **FIGURE 6.61 Adductor Tears: Acute.** Ultrasound images in long axis to the adductor longus tendon in three different patients show retracted full-thickness tears *(arrows)* of the adductor longus (A and B), with adductor brevis (C) and intervening hemorrhage *(curved arrows)*. P, Pubis.

a muscle strain from a stretch injury or a hematoma from direct impact injury may be found (Fig. 6.62). At the adductor insertion onto the posteromedial femur, chronic repetitive stress injury has been termed *thigh splints* or *adductor*

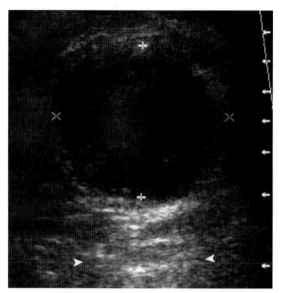

■ **FIGURE 6.62 Adductor Muscle Injury.** Ultrasound image shows a heterogeneous hypoechoic hematoma *(between cursors)* with increased through-transmission *(arrowheads)*.

insertion avulsion syndrome.[75] In this condition, an irregular bone surface can indicate periostitis and possible stress fracture and is typically the site of point tenderness with transducer pressure (Fig. 6.63). Because groin symptoms are often multifactorial, a comprehensive ultrasound evaluation should be considered; inguinal hernia and adductor tendon abnormalities often coexist in patients with femoroacetabular impingement.[16]

RECTUS FEMORIS

Abnormalities may involve the individual direct (Fig. 6.64A) and indirect head origins of the rectus femoris, whereas complete tears of both heads result in a full-thickness tear and retraction (Fig. 6.64B). Injury can also occur at the central myotendinous aponeurosis, which will appear as abnormal hypoechogenicity surrounding the indirect head within the muscle belly (Figs. 6.65 and 6.66).[6] Partial tear can appear as hypoechoic fiber disruption.[73] More distally, the posterior aponeurosis may be injured with resulting hematoma (Fig. 6.67A and B), which may later appear as hyperechoic scar (Fig. 6.67C). A complete tear of the distal rectus femoris is characterized by muscle retraction and may be associated with anechoic fluid (Fig. 6.68). It is not uncommon for patients to present later with a palpable pseudomass, which

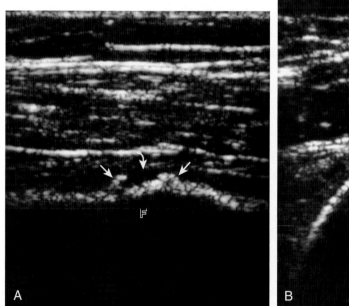

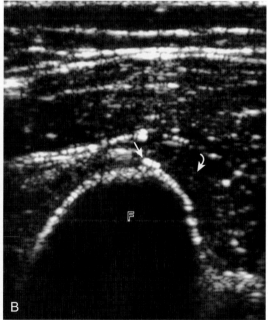

■ **FIGURE 6.63 Thigh Splints (Adductor Insertion Avulsion Syndrome).** Ultrasound images in (A) long axis and (B) short axis to the femoral diaphysis show a cortical irregularity *(arrows)* and adjacent hypoechoic hemorrhage or periostitis *(curved arrows)* at the adductor tendon insertion. *F, Femur. (From Weaver JS, Jacobson JA, Jamadar DA, et al: Sonographic findings of adductor insertion avulsion syndrome with magnetic resonance imaging correlation. J Ultrasound Med 22:403-407, 2003. Reproduced with permission from the American Institute of Ultrasound in Medicine.)*

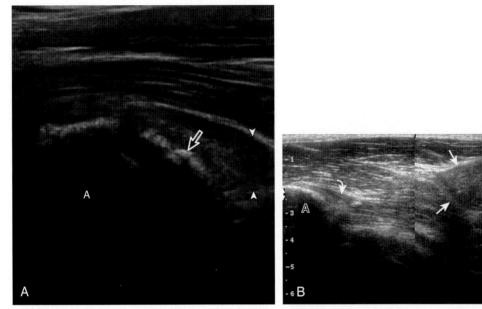

■ **FIGURE 6.64 Rectus Femoris Injury (Proximal).** Ultrasound images from two different patients in long axis to the proximal rectus femoris show (A) cortical avulsion *(open arrow)* of direct head *(arrowheads)* from anterior inferior iliac spine *(A),* and (B) full-thickness tear *(arrows)* retracted from its origin *(curved arrow).*

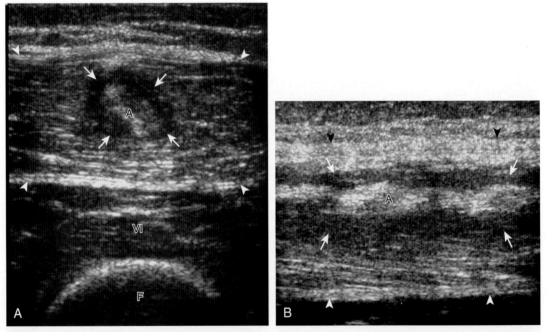

■ **FIGURE 6.65 Rectus Femoris Tear: Central Aponeurosis.** Ultrasound images in (A) short axis and (B) long axis to the rectus femoris show hypoechoic hemorrhage *(arrows)* that surrounds the central aponeurosis *(A)* within the center of the rectus femoris muscle *(arrowheads). F,* Femur; *VI,* vastus intermedius.

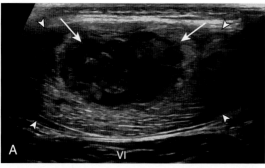
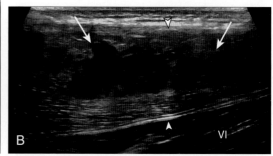

■ **FIGURE 6.66 Rectus Femoris Tear: Central Aponeurosis.** Ultrasound images in (A) short axis and (B) long axis to the rectus femoris show hypoechoic hemorrhage *(arrows)* that disrupts the central aponeurosis within the center of the rectus femoris muscle *(arrowheads)*. *VI,* Vastus intermedius.

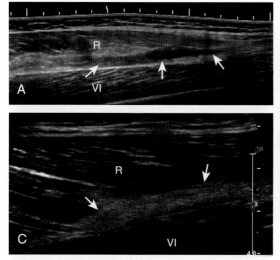
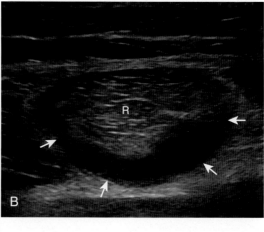

■ **FIGURE 6.67 Rectus Femoris Tear: Posterior Aponeurosis.** Ultrasound images in (A) long axis (with extended field of view) and (B) short axis to the rectus femoris *(R)* show hypoechoic hemorrhage *(arrows)* along the posterior aponeurosis. Ultrasound image (C) in long axis to the rectus femoris *(R)* in a different patient shows hyperechoic scar *(arrows)* from remote injury. *VI,* Vastus intermedius.

■ **FIGURE 6.68 Rectus Femoris Tear (Distal): Full Thickness.** Ultrasound images in two different patients in long axis to the rectus femoris *(R)* show full-thickness disruption *(between arrows)* and tendon retraction *(curved arrow)* producing a palpable mass. Note hypoechoic *(asterisks)* and anechoic organizing hematoma at the site of the tear *(between arrows)*. *VI,* Vastus intermedius.

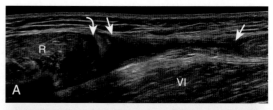
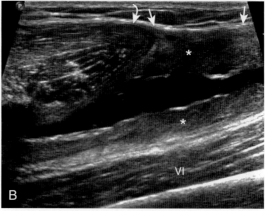

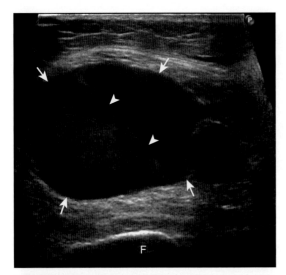

■ FIGURE 6.69 **Quadriceps Hematoma.** Ultrasound image in short axis to the quadriceps musculature shows acute hematoma *(arrows)* with dependent serum hematocrit level *(arrowheads)*. *F,* Femur.

represents the retracted muscle and tendon. A direct impact injury may cause an intramuscular hematoma (Fig. 6.69). Distal quadriceps tendon tears are discussed in Chapter 7.

GLUTEUS MINIMUS AND MEDIUS

The gluteus minimus and medius tendons may also be abnormal at their greater trochanter insertion, ranging from tendinosis (Figs. 6.70 and 6.71) to tendon tear (Figs. 6.72 and 6.73).[58] After surgical repair, an intact tendon may appear hypoechoic with visible suture material (Fig. 6.74). As described earlier, symptoms causing *greater trochanteric pain syndrome* are due to gluteal tendon abnormalities and not an isolated true bursitis.[54-57] The reported sensitivity of ultrasound in the diagnosis of gluteal tendon tears ranges from 79% to 100%.[76] Gluteus medius tendon tears are more common than gluteus minimus tendon tears, and often a bursal abnormality is associated with the

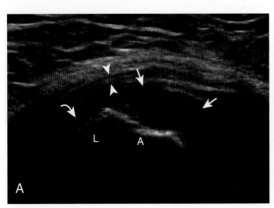

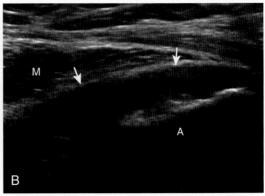

■ FIGURE 6.70 **Gluteus Minimus: Tendinosis.** Ultrasound images (A) short axis and (B) long axis to the gluteus minimus show hypoechoic thickening *(arrows)* *(curved arrow,* gluteus medius tendon; *arrowheads,* iliotibial tract). *A,* Anterior facet; *L,* lateral facet of greater trochanter; *M,* gluteus medius muscle.

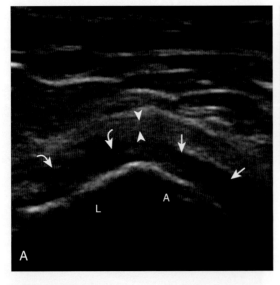

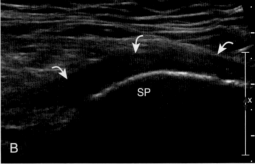

■ FIGURE 6.71 **Gluteus Medius and Minimus: Tendinosis.** Ultrasound images (A) short axis and (B) long axis to the gluteus tendons show hypoechoic thickening of the gluteus medius *(curved arrows)* and minimus *(arrows).* Note involvement of gluteus medius at the superoposterior facet *(SP)* in (B). *A,* Anterior facet; *L,* lateral facet of greater trochanter; *(arrowheads,* iliotibial tract).

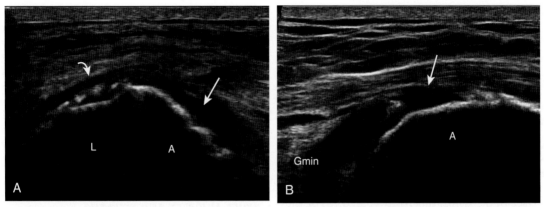

■ **FIGURE 6.72 Gluteus Minimus: Tear.** Ultrasound images in (A) short axis and (B) long axis to the gluteus minimus tendon show anechoic tear *(arrow)* (*curved arrow*, gluteus medius tendon with tendinosis and calcification). *A*, Anterior facet; *L*, lateral facet of greater trochanter; *Gmin*, proximal gluteus minimus muscle.

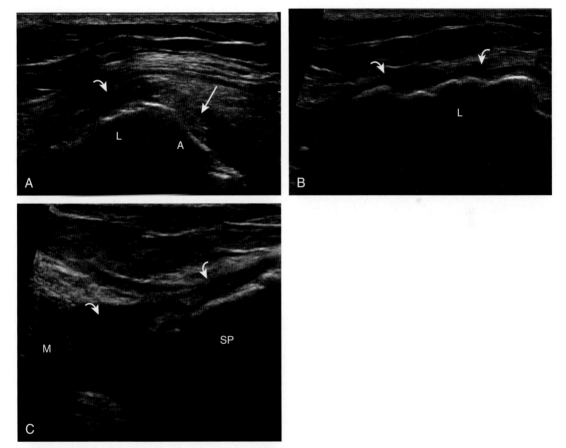

■ **FIGURE 6.73 Gluteus Medius: Tear.** Ultrasound images in (A) short axis and (B and C) long axis to the gluteus medius show absence of the gluteus medius tendon *(curved arrows)* (*arrow*, gluteus minimus tendon). *A*, Anterior facet of greater trochanter; *L*, lateral facet; *SP*, superoposterior facet; *M*, proximal gluteus medius muscle.

tendon tear.[59] Identification of the characteristic bone contours of the greater trochanter is essential for orientation and accurate localization of tendon and soft tissue abnormalities (see Fig. 6.16).[2] Calcific tendinosis of the gluteal tendons is discussed later in this chapter.

HAMSTRINGS

Chronic hamstring injury produces tendinosis, possible partial-thickness tear, and bone irregularity of the ischium.[8,77] Injury may selectively involve the semimembranosus tendon origin at the lateral surface of the ischial tuberosity (Fig. 6.75) or the conjoined biceps femoris–semitendinosus tendon at the superficial surface (Fig. 6.76). Isolated tear of one of the two tendons may also be possible (Fig. 6.77), as well as partial tear and hematoma at the musculotendinous junction (Fig. 6.78). In the setting of a proximal conjoined biceps femoris–semimembranosus tendon tear, intact

sacrotuberous ligament fibers may minimize tendon retraction (Fig. 6.79).[34] Complete tear of the hamstring tendon origin is characterized by absence of tendon fibers and retraction (Fig. 6.80). Chronic injuries may be associated with hyperechoic scar formation, which may affect the adjacent sciatic nerve, and possible pseudotumor appearance at physical examination as a result of muscle retraction (Fig. 6.81).[78] Given close proximity, adductor magnus tendon injury should also be considered when evaluating the hamstrings (Fig. 6.82).

OTHER MUSCLES AND TENDONS

Other muscle and tendon injuries can also involve the sartorius (Fig. 6.83) and proximal tensor fascia latae (Fig. 6.84). Spontaneous muscle hemorrhage has been described with the iliopsoas in the setting of hemophilia and in patients who are anticoagulated (Fig. 6.85), which may appear as heterogeneous muscle enlargement that could simulate a soft tissue tumor (Video 6.17).

Snapping Hip Syndrome

Abnormal snapping conditions with hip movement have been termed *snapping hip syndrome*, which can be divided into intra-articular and extra-articular causes. Intra-articular causes relate to joint processes, such as intra-articular bodies or prior trauma. Extra-articular types include internal (related to iliopsoas) and external (related to iliotibial tract and gluteus maximus) and are ideally evaluated dynamically with ultrasound.[79,80]

Snapping hip syndrome related to the iliopsoas complex occurs anteriorly at the level of the anterior inferior iliac spine.[4] To diagnose this specific condition, a flexed, abducted, and

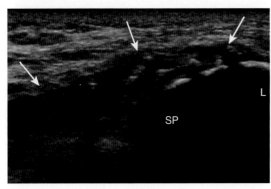

■ FIGURE 6.74 **Gluteus Medius: Repair.** Ultrasound image in long axis to the gluteus medius shows hypoechoic enlarged tendon with internal hyperechoic suture material. *L,* Lateral facet of greater trochanter; *SP,* superoposterior facet.

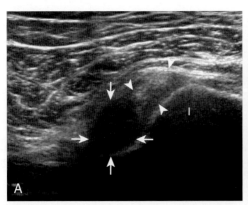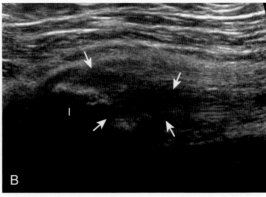

■ FIGURE 6.75 **Semimembranosus: Tendinosis.** Ultrasound images in (A) short axis and (B) long axis to the proximal hamstring tendons show hypoechoic swelling *(arrows)* of the semimembranosus tendon with adjacent cortical irregularity of the ischial tuberosity *(I)* and normal conjoined biceps femoris–semitendinosus tendon *(arrowheads).* Left side of image is lateral in (A).

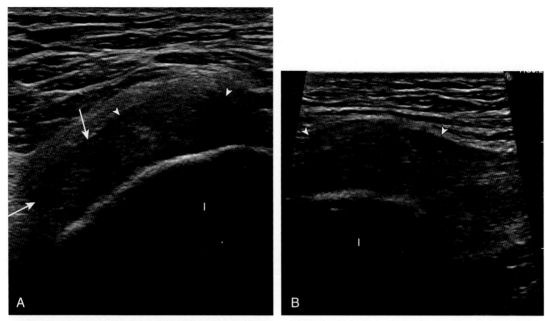

■ **FIGURE 6.76 Conjoined Biceps Femoris–Semitendinosus Tendon: Tendinosis.** Ultrasound images in (A) short axis and (B) long axis to the conjoined biceps femoris–semitendinosus tendon show hypoechoic swelling *(arrowheads)* and normal semimembranosus tendon *(arrows)*. *I*, Ischial tuberosity. Left side of image is lateral in (A).

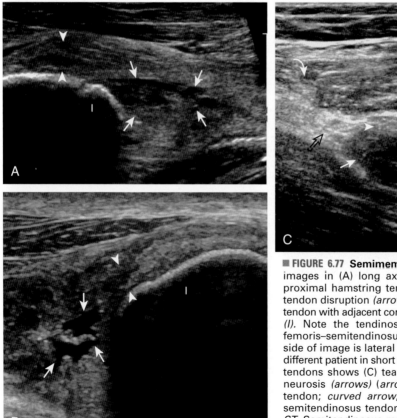

■ **FIGURE 6.77 Semimembranosus: Tear.** Ultrasound images in (A) long axis and (B) short axis to the proximal hamstring tendons show anechoic partial tendon disruption *(arrows)* of the semimembranosus tendon with adjacent cortical irregularity of the ischium *(I)*. Note the tendinosis of the conjoined biceps femoris–semitendinosus tendon *(arrowheads)*. Left side of image is lateral in (B). Ultrasound image in a different patient in short axis to the proximal hamstring tendons shows (C) tear of semimembranosus aponeurosis *(arrows)* *(arrowheads, semimembranosus tendon; curved arrow, conjoined biceps femoris–semitendinosus tendon; open arrow, sciatic nerve)*. *ST*, Semitendinosus muscle.

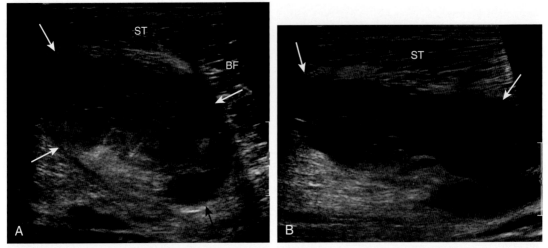

■ **FIGURE 6.78** **Semimembranosus: Tear (Distal).** Ultrasound images in (A) short axis and (B) long axis to the semimembranosus show partial muscle tear and hematoma *(arrows)* with increased posterior through-transmission. *ST,* Semitendinosus; *BF,* biceps femoris.

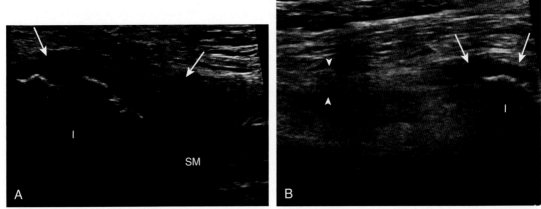

■ **FIGURE 6.79** **Conjoined Biceps Femoris–Semitendinosus Tendon: Tear.** Ultrasound image in (A) long axis shows hypoechoic thickening and small anechoic clefts of conjoined biceps femoris–semitendinosus tendon *(arrows)* with cortical irregularity of ischium *(I).* Ultrasound image in (B) long axis to sacrotuberous ligament *(arrowheads)* shows hypoechoic thickening where its fibers are continuous with the conjoined biceps femoris–semitendinosus tendon.

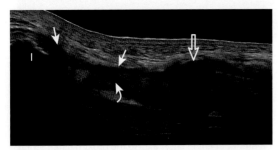

■ **FIGURE 6.80** **Hamstring Tendons: Complete Tear.** Ultrasound image in long axis (with extended field of view) to the hamstrings shows absence of the proximal hamstring tendons *(between arrows)* with distal retraction *(curved arrow)* and avulsion fracture fragment *(open arrow)*. *I,* Ischium.

externally rotated hip (frog-leg position) is straightened during sonographic visualization, or the patient is asked to reproduce the snapping sensation. Normally, the psoas major tendon moves anterior and laterally during the maneuver and returns to normal position when the leg is straightened without muscle interposition deep to the tendon or abrupt snapping. In the abnormal situation, the medial fibers of the iliacus muscle are temporarily entrapped between the psoas major tendon and superior pubic ramus in the flexed, abducted, externally rotated hip. When the leg is straightened, the medial fibers of the iliacus muscle move laterally and the psoas major tendon abruptly moves toward the superior pubic

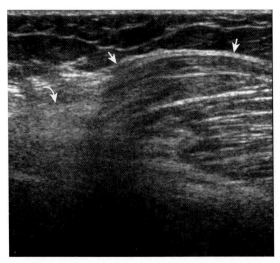

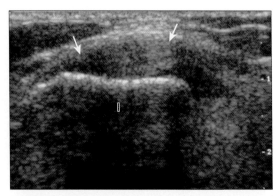

■ FIGURE 6.84 **Tensor Fascia Latae: Tendinosis.** Ultrasound image in long axis to the proximal tensor fascia latae shows hypoechoic thickening *(arrows). I,* Ilium.

■ FIGURE 6.81 **Semimembranosus Tear: Chronic.** Ultrasound image in long axis to the semimembranosus shows chronic tear with pseudomass appearance at the muscle contraction *(arrows)* and adjacent hyperechoic scar tissue *(curved arrow).*

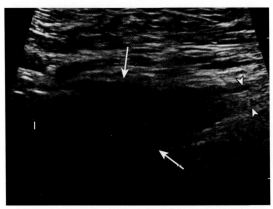

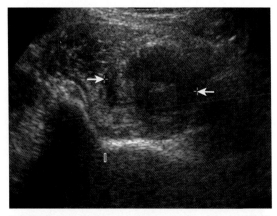

■ FIGURE 6.85 **Iliopsoas: Hemorrhage (Hemophilia).** Ultrasound image in short axis to the iliopsoas shows heterogeneous but predominantly hypoechoic hemorrhage *(arrows). I,* Ilium.

■ FIGURE 6.82 **Adductor Magnus Tear.** Ultrasound image in long axis to the adductor magnus shows hypoechoic enlargement *(arrows)* at the ischial tuberosity *(I).*

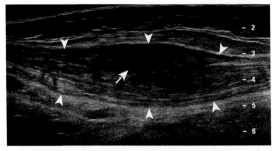

■ FIGURE 6.83 **Sartorius: Partial Tear.** Ultrasound image in long axis to the sartorius muscle shows hypoechoic thickening *(arrowheads)* and anechoic clefts *(arrow)* representing a partial-thickness tear.

ramus producing the snap that is felt though the transducer, correlating with patient symptoms (Fig. 6.86) (Videos 6.18 and 6.19).[4] Snapping of the psoas major tendon may uncommonly occur during the flexion aspect of the maneuver, or may be due to a bifid tendon, or psoas major tendon movement over a paralabral cyst.[4,81] Contrary to prior descriptions, the snapping is usually not related to tendon contact with the iliopectineal eminence.[4]

The external variety of external snapping hip syndrome can result from snapping the gluteus maximus tendon (Video 6.20) and/or iliotibial tract over the greater trochanter with hip flexion and extension (Fig. 6.87) (Video 6.21).[82,83] The patient is asked to reproduce the symptom, and many times the patient has to stand and shift weight on the affected limb, or the patient may lie on the contralateral hip to allow hip flexion and extension. Ultrasound transverse over the greater trochanter shows abnormal abrupt snapping of the

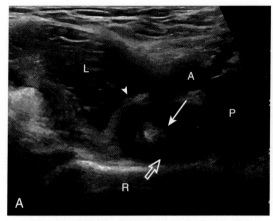
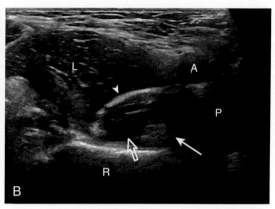

■ **FIGURE 6.86 Snapping Hip Syndrome: Iliopsoas Tendon.** Ultrasound image in short axis to the iliopsoas complex with (A) hip flexion/abduction shows entrapment of the medial fibers of iliacus muscle *(open arrow)* between the psoas major tendon *(arrow)* and superior pubic ramus *(R)*. During hip extension (B), the medial fibers of the iliacus muscle *(open arrow)* move laterally and there is abrupt motion of the psoas major tendon *(arrow)* toward the superior pubic ramus *(R)* producing the snapping symptom. *L*, Lateral fibers of iliacus muscle; *arrowhead*, intermuscular fascia; *P*, psoas major muscle; *A*, femoral artery (left side of images is lateral).

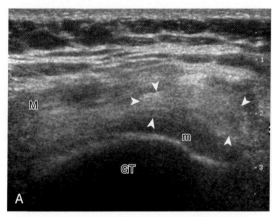
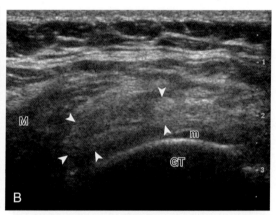

■ **FIGURE 6.87 Snapping Hip Syndrome: Iliotibial Tract.** Ultrasound images in the transverse over the greater trochanter *(GT)* show abrupt motion of the thickened iliotibial tract *(arrowheads)* between (A) active hip extension and (B) flexion. *M*, Gluteus maximus; *m*, gluteus medius (left side of images is posterior).

involved iliotibial tract and/or gluteus maximus muscle, which is often thickened, over the greater trochanter.[82,83]

Calcific Tendinosis

Although more common in the rotator cuff, calcium hydroxyapatite deposition may occur in a number of tendons around the hip, including the gluteus maximus, gluteus medius (Fig. 6.88), and rectus femoris (Fig. 6.89) tendons.[84,85] In this situation, the hyperechoic focus may show posterior acoustic shadowing, and the involved tendon may be abnormally hypoechoic with increased flow on color Doppler imaging. Ultrasound-guided percutaneous lavage and aspiration may be used for treatment.

Diabetic Muscle Infarction

In evaluation of a painful or swollen thigh, one consideration is a condition called *diabetic muscle infarction*, or myonecrosis. Common to the thigh and calf, diabetic muscle infarction occurs in patients with longstanding diabetes, and it may be bilateral. The cause is not completely known, but a possible consideration is vascular occlusive disease. At ultrasound, the involved musculature is hypoechoic and swollen, although muscle fiber architecture is still identified (Fig. 6.90A), severe cases can produce significant heterogeneity (Fig. 6.90B).[86] Subfascial fluid may also be another finding in diabetic muscle infarction. Correlation with laboratory values and the patient's clinical presentation is helpful to exclude infection.

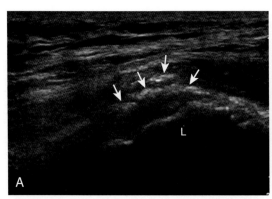

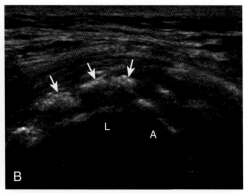

■ FIGURE 6.88 Calcific Tendinosis: Gluteus Medius. Ultrasound images in (A) long axis and (B) short axis to the gluteus medius tendon show hyperechoic and shadowing calcifications *(arrows)*. *A*, Anterior facet of the greater trochanter; *L*, lateral facet of the greater trochanter.

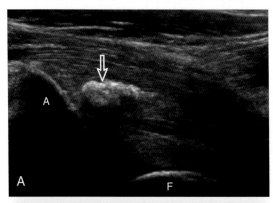

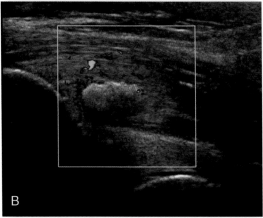

■ FIGURE 6.89 Calcific Tendinosis: Rectus Femoris, Direct Head. Ultrasound (A) gray-scale and (B) power Doppler images in long axis to the rectus femoris tendon show hyperechoic calcification *(open arrow)* with increased blood flow. *A*, Anterior inferior iliac spine; *F*, femoral head.

Pseudohypertrophy of the Tensor Fasciae Latae

The most common effects of chronic denervation are muscle atrophy and fatty replacement. Uncommonly, fatty infiltration of the involved muscle may instead cause muscle enlargement or pseudohypertrophy. This condition commonly involves the tensor fasciae latae muscle in the upper thigh, where it may present clinically as a soft tissue mass, although involvement of other muscles of the lower extremity have been described.[87] At ultrasound, the involved muscle is enlarged, either focally or more commonly diffusely, with increased echogenicity and sound beam attenuation, which is related to reflective interfaces between fat infiltration and muscle fibers (Fig. 6.91). The finding is usually asymmetrical, and it has been described in older individuals in the setting of chronic nerve impingement and partial denervation related to lumbar spine degenerative disease. Chronic peripheral neuropathy may also be a cause, and pseudohypertrophy has been described with muscular dystrophies.[87]

■ PERIPHERAL NERVE ABNORMALITIES

Several peripheral nerve abnormalities occur at the hip and thigh. One nerve entrapment condition specific to the hip involves the lateral femoral cutaneous nerve. As in other entrapment conditions, the involved nerve may demonstrate hypoechoic swelling at the site of entrapment or injury and is symptomatic with transducer pressure (Fig. 6.92) (Video 6.22).[88] The lateral femoral cutaneous nerve is susceptible to injury because of its course and variations in its location as it exits the pelvis at the inguinal ligament, sartorius, or iliac crest.[15,22]

Another peripheral nerve abnormality is nerve transection, which is characterized by nerve discontinuity, a swollen and hypoechoic terminal neuroma at the transection site, and possible retraction if completely disrupted (Fig. 6.93) (Videos 6.23 and 6.24).[89] Neuroma formation

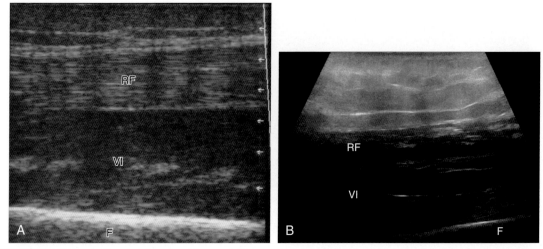

■ **FIGURE 6.90 Diabetic Muscle Infarction.** Ultrasound images in long axis to anterior thigh musculature in two different patients show hypoechoic vastus intermedius *(VI)* and sparing of the rectus femoris *(RF)*. Note (A) continuity of vastus intermedius muscle fibers, and (B) hypoechoic and heterogeneous vastus intermedius with overlying hyperechoic subcutaneous edema.

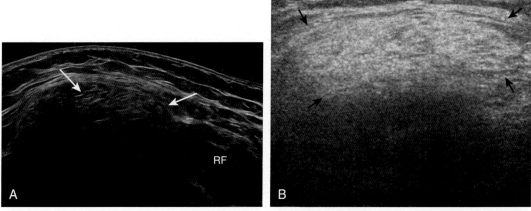

■ **FIGURE 6.91 Tensor Fasciae Latae Pseudohypertrophy.** Ultrasound images in short axis to the tensor fasciae latae in two different patients show abnormal (A) focal and (B) diffuse enlargement with increased echogenicity *(arrows)* from fatty infiltration. *RF,* Rectus femoris.

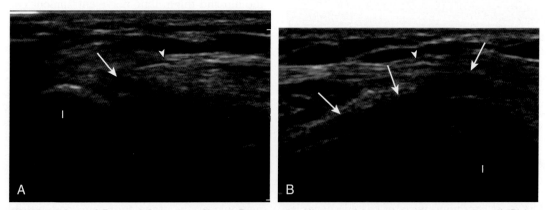

■ **FIGURE 6.92 Lateral Femoral Cutaneous Nerve: Entrapment.** Ultrasound images in (A) short axis and (B) long axis to the lateral femoral cutaneous nerve *(arrows)* show hypoechoic enlargement. Note inguinal ligament *(arrowhead)* and ilium *(I)*.

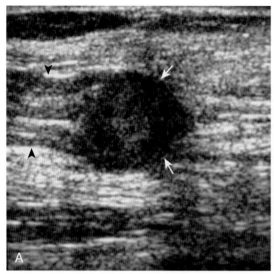

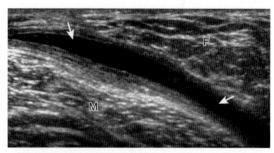

■ FIGURE 6.93 **Peripheral Nerve Transection Neuroma.** Ultrasound images from two different patients in (A) long axis to the sciatic nerve and (B) long axis to the common peroneal nerve show hypoechoic neuroma formation *(arrows)* in continuity with the transected nerve *(arrowheads).*

is an expected finding after nerve transection as part of attempted nerve regeneration. After knee amputation, sonographic evaluation for neuromas is very useful. Ultrasound can diagnose the neuromas and can also identify which neuroma is the cause of patients' symptoms through application of transducer pressure over each neuroma.

■ MISCELLANEOUS CONDITIONS
Morel-Lavallée Lesion

This post-traumatic condition or *Morel-Lavallée lesion* is described at the thigh and proximal hip and is characterized by a fluid collection between the subcutaneous fat and the underlying fascia. As a result of a closed degloving or shearing injury, bridging vascular structures and lymphatics are disrupted causing the fluid collection that is often recurrent. At ultrasound, the anechoic or hypoechoic fluid collection is found between the superficial fat and the underlying fascial tissues at the proximal thigh. Its appearance may be heterogeneous when acute but becomes more homogeneous and flat in shape when chronic, and may contain lobules of fat (Fig. 6.94).[90]

Inguinal Lymph Node

At ultrasound, a normal lymph node is typically oval with a hyperechoic hilum, uniform hypoechoic cortex, and hilar pattern of blood flow (if present) (Fig. 6.95). Asymptomatic inguinal lymph nodes are on average 5 mm short axis,

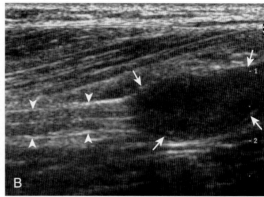

■ FIGURE 6.94 **Morel-Lavallée Lesion.** Ultrasound image over the lateral thigh shows anechoic fluid *(arrows)* between the subcutaneous fat *(F)* and thigh musculature *(M).*

multiple, with consistent identification of an hyperechoic hilum.[91,92] In older individuals, lymph nodes are often smaller as the hypoechoic cortex is diminished.[91] If the short axis measures greater than 1.5 cm or if there is eccentric thickening of the hypoechoic cortex, then an inguinal lymph node is considered abnormal.[93,94] An enlarged lymph node may be benign or malignant, although lymph node size is not a reliable criterion in this differentiation. Benign enlargement may be inflammatory or reactive and is characterized by an enlarged lymph node but still maintaining an oval shape, a hyperechoic hilum, and hilar pattern of blood flow (Fig. 6.96) (Video 6.25). In contrast, a malignant lymph node is characterized by a round shape, absence or narrowing of the echogenic hilum, thickening of the cortex,

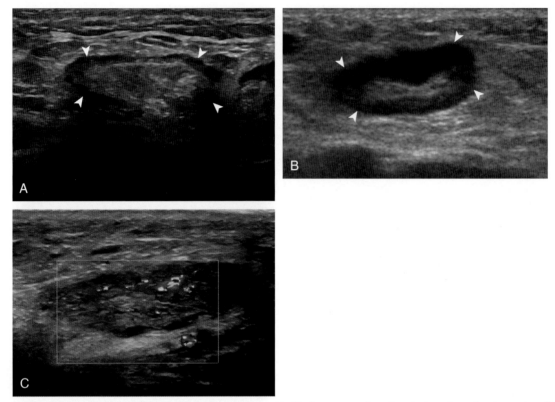

■ **FIGURE 6.95 Lymph Nodes: Normal.** Ultrasound images (A–C) show normal oval groin lymph nodes *(arrowheads)* with echogenic hilum and hypoechoic cortex and a hilar blood flow pattern in (C).

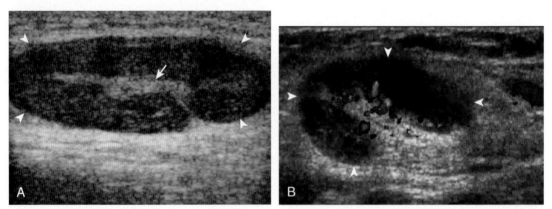

■ **FIGURE 6.96 Lymph Node: Hyperplastic.** Ultrasound images in (A) long axis and (B) short axis with color Doppler show enlargement of a groin lymph node *(arrowheads)*, although with uniform cortical thickening, oval shape, and hilar pattern of vascularity *(arrow, hyperechoic hilum)*.

and a mixed or peripheral blood flow pattern (Fig. 6.97).[94-96] Percutaneous biopsy is often required to determine the cause of lymph node enlargement. While a less common location compared with the sacrococcygeal region, a pilonidal cyst may also be seen in the groin region, which appears hypoechoic with internal hyperechoic linear hair fragments (Fig. 6.98).[97]

Other Soft Tissue Masses

Most soft tissue masses are nonspecific in the thigh and hip region; however, some soft tissue tumors commonly involve the thigh. One benign soft tissue tumor, an intramuscular myxoma, which has a uniformly heterogeneous but overall hypoechoic appearance (Fig. 6.99), may simulate

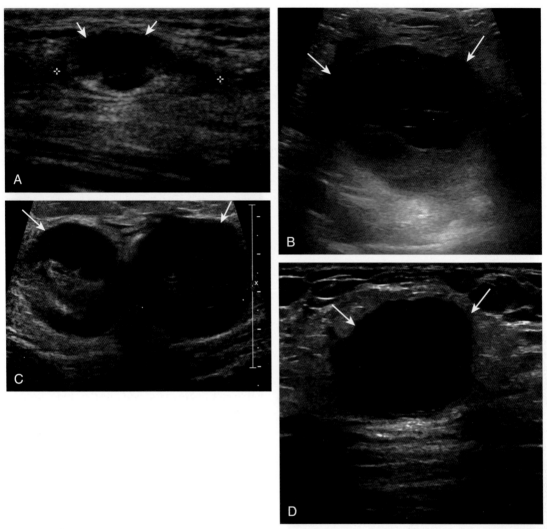

■ **FIGURE 6.97 Lymph Nodes: Malignant.** Ultrasound images from four different patients show (A) focal hypoechoic cortical enlargement *(arrows)* from angiosarcoma metastasis (lymph node length *between cursors*), (B) heterogeneous anechoic and septated enlargement *(arrows)* from sarcoma metastasis; (C) hypoechoic enlargement of two lymph nodes from lymphoma *(arrows)* with partial visualization of each hyperechoic hilum; and (D) marked hypoechoic enlargement from lymphoma with increased through transmission.

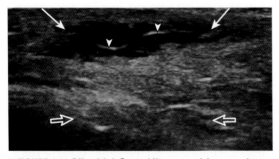

■ **FIGURE 6.98 Pilonidal Cyst.** Ultrasound image shows hypoechoic pilonidal cyst *(arrows)*. Note increased through-transmission *(open arrows)* and hyperechoic linear hair fragment *(arrowheads)*.

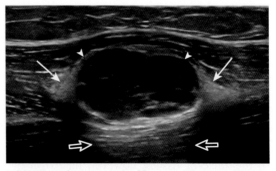

■ **FIGURE 6.99 Intramuscular Myxoma.** Ultrasound image shows heterogeneous but predominantly hypoechoic myxoma *(arrowheads)*. Note increased through-transmission *(open arrows)* and hyperechoic fat caps *(arrows)*.

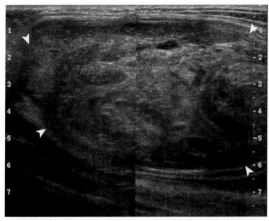

■ FIGURE 6.100 **High-Grade Pleomorphic Sarcoma**. Ultrasound image shows a heterogeneous mass (arrowheads).

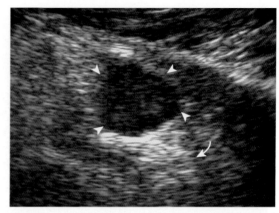

■ FIGURE 6.102 **Metastasis: Lung Cancer**. Ultrasound image shows a well-defined hypoechoic mass (arrowheads) with increased through-transmission (curved arrow).

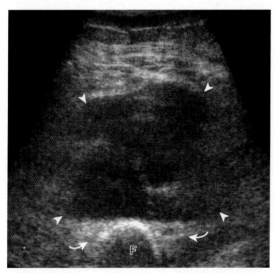

■ FIGURE 6.101 **Lymphoma**. Ultrasound image shows a lobular hypoechoic mass (arrowheads) with increased through-transmission (curved arrows). F, femur.

a complex cyst because it is well defined and oval, often with increased through-transmission.[98] A hyperechoic rim and hyperechoic cap have been described with intramuscular myxomas related to adjacent fatty atrophy and fatty infiltration.[98]

With regard to malignancy, the thigh is a common site for sarcomas (Fig. 6.100), although other primary malignant tumors (Fig. 6.101) and soft tissue metastases (Fig. 6.102) may occur. Such tumors are generally hypoechoic relative to the adjacent tissues; however, heterogeneity is common with larger and more aggressive tumors, especially when they are associated with necrosis and hemorrhage. In addition, many solid soft tissue tumors demonstrate increased

through-transmission. Although increased flow on color Doppler imaging is more common with malignant tumors, such findings may also be seen with benign conditions. After surgery, ultrasound is effective in evaluating for soft tissue sarcoma recurrence (Fig. 6.103).[99,100] In evaluation of a palpable soft tissue mass, one must exclude disorders that may produce a pseudomass appearance, such as pseudohypertrophy of the tensor fasciae latae and chronic retracted tendon or muscle tears, as described earlier.

Hernias

The key to successful evaluation for inguinal region hernias lies in sonographic technique, knowledge of anatomy, and identification of key sonographic landmarks.[17] With the Valsalva maneuver (forced expiration against a closed airway) and possibly scanning with the patient upright, one looks for abnormal movement of intra-abdominal contents from one compartment to another at a key anatomic location. For example, a Spigelian hernia occurs at the lateral margin of the rectus abdominis (Fig. 6.104) (Video 6.26). Most commonly, hyperechoic fat is visualized in the hernia and, less commonly, bowel. It is important to ascertain whether hernias are transient, reducible, or incarcerated.

An indirect inguinal hernia begins at the deep inguinal ring, at the lateral aspect of the external iliac artery just proximal to the origin of the inferior epigastric artery (Fig. 6.105). Intra-abdominal contents enter into the inguinal canal, beginning at the deep inguinal ring, and move superficially and then medially toward the pubic symphysis parallel to the skin surface (Fig. 6.106) (Videos 6.27, 6.28, and 6.29). Evaluation for

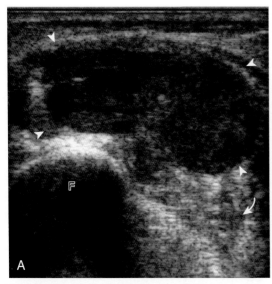

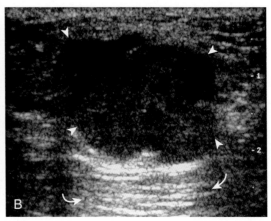

■ FIGURE 6.103 **Recurrent Soft Tissue Malignancy.** Ultrasound images from two separate patients show a lobular hypoechoic mass *(arrowheads)* from (A) undifferentiated pleomorphic sarcoma and (B) high-grade pleomorphic sarcoma recurrence. Note increased through-transmission *(curved arrows)*. F, Femur.

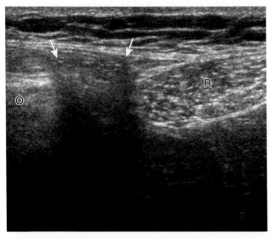

■ FIGURE 6.104 **Spigelian Hernia.** Ultrasound image over the lateral aspect of the right rectus abdominis muscle during the Valsalva maneuver shows movement of intra-abdominal contents *(arrows)* anteriorly between the rectus abdominis *(R)* and oblique musculature *(O)* (left side of image is lateral; right side is toward the midline).

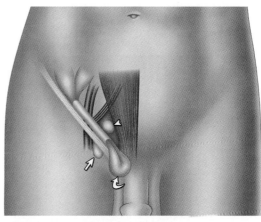

■ FIGURE 6.105 **Inguinal Region Hernias.** Illustration of the male right inguinal region shows the location of indirect inguinal *(curved arrow)*, direct inguinal *(arrowhead)*, and femoral *(arrow)* hernias. *(From Jacobson JA, Khoury V, Brandon CJ: Ultrasound of the Groin: Techniques, Pathology, and Pitfalls. AJR Am J Roentgenol 205:1-11, 2015.)*

indirect hernias must be completed in both long axis and short axis to the inguinal canal; limiting evaluation to long axis may cause one to overlook a hernia that is not included in the imaging plane.[17] This pitfall is avoided with short axis imaging, in which the hernia can be visualized within the inguinal canal adjacent to the spermatic cord or round ligament (Video 6.30). An indirect hernia may extend to the superficial inguinal ring (Fig. 6.107) (Video 6.31) and into the scrotum in males and labia majora in females.[101] Most hernias contain echogenic fat. To differentiate a fat-containing indirect hernia from a lipoma of the spermatic cord (Fig. 6.108) (Video 6.32), a hernia typically moves more with Valsalva maneuver and will distend the deep inguinal ring. Other pathology seen in women in the inguinal canal includes a cyst of the canal of Nuck[102] (Fig. 6.109) due to a patent processus vaginalis and round ligament varicosities seen in pregnancy (Fig. 6.110) (Video 6.33).[17,103] Undescended testicle may also be seen in the inguinal canal in males (Fig. 6.111).

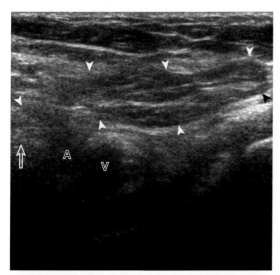

■ FIGURE 6.106 **Indirect Inguinal Hernia.** Ultrasound image parallel to the right inguinal canal during the Valsalva maneuver shows abnormal intra-abdominal contents *(arrowheads)* that extend through the deep inguinal ring *(open arrow)*, located lateral to the external iliac vasculature (*A* and *V*), and then medial parallel to the skin surface (left side of image is lateral).

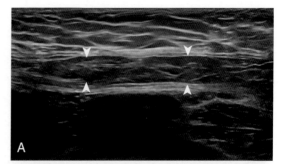

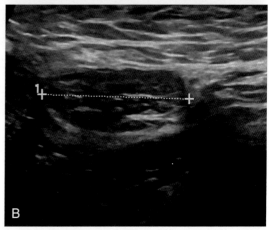

■ FIGURE 6.108 **Lipoma of the Spermatic Cord.** Ultrasound images in (A) long axis and (B) short axis to the spermatic cord show a predominantly hypoechoic lipoma (*between arrowheads* in A and *cursors* in B).

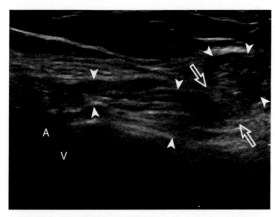

■ FIGURE 6.107 **Indirect Inguinal Hernia.** Ultrasound image parallel to the right inguinal canal during the Valsalva maneuver shows abnormal intra-abdominal contents *(arrowheads)* that extend through the superficial inguinal ring *(open arrows)* (left side of image is lateral).

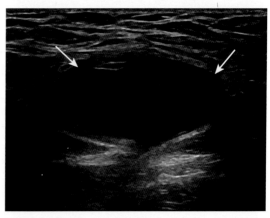

■ FIGURE 6.109 **Cyst of the Canal of Nuck.** Ultrasound image of inguinal canal shows anechoic cyst *(arrows)* with increased through-transmission.

In contrast to the location of an indirect inguinal hernia, a direct inguinal hernia originates medial to the external iliac vessels and moves toward the transducer in an anterior direction with the Valsalva maneuver (Fig. 6.112) (Videos 6.34 and 6.35).[17] It is essential to evaluate for direct hernia both in the sagittal and transverse planes over the Hesselbach triangle. If one limits evaluation to the transverse plane, it is possible to misinterpret the normal abdominal contents moving from a superior to inferior direction into the imaging plane, which can simulate a direct hernia (Video 6.36).[17] Sagittal imaging will differentiate normal movement of abdominal contents inferiorly from a true direct hernia, with the latter showing focal anterior movement.[17]

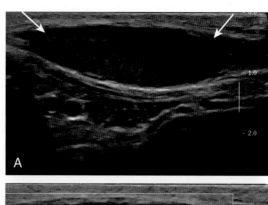

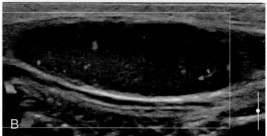

■ FIGURE 6.111 **Undescended Testes.** Ultrasound image of inguinal canal shows (A) hypoechoic undescended testicle with (B) minimal flow on color Doppler imaging.

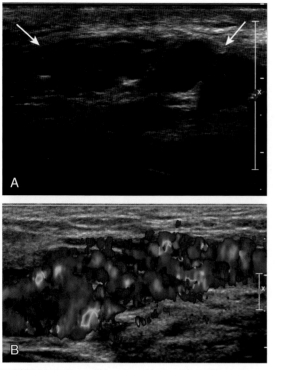

■ FIGURE 6.110 **Round Ligament Varicosities of Pregnancy.** Ultrasound image of inguinal canal shows (A) anechoic lobular channels *(arrows)* with (B) increased flow on color Doppler imaging.

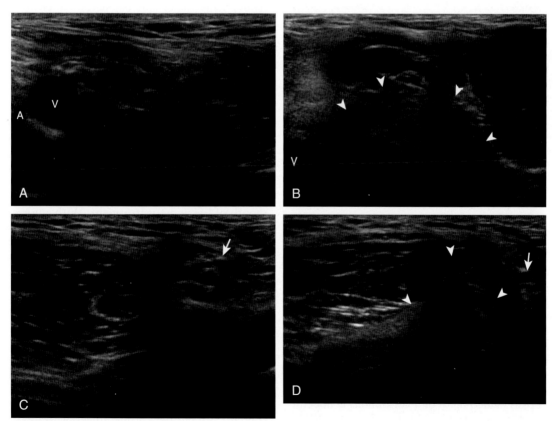

■ FIGURE 6.112 **Direct Inguinal Hernia.** Ultrasound images parallel to the right inguinal canal (A) before and (B) during the Valsalva maneuver show abnormal echogenic intra-abdominal contents *(arrowheads)*, which protrude anteriorly, medial to the external iliac vasculature (*A* and *V*) (left side of image is lateral). Ultrasound images in short axis to the right inguinal canal (C) before and (D) during the Valsalva maneuver show abnormal echogenic intra-abdominal contents *(arrowheads)*, which protrude anteriorly and displace the spermatic cord *(arrow)*.

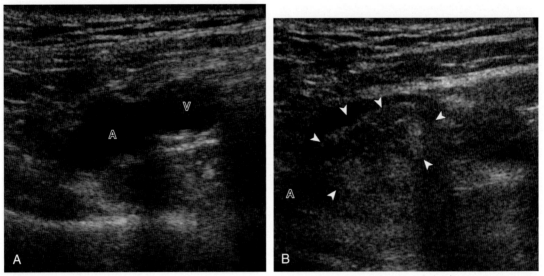

■ FIGURE 6.113 **Femoral Hernia.** Ultrasound images parallel and inferior to the right inguinal ligament (A) before and (B) during the Valsalva maneuver show abnormal intra-abdominal contents *(arrowheads)*, which protrude inferiorly, medially, and adjacent to the femoral vasculature *(A and V)* (left side of image is lateral).

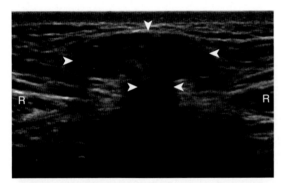

■ FIGURE 6.114 **Ventral Hernia.** Ultrasound image transverse over the anterior abdominal wall shows diastasis of the rectus abdominis and resulting ventral hernia *(arrowheads). R,* Rectus abdominis.

Another type of hernia seen below the level of the inguinal ligament is a femoral hernia, in which intra-abdominal contents move in a superior to inferior direction medial to the femoral vein with the Valsalva maneuver, often compressing the vein when large (Fig. 6.113) (Videos 6.37, 6.38, and 6.39).[104] A ventral hernia occurs in midline through diastasis of the rectus abdominis (Fig. 6.114), at the umbilicus (Fig. 6.115), or through an incision. After surgical repair of a hernia, mesh may be seen either as a linear area of speckled echoes (Fig. 6.116A) (Video 6.40) or a continuous echogenic area with posterior shadowing (Fig. 6.116B).[105] A recurrent indirect hernia will show abnormal movement of abdominal contents into the inguinal

canal (Fig. 6.116B) (Video 6.41). Other pathology of the abdominal region includes abdominal wall hemorrhage in an anticoagulated patient (Fig. 6.117), mass (Fig. 6.118), and intra-abdominal malignancy (Fig. 6.119).

Developmental Dysplasia of the Hip

One screening protocol using ultrasound to detect hip dysplasia depends on the clinical examination.[35] With abnormal clinical examination findings during the Barlow and Ortolani maneuvers, ultrasound is performed in patients younger than 2 weeks of age if the hip is unstable or at 4–6 weeks of age if there is a stable click. Minor physiologic laxity may disappear during the first month of life without treatment. With a normal clinical examination, ultrasound examination is performed at 4–6 weeks if there are risk factors for dysplasia, such as family history, breech presentation, and postural deformity, to name a few. With normal clinical examination and no risk factors present, no ultrasound examination is performed.

As described in the earlier section on ultrasound examination technique, diagnostic criteria for hip dysplasia rely on dynamic evaluation with optional measurements. Findings of hip dysplasia include subluxation or dislocation of the femoral head during the dynamic maneuvers with applied stress (Fig. 6.120). On the coronal image with the hip neutral or slightly flexed, an α angle is normally greater than 60 degrees. When the α angle is less

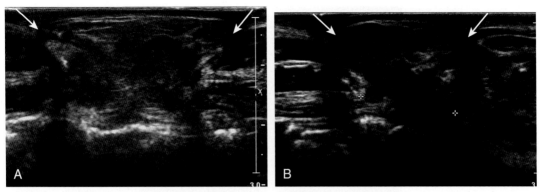

■ FIGURE 6.115 **Umbilical Hernia.** Ultrasound images (A) transverse and (B) sagittal over the umbilicus show focal hernia *(arrowheads)*. Note hernia neck *(between cursors)* in (B).

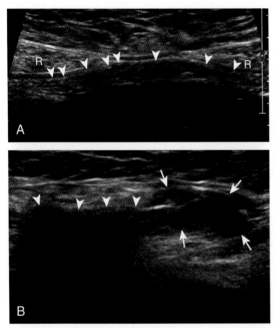

■ FIGURE 6.116 **Mesh Hernia Repair.** Ultrasound images from two separate patients show (A) mesh material *(arrowheads)* beneath the anterior abdominal wall (*R*, rectus abdominis), and (B) echogenic and shadowing mesh material *(arrowheads)* with recurrent indirect right inguinal hernia *(arrows)*.

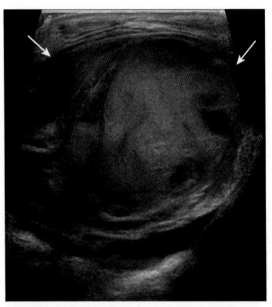

■ FIGURE 6.117 **Rectus Abdominis Hematoma.** Ultrasound image shows a heterogeneous mass within rectus abdominis.

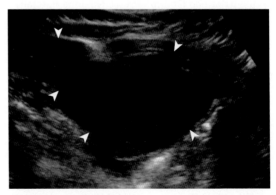

■ FIGURE 6.118 **Ewing Sarcoma of the Abdominal Wall.** Ultrasound image shows a hypoechoic mass of the abdominal wall *(arrowheads)*.

than 50 degrees, the β angle becomes important and is greater than 77 degrees with femoral head subluxation and dislocation.[36] The presence of interposed echogenic fibroadipose tissue between the femoral head and the acetabulum is also noted because this is associated with hip dysplasia. Ultrasound also enables one to evaluate for proximal femoral focal deficiency and to assess for variable degrees of femoral aplasia, including the unossified femoral head cartilage.

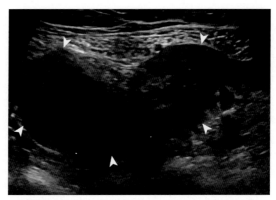

■ FIGURE 6.119 **Ovarian Carcinoma With Omental Involvement.** Ultrasound image shows a hypoechoic mass within the abdomen *(arrowheads)*.

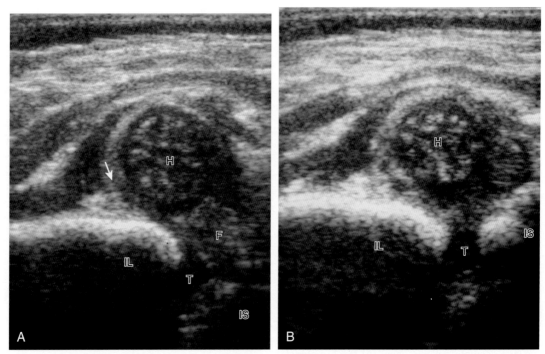

■ FIGURE 6.120 **Developmental Dysplasia of the Hip.** A, Ultrasound image coronal to the hip joint in a neutral position shows dislocation of the femoral head *(H)*, dysplasia of the acetabulum (*IL*, ilium), and increased echogenicity of the deformed labrum *(arrow)*. Note the fibrofatty tissue *(F)* in the acetabulum. B, Ultrasound image coronal and posterior to the hip joint with hip flexion and posteriorly directed stress shows posterior dislocation of the femoral head *(H)*. *IL*, Ilium; *IS*, ischium; *T*, triradiate cartilage.

SELECT REFERENCES

1. Robben SG, Lequin MH, Diepstraten AF: Anterior joint capsule of the normal hip and in children with transient synovitis: US study with anatomic and histologic correlation. *Radiology* 210(2):499–507, 1999.
2. Pfirrmann CW, Chung CB, Theumann NH: Greater trochanter of the hip: attachment of the abductor mechanism and a complex of three bursae—MR imaging and MR bursography in cadavers and MR imaging in asymptomatic volunteers. *Radiology* 221(2):469–477, 2001.
3. Philippon MJ, Michalski MP, Campbell KJ, et al: Surgically relevant bony and soft tissue anatomy of the proximal femur. *Orthop J Sports Med* 2(6): 2325967114535188, 2014.
4. Guillin R, Cardinal E, Bureau NJ: Sonographic anatomy and dynamic study of the normal iliopsoas musculotendinous junction. *Eur Radiol* 19(4):995–1001, 2009.
17. Jacobson JA, Khoury V, Brandon CJ: Ultrasound of the groin: techniques, pathology, and pitfalls. *AJR Am J Roentgenol* 205(3):513–523, 2015.

20. Damarey B, Demondion X, Boutry N: Sonographic assessment of the lateral femoral cutaneous nerve. *J Clin Ultrasound* 37(2):89–95, 2009.

24. Morley N, Grant T, Blount K: Sonographic evaluation of athletic pubalgia. *Skeletal Radiol* 45(5): 689–699, 2016.

34. Bierry G, Simeone FJ, Borg-Stein JP: Sacrotuberous ligament: relationship to normal, torn, and retracted hamstring tendons on MR images. *Radiology* 271(1): 162–171, 2014.

40. Weybright PN, Jacobson JA, Murry KH, et al: Limited effectiveness of sonography in revealing hip joint effusion: preliminary results in 21 adult patients with native and postoperative hips. *AJR Am J Roentgenol* 181(1):215–218, 2003.

55. Long SS, Surrey DE, Nazarian LN: Sonography of greater trochanteric pain syndrome and the rarity of primary bursitis. *AJR Am J Roentgenol* 201(5): 1083–1086, 2013.

64. Hadduck TA, van Holsbeeck MT, Girish G, et al: Value of ultrasound before joint aspiration. *AJR Am J Roentgenol* 201(3):W453–W459, 2013.

66. Ostlere S: How to image metal-on-metal prostheses and their complications. *AJR Am J Roentgenol* 197(3):558–567, 2011.

72. Davis KW: Imaging of the hamstrings. *Semin Musculoskelet Radiol* 12(1):28–41, 2008.

The complete references for this chapter can be found on *www.expertconsult.com.*

KNEE ULTRASOUND

■ KNEE ANATOMY

The knee is a synovial joint that consists of hyaline cartilage articulations between the femur, the tibia, and the patella (Fig. 7.1). The menisci are C-shaped fibrocartilage structures between the femur and the tibia (Fig. 7.1E). A prominent joint recess, the suprapatellar recess or pouch, extends superiorly from the knee joint between the patella and the femur and communicates with the medial and lateral joint recesses, which extend over the medial and lateral aspects of the femoral condyles beneath the patellar retinaculum (Fig. 7.1F).[1] In

the sagittal plane, the quadriceps fat pad is located anteriorly between the suprapatellar recess and quadriceps tendon, and the prefemoral fat pad is located between the suprapatellar recess and the femur. The infrapatellar fat pad of Hoffa is an intra-capsular but extra-synovial fat pad between the anterior knee joint and the patellar tendon.[2] Various bursae exist around the anterior knee joint, including the prepatellar bursa anterior to the patella, the superficial infrapatellar bursa anterior to the distal patellar tendon, and the deep infrapatellar bursa between the patellar tendon and proximal tibia (Fig. 7.1F). Additional bursae are present around the medial knee, including the pes anserine bursa deep to the pes anserinus tendons, and the semimembranosus–tibial collateral ligament bursa, which has an inverted U shape located at the joint line between the medial collateral ligament and the semimembranosus tendon (Fig. 7.1F).[3,4] These latter two bursae do not communicate with the knee joint. A more common bursa is the semimembranosus-medial gastrocnemius bursa, which, when distended, is called a *Baker (or popliteal) cyst*.[5] This bursa communicates to the knee joint in 50% of adults who are older than 50 years and becomes a common recess for joint fluid and intra-articular bodies.[5]

The knee joint is stabilized by a number of ligaments. Medially, the medial collateral ligament extends from the medial femoral condyle to the tibia in the coronal plane. Thin, deep layers of the medial collateral ligament (meniscofemoral and meniscotibial ligaments) extend from the meniscus to the femur and tibia, respectively, whereas a thicker, more superficial layer (tibial collateral ligament) extends from the femur to insert distally on the tibia deep to the pes anserinus.[6] Superficial to the medial collateral ligament is found the deep crural fascia.[6] The lateral or fibular collateral ligament originates from the lateral femur and extends over the popliteus tendon to insert on the lateral aspect of the fibula with the biceps femoris tendon.[7,8] Other supporting structures of the posterolateral knee include the popliteofibular ligament and the arcuate ligament.[8] The popliteofibular ligament extends from the popliteus tendon to the styloid process of the proximal fibula, whereas the arcuate ligament extends from the femur and joint capsule to the

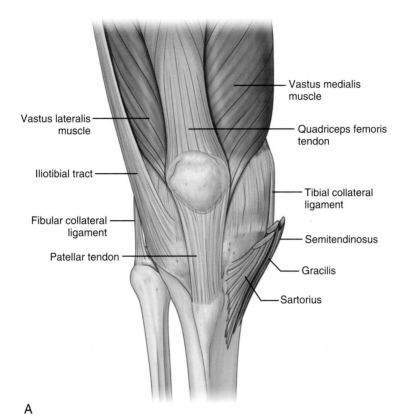

A

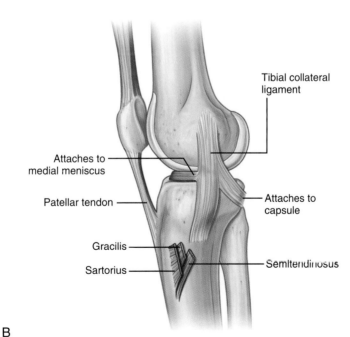

B

■ **FIGURE 7.1 Knee Anatomy.** A, Anterior view of the knee. B, Medial view of knee. C, Lateral view of knee. D, Posterior view of knee. E, Superior view of knee menisci. F, Medial view showing suprapatellar recess and bursae. *(A–E: From Drake R, Vogl W, Mitchell A: Gray's Anatomy for Students. Philadelphia, 2005, Churchill Livingstone; F: Courtesy Daniel Dobbs, Ann Arbor, Michigan.)*

Continued

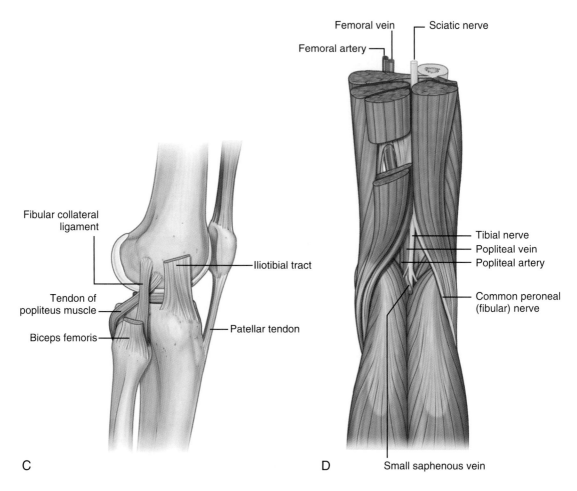

Femoral vein
Sciatic nerve
Femoral artery
Tibial nerve
Popliteal vein
Popliteal artery
Common peroneal (fibular) nerve

Fibular collateral ligament
Iliotibial tract
Tendon of popliteus muscle
Biceps femoris
Patellar tendon

C
D
Small saphenous vein

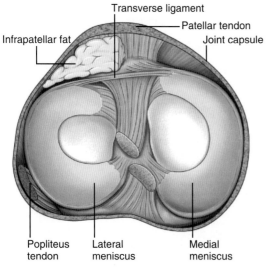

Transverse ligament
Patellar tendon
Infrapatellar fat
Joint capsule

Popliteus tendon
Lateral meniscus
Medial meniscus

E

■ FIGURE 7.1, cont'd

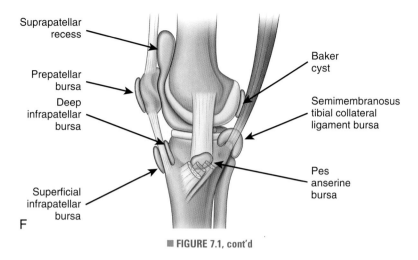

Suprapatellar recess

Prepatellar bursa

Deep infrapatellar bursa

Superficial infrapatellar bursa

F

Baker cyst

Semimembranosus tibial collateral ligament bursa

Pes anserine bursa

■ **FIGURE 7.1,** cont'd

fibula tip as well.[7,8] When a fabella is present, another posterolateral structure is the fabellofibular ligament. An additional ligament, the anterolateral ligament, extends from the lateral femoral epicondyle region to the anterolateral tibia between the tubercle of Gerdy and the fibula, with fibers also attaching to the lateral meniscus.[9,10] The anterior and posterior cruciate ligaments within the intercondylar notch extend from the femur to the proximal tibia as intra-capsular but extra-synovial structures.

With regard to tendons around the knee, anteriorly the quadriceps femoris tendon inserts on the superior patellar pole, although superficial fibers extend over the patella (termed the *prepatellar quadriceps continuation*) to insert on the tibial tuberosity as part of the patellar tendon.[11] The medial and lateral patellar retinaculum extends from each side of the patella to the femur; the medial aspect is reinforced by the medial patellofemoral ligament, which extends from the medial patella to the adductor tubercle region of the medial femoral condyle.[12] The distal aspect of the vastus medialis, termed the *vastus medialis obliquus*, blends with the medial patellar retinaculum to insert onto the medial patella.[12-14] Medially and anteriorly, the sartorius, gracilis, and semitendinosus tendons insert on the tibia near the tibial collateral ligament as the pes anserinus (a helpful mnemonic is "Say Grace before Tea" where S, Sartorius; G, Gracilis; and T, semiTendinosis; or the abbreviation for sergeant as "SGT"). Posterior and proximal to the pes anserinus, the semimembranosus primarily inserts on the tibia just beyond the tibia articular surface, although the distal anatomy is quite complex.[11] Posteriorly, the medial and lateral heads of the gastrocnemius originate from the posterior aspect of the femoral condyles. Laterally, the biceps femoris tendon and

lateral collateral ligament attach to the lateral margin of the fibular head.[7] The direct arm of the long head of the biceps femoris tendon inserts on the lateral aspect of the fibula with the lateral collateral ligament, whereas the anterior arm of the long head biceps femoris inserts more anterior on the fibula. The short head of the biceps femoris also has two insertions: the direct arm insertion on the proximal fibula medial to the long head and the anterior arm insertion on the proximal tibia.[8] The popliteus tendon originates at the lateral aspect of the femur, lies within a groove or sulcus of the lateral femur, and courses obliquely with its muscle belly located between the posterior aspect of the tibia and the tibial artery and vein. Anterolaterally, the iliotibial tract or band inserts on the tubercle of Gerdy of the proximal tibia.

With regard to the peripheral nerves, the sciatic nerve bifurcates as the tibial nerve, which extends distally posterior to the popliteal artery and vein, and the common peroneal nerve, which courses laterally parallel and posterior to the biceps femoris tendon. The common peroneal or fibular nerve curves anteriorly around the fibular neck deep to the peroneus longus origin and bifurcates as the superficial peroneal nerve, which courses along the peroneal musculature, and the deep peroneal nerve, which continues to the interosseous membrane and follows the anterior tibial artery between the tibia and fibula.

■ ULTRASOUND EXAMINATION TECHNIQUE

Table 7.1 is a checklist for a knee ultrasound examination. Examples of diagnostic knee ultrasound reports are shown in Boxes 7.1 and 7.2.

TABLE 7.1 Knee Ultrasound Examination Checklist

Location of Interest	Structures/Pathologic Features
Anterior	Quadriceps tendon Patella Patellar tendon Patellar retinaculum Suprapatellar recess Medial and lateral recesses Anterior knee bursae Femoral articular cartilage
Medial	Medial collateral ligament Medial meniscus: body and anterior horn Pes anserinus
Lateral	Iliotibial tract Lateral collateral ligament Biceps femoris Common peroneal nerve Anterolateral ligament Popliteus Lateral meniscus: body and anterior horn
Posterior	Baker cyst Menisci: posterior horns Posterior cruciate ligament Anterior cruciate ligament Neurovascular structures

BOX 7.1 Sample Diagnostic Knee Ultrasound Report: Normal, Complete

Examination: Ultrasound of the Right Knee
Date of Study: March 11, 2016
Patient Name: Meg White
Registration Number: 8675309
History: Trauma
Findings: The extensor mechanism, including the quadriceps tendon, patella, and patellar tendon, is normal without bursal abnormalities. No significant joint effusion or synovial hypertrophy. The medial collateral and lateral collateral ligaments are normal. Unremarkable iliotibial tract, biceps femoris, popliteus tendon, and common peroneal nerve. No Baker cyst. Limited evaluation of the menisci is unremarkable.
Impression: Unremarkable ultrasound examination of the right knee.

General Comments

Ultrasound examination of the majority of the knee structures is completed with the patient supine; the posterior structures are best evaluated with the patient prone. A high-frequency transducer of at least 10 MHz is typically used, with the exception of the posterior knee, for which

BOX 7.2 Sample Diagnostic Knee Ultrasound Report: Abnormal, Complete

Examination: Ultrasound of the Right Knee
Date of Study: March 11, 2016
Patient Name: Frank Ricard
Registration Number: 8675309
History: Pain, evaluate for cyst
Findings: The extensor mechanism, including the quadriceps tendon, patella, and patellar tendon, is normal. There is a moderate-sized joint effusion and no synovial hypertrophy or intra-articular body. The medial and lateral collateral ligaments are normal, as is the iliotibial tract, biceps femoris, popliteus tendon, and common peroneal nerve. There is medial compartment joint space narrowing and osteophyte formation with mild extrusion of the body of the medial meniscus, which is abnormally hypoechoic. No parameniscal cyst. There is a Baker cyst measuring $2 \times 2 \times 6$ cm. Abnormal hypoechogenicity is noted at the inferior margin of the Baker cyst. There is also a hypoechoic cleft involving the posterior horn of the medial meniscus, which extends to the articular surface.
Impression:
1. Baker cyst with evidence for rupture.
2. Medial compartment osteoarthritis with moderate joint effusion.
3. Suspect posterior horn medial meniscal tear. Consider MRI for confirmation if indicated.

a transducer of less than 10 MHz may be needed to penetrate the deep soft tissues. Evaluation of the knee may be focused over the area that is clinically symptomatic or that is relevant to the patient's history. Regardless, a complete examination of all areas should always be considered and is recommended for one to become familiar with normal anatomy and normal variants and to develop a quick and efficient sonographic technique.

Anterior Evaluation

The primary structures evaluated from the anterior approach are the quadriceps tendon, the patella, the patellar tendon, the patellar retinaculum, the suprapatellar recess, the medial and lateral recesses, and the bursae around the anterior knee. Examination is begun in the sagittal plane proximal to the patella (Fig. 7.2A). This plane demonstrates the normal hyperechoic and fibrillar appearance of the quadriceps tendon (Fig. 7.2B). Slight flexion of the knee with a posterior pad or roll is helpful as this position straightens and tenses the extensor mechanism to reduce tendon anisotropy. Often,

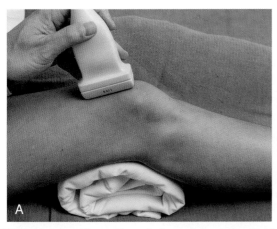

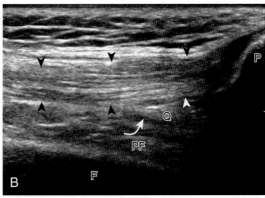

■ **FIGURE 7.2 Quadriceps Femoris: Long Axis.** A, Sagittal imaging over anterior knee proximal to the patella shows (B) the quadriceps tendon *(arrowheads)*, quadriceps fat pad *(Q)*, prefemoral fat pad *(PF)*, and collapsed joint recess *(curved arrow). F*, Femur; *P*, patella.

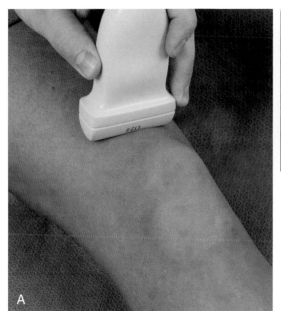

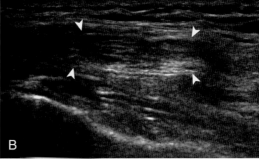

■ **FIGURE 7.3 Quadriceps Femoris: Short Axis.** A, Transverse imaging over anterior knee proximal to patella shows (B) the quadriceps tendon *(arrowheads)*.

the trilaminar appearance of the quadriceps tendon can be appreciated, with the rectus femoris as the anterior layer, the combined vastus medialis and intermedius as the middle layer, and the vastus intermedius as the deepest layer (see Quadriceps Femoris Injury). The quadriceps tendon is also evaluated in short axis (Fig. 7.3). Returning to the quadriceps tendon in long axis, the suprapatellar recess is identified deep to the quadriceps tendon and evaluated for anechoic or hypoechoic joint fluid, which would separate the quadriceps fat

pad (located superficial) from the prefemoral fat pad (located deep) (Fig. 7.2). Slight knee flexion also shifts fluid from other parts of the knee joint into the suprapatellar recess.[15,16] The transducer is then moved inferiorly below the patella in the sagittal plane to visualize the hyperechoic, fibrillar, and uniform patellar tendon (Fig. 7.4). The infrapatellar fat pad of Hoffa appears minimally hyperechoic or isoechoic to muscle deep to the patellar tendon. The transducer should also be floated on a layer of gel over the patella and

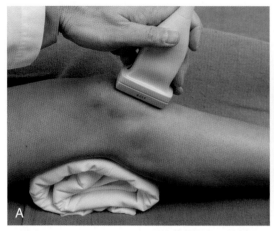
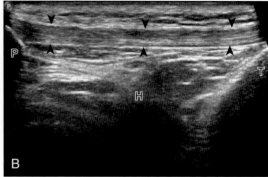

■ **FIGURE 7.4 Patellar Tendon: Long Axis.** A, Sagittal imaging over anterior knee distal to the patella shows (B) the patellar tendon *(arrowheads)* and Hoffa fat pad *(H)*. *P*, Patella; *T*, tibia.

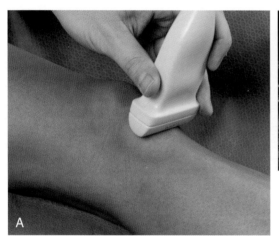
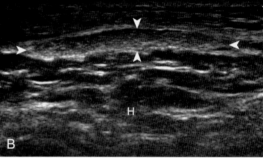

■ **FIGURE 7.5 Patellar Tendon: Short Axis.** A, Transverse imaging over anterior knee distal to patella shows (B) the patellar tendon *(arrowheads)* and Hoffa fat pad *(H)*.

proximal patellar tendon to evaluate for patellar fracture, as well as prepatellar bursal fluid, because the latter may be easily redistributed out of view with the slightest transducer pressure. The region around the distal patellar tendon is also evaluated for superficial and deep infrapatellar bursal fluid; minimal fluid in the latter is considered physiologic (see Other Bursae). Although long axis is most important in evaluation of extensor mechanism abnormalities, imaging should also be completed in short axis to ensure a thorough evaluation, especially with the patellar tendon, where a focal abnormality may not be located in midline (Fig. 7.5).

The transducer is then moved to both the medial and lateral margins of the patella in the transverse plane (Fig. 7.6). The thin hyperechoic patellar retinaculum is visualized as well as potential distention of the medial and lateral joint recesses, which is more apparent when the knee is completely extended. One must be careful not to displace joint fluid from view with transducer pressure (see Joint Effusion and Synovial Hypertrophy). The patellar retinaculum may demonstrate three defined layers.[12] Within the medial patellar retinaculum, the medial patellofemoral ligament may be identified as a hyperechoic, compact fibrillar structure, which extends from the adductor tubercle of the femur to the patella. Finally, with the knee in flexion, the hypoechoic hyaline cartilage that covers the trochlea of the anterior femur can be visualized in

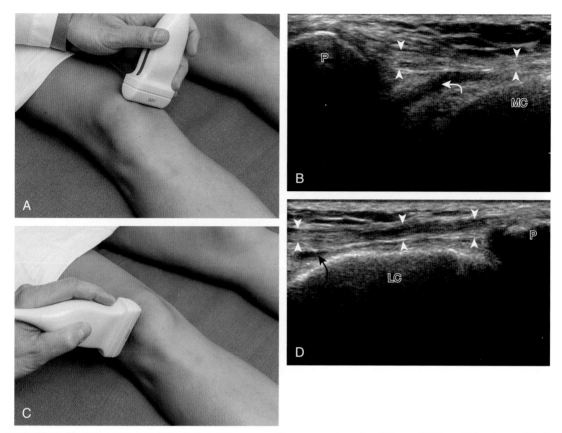

■ **FIGURE 7.6 Medial and Lateral Knee Joint Recesses.** Transverse imaging (A) medial to patella shows (B) the medial patellar retinaculum, which contains the medial patellofemoral ligament *(arrowheads)*. Transverse imaging (C) lateral to patella shows (D) the lateral patellar retinaculum *(arrowheads)* (*curved arrow*, collapsed joint recess). *LC,* Lateral femoral condyle; *MC,* medial femoral condyle; *P,* patella.

the transverse plane superior to the patella (Fig. 7.7A and B), and the hypoechoic hyaline cartilage covering the anterior and central aspects of the femoral condyles can be seen in the parasagittal plane (Fig. 7.7C).[17,18] With knee flexion, the anterior aspect of the anterior cruciate ligament can be visualized in the oblique sagittal plane with the transducer angled from the intercondylar notch to the medial tibia.

Medial Evaluation

For medial knee evaluation, the patient remains supine and rotates the hip externally to gain access to the medial structures. The structures of interest include the medial collateral ligament (composed of several layers), the body and anterior horn of the medial meniscus, and the pes anserinus.[6] To begin, the transducer is placed in the coronal plane along the medial joint line, which is identified by the bone contours of the femoral condyle and the proximal tibia (Fig. 7.8A).[19] The hyperechoic and

fibrillar superficial layer of the medial collateral ligament (or tibial collateral ligament) is easily identified in long axis (Fig. 7.8B), which extends from the medial femoral condyle distally and to the proximal tibial metaphysis. With rotation of the transducer short axis to the tibial collateral ligament, the anteroposterior extent of this structure can be appreciated (Fig. 7.9A and B). By toggling the transducer along the long axis of the tibial collateral ligament, the borders of the ligament can be better appreciated because the ligament fibers become hypoechoic as a result of anisotropy and the adjacent soft tissues remain hyperechoic (Fig. 7.9C). Returning to the coronal plane or long axis to the tibial collateral ligament, the thinner hyperechoic deep layers of the medial collateral ligament, also called the *meniscofemoral* and *meniscotibial ligaments*, are identified from the meniscus to the femur and tibia, respectively (Fig. 7.8B). The fibrocartilage meniscus is identified as a triangular hyperechoic structure between the femur and the tibia. The transducer is then

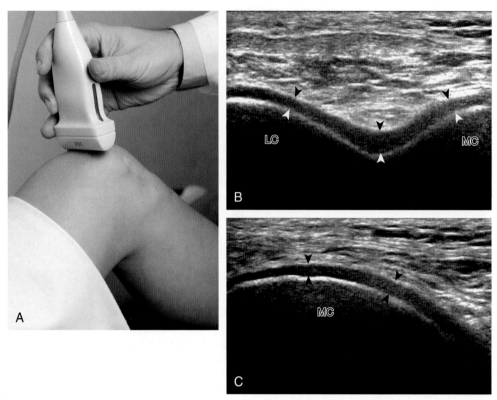

■ **FIGURE 7.7 Trochlear and Femoral Condyle Cartilage.** A, With knee flexion, (B) transverse imaging and (C) parasagittal imaging show hypoechoic hyaline cartilage *(arrowheads)*. *LC*, Lateral femoral condyle; *MC*, medial femoral condyle.

moved anteriorly from the coronal plane to the oblique-sagittal plane to visualize the anterior horn of the medial meniscus.

Returning back to the coronal plane long axis to the tibial collateral ligament, the transducer is moved distally beyond the joint line along the tibial collateral ligament and slightly anterior to visualize its attachment on the tibia, approximately 4–5 cm beyond the joint line (Fig. 7.10A). Here, the pes anserinus can be seen as three hyperechoic tendons superficial to the tibial collateral ligament that converge onto the tibia. Toggling the transducer is often helpful because this will cause the tendons of the pes anserinus superficial to the tibial collateral ligament to appear hypoechoic from anisotropy and be more conspicuous. By turning the transducer to the oblique-axial plane along the long axis of each pes anserinus tendon, the individual sartorius, gracilis, and semitendinosus tendons can be seen; they extend to their tibial attachment as the pes anserinus (Fig. 7.10B). The more proximal aspects of the pes anserinus tendons can also be visualized when the posterior knee is evaluated. One potential pitfall in evaluation of the posterior aspect of the medial meniscus

body is misinterpretation of the adjacent semimembranosus tendon anisotropy as a parameniscal cyst. Identification of a hypoechoic round structure just distal to the meniscus with an associated osseous groove represents anisotropy of the semimembranosus tendon at its tibial insertion (Fig. 7.11). The normal semimembranosus tendon may be confirmed with the transducer repositioned long axis and perpendicular to the tendon to demonstrate the normal hyperechoic and fibrillar echotexture.

Lateral Evaluation

For evaluation of the lateral knee structures, the leg is internally rotated, or the patient rolls partly onto the contralateral side. Structures of interest laterally include the iliotibial tract (or band), the lateral (or fibular) collateral ligament, the biceps femoris tendon, the anterolateral ligament, the supporting structures of the posterolateral corner of the knee, and the common peroneal nerve. To begin, the transducer may be initially placed over the anterior knee long axis to the patellar tendon. The transducer is then moved laterally (Fig. 7.12A)

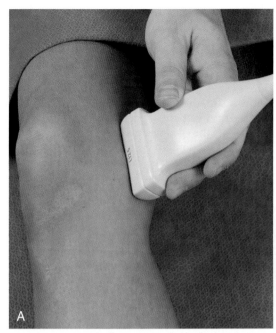

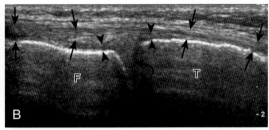

■ FIGURE 7.8 **Medial Knee Evaluation: Coronal Plane.** A, Coronal imaging at the medial joint line shows (B) the superficial *(arrows)* and deep *(arrowheads)* layers of the medial collateral ligament *(curved arrow,* body of medial meniscus). *F,* Femur; *T,* tibia.

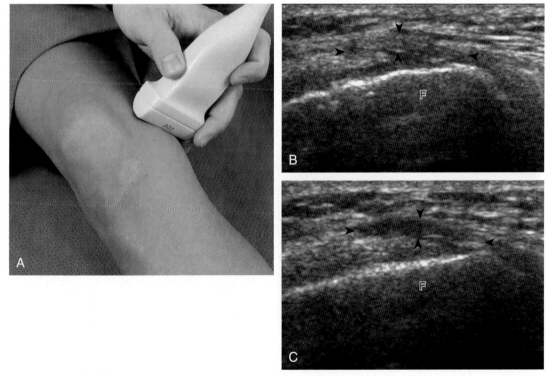

■ FIGURE 7.9 **Medial Knee Evaluation: Transverse Plane.** A, Transverse imaging (B) without and (C) with anisotropy shows the medial collateral ligament *(arrowheads). F,* Femur.

and the next fibrillar structure identified is the iliotibial tract or band, which inserts on the Gerdy tubercle of the proximal tibia, which may also be identified via palpation (Fig. 7.12B). The transducer is then moved proximally to evaluate the tissues between the iliotibial tract and the distal

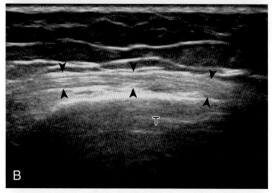

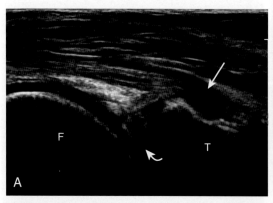

■ FIGURE 7.10 Distal Medial Collateral Ligament and Pes Anserinus. Coronal imaging distal to knee joint shows (A) the superficial layer of the medial collateral ligament *(arrowheads)* and the tendons of the pes anserinus *(arrows)* (*T*, tibial metaphysis). B, Imaging in long axis to semitendinosus proximal to pes anserinus shows normal tendon *(arrowheads).*

femur for disorders related to iliotibial band friction syndrome.

Next, the transducer is moved laterally to the coronal plane over the lateral femoral condyle to identify an important bone landmark, which is the groove or sulcus for the popliteus tendon.[19] At this site, the femoral attachment of the lateral collateral ligament is identified at the proximal ridge of the groove, as well as the adjacent popliteus tendon. To visualize the lateral collateral ligament in long axis, the proximal aspect of the transducer is then fixed to the femur at this site while the distal aspect is rotated posteriorly toward the fibular head (Fig. 7.13A). In this position, the hyperechoic and fibrillar echotexture of the lateral collateral ligament is seen, which extends from the lateral femoral condyle to the lateral aspect of the fibular head (Fig. 7.13B and C). The proximal aspect of the lateral collateral ligament extends over the popliteus tendon located within the femoral groove. The distal insertion on the fibula may appear thickened and heterogeneous owing to the bifurcating distal biceps femoris tendon seen both superficial and deep to the lateral collateral ligament (Fig. 7.13C).[20] If the knee is in valgus angulation, the lateral collateral ligament may have a wavy appearance with anisotropy. This effect can be minimized with the patient positioned so that the opposite knee is flexed under the knee being examined, or with a pillow placed between the knees, which places the knee in slight varus angulation.

After the transducer is moved along the lateral collateral ligament to its fibular attachment, the distal aspect of the transducer is fixed to the fibular head while the proximal aspect is rotated posteriorly to the coronal plane (Fig. 7.14A) to bring the biceps femoris tendon into view; this tendon

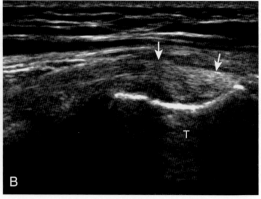

■ FIGURE 7.11 Semimembranosus: Pseudocyst Appearance. Coronal-oblique imaging at the posteromedial joint line shows (A) a hypoechoic round area *(arrow)*, which represents anisotropy of the distal semimembranosus tendon at its tibial attachment. B, This area *(arrows)* becomes hyperechoic and fibrillar with repositioning of the transducer. Note characteristic bone contour of tibia *(T)* at semimembranosus tendon attachment (*curved arrow*, medial meniscus degeneration). *F,* Femur.

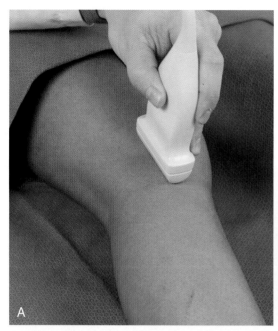

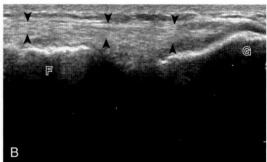

■ **FIGURE 7.12 Iliotibial Tract: Long Axis.** A, Coronal imaging between lateral joint line and patellar tendon shows (B) the iliotibial tract *(arrowheads)*. *F*, Femur; *G*, Gerdy tubercle of tibia.

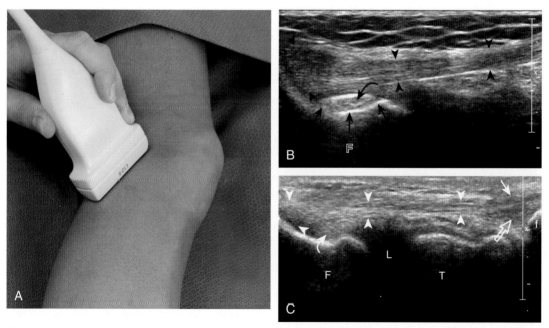

■ **FIGURE 7.13 Lateral Collateral Ligament.** A, Coronal-oblique imaging shows (B and C) characteristic contours *(arrows)* of the femur *(F)* adjacent to the popliteus tendon *(curved arrow)* and proximal lateral collateral ligament *(arrowheads)*. Note superficial *(arrow)* and deep *(open arrow)* heads of bifurcating biceps femoris tendon in C. *f*, Fibula; *L*, lateral meniscus; *T*, tibia.

is differentiated from ligament by the less compact fibrillar echotexture and the associated hypoechoic muscle more proximally (Fig. 7.14B). Both the lateral collateral ligament and the biceps femoris tendon insert onto the lateral aspect of the proximal fibula. The distal biceps femoris may appear heterogeneous as fibers bifurcate both superficial and deep to the lateral collateral ligament at the fibula, which should not be mistaken for tendinosis (see Fig. 7.13C).[20] The transducer

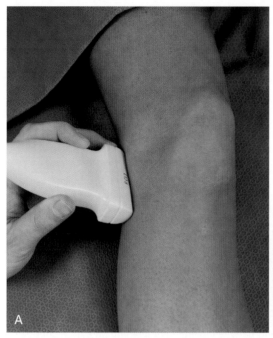
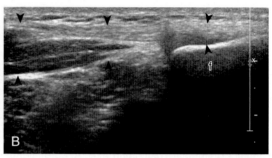

■ FIGURE 7.14 **Biceps Femoris.** A, Coronal imaging shows (B) the biceps femoris *(arrowheads)*. f, Fibula.

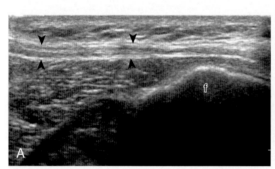
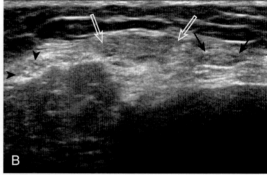

■ FIGURE 7.15 **Common Peroneal Nerve.** Coronal imaging posterior to biceps femoris shows (A) the common peroneal nerve *(arrowheads)* (f, fibula). Transverse imaging proximal to the fibula shows (B) the lateral collateral ligament *(arrows)*, biceps femoris *(open arrows)*, and common peroneal nerve *(arrowheads)* in short axis (left side of image is posterior).

placement for evaluating the iliotibial tract, lateral collateral ligament, and biceps femoris has the configuration of a "Z."

As the transducer is then moved posteriorly from the biceps femoris in the coronal plane, the relatively hypoechoic and striated appearance of the common peroneal nerve can be seen in long axis (Fig. 7.15A), although peripheral nerves are more conspicuous when visualized in short axis (Fig. 7.15B). Evaluation proximal to the fibula is best evaluated in short axis from a posterior approach with the patient prone, which shows the relative locations of the lateral collateral

ligament, the biceps femoris, and the common peroneal nerve (Fig. 7.15B).

To evaluate the anterolateral ligament, the transducer is placed over the anterolateral tibia approximately midway between the Gerdy tubercle and the fibula and angled toward the proximal lateral collateral ligament origin (Fig. 7.16A).[9] The anterolateral ligament will be seen as a linear hyperechoic structure attaching to the lateral meniscus and the proximal femur from the tibia (Fig. 7.16B) (Video 7.1).[9]

Returning to the popliteus groove in the lateral femoral condyle in the coronal plane, the popliteus

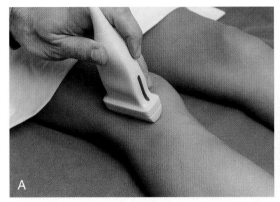
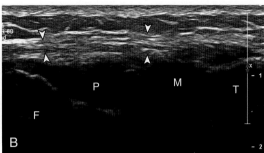

■ FIGURE 7.16 **Anterolateral Ligament.** Coronal-oblique imaging (A) midway between Gerdy tubercle and fibula shows (B) the anterolateral ligament *(arrowheads)* (*F*, femur; *T*, tibia). Note popliteus *(P)* and lateral meniscus *(M)*, which appear hypoechoic from anisotropy.

tendon may be followed as it curves posteriorly around the knee joint. The adjacent hyperechoic fibrocartilage body and anterior horn of the lateral meniscus may also be evaluated. Because of the curved course of the popliteus tendon, this tendon is assessed in segments to avoid misinterpretation of hypoechoic anisotropy as tendon abnormality (Fig. 7.17A). The popliteus muscle is best evaluated from a posterior approach, in which the muscle belly is located between the tibia and the tibial vessels (see Posterior Evaluation). Finally, a hyperechoic extension from the popliteus tendon at the joint line may be seen, which attaches to the fibular styloid, called the *popliteofibular ligament* (Fig. 7.17B).[21] Other supporting structures of the posterolateral corner, such as the arcuate ligament and the possible fabellofibular ligament, are difficult to identify.

Posterior Evaluation

To evaluate the posterior structures of the knee, the patient is turned prone. The structures and pathology of interest include a Baker (or popliteal) cyst, the posterior horns of the menisci, the cruciate ligaments, and the neurovascular structures of the posterior knee. Examination begins with evaluation for a Baker cyst. The key bone landmark is the rounded surface of the medial femoral condyle with a layer of hypoechoic hyaline cartilage. To identify this site, the transducer may be placed over the central aspect of the posterior knee in the transverse plane to identify the neurovascular structures and bone landmarks of the intercondylar notch (Fig. 7.18). The transducer is then moved medially to identify the medial femoral condyle (Fig. 7.19). At this site, the medial head of the gastrocnemius and semimembranosus tendons are seen, with the latter seen more medially. These are the key soft tissue landmarks as a Baker cyst must display a channel or neck between these two tendons. The semitendinosus tendon

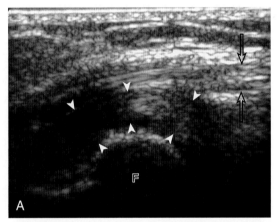
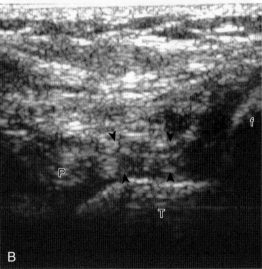

■ FIGURE 7.17 **Popliteus and Popliteofibular Ligament.** Imaging long axis to the proximal popliteus tendon shows (A) the popliteus tendon *(arrowheads)* and lateral collateral ligament *(open arrows)* (*F*, femur). Coronal imaging shows (B) the popliteofibular ligament *(arrowheads)* between the popliteus tendon *(P)* and the fibula *(f)*. *T*, Tibia. *(B, From: Sekiya JK, Jacobson JA, Wojtys EM: Sonographic imaging of the posterolateral structures of the knee: findings in human cadavers. Arthroscopy 18:872-881, 2002.)*

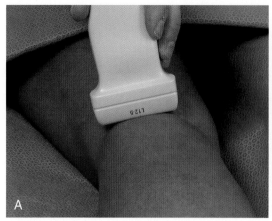

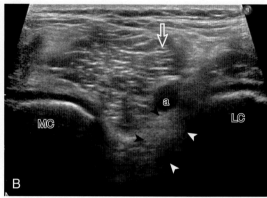

■ **FIGURE 7.18 Posterior Knee Evaluation.** A, Transverse imaging over the posterior distal femur shows (B) medial *(MC)* and lateral *(LC)* femoral condyles, popliteal artery *(a)*, tibial nerve *(open arrow)*, and anterior cruciate ligament *(arrowheads)* in the lateral aspect of the intercondylar notch.

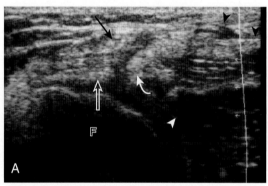

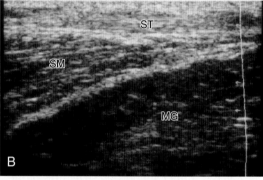

■ **FIGURE 7.19 Posterior Knee Evaluation: Baker Cyst.** Transverse (A) and sagittal (B) imaging centered over medial femoral condyle *(F)* shows the medial head of gastrocnemius muscle *(arrowheads, MG)* and tendon *(curved arrow)* as well as the semimembranosus tendon *(open arrow)* and semitendinosus tendon *(arrow, ST)* (left side of image is medial). *SM,* Semimembranosus muscle.

is also identified immediately superficial to the semimembranosus tendon. To assist in identifying these tendons, the transducer can be toggled to create anisotropy, which causes the tendons to become hypoechoic (Fig. 7.20) (Video 7.2). In addition, toggling the transducer can correct for anisotropy and avoid the pitfall of mistaking a hypoechoic tendon from anisotropy as a Baker cyst (Fig. 7.20A).[5] The course of the medial head of the gastrocnemius tendon is not parallel to that of the semimembranosus tendon; therefore, it may be difficult to have both tendons appear hyperechoic in the same plane. If a Baker cyst is identified, the transducer is then turned in the sagittal plane to evaluate the extent of the Baker cyst and to assess for rupture. The semitendinosus can also be imaged from this point distally to its insertion at the pes anserinus.

The transducer is then moved over the medial aspect of the posterior knee in the sagittal plane to again identify the posterior femoral condyle (Fig. 7.21A). At this location, the posterior horn of the medial meniscus is evaluated; this structure normally appears hyperechoic and triangular (Fig. 7.21B). A lower-frequency transducer (less than 10 MHz) may be required to visualize the meniscus. At the medial aspect of the medial meniscus posterior horn, the semimembranosus can be seen as it inserts on the posteromedial tibial cortex, just beyond the meniscus at a prominent concavity or sulcus in the bone. With anisotropy, the normal semimembranosus tendon may appear hypoechoic and may potentially simulate a parameniscal cyst (see Fig. 7.11).

The transducer is then moved toward the midline in the sagittal plane, and the posterior cruciate ligament is seen with its attachment to the posterior tibia, identified by characteristic bone contours (Fig. 7.21C). The normal posterior cruciate ligament may appear artifactually hypoechoic as a result of anisotropy, but its thickness should be uniform and less than 1 cm.[22] Anisotropy of the

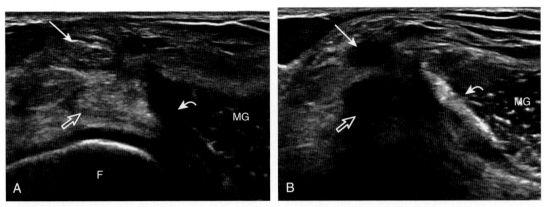

■ FIGURE 7.20 **Semimembranosus Anisotropy: Pseudo-Baker Cyst.** Transverse imaging (A and B) shows differential anisotropy of the semimembranosus *(open arrow)*, semitendinosus *(arrow)*, and medial head of gastrocnemius tendon *(curved arrows)*, the latter of which may simulate a small Baker cyst in (A). *F,* Femur; *MG,* medial head of gastrocnemius muscle.

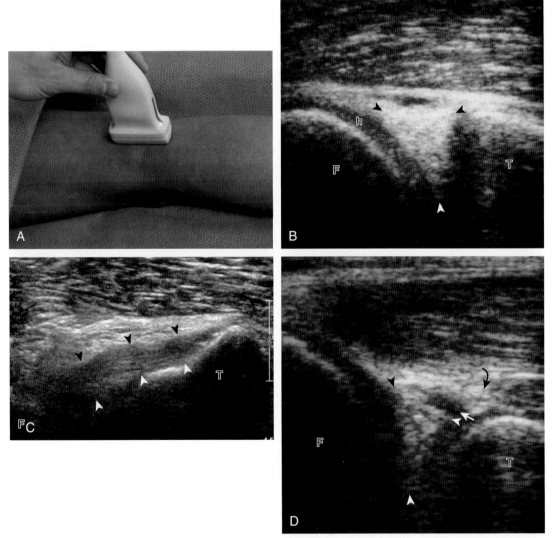

■ FIGURE 7.21 **Posterior Knee Evaluation: Menisci and Posterior Cruciate Ligament.** A, Parasagittal imaging over the posterior medial knee shows (B) the posterior horn of the medial meniscus *(arrowheads)* (*h*, hyaline articular cartilage). Sagittal imaging in midline shows (C), the posterior cruciate ligament *(arrowheads)*. Lateral parasagittal imaging shows (D) the posterior horn of the lateral meniscus *(arrowheads)*, popliteus tendon *(curved arrow)*, and popliteus tension sheath *(arrow)*. *F,* Femur; *T,* tibia.

posterior cruciate ligament may be reduced with the heel-toe maneuver or the use of beam steering (available on some ultrasound machines). The transducer is then moved laterally to assess the posterior horn of the lateral meniscus, although accurate identification of pathology is difficult in this location because the popliteus tendon and sheath cross at the peripheral aspect of the lateral meniscus (Fig. 7.21D).

The transducer is then turned to the transverse plane and positioned over the intercondylar notch (see Fig. 7.18A). Normally, this space should be hyperechoic, which contains the anterior cruciate ligament along the lateral aspect and the adjacent hyperechoic fat (see Fig. 7.18B).[23] Identification of the anterior cruciate ligament may be improved by toggling the transducer because the normal ligament becomes hypoechoic relative to the adjacent hyperechoic fat as a result of anisotropy. Finally, the popliteal artery and vein are evaluated in short axis and long axis. The muscle belly of the popliteus is located between these vessels and the tibia. The tibial nerve can be followed proximally to its junction with the common peroneal

nerve at the sciatic nerve, which is evaluated with the posterior thigh. Although the sciatic nerve demonstrates a honeycomb appearance from hypoechoic nerve fascicles and surrounding hyperechoic connective tissue, the smaller peripheral nerve branches may consist of only a few hypoechoic fascicles.

■ JOINT ABNORMALITIES

Joint Effusion and Synovial Hypertrophy

Increased joint fluid in the knee is characterized by anechoic or hypoechoic distention of the knee joint recesses. Evaluation of the anterior knee joint recesses, namely the suprapatellar recess, and medial and lateral recesses are most accessible. With 30 degrees of knee flexion, there is preferential distention of the suprapatellar recess with joint fluid that extends superiorly from the central joint compartment (Fig. 7.22; see Fig. 7.1F).[16] Suprapatellar recess distention will separate the quadriceps and prefemoral fat pads, and extend

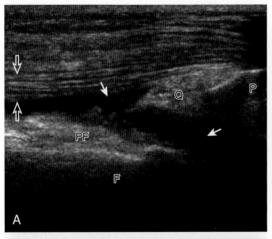

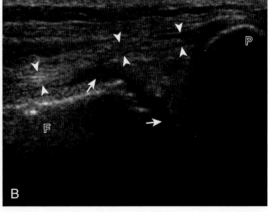

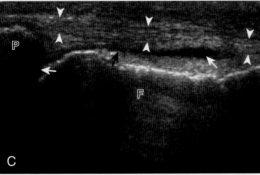

■ **FIGURE 7.22 Joint Effusion: Knee Flexion.** Ultrasound images with knee in slight flexion (A) long axis to the quadriceps tendon and transverse over the (B) medial and (C) lateral patellar retinacula show hypoechoic joint recess distention *(arrows)*. Note preferential distention deep to quadriceps tendon *(open arrows)* and separation of the quadriceps *(Q)* and prefemoral *(PF)* fat pads *(arrowheads, patellar retinaculum)*. *F*, Femur; *P*, patella.

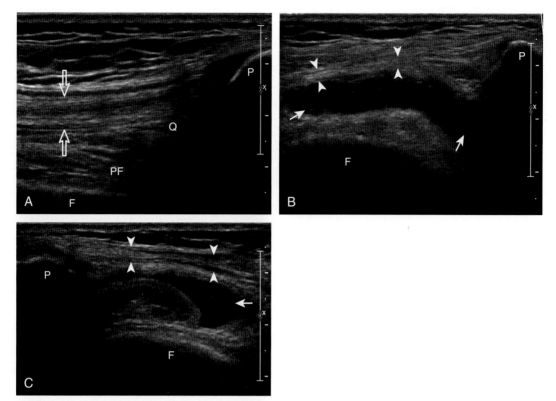

■ FIGURE 7.23 Joint Effusion: Knee Extension. Ultrasound images with knee in full extension (A) long axis to the quadriceps tendon and transverse over (B) the lateral and (C) medial patellar retinacula show hypoechoic joint recess distention *(arrows)*. Note preferential distention lateral and medial to the patella (P) *(arrowheads,* patellar retinaculum; *open arrows,* quadriceps tendon). *F,* Femur; *PF,* prefemoral fat pad; *Q,* quadriceps fat pad.

superiorly and anteriorly to contact the quadriceps tendon.[1] Often small amounts of fluid may only be seen superolateral to the patella in the suprapatellar recess, where detection may be improved with quadriceps muscle contraction.[24] This is an ideal location for ultrasound-guided aspiration or injection.[25] In knee extension, joint recess distention may be seen only medial or more likely lateral to the patella in the transverse plane without distention of the suprapatellar recess (Fig. 7.23).[15] Larger joint effusions will typically distend all three recesses. When imaging the medial and lateral recesses, transducer pressure should be minimized to avoid collapse of the joint recess and displacement of the joint fluid out of view (Video 7.3). Joint fluid may also collect in the popliteus tendon sheath or in a Baker cyst when communication exists with the posterior knee joint.[5] The lateral perimeniscal recesses may also distend, which should not be mistaken for parameniscal cyst (Fig. 7.24).[1] A superior patellar plica, which is located in the transverse plane through the suprapatellar recess superior to the patella, may uncommonly completely separate the suprapatellar recess into two compartments (Fig. 7.25).[26] In the setting of an intra-articular fracture, several

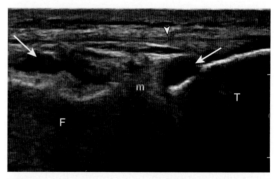

■ FIGURE 7.24 Lateral Perimeniscal Recess. Ultrasound image over the anterolateral knee shows anechoic joint effusion *(arrows)* adjacent to the anterior horn of the lateral meniscus *(m)*. Note iliotibial tract *(arrowhead)*. *F,* Femur; *T,* tibia.

layers of varying echogenicity within the joint may be visible as a lipohemarthrosis (Fig. 7.26).[27]

The causes of joint effusion are many; however, ultrasound including color or power Doppler imaging cannot distinguish between aseptic and septic effusion (Figs. 7.27 and 7.28). If joint recess distention is not anechoic but rather hypoechoic, isoechoic, or hyperechoic to subcutaneous fat,

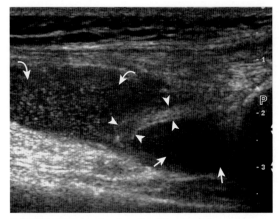

■ **FIGURE 7.25 Superior Patellar Plica.** Ultrasound image long axis to the quadriceps tendon shows the superior plica *(arrowheads)* that separates the superior aspect of the suprapatellar recess *(curved arrow, distended with hypoechoic complex fluid)* from the knee joint *(arrows, distended with anechoic simple fluid). P,* Patella.

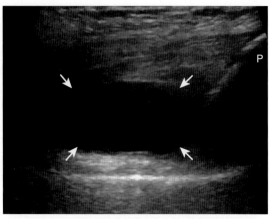

■ **FIGURE 7.27 Joint Effusion: Infection.** Ultrasound image long axis to quadriceps tendon shows hypoechoic distention of the suprapatellar recess *(arrows)*. Note increased through-transmission. *P,* Patella.

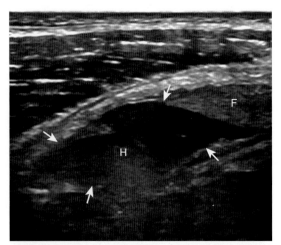

■ **FIGURE 7.26 Lipohemarthrosis.** Ultrasound image over lateral aspect of suprapatellar recess shows layering of echogenic fat *(F)* superficial to intra-articular hemorrhage *(arrows)* and more dependent hematocrit level separating serum from blood cells *(H)*.

then considerations include complex fluid versus synovial hypertrophy. Compressibility of the joint recess, redistribution of recess contents, or swirling of the contents with compression or joint movement, and lack of internal flow on color Doppler imaging all suggest complex fluid rather than synovial hypertrophy (Video 7.4).[28] The differential diagnosis for complex fluid includes infection (Fig. 7.28), gout,[29,30] hemorrhage (Fig. 7.29), and lipohemarthrosis (see Fig. 7.26). If there is concern for infection, percutaneous aspiration should be considered.

Inflammatory synovial hypertrophy may be associated with cortical erosions, characterized by cortical irregularity and discontinuity visualized

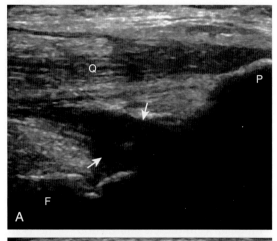

■ **FIGURE 7.28 Joint Effusion: Infection.** Ultrasound images (A) long axis and (B) short axis to quadriceps tendon *(Q)* from two different patients show complex fluid and synovial hypertrophy distending the suprapatellar recess from *Pseudomonas* and fungal infection, respectively. *F,* Femur; *P,* patella; *Q,* quadriceps tendon; *A,* total knee arthroplasty.

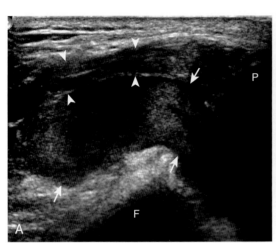

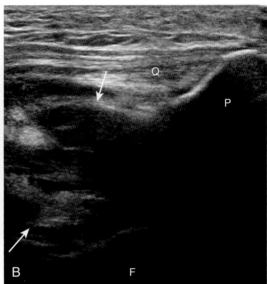

■ FIGURE 7.29 **Intra-Articular Hemorrhage**. Ultrasound images in two different patients show mixed-echogenicity hemorrhagic joint fluid *(arrows)* distending the (A) lateral recess and (B) suprapatellar recess. Note (A) abnormally thickened lateral patellar retinaculum *(arrowheads)*. *F*, Femur; *P*, patella; *Q*, quadriceps.

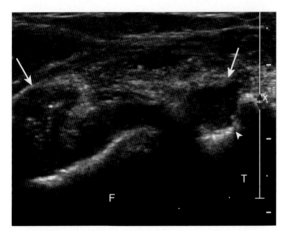

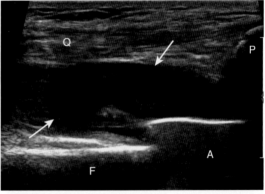

■ FIGURE 7.30 **Rheumatoid Arthritis**. Ultrasound image in coronal plane over medial knees shows hypoechoic synovial hypertrophy *(arrows)* with cortical erosion *(arrowhead)*. *F*, Femur; *T*, tibia. There was no flow on color Doppler imaging.

■ FIGURE 7.31 **Seronegative Arthritis**. Ultrasound image in sagittal plane over anterior knee shows hypoechoic to isoechoic synovial hypertrophy and anechoic effusion *(arrows)*. Note echogenic surface of total knee arthroplasty *(A)* with posterior reverberation artifact. *F*, Femur; *P*, patella; *Q*, quadriceps.

in two planes, often associated with increased blood flow on color Doppler imaging. Although synovial hypertrophy may also result from inflammation, such as chronic infection (see Fig. 7.28), rheumatoid arthritis (Fig. 7.30), seronegative arthritis (Fig. 7.31), crystal deposition (Fig. 7.32), and particle disease from arthroplasty wear (Fig. 7.33), synovial proliferative disorders such as pigmented villonodular synovitis[31] (Fig. 7.34), lipoma arborescens,[32,33] and synovial chondromatosis[34] are other considerations, with possible hyperechoic foci seen in the last condition when

calcified. The differential diagnosis for mixed hyperechoic and hypoechoic tissue associated with the suprapatellar recess with compressible vascular channels is synovial hemangioma (see Vascular Abnormalities).[35] Localized nodular synovitis may also occur in the knee joint recesses, and it typically appears hypoechoic and noncompressible with possible increased through-transmission (Fig. 7.35).[36] Dynamic imaging may demonstrate snapping of synovial hypertrophy (Video 7.5).[37] In the setting of a total knee arthroplasty, abnormal synovial hypertrophy may cause snapping, termed

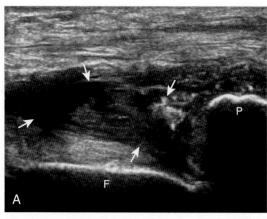

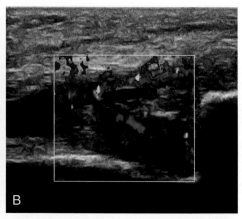

■ **FIGURE 7.32 Pseudogout (Calcium Pyrophosphate Dihydrate Deposition Disease).** Ultrasound images (A and B) long axis to quadriceps tendon show heterogeneous distention of the suprapatellar recess *(arrows)* from synovial hypertrophy and complex fluid with increased flow on color Doppler imaging. *F,* Femur; *P,* patella.

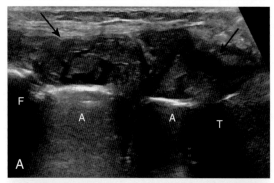

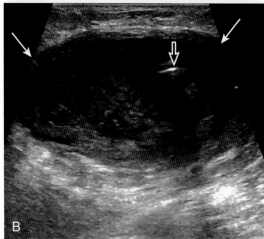

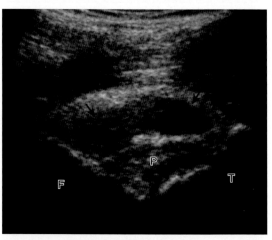

■ **FIGURE 7.34 Pigmented Villonodular Synovitis.** Ultrasound image in the sagittal plane over the posterior knee shows hypoechoic synovial hypertrophy *(arrows)* adjacent to posterior cruciate ligament *(P).* *F,* Femur; *T,* tibia.

■ **FIGURE 7.33 Particle Disease.** Ultrasound image in coronal plane over medial knee (A) shows hypoechoic to isoechoic synovial hypertrophy and anechoic fluid *(arrows).* Note echogenic surface of total knee arthroplasty (A) with posterior reverberation artifact (*F,* femur; *T,* tibia). Ultrasound image of Baker cyst (B) shows similar synovial hypertrophy *(arrows)* with internal metal debris *(open arrow).*

patellar clunk syndrome (Fig. 7.36) (Video 7.6).[38] Within joint fluid, intra-articular bodies may be identified, commonly in a Baker cyst (see Baker Cyst) or suprapatellar recess (Fig. 7.37). Such intra-articular bodies may be hypoechoic if cartilaginous or echogenic with shadowing if calcified or ossified and may be mobile with dynamic imaging (Video 7.7). When an intra-articular body is identified, the hyaline articular cartilage should be evaluated for a donor site (Fig. 7.38).

Cartilage Abnormalities

One common cause of joint effusion is a cartilage abnormality. Meniscal degeneration may appear as heterogeneous or internal hypoechogenicity,

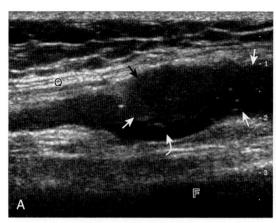

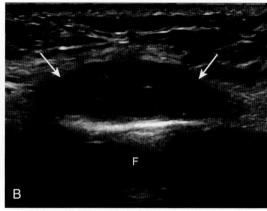

FIGURE 7.35 Localized Nodular Synovitis. Ultrasound images from two different patients show hypoechoic synovial hypertrophy *(arrows)* within the suprapatellar recess (A) and lateral recess (B). Note joint effusion *(curved arrow in A)*. *F*, Femur; *Q*, quadriceps tendon.

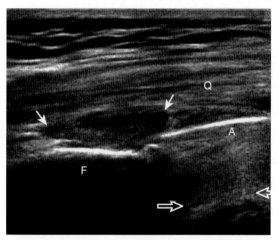

FIGURE 7.36 Patellar Clunk Syndrome. Ultrasound image long axis to quadriceps tendon *(Q)* shows hypoechoic synovial hypertrophy *(arrows)*, which moved and produced a snapping sensation with knee flexion and extension. Note hyperechoic metal component of total knee arthroplasty *(A)* with hyperechoic posterior reverberation *(open arrows)*, and native femur *(F)* with shadowing (right side of image is distal).

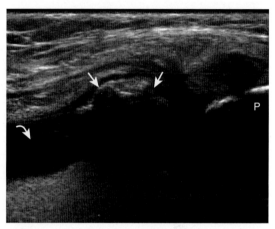

FIGURE 7.37 Intra-Articular Body. Ultrasound image long axis to quadriceps tendon shows hyperechoic and shadowing ossified intra-articular body *(arrows)* within the suprapatellar recess. Note anechoic joint fluid *(curved arrow)*. *P*, Patella.

whereas a meniscal tear appears as a well-defined anechoic or hypoechoic cleft that extends to the articular surface, or possibly meniscal irregularity and truncation (Fig. 7.39). Sensitivity and specificity for diagnosis of meniscal tears using ultrasound have been described as 88% and 85%, respectively.[39,40] Because ultrasound evaluation of the menisci is limited due to incomplete visualization and inadequate delineation of displaced tears, MRI remains the imaging method of choice for evaluation of the menisci. However, evaluation of the menisci can be accomplished in minutes, and pathologic features may be seen, including displacement of meniscal tissue during knee movement visualized dynamically (Videos 7.8 and

7.9).[37,41] The posterior horn of the medial meniscus is the most common site for tears, so evaluation should be at least considered at this site.

Parameniscal cysts can be diagnosed at ultrasound with a reported accuracy of 88% and are associated with an adjacent meniscal tear, although parameniscal cysts adjacent to the anterior horn of the lateral meniscus are less likely to have an associated meniscal tear.[42,43] Parameniscal cysts are usually multilocular and non-compressible, characteristically located at the joint line at the base of the meniscus.[43] Whereas some parameniscal cysts are anechoic with increased through-transmission (Fig. 7.40), others are complex cysts and hypoechoic (Fig. 7.41).[44] A medial parameniscal cyst may extend some distance from the meniscal tear, so the possible diagnosis of parameniscal cyst should be considered with any

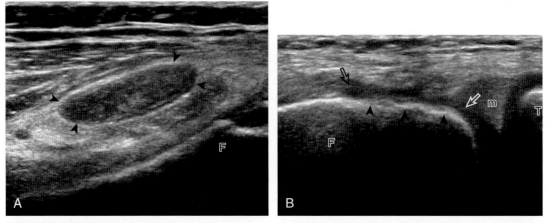

■ **FIGURE 7.38 Intra-Articular Body.** Ultrasound image over the lateral aspect of the suprapatellar recess shows (A) a well-defined hypoechoic non-calcified intra-articular body *(arrowheads)*. Ultrasound image over the anterior aspect of the medial femoral condyle (B) shows cortical irregularity *(arrowheads)* and a cartilage defect *(between open arrows)*. F, Femur; *m*, medial meniscus; *T*, tibia.

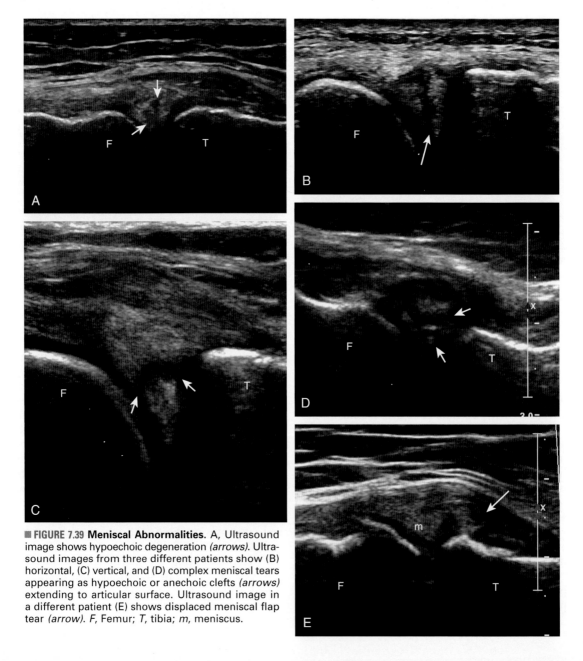

■ **FIGURE 7.39 Meniscal Abnormalities.** A, Ultrasound image shows hypoechoic degeneration *(arrows)*. Ultrasound images from three different patients show (B) horizontal, (C) vertical, and (D) complex meniscal tears appearing as hypoechoic or anechoic clefts *(arrows)* extending to articular surface. Ultrasound image in a different patient (E) shows displaced meniscal flap tear *(arrow)*. F, Femur; *T*, tibia; *m*, meniscus.

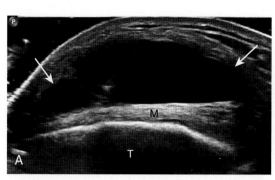

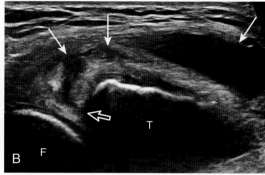

■ **FIGURE 7.40 Parameniscal Cyst: Medial.** Ultrasound image in coronal plane over medial knee (A) shows multilocular anechoic parameniscal cyst *(arrows)* with increased through-transmission. Ultrasound image over posterior horn of medial meniscus (B) shows hypoechoic meniscal tear *(open arrows)* communicating with parameniscal cyst *(arrows)*. *F,* Femur; *T,* tibia; *M,* medial collateral ligament.

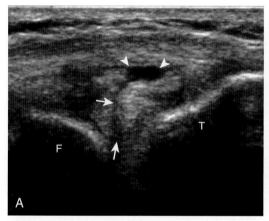

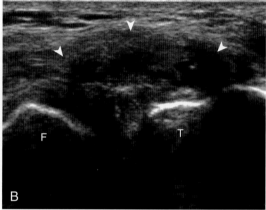

■ **FIGURE 7.41 Parameniscal Cyst: Lateral.** Coronal ultrasound image over body of lateral meniscus shows (A) hypoechoic meniscal tear *(arrow)* in connection with anechoic parameniscal cyst *(arrowheads)*. Ultrasound image posterior to (A) shows (B) hypoechoic heterogeneous appearance of parameniscal cyst *(arrowheads)*. *F,* Femur; *T,* tibia.

multilocular cyst around the knee, and possible meniscal extension should always be sought. As a potential pitfall, the normal semimembranosus tendon insertion on the tibia should not be misinterpreted as a parameniscal cyst; this tendon often appears oval and hypoechoic in evaluation of the posterior horn medial meniscus as a result of anisotropy given the oblique course of the tendon (see Fig. 7.11).

In addition to meniscal tear and degeneration, other meniscal pathology includes meniscal extrusion in the setting of osteoarthritis, often associated with pain (Fig. 7.42).[45] Abnormal displacement of the meniscus relative to the tibia is often appreciated in the coronal plane deep to the tibial collateral ligament, where associated edema of the tibial collateral ligament is possible.[46] In contrast to extrusion of the medial meniscus, extrusion of the anterior horn and body of the lateral meniscus may be a variation of normal.[47]

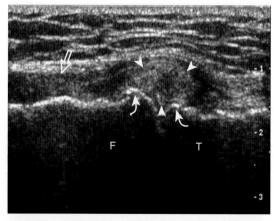

■ **FIGURE 7.42 Meniscal Extrusion.** Coronal ultrasound image over the medial joint shows abnormal hypoechoic meniscus *(arrowheads)* with joint space narrowing and meniscal extrusion medial to the tibia *(T)* (*curved arrows,* osteophytes). *F,* Femur. Note hypoechoic thickening of medial collateral ligament *(open arrow)*.

One hallmark of osteoarthritis is the osteophyte, which can be reliably assessed at the knee with ultrasound.[48]

Other cartilage abnormalities may involve the hyaline articular cartilage, such as cartilage thinning or defect (Fig. 7.43; see Fig. 7.38B).[17,48,49] In the setting of osteoarthritis, femoral articular cartilage thickness is best assessed in knee flexion in the parasagittal plane and correlates with MRI to a better degree than imaging of the trochlear cartilage in the transverse plane.[18] If an intra-articular body is identified, the hyaline cartilage should be evaluated for a defect as a potential donor site.[50,51] Another cartilage abnormality relates to calcification, which can involve both the fibrocartilage meniscus (Fig. 7.44) and the hyaline articular cartilage (Fig. 7.45). Calcification

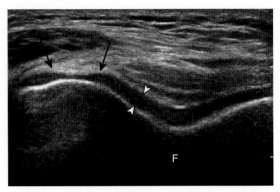

■ FIGURE 7.43 **Cartilage Defect.** Ultrasound image in the transverse plane over the distal femur shows focal hyaline cartilage loss *(arrows)* of trochlea. Note normal hypoechoic hyaline cartilage *(arrowheads)*. F, Femur.

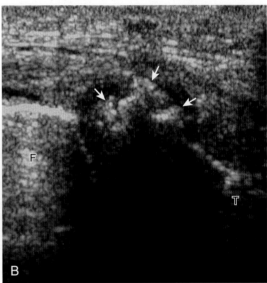

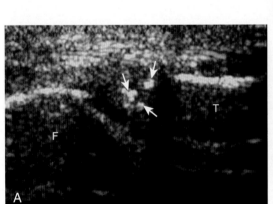

■ FIGURE 7.44 **Chondrocalcinosis: Pseudogout.** A and B, Ultrasound images of the medial meniscus in two different patients show hyperechoic and shadowing chondrocalcinosis *(arrows)* within the meniscus. *F,* Femur; *T,* tibia.

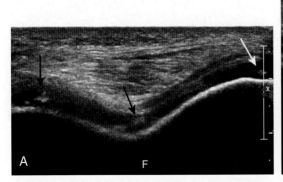

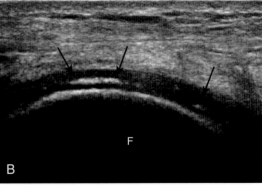

■ FIGURE 7.45 **Chondrocalcinosis: Pseudogout.** Ultrasound images of the (A) trochlea and (B) anterior femoral condyle show hyperechoic calcification *(arrows)* within the hypoechoic hyaline cartilage.

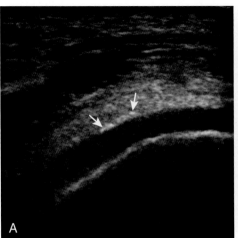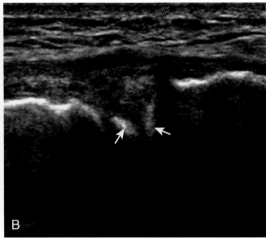

■ **FIGURE 7.46 Gout.** Ultrasound images show hyperechoic monosodium urate crystals *(arrows)* on surface of (A) anterior femoral condyle hyaline cartilage and (B) medial meniscus body.

deposition within cartilage is seen as hyperechoic foci and occurs in pseudogout (calcium pyrophosphate dihydrate crystal deposition disease), among other conditions.[52,53] The anterior femoral cartilage is evaluated with the knee flexed in transverse and parasagittal planes, as well as the posterior femoral cartilage (Video 7.10). In contrast to chondrocalcinosis, monosodium urate crystals with gout are seen on the surface of the cartilage (Fig. 7.46), which can be seen coating the meniscus (Video 7.11) and hyaline cartilage; the latter, termed the *double contour sign*, disappears when serum urate levels are below 6 mg/dL.[30,53-55]

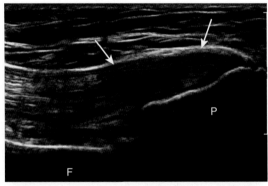

■ **FIGURE 7.47 Quadriceps Tendinosis.** Ultrasound image long axis to the quadriceps tendon shows hypoechoic thickening of the distal quadriceps tendon *(arrows)* without disruption of tendon fibers. *F,* Femur; *P,* patella.

■ TENDON AND MUSCLE ABNORMALITIES

Quadriceps Femoris Injury

Ultrasound is well suited to evaluate the extensor mechanism of the knee because the tendons are superficial and relatively large.[56,57] With regard to the quadriceps tendon, tendinosis is characterized by a hypoechoic tendon with possible increased thickness (Fig. 7.47).[58] Calcifications may also be possible as well as increased flow on color or power Doppler imaging, which often correlates with patient symptoms.[58] Continuous tendon fibers without a tendon defect excludes tendon tear. The term *tendinosis* is used rather than *tendinitis* because this condition primarily represents a degenerative process without acute inflammatory cells. Superimposed partial-thickness tears appear as well-defined hypoechoic or anechoic clefts or incomplete disruption of tendon fibers.[56,57]

Partial-thickness tears of the quadriceps tendon may selectively involve only one or two of the

three layers while sparing other layers of the quadriceps tendon (Fig. 7.48). Full-thickness tears are characterized by complete tendon disruption, tendon retraction, joint fluid that tracks from the suprapatellar recess through the tendon defect, and secondary wavy appearance of the patellar tendon resulting from a low-lying patella (Fig. 7.49).[59] A retracted tendon stump may show posterior refraction shadowing, or it may be associated with a hyperechoic bone avulsion fragment. A displaced avulsion fracture fragment from the superior patellar pole may be seen in both partial-thickness and full-thickness quadriceps tendon tears.[57] Dynamic imaging during evaluation of the quadriceps tendon is often helpful in the diagnosis of a full-thickness tear because lack of tendon movement or translation across the

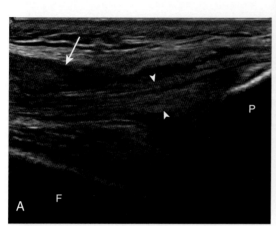
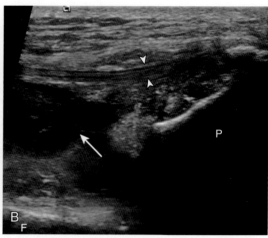

■ **FIGURE 7.48 Quadriceps Partial-Thickness Tears.** Ultrasound image long axis to the quadriceps tendon shows (A) retracted tear of the rectus femoris of the quadriceps tendon *(arrow)* with an intact vastus medialis, lateralis, and intermedius layers *(arrowheads)*. Ultrasound image in another patient (B) shows retracted tear of the vastus medialis, lateralis, and intermedius *(arrow)* with intact rectus femoris layer *(arrowheads)*. *F*, Femur; *P*, patella.

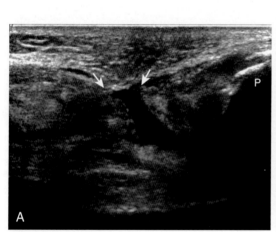
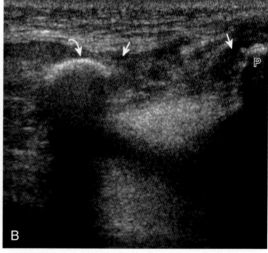

■ **FIGURE 7.49 Quadriceps Full-Thickness Tears.** Ultrasound images long axis to the quadriceps tendon from two patients show complete disruption of the quadriceps tendon *(arrows)*. Note superior patellar pole bone avulsion *(curved arrow)* in B. *F*, Femur; *P*, patella.

abnormal tendon segment, or movement of the tendon stump (Video 7.12) or avulsion fragment away from the patella (Video 7.13) indicates complete tear.[56] Dynamic imaging can be accomplished by slightly flexing the knee or manually pressing inferiorly on the patella. This method is helpful with a subacute tear, when hemorrhage may fill the torn tendon gap with echogenic material, and also with a chronic tear, in which a complete tear may demonstrate partial healing. Ultrasound is able to diagnose full-thickness and

high-grade partial-thickness quadriceps tendon tears with 100% accuracy.[56]

Patellar Tendon Injury

Tendinosis and partial-thickness tears may also involve the proximal patellar tendon, also termed *jumper's knee* (Fig. 7.50). At ultrasound, tendinosis is characterized by abnormal hypoechogenicity with possible tendon enlargement, although continuous tendon fibers remain visible.[58,60] The

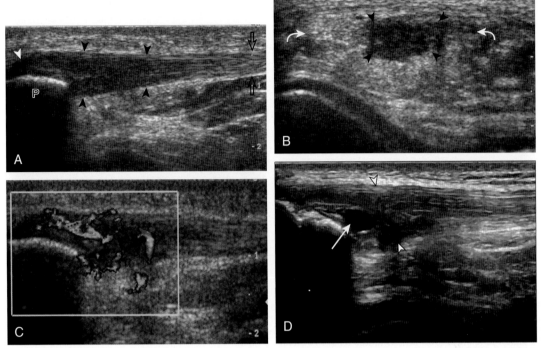

■ FIGURE 7.50 Patellar Tendon Tendinosis. Ultrasound images (A) long axis and (B) short axis to proximal patellar tendon show hypoechoic tendon swelling with intact fibers *(arrowheads)*. Note the normal distal patellar tendon thickness *(open arrows)* in A and width of the patellar tendon *(curved arrows)* in B. Corresponding long axis color Doppler image is shown in C (*P*, patella). Ultrasound image from another patient (D) shows tendinosis *(arrowheads)* and more focal hypoechoic mucoid degeneration *(arrow)*.

presence of more clearly defined hypoechoic or anechoic clefts suggests a superimposed interstitial tear. Marked hyperemia from neovascularity may be seen with color and power Doppler imaging, which is associated with a higher level of pain.[61] In the setting of a full-thickness patellar tendon tear, there is complete tendon fiber discontinuity and refraction shadowing at the retracted torn tendon stumps (Fig. 7.51) (Video 7.14). Dynamic imaging may be used to confirm tendon discontinuity and to identify tendon retraction in the setting of a full-thickness tendon tear by minimally flexing the knee or by manually pressing superiorly on the patella (Video 7.15). Another pathologic process of the patellar tendon is *Osgood-Schlatter disease*, a painful condition that affects the distal patellar tendon insertion from repetitive trauma in an adolescent that is characterized by hypoechoic enlargement of the distal patellar tendon and the non-ossified cartilage, and possible fragmentation of the tibial tuberosity (Fig. 7.52).[62] Similar changes may involve the proximal patellar tendon at the inferior pole of the patella, termed *Sinding-Larsen-Johansson disease*.[62] A central defect or persistent hypoechoic area in the central patellar tendon may be seen when this segment of the tendon is used for anterior cruciate ligament

reconstruction (Fig. 7.53).[63] After total knee arthroplasty, the patellar tendon may be swollen as an expected finding.[64]

Other Knee Tendon Injuries

Other tendon abnormalities around the knee are less common. However, tendinosis may involve the semimembranosus (Fig. 7.54) or biceps femoris. Normal bifurcation of the distal biceps femoris tendon around the lateral collateral ligament should not be confused with tendinosis (see Fig. 7.13C).[20] One other disorder that deserves mention is iliotibial friction band syndrome.[65,66] In this condition, chronic and repetitive contact between the iliotibial tract or band and the lateral femoral condyle may produce hypoechoic edema, inflammation, and possibly adventitious bursa formation deep to the iliotibial tract, with a possible thickened iliotibial tract (Fig. 7.55). Extension of lateral recess joint fluid deep to the iliotibial tract should not be confused with bursa formation.[67] Acute trauma may also cause injury to the iliotibial tract (Fig. 7.56). Although unrelated to trauma, uncommonly abnormal snapping of the semitendinosus can be demonstrated dynamically with ultrasound (Videos 7.16 and 7.17).

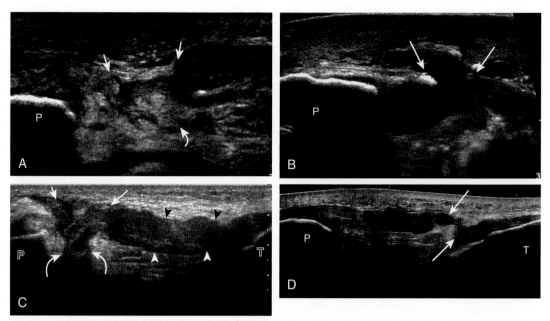

■ **FIGURE 7.51 Patellar Tendon Full-Thickness Tears.** Ultrasound images (A–D) long axis to the patellar tendon from four patients show complete disruption of the patellar tendon *(arrows)* with refraction shadowing *(curved arrows)* deep to the torn tendon stumps. Note tendon retraction, heterogeneous hemorrhage, and diffuse thickening of the distal patellar tendon *(arrowheads)* in C. *P*, Patella; *T*, tibia.

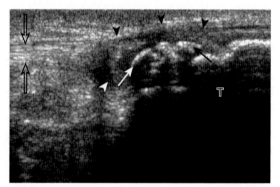

■ **FIGURE 7.52 Osgood-Schlatter Disease.** Ultrasound image long axis to the distal patellar tendon shows hypoechoic thickening *(arrowheads)* with tibial tuberosity bone fragmentation *(arrows)*. Pain was present with transducer pressure. Note the normal proximal patellar tendon *(open arrows)*. *T*, Tibia.

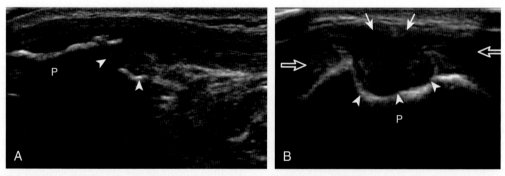

■ **FIGURE 7.53 Postoperative Patellar Tendon: Anterior Cruciate Ligament (ACL) Reconstruction.** Ultrasound images (A) long axis and (B) short axis to patellar tendon show post-surgical defect in the inferior patella *(arrowheads)* and absence of the central third of the patellar tendon *(arrows)* for ACL reconstruction. Note full width of patellar tendon *(open arrows)* in B. *P*, Patella.

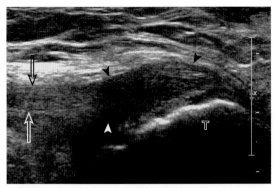

■ **FIGURE 7.54 Tendinosis: Semimembranosus.** Ultrasound image long axis to the distal semimembranosus tendon shows hypoechoic thickening *(arrowheads)* *(open arrows, normal proximal semimembranosus tendon).* *T*, Tibia.

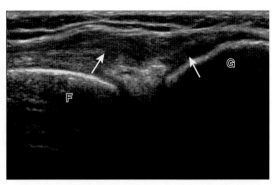

■ **FIGURE 7.56 Iliotibial Tract Tear.** Ultrasound image long axis to iliotibial tract shows tear *(arrows)* with heterogeneous hemorrhage. *F*, Femur; *G*, Gerdy tubercle of tibia.

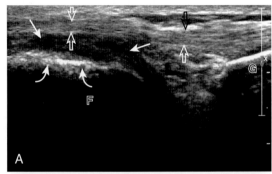

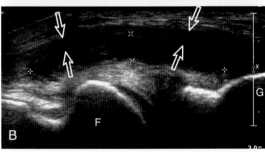

■ **FIGURE 7.55 Iliotibial Band Friction Syndrome.** Ultrasound images long axis to the iliotibial tract in two different patients show (A) hypoechoic soft tissue thickening *(arrows)* and (B) heterogeneous but hypoechoic bursa *(between cursors)* deep to the iliotibial tract *(open arrows)*. Note bone irregularity of the femur in A *(curved arrows)*. *F*, Femur; *G*, Gerdy tubercle of tibia.

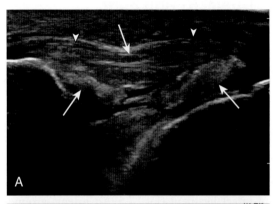

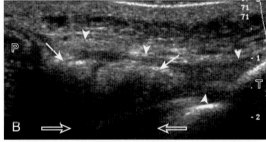

■ **FIGURE 7.57 Gout: Patellar Tendon Tophus.** Ultrasound images from two different patients (A and B) show hyperechoic tophi *(arrows)* within the patellar tendon *(arrowheads)*. Note (B) posterior acoustic shadowing *(open arrows)* from sound beam attenuation of noncalcified tophus. *P*, Patella; *T*, tibia.

Gout

In the setting of gout, the patellar tendon (Fig. 7.57) (Videos 7.18 and 7.19) and popliteus tendon (Fig. 7.58) (Videos 7.20 and 7.21) are prone to involvement; therefore, these sites should be included when evaluating for inflammatory arthritis. Even with asymptomatic hyperuricemia, involvement of the distal patellar tendon is not uncommon.[68] At ultrasound, a gouty tophus appears hyperechoic and amorphous, with punctate internal echoes,

often with an anechoic or hypoechoic halo.[30,54,69,70] A tophus is often more difficult to delineate in a tendon given that both are hyperechoic; however, real-time imaging shows lack of fibrillar echotexture within the tophus. Shadowing may also be seen deep to the tophus, which is more often due to sound beam attenuation than true shadowing from calcification of the tophus (Fig. 7.57B) (Video 7.22). Hyperemia may also be present, as may adjacent cortical erosion (Fig. 7.58B), and soft tissue extension of the tophus.

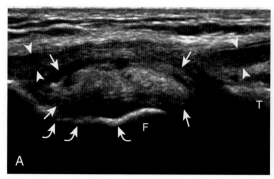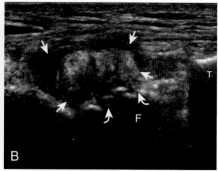

■ **FIGURE 7.58 Gout: Popliteus Tendon Tophus.** Ultrasound images (A and B) long axis to the proximal popliteus tendon in two different patients show hyperechoic tophi with hypoechoic halo *(arrows)*. Note erosions of lateral femur *(curved arrows)* *(arrowheads,* lateral collateral ligament). *F,* Femur; *T,* tibia.

■ LIGAMENT AND BONE ABNORMALITIES

Medial Collateral Ligament

Sonographic evaluation of the ligaments around the knee is most effective for the superficially located ligaments, such as the medial collateral and lateral collateral ligaments. Transducer position long axis to a ligament is the most important plane, although any abnormality is also assessed short axis to the ligament as well. With regard to the tibial collateral ligament, a grade 1 sprain is characterized by adjacent hypoechoic or anechoic fluid but an intact ligament (Fig. 7.59A). Edema around the tibial collateral ligament may not be traumatic because it may be secondary to meniscal extrusion and osteoarthritis (see Fig. 7.42).[46] With a grade 2 injury or partial-thickness tear, the normally hyperechoic and compact fibrillar echotexture is replaced by abnormal hypoechogenicity and possible adjacent hypoechoic or anechoic fluid. With a grade 3 injury or full-thickness tear, there is complete disruption of the ligamentous fibers with heterogeneous hemorrhage and fluid (Fig. 7.59B). Overall, a tibial collateral ligament injury is suggested when greater than 6 mm thick at the femoral attachment or greater than 3.6 mm thick at the tibial attachment.[71] Dynamic imaging may also be used to assess the integrity of the medial collateral ligament because medial joint space widening with valgus stress less than 5 mm represents a grade 1 injury, 5–10 mm represents a grade 2 injury, and greater than 10 mm indicates a grade 3 injury.[71] Shadowing calcification or ossification at the proximal aspect of the medial collateral ligament indicates prior tear, termed Pelligrini-Stieda (Fig. 7.59B). Increased thickness of the tibial collateral ligament with intact fibers and no symptoms is compatible with a remote injury (Fig. 7.59C) or prior total knee arthroplasty.[64] Because the tibial collateral ligament is a relatively flat structure, the entire anterior to posterior extent must be evaluated in short axis. It is not uncommon to have complete fiber discontinuity involving the anterior fibers but with intact fibers posteriorly. A bursa may also be found between the superficial and deep layers of the medial collateral ligament.[72]

Lateral Collateral Ligament

The lateral collateral ligament is an important structure that is a part of the posterolateral ligamentous complex.[21] Injuries may create a thickened, hypoechoic appearance or complete discontinuity (Fig. 7.60).[73] Distal ligamentous avulsions may be associated with a hyperechoic fibular fracture fragment. In this situation, the ligament is structurally intact but functionally completely torn. Other supporting structures of the posterolateral corner include the popliteo-fibular ligament. Because this ligament may be difficult to visualize, it is often helpful to use other signs of posterolateral corner injury, such as lateral collateral ligament tear and abnormal widening of the lateral joint space with varus stress, where lateral joint space of more than 10.5 mm can predict those who will require posterolateral corner repair or reconstruction.[73]

Cruciate and Other Ligaments

With regard to the anterior cruciate and posterior cruciate ligaments, each can be partially visualized at sonography, but MRI is considered the imaging method of choice in their evaluation. At sonography, the posterior cruciate ligament is considered abnormal if it is hypoechoic or anechoic with a thickness greater than 1 cm (Fig. 7.61).[22] A torn posterior cruciate ligament may be focally disrupted or diffusely enlarged.[74] Hyperechoic bone avulsions from the posterior aspect of the tibia are also possible.[75] An anterior cruciate ligament

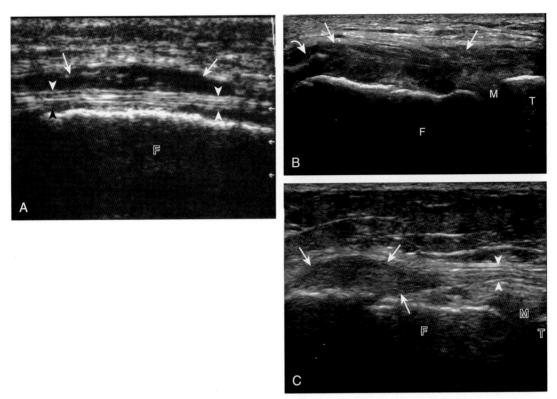

■ **FIGURE 7.59 Medial Collateral Ligament Injury.** Ultrasound images long axis to the medial collateral ligament in three different patients show (A) anechoic fluid *(arrows)* superficial to the intact tibial collateral ligament *(arrowheads)* (grade 1 injury), (B) full-thickness tear *(arrows)* (grade 3 injury) with Pelligrini-Stieda calcification *(curved arrow)*, and (C) hypoechoic thickening of the proximal tibial collateral ligament *(arrows)* from remote injury with normal distal ligament *(arrowheads)*. *F*, Femur; *M*, medial meniscus body; *T*, tibia.

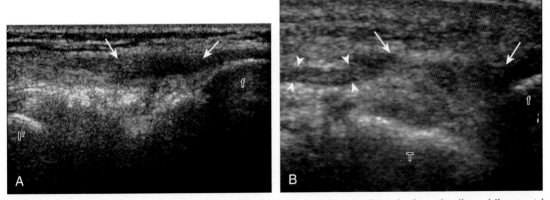

■ **FIGURE 7.60 Lateral Collateral Ligament Tears.** Ultrasound images long axis to the lateral collateral ligament in two different patients show (A) hypoechoic thickening *(arrows)* at the fibula *(f)* consistent with high-grade partial-thickness tear and (B) full-thickness tear *(arrows)* with proximal ligament edema and laxity *(arrowheads)*. *F*, Femur; *T*, tibia.

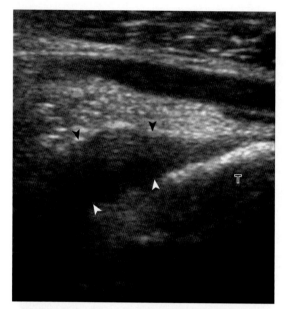

■ FIGURE 7.61 **Posterior Cruciate Ligament Tear.** Ultrasound images long axis to the posterior cruciate ligament shows hypoechoic thickening of the posterior cruciate ligament *(arrowheads)*. *F,* Femur; *T,* tibia.

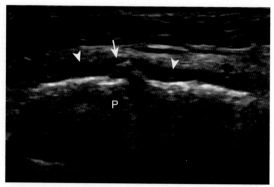

■ FIGURE 7.62 **Fracture: Patella.** Ultrasound image transverse over patella shows cortical discontinuity *(arrow)* and adjacent edema or hemorrhage *(arrowheads)*. *P,* Patella.

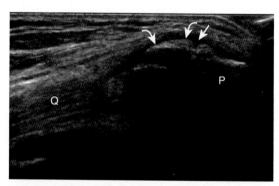

■ FIGURE 7.63 **Bipartite Patella.** Ultrasound image in the sagittal plane over the lateral patella shows the separate patellar bone segment *(curved arrows)* and synchondrosis *(arrow)* with native patella *(P)*. *Q,* Quadriceps tendon.

tear is diagnosed at ultrasound when the normally hyperechoic ligament in the lateral aspect of the intercondylar notch (see Fig. 7.18B), when imaged transversely, is abnormally hypoechoic or anechoic.[23,76] Dynamic stress views have also been used in conjunction with ultrasound to identify abnormal anterior tibial translation as an indirect sign of anterior cruciate ligament tear.[77] Although evaluation for anterior and posterior cruciate ligament tears is limited with ultrasound, ganglion cysts associated with the cruciate ligaments (discussed later) may extend posteriorly and can be visible at sonography.[78] When an anterior cruciate ligament tear is suspected, evaluation should also include the anterolateral ligament and possible avulsion fracture from the proximal tibia (Segond fracture).[79]

Osseous Injury

With regard to ultrasound of bone, the osseous surfaces have a characteristic contour that is important for orientation, especially when evaluating ligaments. The normal bone cortex is smooth and continuous. Any focal step-off deformity, especially if point tenderness with transducer pressure, should raise concern for fracture (Fig. 7.62).[80,81] With regard to the patella, a bipartite or tripartite patella, which is a normal variation, should not be misinterpreted as a fracture.[82] Unlike a fracture, this normal variation is isolated to the upper outer quadrant of the patella, has more

irregular osseous margins, and is often asymptomatic; correlation with radiography is also important (Fig. 7.63).

■ BURSAE AND CYSTS
Baker Cyst

Besides parameniscal cysts described in the preceding section, other cystic abnormalities are often seen around the knee (see Fig. 7.1F). One of the most common is distention of the gastrocnemio-semimembranosus bursa, which results in Baker (or popliteal) cyst.[5] Although distention of this bursa may occur from local irritation or inflammation, more commonly it becomes distended with joint fluid through communication with the knee joint. Present in 50% of adults who are older than 50 years, this communication is acquired by a combination of degenerative weakening of the intervening capsule, and increased intra-articular pressure and joint

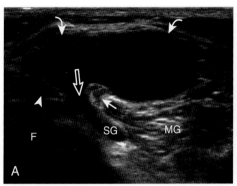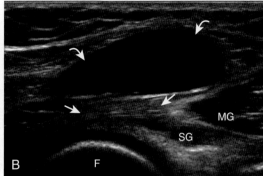

■ **FIGURE 7.64 Baker Cyst.** Ultrasound images transverse (A) and sagittal (B) over the posterior medial knee show anechoic distention of the gastrocnemio-semimembranosus bursa *(curved arrows)*. Note the communication to the knee joint *(open arrow)* between the semimembranosus tendon *(arrowhead)* and the medial head of the gastrocnemius tendon *(arrows)* and muscle *(MG)* via the subgastrocnemius bursa *(SG)*. F, Medial femoral condyle.

fluid from internal derangement.[5] In the pediatric population, Baker cyst communication to the knee joint is present in the majority of cases and may be associated with underlying arthritis or joint hypermobility.[83] Accurate diagnosis of Baker cyst relies on identification of the characteristic channel or neck between the semimembranosus and the medial head of the gastrocnemius tendons which connects the bursa to the knee joint via the subgastrocnemius bursa.[5] The result is a C-shaped fluid collection, concave lateral, which wraps around the medial head of the gastrocnemius tendon and muscle (Fig. 7.64).

A Baker cyst may be distended with anechoic or hypoechoic fluid. The presence of isoechoic or hyperechoic material within a Baker cyst may represent complex fluid, hemorrhage, or synovial hypertrophy (inflammatory or the result of proliferative synovial conditions such as pigmented villonodular synovitis) (Fig. 7.65; see Fig. 7.33). Intra-articular bodies (with shadowing if calcified) are also commonly present within a Baker cyst (Fig. 7.65D and E; see Fig. 7.33B). The inferior margin of the Baker cyst should also be evaluated in the sagittal plane, which is normally well defined and smooth. The presence of anechoic or hypoechoic fluid beyond the confines of the Baker cyst suggests acute or subacute rupture, which can produce diffuse edema or reactive cellulitis that typically is located superficial to the medial head of the gastrocnemius muscle and may extend to the ankle (Fig. 7.66A). Focal soft tissue at the inferior margin indicates remote rupture (Fig. 7.66B). A more extensive ruptured Baker cyst may result in a heterogeneous mass-like area in the calf, usually superficial to the medial head of the gastrocnemius muscle (Fig. 7.67). In this situation, a ruptured Baker cyst must be differentiated from a soft tissue neoplasm; identification of the Baker cyst communication to the knee joint between the medial head of the gastrocnemius and semi-membranosus tendons is critical in this differentiation.[5] Extension of a Baker cyst deep to the calf musculature is uncommon, and extension within the muscle is rare, so such findings should raise concern for another etiology, such as sarcoma. Ultrasound-guided aspiration and steroid injection of Baker cyst may be considered, although re-accumulation of fluid from the knee joint is possible (see Chapter 9).

Other Bursae

Several other bursae around the knee in addition to Baker cysts may become distended (see Fig. 7.1F). Medially and anteriorly, the pes anserine bursa is located deep to the pes anserinus adjacent to the medial tibia, but it may be extensive when distended (Fig. 7.68).[3] Symptoms referable to the pes anserinus rarely correspond to a tendon or bursal abnormality but rather are associated with knee osteoarthritis.[84] Rarely, the sartorius tendon may be identified snapping over a distended pes anserine bursa causing symptoms (Video 7.23). Posterior and superior to the pes anserinus and at the joint line, the semimembranosus–tibial collateral ligament bursa takes the form of an inverted U shape as it wraps around the semi-membranosus tendon (Fig. 7.69).[4] The prepatellar bursa is located anterior to the patella and proximal patellar tendon and is most often multi-compartmental (Fig. 7.70).[85] When evaluating the prepatellar bursa, transducer pressure should be minimized so as not to displace fluid from view (Video 7.24). The superficial infrapatellar bursa (Fig. 7.71) and deep infrapatellar bursa (Fig. 7.72) are located around the distal patellar tendon, the latter of which normally contains minimal fluid (Fig. 7.72A).[86] Bursae may also form at points of abnormal mechanical friction or contact, such as

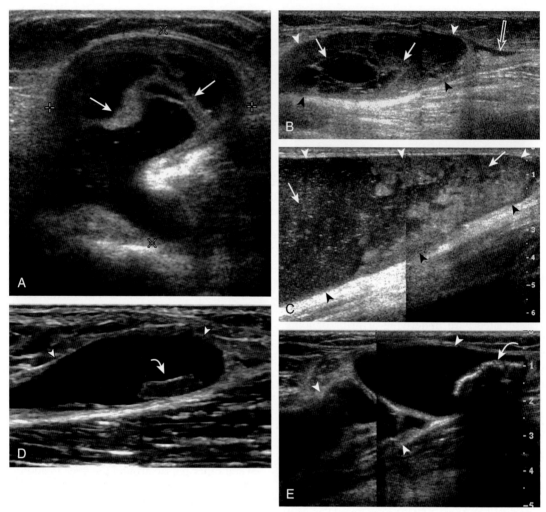

■ **FIGURE 7.65 Complex Baker Cysts**. Ultrasound images transverse (A) and sagittal (B–E) over the posterior medial knee from five different patients show heterogeneous and variable echogenicity *(arrows)* within Baker cysts *(cursors* or *arrowheads)* from complex fluid, hemorrhage, and synovitis. Note Baker cyst rupture *(open arrow)* in B, hypoechoic hyaline cartilage body *(curved arrow)* in D, and an ossified intra-articular body with posterior acoustic shadowing *(curved arrow)* in E that was mobile with transducer pressure.

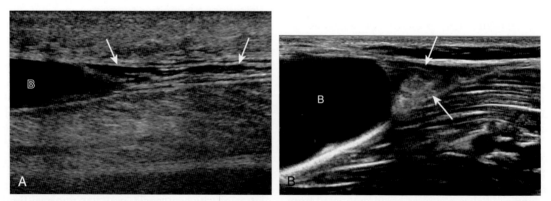

■ **FIGURE 7.66 Ruptured Baker Cysts**. Ultrasound images sagittal over the posterior medial knee from two patients show (A) anechoic fluid *(arrows)* and (B) hypoechoic to isoechoic soft tissue *(arrows)* at the inferior margin of the Baker cyst *(B)*, from acute and remote rupture, respectively.

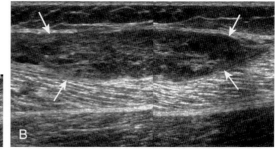

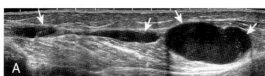

■ FIGURE 7.67 **Ruptured Baker Cysts.** Sagittal ultrasound images in two different patients show (A) loculated hypoechoic fluid *(arrows)* and (B) hypoechoic to isoechoic hematoma *(arrows)* superficial to the medial head of the gastrocnemius. In each case, proximal communication to the posterior knee joint was demonstrated.

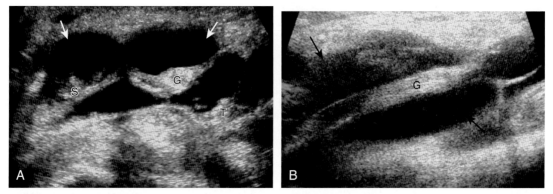

■ FIGURE 7.68 **Pes Anserine Bursa.** Ultrasound images (A) short axis and (B) long axis to the gracilis tendon *(G)* show anechoic distention of the pes anserine bursa *(arrows)*. *S*, Sartorius; *T*, semitendinosus.

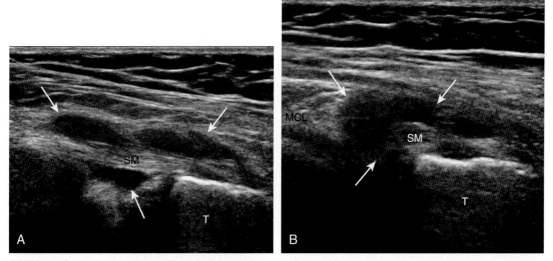

■ FIGURE 7.69 **Semimembranosus–Tibial Collateral Ligament Bursa.** Ultrasound images (A) long axis and (B) short axis to the semimembranosus tendon *(SM)* show hypoechoic fluid *(arrows)*, which distends the semimembranosus–tibial collateral ligament bursa. Note location between the semimembranosus and tibial collateral ligament *(MCL)*. *T*, Tibia.

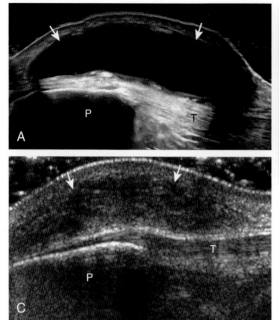
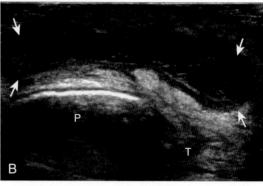

■ **FIGURE 7.70 Prepatellar Bursa.** Ultrasound images long axis to the proximal patellar tendon over distal patella in three different patients show prepatellar bursal distention *(arrows)* from (A) anechoic fluid (aseptic), (B) hypoechoic heterogeneous synovial hypertrophy and complex fluid (infection), and (C) isoechoic hemorrhage (*P*, patella; *T*, patellar tendon). Note that the transducer is floated on a thick layer of gel in A and C.

after knee amputation, termed *adventitious bursa* (Fig. 7.73).[87] A bursa may be distended with anechoic or hypoechoic fluid, although complex fluid, hemorrhage, or synovial hypertrophy may range from hypoechoic to hyperechoic, with possible increased flow on color or power Doppler imaging.

Causes of bursal distention include trauma, inflammation (such as infection, rheumatoid arthritis, and gout), and synovial proliferative disorders. Echogenic gas may be seen in the setting of infection (Video 7.25). The presence of pain with transducer pressure and hyperemia on color or power Doppler imaging suggest true inflammation or bursitis rather than mechanical or reactive bursal fluid. Knowledge of these common bursae allows one to distinguish an abnormal bursa from a nonspecific fluid collection or abscess. Unlike a Baker cyst, the previously described bursae do not normally communicate to the knee joint; therefore, ultrasound-guided percutaneous aspiration and injection may be warranted.

Ganglion Cysts

Ganglion cysts have a propensity to be located at several areas around the knee.[88] The exact cause of ganglion cysts is not known, but synovial herniation, tissue degeneration, and tissue response to trauma are possibilities.[88] One common site is

around the cruciate ligaments, where a ganglion cyst may extend into the soft tissue and bone (Fig. 7.74).[78] Ganglion cysts may also occur posteriorly at the gastrocnemius tendon origins (Fig. 7.75) and anteriorly in the Hoffa infrapatellar fat pad (Fig. 7.76).[88,89] At ultrasound, ganglion cysts characteristically demonstrate lobular margins and internal septations with a multilocular appearance and are non-compressible. Ganglion cysts may be anechoic, with increased through-transmission, or hypoechoic, without increased through-transmission when small. Percutaneous aspiration reveals thick and clear gelatinous fluid. The differential diagnosis of a soft tissue multilocular cyst is a parameniscal cyst, with the latter located around the joint line, which extends from a meniscal tear. If a large cyst-appearing abnormality is identified at ultrasound that is not multilocular (such as a ganglion cyst) and not in the expected location of a bursa, then a hypoechoic solid neoplasm must be considered. Intraneural ganglion cysts of the peroneal nerve are discussed in the next section of this chapter.

■ PERIPHERAL NERVE ABNORMALITIES

Ultrasound evaluation of the knee includes imaging of peripheral nerves. The common peroneal nerve

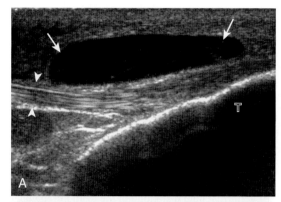

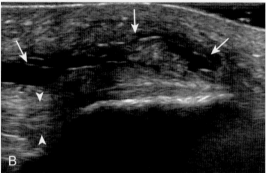

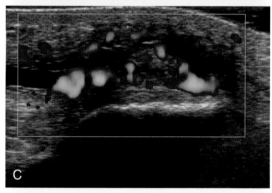

■ FIGURE 7.71 **Superficial Infrapatellar Bursa.** Ultrasound image (A) long axis to the distal patellar tendon *(arrowheads)* shows predominantly hypoechoic distention of the superficial infrapatellar bursa *(arrows)* with internal linear echoes resulting from sterile complex fluid and hemorrhage. B, Long axis ultrasound image in a different patient shows complex fluid and variable echogenicity synovial hypertrophy *(arrows)* with increased blood flow on (C) power Doppler imaging *(arrowheads,* patellar tendon). *T,* Tibia.

near the fibula is predisposed to pathology, which includes direct injury or entrapment between the peroneus longus muscle and fibula (Fig. 7.77) (Video 7.26).[90] The findings of peripheral nerve entrapment include hypoechoic swelling of the involved nerve at and just proximal to the site of entrapment, with transition to normal-appearing nerve distally. Transducer pressure over the abnormal nerve often elicits symptoms.[91]

An intraneural ganglion cyst characteristically involves the peroneal nerve (Fig. 7.78). More common in patients with a high body mass index, joint fluid from the proximal tibiofibular joint may extend to the common peroneal nerve via the articular branch to create the intraneural ganglion cyst.[92] Such cysts originate near the fibular neck but can extend proximally to the level of the sciatic nerve and beyond, both proximal in the sciatic nerve and distal in the tibial nerve.[93] At ultrasound, intraneural peroneal nerve ganglion cysts are hypoechoic and often multilocular and track along the course of the involved nerves.[92] As with any peripheral nerve disorder, the distal musculature should be evaluated for signs of denervation (increased echogenicity) and possible atrophy (Fig. 7.79). Intraneural ganglion cysts have been described in 18% of patients with isolated peroneal mononeuropathy.[91] The common peroneal nerve may also be compressed from an adjacent ganglion cyst that is not intraneural in location (Video 7.27).

One additional application for peripheral nerve evaluation is after knee amputation for evaluation of a neuroma. After nerve transection, a neuroma is an expected finding as the nerve attempts to regenerate.[94] Ultrasound can locate each neuroma and importantly determine which neuroma is responsible for symptoms through transducer palpation. Neuromas will appear hypoechoic in continuity with the involved peripheral nerve (Fig. 7.80).[95] Deeper neuromas may be difficult to identify in the presence of surrounding muscle atrophy, which attenuates the ultrasound beam. Peripheral nerve sheath tumors are discussed in Chapter 2.

■ VASCULAR ABNORMALITIES

Evaluation of the posterior knee should always include assessment of the popliteal vasculature. The differential diagnosis for a cyst in the popliteal region includes aneurysm and pseudoaneurysm, with the latter showing the characteristic to-and-fro appearance of blood flow from the adjacent vessel into a pseudoaneurysm with color Doppler imaging (Fig. 7.81).[96] A soft tissue hematoma may also manifest as a soft tissue mass (Fig. 7.82), where soft tissue neoplasm must also be considered (Fig. 7.83). The popliteal vein also should be assessed for thrombosis, which causes the popliteal vein to be non-compressible without flow (Fig. 7.84) (Video 7.28).[97] The differential diagnosis for a cyst adjacent to the popliteal artery also includes adventitial cystic disease of the popliteal artery (Fig. 7.85).[98] Although vascular

Text continued on p. 327

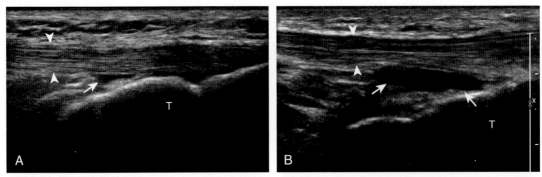

■ **FIGURE 7.72 Deep Infrapatellar Bursa.** Ultrasound images long axis to the distal patellar tendon *(arrowheads)* in two different patients show (A) physiologic distention and (B) abnormal fluid distention of the deep infrapatellar bursa *(arrows)*. *T*, Tibia.

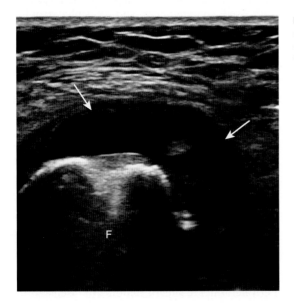

■ **FIGURE 7.73 Adventitious Bursa.** Sagittal ultrasound image over the distal femur *(F)* amputation site shows hypoechoic adventitious bursa formation *(arrows)* with internal synovial hypertrophy.

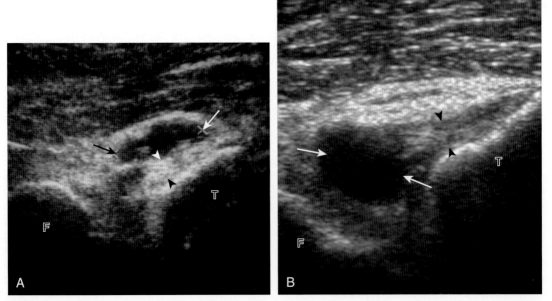

■ **FIGURE 7.74 Ganglion Cysts: Cruciate Ligaments.** Sagittal ultrasound images over posterior knee long axis to posterior cruciate ligament *(PCL)* in two different patients show hypoechoic ganglion cysts *(arrows)* *(arrowheads, PCL)*. *F*, Femur; *T*, tibia.

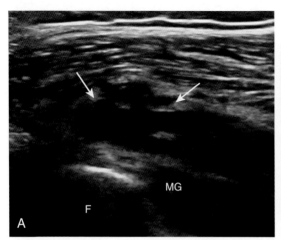

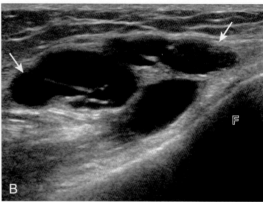

■ **FIGURE 7.75 Ganglion Cysts: Gastrocnemius Tendon.** Sagittal ultrasound images over posterior knee long axis to gastrocnemius tendons in two different patients (A and B) show anechoic multilobular gastrocnemius origin ganglion cysts *(arrows)*. Note posterior through-transmission in B. *F*, Femur; *MG*, medial head of gastrocnemius.

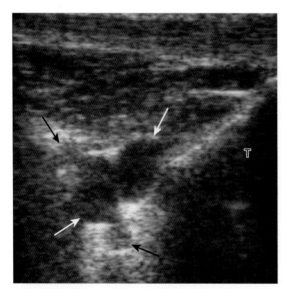

■ **FIGURE 7.76 Ganglion Cyst: Hoffa Fat Pad.** Ultrasound image long axis to patellar tendon shows hypoechoic multilobular cyst *(arrows)* in Hoffa fat pad (*T*, tibia) with increased through-transmission.

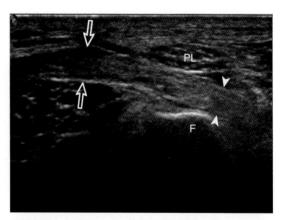

■ **FIGURE 7.77 Common Peroneal Nerve Entrapment.** Ultrasound image long axis to the common peroneal nerve shows proximal hypoechoic enlargement *(open arrows)* with transition to normal appearance distally *(arrowheads)* at compression site between peroneus longus *(PL)* and fibula *(F)*.

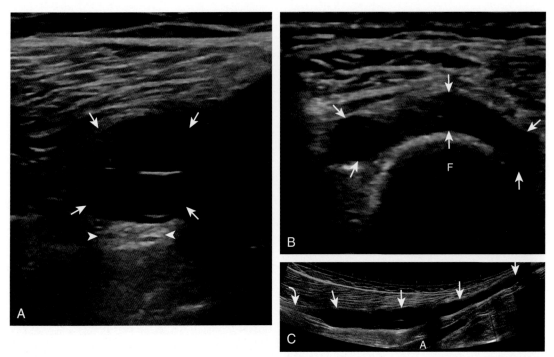

■ FIGURE 7.78 **Intraneural Ganglion Cyst: Common Peroneal Nerve.** Ultrasound image (A) short axis to common peroneal nerve *(arrowheads)* shows lobulated anechoic intraneural ganglion cyst *(arrows)*. Ultrasound image (B) transverse to fibula shows hypoechoic cyst *(arrows)* coursing around fibular neck *(F)*. Extended field of view ultrasound image (C) shows full extent (16 cm) of ganglion cyst *(arrows)* to involve the sciatic nerve *(curved arrow)*. *A,* Popliteal artery.

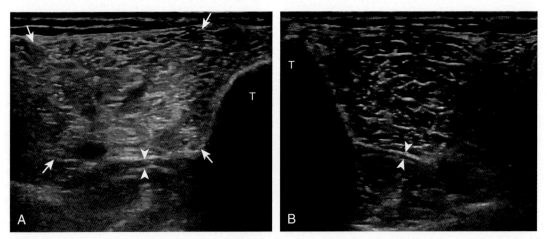

■ FIGURE 7.79 **Muscle Denervation: Anterior Compartment of Leg.** Ultrasound image (A) shows increased echogenicity of the anterior compartment musculature *(arrows)* compared with contralateral asymptomatic side (B) *(arrowheads,* interosseous membrane). *T,* tibia.

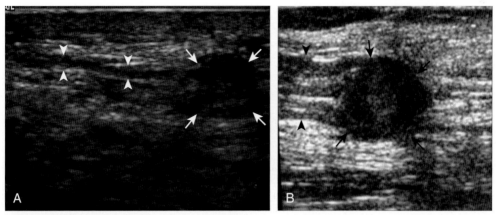

■ FIGURE 7.80 **Amputation Neuromas.** Ultrasound images in two different patients long axis to (A) a peripheral nerve branch and (B) sciatic nerve after knee amputation shows hypoechoic neuromas *(arrows)* in continuity with the associated nerves *(arrowheads)*.

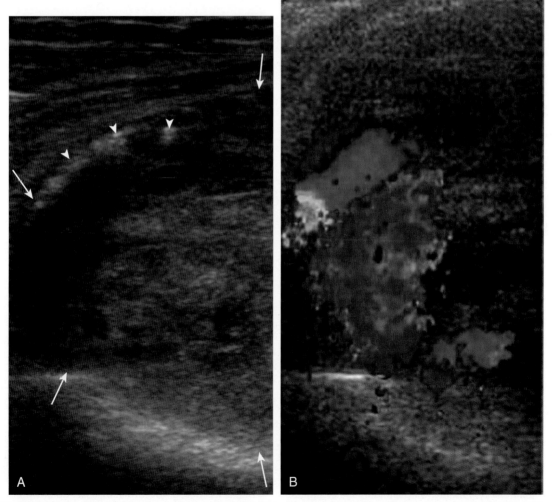

■ FIGURE 7.81 **Popliteal Artery Pseudoaneurysm.** Sagittal ultrasound images over the posterior knee show (A) a heterogeneous mass-like area *(arrows)* with peripheral calcifications *(arrowheads)*. Color Doppler image shows (B) pulsatile blood flow into the pseudoaneurysm.

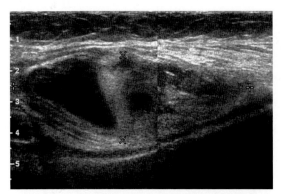

■ FIGURE 7.82 **Soft Tissue Hematoma.** Ultrasound image shows a heterogeneous mixed-echogenicity mass-like area *(cursors)* from soft tissue hemorrhage.

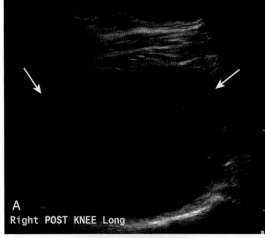

■ FIGURE 7.83 **Lymphoma.** Ultrasound image in sagittal plane over posterior knee (A) shows hypoechoic solid mass *(arrows)* that surrounds the popliteal artery, shown with flow on transverse color Doppler image (B).

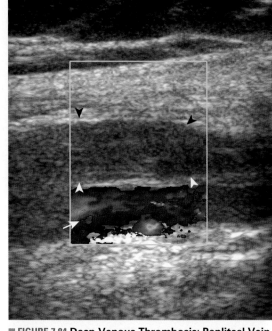

■ FIGURE 7.84 **Deep Venous Thrombosis: Popliteal Vein.** Ultrasound image long axis to popliteal vein *(arrow-heads)* shows abnormal hypoechogenicity from thrombus, which was non-compressible with no flow on color Doppler imaging *(arrow, normal popliteal artery)*.

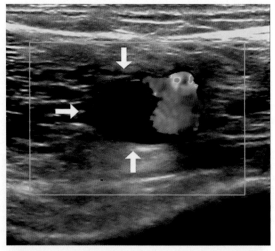

■ FIGURE 7.85 **Cystic Adventitial Disease.** Color Doppler image in transverse plane over posterior knee shows anechoic cyst *(arrows)* in direct contact with the popliteal artery, which shows flow.

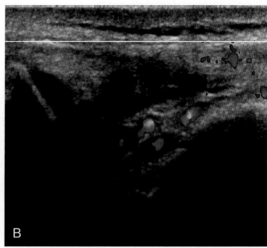

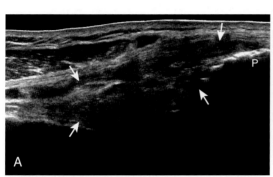

■ **FIGURE 7.86 Synovial Hemangioma.** Ultrasound image (A) in the sagittal plane over the suprapatellar recess and color Doppler image (B) in the transverse plane over medial patella and medial joint recess shows mixed hyperechoic and hypoechoic hemangioma *(arrows)* with compressible vascular channels. *F*, Femur; *P*, patella.

malformations are discussed in Chapter 2, synovial hemangioma deserves mention here in that it most commonly involves the suprapatellar recess of the knee, appearing as mixed hyperechoic and hypoechoic tissue with compressible vascular channels (Fig. 7.86).[35]

SELECTED REFERENCES

1. Fenn S, Datir A, Saifuddin A: Synovial recesses of the knee: MR imaging review of anatomical and pathological features. *Skeletal Radiol* 38(4): 317–328, 2009.
5. Ward EE, Jacobson JA, Fessell DP, et al: Sonographic detection of Baker's cysts: comparison with MR imaging. *AJR Am J Roentgenol* 176(2):373–380, 2001.
19. De Maeseneer M, Vanderdood K, Marcelis S, et al: Sonography of the medial and lateral tendons and ligaments of the knee: the use of bony landmarks as an easy method for identification. *AJR Am J Roentgenol* 178(6):1437–1444, 2002.
28. Wakefield RJ, Balint PV, Szkudlarek M, et al: Musculoskeletal ultrasound including definitions for ultrasonographic pathology. *J Rheumatol* 32(12): 2485–2487, 2005.
30. Thiele RG: Role of ultrasound and other advanced imaging in the diagnosis and management of gout. *Curr Rheumatol Rep* 13(2):146–153, 2011.
37. Marchand AJ, Proisy M, Ropars M, et al: Snapping knee: imaging findings with an emphasis on dynamic sonography. *AJR Am J Roentgenol* 199(1): 142–150, 2012.
60. Khan KM, Bonar F, Desmond PM, et al: Patellar tendinosis (jumper's knee): findings at histopathologic examination, US, and MR imaging. Victorian Institute of Sport Tendon Study Group. *Radiology* 200(3):821–827, 1996.
90. Grant TH, Omar IM, Dumanian GA, et al: Sonographic evaluation of common peroneal neuropathy in patients with foot drop. *J Ultrasound Med* 34(4):705–711, 2015.
95. Tagliafico A, Altafini L, Garello I, et al: Traumatic neuropathies: spectrum of imaging findings and postoperative assessment. *Semin Musculoskelet Radiol* 14(5):512–522, 2010.
93. Spinner RJ, Desy NM, Amrami KK: Sequential tibial and peroneal intraneural ganglia arising from the superior tibiofibular joint. *Skeletal Radiol* 37(1):79–84, 2008.

The complete references for this chapter can be found on *www.expertconsult.com.*

CHAPTER 8

ANKLE, FOOT, AND LOWER LEG ULTRASOUND

■ ANKLE AND FOOT ANATOMY

Osseous Anatomy

The ankle joint is a hinged synovial articulation between the talus and the distal tibia and fibula

(Fig. 8.1). Inferiorly, the talus articulates with the calcaneus through three facets, joined by the cervical and interosseous talocalcaneal ligaments located in a cone-shaped region termed the *sinus tarsi*, which opens laterally.[1] The *Chopart joint* represents the articulations between the talus and navicular, and the calcaneus and cuboid bones, respectively. The navicular, in turn, articulates with the medial, middle, and lateral cuneiforms, which then articulate with the first through third metatarsals. The fourth and fifth metatarsals articulate directly with the cuboid bone, and the tarsometatarsal articulations collectively are called the *Lisfranc joint*. The metacarpophalangeal joints are stabilized by collateral ligaments as well as the fibrocartilage connective tissue plantar plates.[2] Phalangeal bones extend beyond the metatarsals.

Muscle, Tendon, and Nerve Anatomy

ANTERIOR ANATOMY

Anteriorly, from medial to lateral, are the tibialis anterior (origin: proximal tibia and interosseous membrane; insertion: base of first metatarsal and medial cuneiform), the extensor hallucis longus (origin: fibula and interosseous membrane; insertion: distal phalanx of the first digit), and the extensor digitorum longus tendons (origin: tibia, fibula, and interosseous membrane; insertion: phalanges of the second through fifth digits) (see Fig. 8.1A–C). An anatomic bursa, called the *Gruberi bursa*, is located between the extensor digitorum longus and talar ridge and may extend into the sinus tarsi.[3] The peroneus tertius extends from the fibula and interosseous membrane to the base of the fifth metatarsal. The anterior tendons are held in place by the superior and inferior extensor retinacula. The anterior tibial artery courses beneath the superior extensor retinaculum and becomes the dorsalis pedis artery, located between the extensor hallucis and extensor digitorum longus tendons. The deep peroneal nerve follows the anterior tibial artery and dorsal pedis and bifurcates as medial and lateral branches anterior to the ankle.

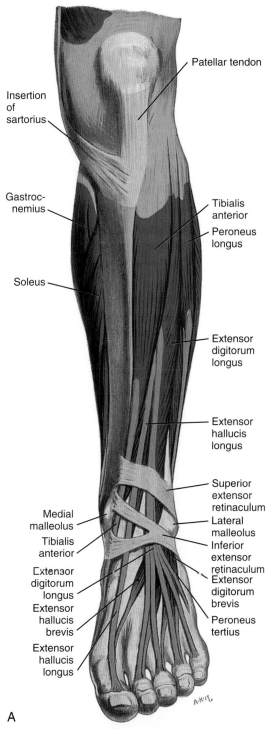

Patellar tendon

Insertion
of
sartorius

Gastroc-
nemius

Tibialis
anterior

Peroneus
longus

Soleus

Extensor
digitorum
longus

Extensor
hallucis
longus

Superior
extensor
retinaculum

Medial
malleolus

Lateral
malleolus

Tibialis
anterior

Inferior
extensor
retinaculum

Extensor
digitorum
longus

Extensor
digitorum
brevis

Extensor
hallucis
brevis

Peroneus
tertius

Extensor
hallucis
longus

A

■ **FIGURE 8.1 Leg, Ankle, and Foot Anatomy.** A, Anterior view of left leg. B, Medial view of left leg. C, Medial view of left ankle. D, Lateral view of left ankle. E, Posterior view of calf. F, Medial ankle and midfoot ligaments. G, Lateral ankle and midfoot ligaments. H, Plantar aspect of left foot. *(A and E: From Schaefer EA, Symington J, Bryce TH, editors:* Quain's Anatomy, *ed 11, London, 1915, Longmans, Green, with permission from Pearson Education; B, C, D, and H: From Standring S:* Gray's Anatomy: The Anatomical Basis of Clinical Practice, *ed 39, Edinburgh, 2005, Churchill Livingstone; F and G, Modified from Netterimages.com, # 4568, Elsevier, Inc.)*

Continued

MEDIAL ANATOMY

Medially, from anterior to posterior, are the tibialis posterior (origin: tibia, fibula, and interosseous membrane; insertion: navicular, cuneiforms, and second through fourth metatarsals), the flexor digitorum longus (origin: tibia; insertion: distal phalanges of second through fifth digits), and the flexor hallucis longus tendons (origin: fibula; insertion: base of distal phalanx of first digit) (see Fig. 8.1A–D). Between the flexor digitorum and flexor hallucis longus tendons at the posterior ankle are the tibial nerve and posterior tibial artery and veins. The order of structures from anterior to posterior from the medial malleolus can be remembered with the phrase "Tom, Dick, And Very Nervous Harry" (T, Tibialis posterior tendon; D, flexor Digitorum longus tendon; A, posterior tibial Artery; V, posterior tibial Veins; N, tibial Nerve; and H, flexor Hallucis longus tendon). The flexor retinaculum extends from the medial malleolus to the calcaneus superficial to the medial tendons and tibial nerve, which forms the roof of the tarsal tunnel. The tibial nerve divides into medial and lateral plantar nerves and a smaller medial calcaneal nerve.[4] The inferior calcaneal

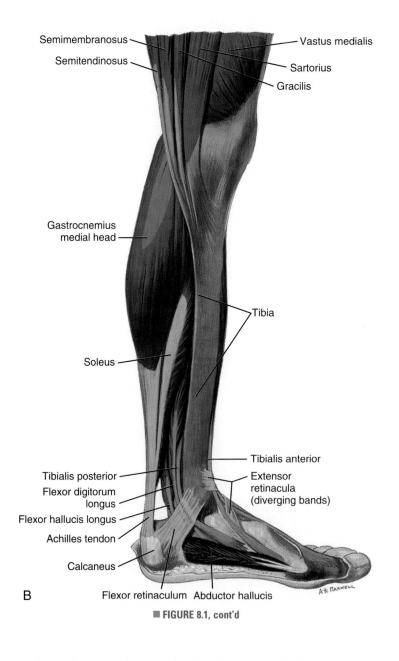

B

■ **FIGURE 8.1, cont'd**

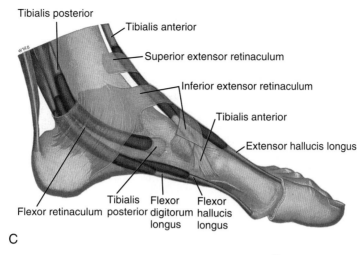

Tibialis posterior
Tibialis anterior
Superior extensor retinaculum
Inferior extensor retinaculum
Tibialis anterior
Extensor hallucis longus

Flexor retinaculum
Tibialis posterior
Flexor digitorum longus
Flexor hallucis longus

C

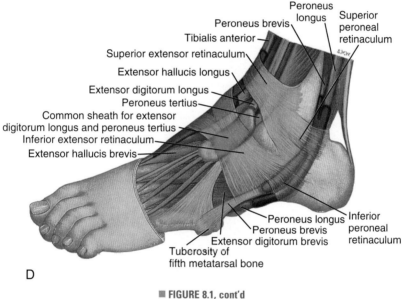

Peroneus longus
Peroneus brevis
Superior peroneal retinaculum
Tibialis anterior
Superior extensor retinaculum
Extensor hallucis longus
Extensor digitorum longus
Peroneus tertius
Common sheath for extensor digitorum longus and peroneus tertius
Inferior extensor retinaculum
Extensor hallucis brevis

Peroneus longus
Peroneus brevis
Extensor digitorum brevis
Tuberosity of fifth metatarsal bone
Inferior peroneal retinaculum

D

■ FIGURE 8.1, cont'd

Continued

nerve usually originates from the lateral plantar branch and courses between the abductor hallucis and quadratus plantae muscles and then plantar to the calcaneus.[5,6] The medial and lateral plantar nerves continue toward the digits as the common plantar digital nerves and then as the proper plantar digital nerves. More distally under the mid-foot, the flexor digitorum and flexor hallucis longus tendons cross each other, a configuration termed the *knot of Henry*. The flexor digitorum brevis and flexor hallucis brevis muscles are located in the plantar aspect of the foot.

LATERAL ANATOMY

Laterally, the peroneus brevis (origin: distal fibula; insertion: fifth metatarsal base) and peroneus longus tendons (origin: proximal fibula and tibial condyle; insertion: first metatarsal base and medial cuneiform) are found posterior to the fibula (see Fig. 8.1A, B, D, and E). The musculotendinous junction of the peroneus longus is more superior to that of the peroneus brevis; at the level of the distal fibula, the peroneus brevis muscle and tendon are found medial and anterior to the tendon of the peroneus longus. More distally, the peroneus brevis tendon is typically in contact with the posterior fibular or retromalleolar groove. The normal peroneus muscle belly should taper so that only tendon is present at the fibula tip.[7] The peroneal tendons are held in place by the superior and inferior peroneal retinacula.[8] The peroneal tendons then course anteriorly on each side of the peroneal tubercle of the calcaneus and extend to their insertions. As a normal variant, an accessory tendon called the *peroneus quartus*

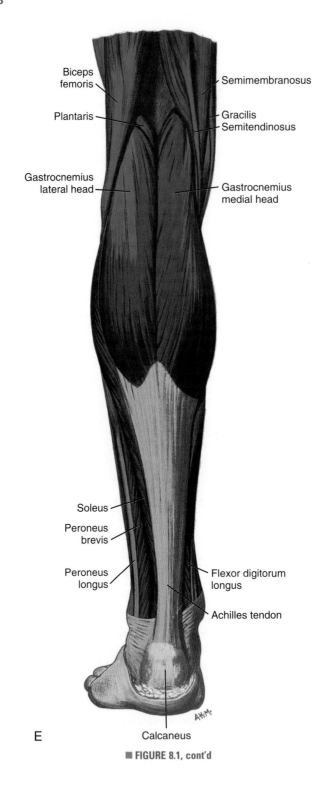

Biceps
femoris

Plantaris

Gastrocnemius
lateral head

Semimembranosus

Gracilis
Semitendinosus

Gastrocnemius
medial head

Soleus

Peroneus
brevis

Peroneus
longus

Flexor digitorum
longus

Achilles tendon

E   Calcaneus

■ FIGURE 8.1, cont'd

may be found posterior to the fibula; this tendon most commonly originates from the peroneus brevis and inserts on the lateral aspect of the calcaneus at the retrotrochlear eminence.[9] Over the lateral aspect of the calcaneus, the extensor digitorum brevis muscle originates from the calcaneus and extensor retinaculum and inserts distally on the second through fourth phalanges. Approximately 9 cm proximal to the lateral malleolus, the deep branch of the peroneal nerve can

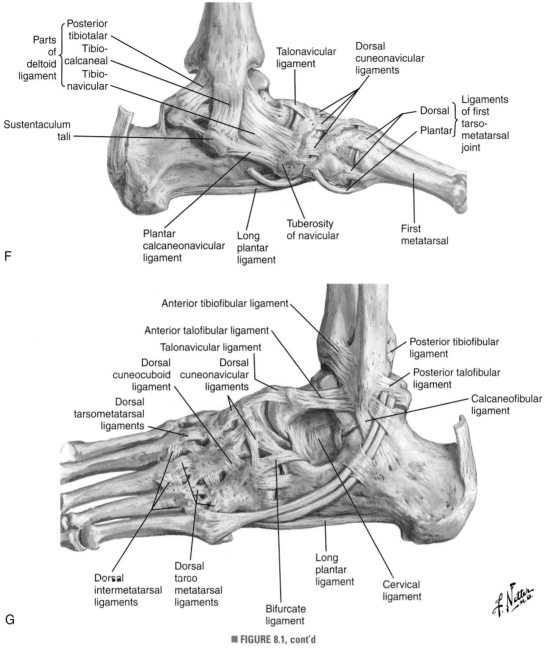

F

G

■ FIGURE 8.1, cont'd

Continued

be seen emerging from between the peroneus longus and extensor digitorum muscles, then piercing the superficial crural fascia to become subcutaneous in location.[10]

POSTERIOR ANATOMY

Posteriorly in the calf, the medial and lateral heads of the gastrocnemius muscle converge with the soleus to form the Achilles tendon, which inserts onto the calcaneus (see Fig. 8.1B and E).[11] The plantaris muscle originates from the lateral femur,

courses obliquely through the popliteal region, continues as a thin tendon between the muscle bellies of the medial head of the gastrocnemius and soleus muscles, courses distally at the medial aspect of the Achilles tendon, and then inserts onto the calcaneus or less commonly the Achilles tendon.[11] Collectively, the gastrocnemius, Achilles, and plantaris are referred to as the triceps surae.[11] The sural nerve can be found at the level of the ankle within the subcutaneous fat adjacent to the lesser saphenous vein centered between the Achilles tendon and peroneal tendons.[12] At the plantar

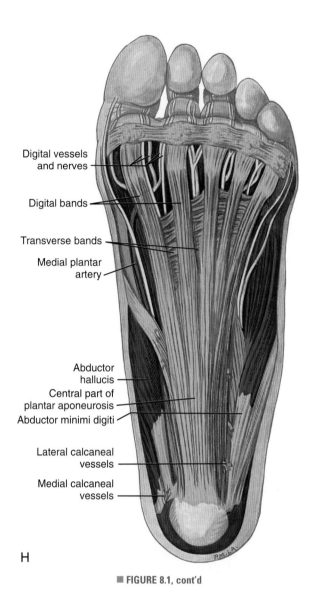

Digital vessels
and nerves

Digital bands

Transverse bands

Medial plantar
artery

Abductor
hallucis

Central part of
plantar aponeurosis

Abductor minimi digiti

Lateral calcaneal
vessels

Medial calcaneal
vessels

H

■ **FIGURE 8.1, cont'd**

aspect of the calcaneus, the plantar aponeurosis originates from the medial calcaneus and extends distally as medial, central, and lateral cords (see Fig. 8.1H). The central cord envelops the flexor digitorum brevis muscle.

Ligamentous Anatomy

The stabilizing structures of the lateral ankle include the anterior talofibular ligament (most commonly consisting of two bands),[13] which extends from the fibula to the talus in the transverse plane; the calcaneofibular ligament, which extends from the fibula inferiorly and posteriorly to the calcaneus deep to the peroneal tendons; and the posterior talofibular ligament, which extends from the fibula to the posterior aspect of

the tibia in the transverse plane (see Fig. 8.1G).[14] In addition, the anterior and posterior tibiofibular ligaments extend laterally and inferiorly in an oblique fashion from the tibia to the fibula. An accessory anterior tibiofibular ligament may be present, also called *Bassett ligament*.[15]

At the medial aspect of the ankle, the deltoid ligament is found, consisting of deep (anterior tibiotalar and posterior tibiotalar) and superficial (tibiocalcaneal, tibionavicular, tibiospring, and tibiotalar) components (see Fig. 8.1F).[16] The spring ligament complex consists of superomedial, medioplantar, and inferoplantar calcaneonavicular ligaments.[17] In addition to other small ligaments that connect the various tarsal bones and are named by their osseous attachments, the Lisfranc ligament proper is a strong ligament that connects obliquely from the medial cuneiform to the base of the second metatarsal bone.[18] The bifurcate ligament extends from the calcaneus to the navicular and cuboid bones at the lateral aspect of the mid-foot.

■ ULTRASOUND EXAMINATION TECHNIQUE

Table 8.1 is a checklist for ankle, calf, and forefoot ultrasound examination. Examples of diagnostic ankle ultrasound reports are shown in Boxes 8.1 and 8.2.

General Comments

Ultrasound examination of the ankle and foot is comfortably completed with the patient supine and the foot and ankle on the examination table. Although limited examination of the distal Achilles and plantar aponeurosis may be completed in supine position with external rotation of the leg to gain access to these structures, a more thorough examination of the posterior ankle is best accomplished with the patient prone. This is essential when the clinical indication is to assess for Achilles tendon or calf abnormalities. A high-frequency

transducer of at least 10 MHz is typically used because most of the structures are superficial. In general, the ankle tendons are first evaluated in short axis (with Achilles being the exception) to identify each structure and for orientation. Following this, evaluation of each tendon in long axis is completed. Evaluation of the calf, ankle, and foot may be initially focused over the area that is clinically symptomatic or that is relevant to the patient's history. Regardless, a complete examination should always be considered and is suggested for one to become familiar with normal anatomy and normal variants, to develop a quick and efficient sonographic technique, and to appreciate subtle or early pathologic changes. An evaluation that is too focused may not include important pathology, especially if clinical history or physical examination findings are vague or incorrect. In addition, it is essential that evaluation include any area of focal symptoms as directed by the patient. This is often a clue to locate pathologic processes, such as a stress fracture, that may not have been assessed in the imaging protocol. This approach is important in the foot, where there are many structures closely associated that may produce similar symptoms.

Anterior Ankle Evaluation

The primary structures evaluated from the anterior approach are the anterior ankle joint recess, the tibialis anterior, the extensor hallucis longus, the

TABLE 8.1 Ankle, Calf, and Forefoot Ultrasound Examination Checklist

Location	Structures of Interest
Ankle: anterior	Anterior tibiotalar joint recess Tibialis anterior Extensor hallucis longus Dorsal pedis artery Superficial peroneal nerve Extensor digitorum longus
Ankle: medial	Tibialis posterior Flexor digitorum longus Tibial nerve Flexor hallucis longus Deltoid ligament
Ankle: lateral	Peroneus longus and brevis Anterior talofibular ligament Calcaneofibular ligament Anterior tibiofibular ligament
Ankle: posterior	Achilles tendon Posterior bursae Plantar fascia
Calf	Soleus Medial and lateral heads of gastrocnemius Plantaris Achilles tendon
Forefoot	Dorsal joint recesses Morton neuroma Tendons and plantar plate

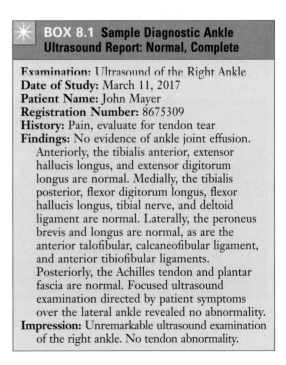

BOX 8.1 Sample Diagnostic Ankle Ultrasound Report: Normal, Complete

Examination: Ultrasound of the Right Ankle
Date of Study: March 11, 2017
Patient Name: John Mayer
Registration Number: 8675309
History: Pain, evaluate for tendon tear
Findings: No evidence of ankle joint effusion. Anteriorly, the tibialis anterior, extensor hallucis longus, and extensor digitorum longus are normal. Medially, the tibialis posterior, flexor digitorum longus, flexor hallucis longus, tibial nerve, and deltoid ligament are normal. Laterally, the peroneus brevis and longus are normal, as are the anterior talofibular, calcaneofibular ligament, and anterior tibiofibular ligaments. Posteriorly, the Achilles tendon and plantar fascia are normal. Focused ultrasound examination directed by patient symptoms over the lateral ankle revealed no abnormality.
Impression: Unremarkable ultrasound examination of the right ankle. No tendon abnormality.

BOX 8.2 Sample Diagnostic Ankle Ultrasound Report: Abnormal, Complete

Examination: Ultrasound of the Right Ankle
Date of Study: March 11, 2017
Patient Name: Ron Burgundy
Registration Number: 8675309
History: Pain, evaluate for tendon tear
Findings: There is a small ankle joint effusion. No synovial hypertrophy. Laterally, there is abnormal anechoic fluid and hypoechoic synovial hypertrophy surrounding the peroneal tendons at the level of the distal fibula. A longitudinal tear is seen in the peroneus brevis. The superior peroneal retinaculum is torn at the fibula, and peroneal tendon dislocation occurs with dynamic evaluation in ankle dorsiflexion and eversion. No low-lying peroneus brevis muscle. Otherwise, the anterior talofibular, calcaneofibular ligament, and anterior tibiofibular ligaments are normal.

Anteriorly, the tibialis anterior, extensor hallucis longus, and extensor digitorum longus are normal. Medially, the tibialis posterior, flexor digitorum longus, flexor hallucis longus, tibial nerve, and deltoid ligament are normal.

Posteriorly, the Achilles tendon and plantar fascia are normal. Focused ultrasound examination directed by patient symptoms over the lateral ankle corresponded to the peroneal tendon tear.

Impression:
1. Longitudinal split tear of the peroneus brevis and tenosynovitis.
2. Superior peroneal retinaculum tear and transient anterolateral dislocation of the peroneal tendons with dynamic imaging.
3. Small ankle joint effusion.

dorsalis pedis artery and superficial peroneal nerve, and the extensor digitorum longus. The transducer is first placed in the sagittal plane at the level of the tibiotalar joint with the foot in mild plantar flexion (Fig. 8.2A). The hyperechoic bone landmarks of the distal tibia and proximal talus are used for orientation, and the anterior ankle joint recess is evaluated for joint abnormality (Fig. 8.2B). The transducer should be moved medial and lateral in the parasagittal plane for complete evaluation; small amounts of joint fluid may only be seen lateral near the anterior talofibular ligament.

To evaluate the anterior tendons, the transducer is placed transversely at the level of the ankle joint (Fig. 8.3A). Beginning evaluation short axis to the tendons allows identification of all anterior tendons for orientation. The tibialis anterior tendon is the largest, located most medially, with the typical hyperechoic and fibrillar echotexture (Fig. 8.3B). One may toggle the transducer (see Fig. 1.3B) to assist in identification of the tendons in short axis. This maneuver causes the normally hyperechoic tendon to appear artifactually hypoechoic from anisotropy, which will make the tendon more conspicuous surrounded by the hyperechoic fat (Fig. 8.3C). Lateral to the tibialis anterior is the extensor hallucis longus (Fig. 8.3D). The muscle belly of this structure extends more inferiorly compared with the other anterior tendons, and this hypoechoic muscle tissue should not be mistaken for tenosynovitis. The adjacent anterior tibial artery is seen as it crosses from medial to lateral deep to the extensor hallucis longus, which continues as the dorsal pedis artery once beyond the superior extensor

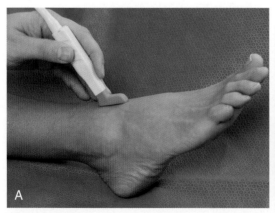 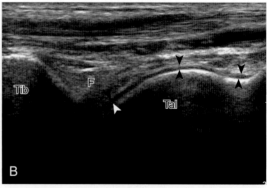

■ **FIGURE 8.2 Anterior Ankle: Joint Recess.** A, Sagittal imaging over the ankle joint shows (B) the normal hyperechoic anterior fat pad *(F)* between the tibia *(Tib)* and talus *(Tal)*. Note hypoechoic hyaline articular cartilage *(arrowheads)*, which shows the full anterior extent of the anterior ankle joint recess. Bone contours appear hyperechoic when imaged perpendicular to sound beam, which is improved by toggling the transducer.

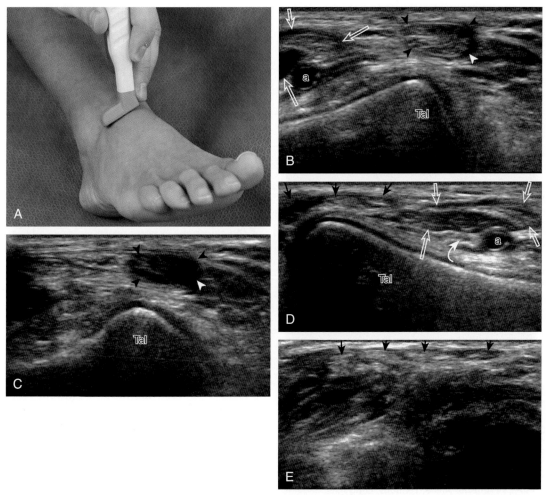

■ FIGURE 8.3 **Anterior Ankle: Tendons, Short Axis.** A, Transverse Imaging over the ankle shows (B) the tibialis anterior *(arrowheads)* and the extensor hallucis longus *(open arrows)* (right side of image is medial). Toggling the transducer shows (C) improved conspicuity of the tibialis anterior tendon *(arrowheads)* owing to anisotropy. Transverse imaging lateral to B shows (D and E) the extensor hallucis longus muscle and tendon *(open arrows)* and the extensor digitorum longus *(arrows)* *(curved arrow,* deep peroneal nerve lateral to anterior tibial artery; left side of images are lateral). *a,* Dorsalis pedis artery; *Tal,* talus.

retinaculum. The next lateral structure is the extensor digitorum longus with its multiple tendons that extend distally to the digits (Fig. 8.3D and E). A Gruberi bursa may be seen between the extensor digitorum tendons and the talus.[3] The peroneus tertius is found lateral to extensor digitorum longus and extends to the fifth metatarsal base. Each of these structures should then be evaluated in long axis from proximal to the ankle joint to at least the mid-foot region, the extent of which can be guided by physical examination findings or patient history (Fig. 8.4). The deep peroneal nerve is identified medial to the anterior tibial artery proximal to the ankle joint (Fig. 8.5), where it then crosses over and is lateral (Fig. 8.3D) to the anterior tibial artery more distally.

Medial Ankle Evaluation

For medial evaluation, the supine patient externally rotates the leg or rolls partially onto the ipsilateral side to gain access to the medial aspect of the ankle. Ultrasound examination begins in the transverse plane over the medial malleolus (Fig. 8.6A). The hyperechoic and shadowing surface of the tibia is seen, and the transducer is moved posteriorly. The first tendon identified is the tibialis posterior tendon in short axis (Fig. 8.6B). One may toggle the transducer (see Fig. 1.3B) to assist in identification of the tendons in short axis, which causes the tendon to appear hypoechoic from anisotropy and improves conspicuity compared with the adjacent hyperechoic fat (Fig. 8.6C). The transducer is then moved posteriorly

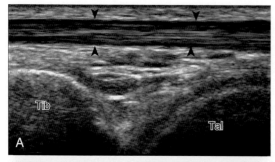

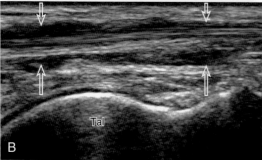

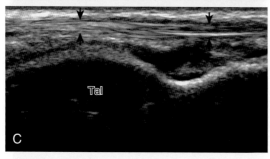

■ **FIGURE 8.4 Anterior Ankle: Tendons, Long Axis.** Sagittal imaging shows (A) the tibialis anterior tendon *(arrowheads)*, (B) the extensor hallucis longus muscle and tendon *(open arrows)*, and (C) one of the extensor digitorum longus tendons *(arrows)* (right side of image is distal). *Tal*, Talus; *Tib*, tibia.

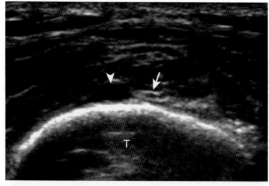

■ **FIGURE 8.5 Anterior Ankle: Deep Peroneal Nerve.** Ultrasound image in the axial plane at level of distal tibia *(T)* shows deep peroneal nerve *(arrow)* medial to anterior tibial artery *(arrowhead)*. The anterior tibial veins are compressed and not visible.

to identify the flexor digitorum longus tendon, the posterior tibial artery and veins, the tibial nerve, and then the flexor hallucis longus tendon in order from anterior to posterior (Fig. 8.6D). The tibialis posterior tendon is typically twice the size of the adjacent flexor digitorum longus tendon. The thin and hyperechoic flexor retinaculum can also be identified superficial to the tendons, and it attaches to the tibia.

Evaluation is continued distally with the transducer short axis to each tendon; the transducer is rotated to the coronal plane as each tendon is followed distally (Fig. 8.7A). Anisotropy is again used to help delineate each tendon in short axis (Fig. 8.7B and C). At the medial aspect of the calcaneus, a bony protuberance called the *sustentaculum tali* protrudes medially to articulate with the talus as the middle facet of the anterior subtalar joint. The medial tendons have characteristic locations relative to the sustentaculum tali (Fig. 8.7B). The tibialis posterior tendon is dorsal and superficial, the flexor digitorum longus lies immediately superficial, and the flexor hallucis longus tendon lies plantar to the sustentaculum tali in a bony groove of the calcaneus.

In the supramalleolar region, the tibial nerve is located between the flexor digitorum longus and flexor hallucis longus tendons. In cross section, the individual hypoechoic nerve fascicles surrounded by hyperechoic connective tissue take on a honeycomb appearance (see Fig. 8.6D), whereas in long axis a fascicular pattern is appreciated that, in contrast to adjacent tendons, is coarser in echotexture (see Fig. 8.10B). In the supramalleolar region, a small medial calcaneal nerve arising from the tibial nerve can be identified; this branch courses directly inferior, medial to the calcaneus and remains superficial (Fig. 8.8A). The tibial nerve then divides into medial and lateral plantar branches, which continue under the mid-foot to give off the common plantar digital nerves and then the proper plantar digital branches. The inferior calcaneal nerve usually originates from the lateral plantar branch of the tibial nerve and courses between the abductor hallucis and quadratus plantae muscles and then plantar to the calcaneus (Fig. 8.8B).[5]

To assess the medial tendons in long axis, the transducer is then moved back to the level of the distal tibia over the tibialis posterior tendon and is turned 90 degrees (Fig. 8.9A and B). As the transducer follows the course of the tibialis posterior tendon in long axis, the transducer moves from a coronal plane relative to the body to the axial plane (Fig. 8.9C–F). At the navicular bone, it is common to visualize mild thickening and decreased echogenicity of the distal tibialis posterior tendon, related to its insertion on the

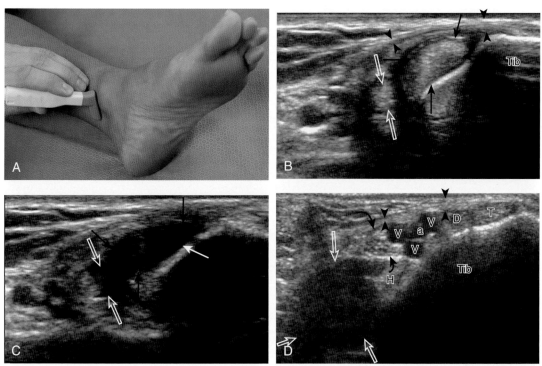

■ FIGURE 8.6 **Medial Ankle: Tendons, Short Axis, Proximal.** A, Transverse imaging superior and posterior to the medial malleolus shows (B) the tibialis posterior *(arrows)* and the flexor digitorum longus *(open arrows)* tendons *(arrowheads*, flexor retinaculum; right side of image is anterior). Toggling the transducer shows (C) improved conspicuity of the tibialis posterior *(arrows)* and flexor digitorum longus *(open arrows)* tendons owing to anisotropy. Transverse imaging posterior to B shows (D) the tibialis posterior tendon *(T)*, flexor digitorum longus tendon *(D)*, posterior tibial artery *(a)* and veins *(V)*, tibial nerve *(curved arrows)*, and flexor hallucis longus tendon *(H)* and muscle *(open arrows)* *(arrowheads*, flexor retinaculum). *Tib,* Tibia.

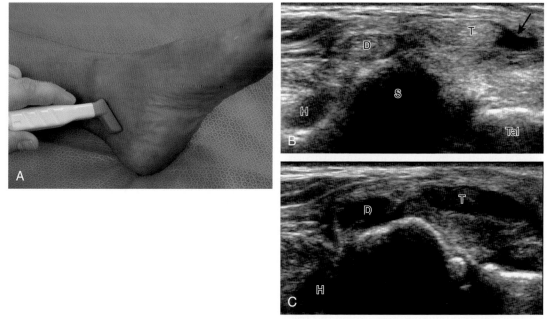

■ FIGURE 8.7 **Medial Ankle: Tendons, Short Axis, Distal.** A, Coronal imaging inferior to medial malleolus shows (B) the tibialis posterior tendon *(T)* with physiologic tenosynovial fluid *(arrow)*, the flexor digitorum longus *(D)*, and flexor hallucis longus *(H)* tendons, which become more conspicuous with anisotropy (C) (left side of images are plantar). *S,* Sustentaculum tali of the calcaneus; *Tal,* talus.

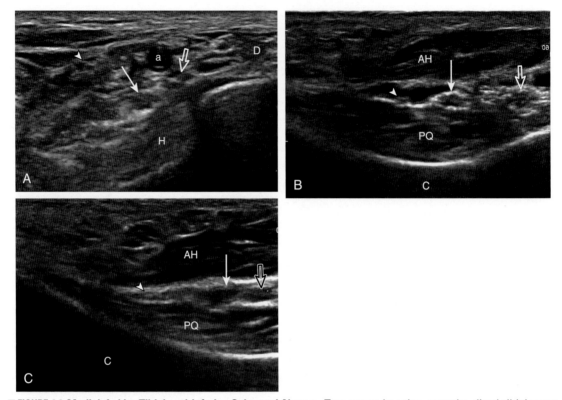

navicular and anisotropy from the tibialis posterior tendon fibers that course plantar to the navicular to insert at the cuneiforms and the second through fourth metatarsals (Fig. 8.9F). It is also common to see a small amount of fluid within the tendon sheath of the tibialis posterior tendon just beyond the medial malleolus, usually seen only along one side of the tendon (see Fig. 8.7B); asymptomatic fluid should not be present at the navicular where a tendon sheath is absent.[19] An accessory navicular bone may be seen within the distal tibialis posterior tendon near the navicular bone (see Fig. 8.80). To assess the flexor digitorum longus tendon, examination again begins transversely at the level of the medial malleolus, followed by assessment in long axis and distally (Fig. 8.10A). Similarly, the flexor hallucis longus tendon can be assessed first in short axis and then in long axis (Fig. 8.10B). As the flexor digitorum longus and flexor hallucis longus tendons are followed distally beneath the mid-foot, the two tendons cross, called the *knot of Henry* (Fig. 8.10C).

After assessment of the medial tendons, the components of the deltoid ligament complex are evaluated. The transducer is initially placed in the coronal plane at the medial malleolus (Fig. 8.11A) and angled slightly posterior. At this location, a superficial hyperechoic and fibrillar tibio-calcaneal ligament is identified, extending from the tibia to the sustentaculum tali (Fig. 8.11B).[16] The transducer is then moved slightly anterior and back into the coronal plane to visualize the tibiospring ligament (Fig. 8.11C), with its fibers coursing from the superficial medial malleolus to the spring ligament, which is anterior to the sustentaculum and deep to the tibialis posterior tendon. Deep to the tibiotalar ligament at this transducer position is the deep anterior tibiotalar ligament (Fig. 8.11C). Next, the transducer is moved and angled anteriorly from the medial malleolus to visualize the tibionavicular component (Fig. 8.11D). The transducer is then placed over the posterior aspect of the medial malleolus and rotated posteriorly with the foot in dorsiflexion to visualize the superficial and larger deep layers of the posterior tibiotalar components of the deltoid ligament that are deep to the tibialis posterior tendon (Fig. 8.11E).[16,20]

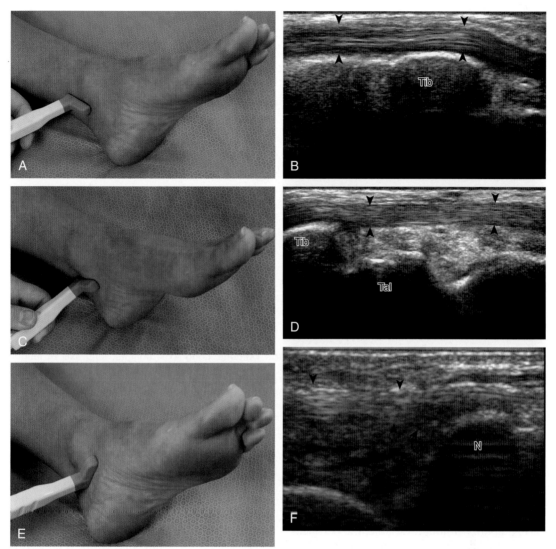

■ **FIGURE 8.9 Medial Ankle: Tibialis Posterior Tendon, Long Axis.** Imaging long axis to tibialis posterior tendon *(arrowheads)* (A and B) proximally, (C and D) at the level of the medial malleolus, and (E and F) distally (right side of image is distal). Note hypoechoic appearance *(curved arrow)* of distal tibialis posterior tendon at navicular in F. *N,* Navicular; *Tal,* talus; *Tib,* tibia.

The spring ligament complex consists of superomedial, medioplantar, and inferoplantar calcaneonavicular ligaments.[17] The superomedial component is easily identified when evaluating the distal tibial posterior tendon in short axis, seen as a hyperechoic and fibrillar structure in between the posterior tibial tendon and navicular (Fig. 8.12A). At this site, the superomedial component is approximately a similar diameter and courses oblique to the tibialis posterior tendon. The superomedial component of the spring ligament can then be imaged in long axis by rotating the transducer to the axial plane to visualize the sustentaculum tali and navicular (Fig. 8.12B).[21]

Lateral Ankle Evaluation

Structures of interest include the peroneal tendons and the lateral ligamentous structures of the ankle. Examination begins in the supramalleolar region in the transverse plane, directly posterior to the fibula in the retromalleolar groove or sulcus (Fig. 8.13A). At this location, the muscle belly and tendon of the peroneus brevis are identified in short axis (Fig. 8.13B). The adjacent peroneus longus tendon is also seen, characterized by lack of a muscle belly at this level. With movement of the transducer from superior to inferior, the normal peroneus brevis muscle belly will taper; only the peroneus brevis and longus tendons

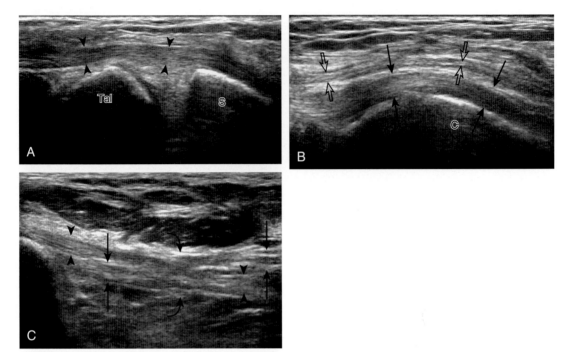

■ **FIGURE 8.10 Medial Ankle: Flexor Digitorum and Hallucis Tendons, Long Axis.** Imaging long axis to tendons shows (A) the flexor digitorum longus *(arrowheads)*, (B) the flexor hallucis longus tendon *(arrows)*, and (C) the crossing of these two tendons under the midfoot called the knot of Henry *(curved arrows)*. Note the tibial nerve and one of its branches in B *(open arrows)*. C, Calcaneus; S, sustentaculum talus of calcaneus; *Tal,* talus.

should be visible at the extreme fibula tip (Fig. 8.14). If the peroneus brevis muscle is present beyond the fibular tip, this normal variation is termed a *low-lying* muscle belly of the peroneus brevis and may be associated with tendon tear (see Fig. 8.98).[7] Although variable, the peroneus brevis is usually directly against the posterior cortex of the fibula ("B against bone"), with the adjacent peroneus longus tendon more posterior. The thin and hyperechoic superior peroneal retinaculum can be seen extending over the tendons to insert on the posterolateral margin of the fibula.

Distal assessment is continued short axis to the peroneal tendons. Toggling the transducer is a helpful maneuver to identify the tendons in short axis, which causes the tendons to appear hypoechoic from anisotropy and improves conspicuity compared with the adjacent hyperechoic fat (see Fig. 1.12). As the transducer crosses the oblique plane between the tip of the fibula and the posterior aspect of the heel, the normal calcaneofibular ligament can be seen deep to the peroneal tendons (see Fig. 8.14). As the peroneal tendons are followed in short axis, the transducer becomes positioned in the coronal plane (Fig. 8.15A). At the lateral aspect of the calcaneus, a bony prominence of variable size called the

peroneal tubercle is present (Fig. 8.15B). At this site, the peroneus brevis and longus tendons diverge into different directions. Because of their different respective orientations at the peroneal tubercle, it is difficult to image both tendons in short axis without one tendon appearing artifactually hypoechoic from anisotropy (Fig. 8.15B). With minimal clockwise and counterclockwise transducer rotation and toggling, anisotropy of each tendon can be eliminated (Fig. 8.15C). The peroneus brevis can be followed distally to its insertion on the fifth metatarsal base, and the peroneus longus similarly can be imaged under the mid-foot and forefoot to its insertion on the medial cuneiform and first metatarsal base, if clinically relevant.

Imaging in short axis is essential in evaluation of the peroneal tendons because this is the optimal plane to visualize the longitudinal split tears. Dynamic maneuvers should also be used in evaluation of the peroneal tendons to assess for subluxation or dislocation lateral and anterior to the fibula. This is accomplished with placement of the transducer in the transverse plane posterior to the distal fibula, and the patient is asked either to reproduce symptoms or to actively move the ankle into dorsiflexion and eversion. Excessive transducer pressure should be avoided throughout

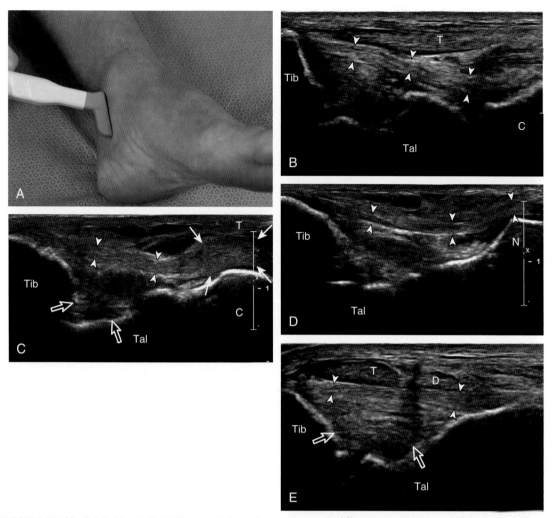

■ **FIGURE 8.11 Medial Ankle: Deltoid Ligament Complex.** A, Coronal oblique imaging at medial malleolus shows (B) the tibiocalcaneal ligament *(arrowheads)*. Moving and rotating the transducer anteriorly into the coronal plane (C), the tibiospring ligament is seen *(arrowheads)* attaching to spring ligament *(arrows)*. The deep anterior tibiotalar ligament *(open arrows)* is also seen. Moving and rotating the transducer anterior further (D), the tibionavicular *(arrowheads)* ligament is identified. With the transducer placed over the posterior aspect of the medial malleolus and angled posteriorly (E), the superficial *(arrowheads)* and deep *(open arrows)* posterior tibiotalar ligaments are seen deep to the tibialis posterior tendon *(T)*. C, Sustentaculum tali of calcaneus; *N*, navicular; *Tal*, talus; *Tib*, tibia; *D*, flexor digitorum longus.

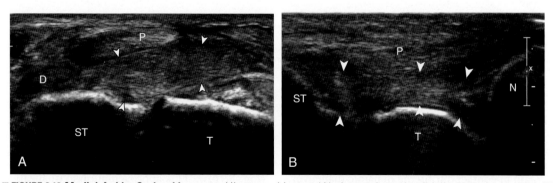

■ **FIGURE 8.12 Medial Ankle: Spring Ligament.** Ultrasound image (A) short axis to the tibialis posterior tendon *(P)* shows the superomedial calcaneonavicular ligament *(arrowheads)* adjacent to talus *(T)*. Slight angulation of transducer to transverse plane shows (B) the spring superomedial calcaneonavicular ligament in long axis *(arrowheads)*. *N*, Navicular; *ST*, sustentaculum tali.

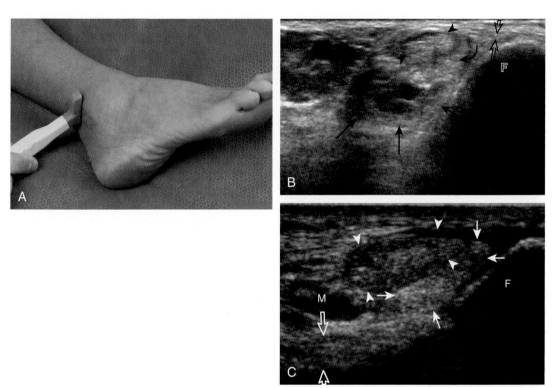

■ FIGURE 8.13 **Lateral Ankle: Peroneal Tendons, Short Axis, Proximal.** A, Transverse imaging superior and posterior to the lateral malleolus shows (B) the peroneus longus tendon *(arrowheads)*, and the peroneus brevis muscle *(arrows)* and tendon *(curved arrow)* (*open arrows,* superior peroneal retinaculum; right side of image is anterior). Transverse imaging near the fibular tip shows (C), the peroneus longus tendon *(arrowheads)*, and the peroneus brevis tendon *(arrows)* and muscle (M) (*open arrows,* posterior talofibular ligament). *F,* Fibula.

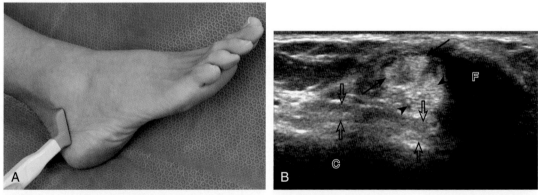

■ FIGURE 8.14 **Lateral Ankle: Peroneal Tendons, Short Axis, at Calcaneofibular Ligament.** A, Coronal-oblique imaging shows (B) the peroneus longus *(arrows)* and peroneus brevis *(arrowheads)* tendons, and calcaneofibular ligament *(open arrows)*. *C,* Calcaneus; *F,* fibula.

the dynamic examination so as not to inhibit abnormal movement of the peroneal tendons. Stabilizing the transducer with two hands is often necessary to minimize transducer pressure yet remain in contact during the dynamic maneuver. The peroneal tendons should normally remain posterior to the fibula with an intact superior peroneal retinaculum.

For assessment of the peroneal tendons in long axis, one again returns to the supramalleolar region and places the transducer over the posterior aspect of the distal fibula in the oblique-sagittal plane (Fig. 8.16A). This approach allows visualization of the peroneus brevis and longus tendons in one imaging plane (Fig. 8.16B). As the transducer is moved distally, the tendons begin to diverge distal

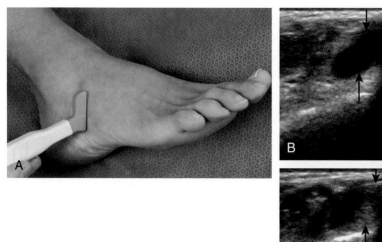

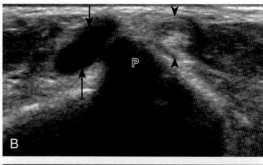

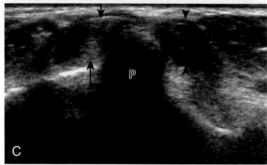

■ **FIGURE 8.15 Lateral Ankle: Peroneal Tendons, Short Axis, Distal.** A, Coronal imaging shows (B and C) the peroneus longus *(arrows)* and peroneus brevis *(arrowheads)* tendons with differential anisotropy related to toggling of transducer. *P,* Peroneal tubercle.

to the fibula within their own tendon sheaths (Fig. 8.16C and D). At this point, the peroneus longus and brevis are followed individually (Fig. 8.16E). The peroneus longus courses deep toward the cuboid, where it commonly demonstrates anisotropy (Fig. 8.16F). An echogenic os peroneum, a normal sesamoid bone, may be seen within the peroneus longus tendon.[22] More distal assessment of the peroneus longus may be completed if symptoms warrant. The peroneus brevis tendon can be followed distally from the fibula to its insertion on the base of the fifth metatarsal (Fig. 8.16G).

The first lateral ankle ligament to be assessed is the anterior talofibular ligament.[20] If the distal fibular tip can be palpated, the transducer is simply placed in the transverse plane over and anterior to the fibula, identifying the characteristic bone contours of the fibula and talus (Fig. 8.17A). In this position, the anterior talofibular ligament often appears hypoechoic from anisotropy from the oblique course of the ligament toward the talus (Fig. 8.17B). The transducer is then angled (heel-toe maneuver) so that the ligament fibers are perpendicular to the sound beam, to eliminate anisotropy, and the normal compact fibrillar ligament will be seen (Fig. 8.17C) (Video 8.1). Anisotropy is used to one's advantage because initial identification of the anterior talofibular ligament is enhanced; the hypoechoic ligament is more conspicuous adjacent to the hyperechoic

fat. If the distal fibular cannot be palpated, another method to find the anterior talofibular ligament is to initially place the transducer over the lateral fibula more superiorly in the transverse plane. The transducer is then moved inferiorly and once the extreme distal fibula tip is reached, the transducer is moved slightly superiorly and anteriorly in the transverse plane to visualize the talus. One potential pitfall is imaging superior to the anterior talofibular ligament and presuming the ligament is absent. This pitfall can be avoided by identifying the extreme distal tip of the fibular as a key bone landmark.

To evaluate the calcaneofibular ligament in long axis, one may palpate the fibular tip and place the transducer along an oblique-coronal plane from the fibular tip to the posterior heel. At this site, the calcaneofibular ligament is identified as a compact fibrillar structure between the peroneal tendons and calcaneus (Fig. 8.18A and B). In ankle dorsiflexion, the calcaneofibular ligament becomes taut reducing anisotropy. The calcaneofibular ligament is often incidentally seen during evaluation of the peroneal tendons (see Fig. 8.14B). In short axis (Fig. 8.18C), the normal calcaneofibular ligament can appear hypoechoic from anisotropy (Fig. 8.18D) and potentially simulate a cyst associated with the peroneal tendons.

To evaluate the anterior inferior tibiofibular ligament, the imaging plane is similar to that of

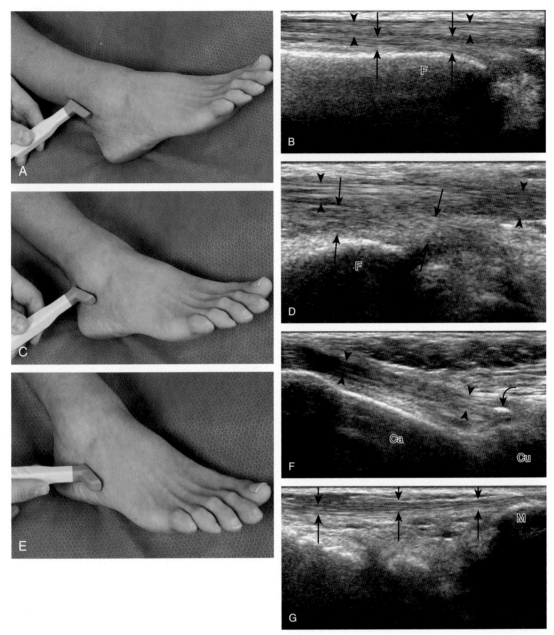

■ FIGURE 8.16 **Lateral Ankle: Peroneal Tendons, Long Axis.** Imaging of peroneal tendons in long axis (A and B) proximal, (C and D) at the level of the lateral malleolus, and (E to G) distal shows the peroneus longus *(arrowheads)* and peroneus brevis *(arrows)* tendons (right side of image is distal). Note the os peroneum *(curved arrow)* within the peroneus longus tendon *(arrowheads)* in F. *Ca,* Calcaneus; *Cu,* cuboid; *F,* fibula; *M,* fifth metatarsal.

the calcaneofibular ligament, but more superior between the fibula and tibia. In fact, after evaluation of the calcaneofibular ligament, the transducer may simply be moved superiorly along the same plane to the other side of the fibula to visualize the bone contours of the fibula and tibia (Fig. 8.19A and B). The normal anterior tibiofibular ligament will appear as a uniform hyperechoic fibrillar structure. Another manner

in identifying the anterior inferior tibiofibular ligament is to begin evaluation at the anterior talofibular ligament; fix the transducer over the fibula, and rotate the transducer so that the medial aspect moves superiorly from the talus to the tibia in an oblique plane. An accessory anterior inferior tibiofibular ligament *(Bassett ligament)* may also be identified as a discrete ligament bundle inferior and adjacent to the anterior inferior tibiofibular

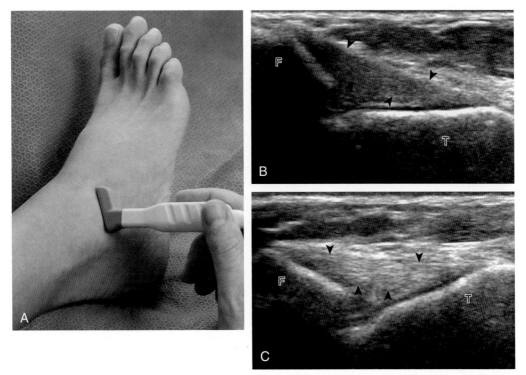

■ FIGURE 8.17 **Lateral Ankle: Anterior Talofibular Ligament.** A, Axial imaging anterior to the tip of the fibula shows (B) the anterior talofibular ligament in long axis *(arrowheads),* which appears hypoechoic from anisotropy. Note that the outer border of the hypoechoic ligament is made conspicuous adjacent to the hyperechoic fat. Heel-to-toe maneuver shows (C) the normal compact and fibrillar echotexture of the anterior talofibular ligament *(arrowheads).* *F,* Fibula; *T,* talus.

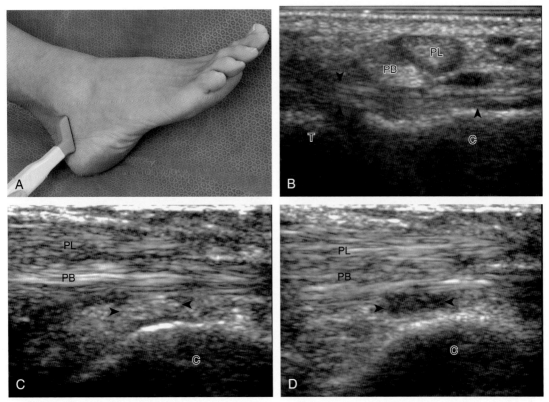

■ FIGURE 8.18 **Lateral Ankle: Calcaneofibular Ligament.** A, Coronal-oblique imaging between the fibular tip and the heel shows (B) the calcaneofibular ligament in long axis *(arrowheads).* The transducer is turned 90 degrees (C) to visualize the calcaneofibular ligament in short axis *(arrowheads),* which demonstrates (D) and corrects anisotropy by toggling the transducer. *C,* Calcaneus; *PB,* peroneus brevis tendon; *PL,* peroneus longus tendon; *T,* talus.

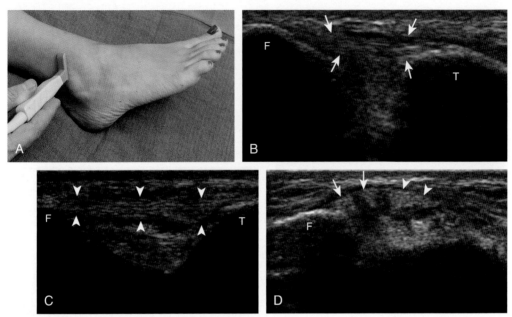

■ **FIGURE 8.19 Lateral Ankle: Anterior Inferior Tibiofibular Ligament.** A, Oblique imaging between the distal tibia and fibula shows (B) the anterior tibiofibular ligament *(arrows)*. Imaging parallel and just inferior to (B) shows (C) accessory anterior inferior tibiofibular ligament *(arrowheads)*. D, Imaging in short axis shows multiple fascicles of anterior inferior tibiofibular ligament *(arrows)* and accessory anterior inferior tibiofibular ligament *(arrowheads)*. *F,* Fibula; *T,* tibia.

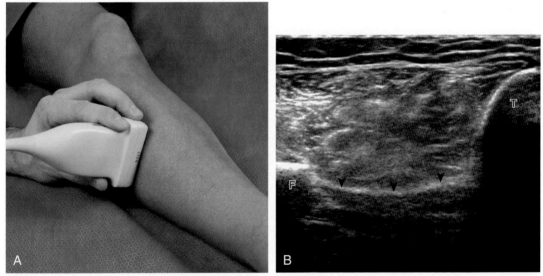

■ **FIGURE 8.20 Lower Leg: Interosseous Membrane.** A, Transverse imaging between the tibia and fibula shows (B) the interosseous membrane *(arrowheads)*. *F,* Fibula; *T,* tibia.

ligament, slightly more horizontal and spanning a greater distance between tibia and fibula often adjacent to the talus (Fig. 8.19C).[15] Variability exists in the number of bundles or fascicles in the inferior tibiofibular ligament (Fig. 8.19D).[23,24]

In the setting of an anterior tibiofibular ligament tear, the interosseous membrane should also be evaluated between the tibia and the fibula.[25] At

ultrasound, the interosseous membrane appears as a thin and hyperechoic often bilaminar structure extending from the tibia to the fibula and best evaluated in the transverse plane perpendicular to the sound beam (Fig. 8.20).[25] The interosseous membrane extends inferiorly and becomes thickened as the interosseous ligament superior to the tibiotalar joint. The combination of the interosseous ligament, the anterior and posterior inferior tibiofibular ligaments, and the posteriorly located inferior transverse ligament stabilizes the ankle syndesmosis or articulation.[23] Although visible, the posterior talofibular and posterior inferior tibiofibular ligaments are not routinely evaluated but may be assessed if clinically relevant (Fig. 8.21).[20]

Posterior Ankle and Heel Evaluation

If the patient has no symptoms posteriorly and one wants simply to screen the distal Achilles tendon and plantar aponeurosis for abnormalities, the patient can externally rotate the leg while supine to gain limited access to the posterior ankle. However, for a thorough examination, the patient should lie prone with the foot extending beyond the examination table to assess the calf and posterior ankle. Dorsiflexion of the ankle elongates the Achilles tendon and reduces anisotropy. The Achilles tendon is easily evaluated as the transducer is placed in the sagittal plane long axis to the

tendon fibers from a posterior approach (Fig. 8.22A). In long axis, the Achilles tendon should be uniform in thickness (Fig. 8.22B and C). The transducer is then turned 90 degrees for evaluation in short axis; in this plane, the anterior margin

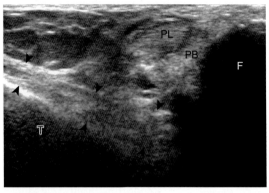

■ FIGURE 8.21 **Lateral Ankle: Posterior.** Transverse imaging between posterior aspects of the talus *(T)* and fibula *(F)* shows the posterior talofibular ligament *(arrowheads)*. *PB,* Peroneus brevis; *PL,* peroneus longus.

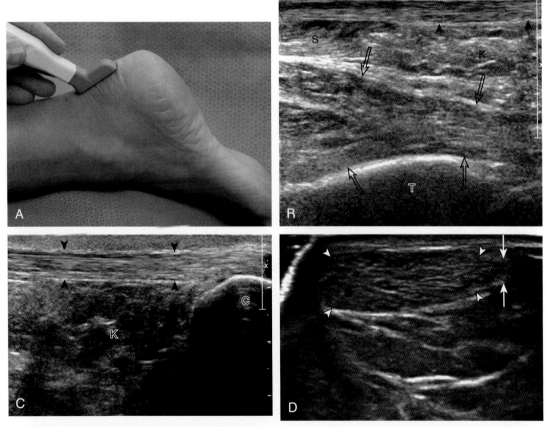

■ FIGURE 8.22 **Posterior Ankle/Heel: Achilles Tendon.** A, Sagittal imaging over the posterior ankle shows (B and C) the Achilles tendon in long axis *(arrowheads)* *(open arrows,* flexor hallucis longus muscle). Transverse imaging shows (D) the Achilles tendon *(arrowheads)* and plantaris tendon *(arrow)* in short axis (right side of image is medial). *C,* Calcaneus; *K,* Kager fat pad; *S,* distal soleus muscle; *T,* tibia.

of the Achilles tendon is predominantly flat or concave and should not be diffusely convex posterior (Fig. 8.22D). When imaged from superior to inferior in short axis, the Achilles tendon fibers rotate 90 degrees, with the gastrocnemius component lateral and the soleus medial.[26] The plantaris tendon can be identified directly medial to the Achilles tendon (Fig. 8.22D) but is often difficult to visualize when normal given its small diameter and is best appreciated in the setting of an Achilles tendon tear. The plantaris tendon may be absent in up to 20% of individuals.[11] Anterior to the Achilles tendon is a normally heterogeneous *Kager fat pad*. Distally, the retrocalcaneal bursa is seen between the calcaneus and Achilles tendon where minimal distention (up to 2.5 mm anteroposterior) is considered normal.[19] In evaluation of the retro-Achilles bursa, located superficial to the distal Achilles tendon, a thick layer of gel as a standoff without transducer pressure should be used so as not to efface the bursa and displace fluid out of the field of view. The sural nerve can be visualized in the subcutaneous fat adjacent to the lesser saphenous nerve midway between the Achilles tendon and the lateral malleolus (Fig. 8.23).

The transducer is then moved over the plantar aspect of the heel to evaluate the plantar aponeurosis (Fig. 8.24A). The transducer is initially placed in the sagittal plane over the calcaneus and moved slightly medial to visualize the plantar aponeurosis in long axis, which appears hyperechoic, uniform, and 4 mm or less in thickness at the calcaneal attachment (Fig. 8.24B).[27] Any identified disorder is also assessed in short axis. More distal assessment of the plantar aponeurosis can be carried out if symptoms or history warrants such evaluation.

Evaluation of the Calf

Structures of interest in the posterior calf include the soleus, the medial and lateral heads of the gastrocnemius, and the plantaris. Evaluation may begin in the transverse plane over the posterior

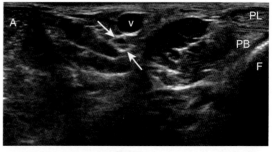

■ FIGURE 8.23 **Posterior Ankle: Sural Nerve.** Ultrasound image shows sural nerve *(arrow)* within subcutaneous fat adjacent lesser saphenous vein *(v)* between Achilles tendon *(A)* and peroneus longus *(PL)* and brevis *(PB)*.

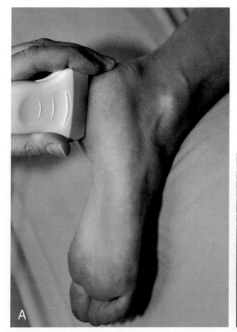
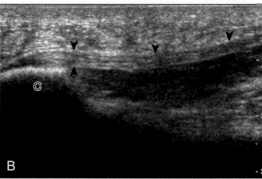

■ FIGURE 8.24 **Posterior Ankle/Heel: Plantar Aponeurosis.** A, Sagittal imaging of the plantar heel just medial to midline of foot shows (B) hyperechoic and fibrillar plantar aponeurosis *(arrowheads)* (right side of image is distal). *C*, Calcaneus.

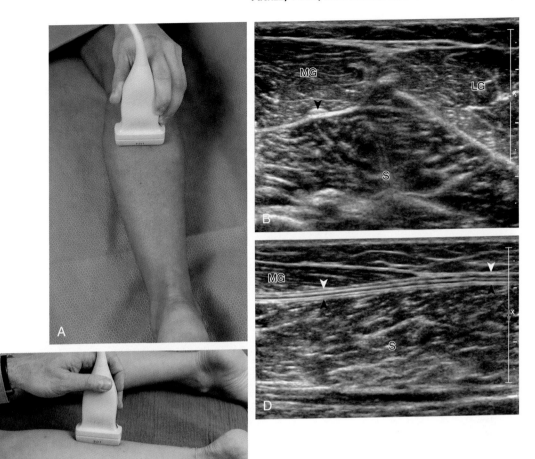

■ **FIGURE 8.25 Calf.** A, Transverse imaging over the proximal calf shows (B) the medial head *(MG)* and the lateral head *(LG)* of the gastrocnemius and soleus *(S)* muscles in short axis. C, Parasagittal imaging medially shows (D) the medial head of the gastrocnemius *(MG)* in long axis, which tapers distally over the soleus *(S)*. Note the plantaris *(arrowheads)*.

mid-calf (Fig. 8.25A). At this location, the medial and lateral heads of the gastrocnemius muscle are identified superficial to the larger soleus muscle (Fig. 8.25B). The transducer is then centered over the medial head of the gastrocnemius and moved distally until the muscle tapers. The transducer is turned 90 degrees to visualize the normal tapering appearance of the medial gastrocnemius head over the soleus in long axis, a very common site of injury (Fig. 8.25C and D). The lateral head of the gastrocnemius can be evaluated in a similar manner. The entire calf should be evaluated for pathologic processes, although the patient often indicates a site of symptoms to focus evaluation. The thin, hyperechoic plantaris tendon, when present, can be seen in the posterior calf deep to the gastrocnemius muscle.[11] Initially, the plantaris crosses midline posterior to the knee joint and then moves medial directly between the muscle bellies of the medial head of the gastrocnemius and soleus muscles (see Fig. 8.24B). Distally, the medial and lateral heads of the gastrocnemius combine with the soleus to form the Achilles tendon. The plantaris tendon courses along the medial aspect of the Achilles tendon to insert on the calcaneus or less commonly the Achilles.

Evaluation of the Forefoot

Evaluation of the distal aspect of the foot is largely guided by the patient's symptoms or history. Tendons around the digits, joint processes, soft tissue fluid collections, and masses can be assessed with ultrasound. If indicated, the forefoot can be assessed for intermetarsal bursal distention as well as Morton neuroma.[28] This is accomplished by placement of the transducer in the coronal plane on the body or short axis to the metatarsals, over

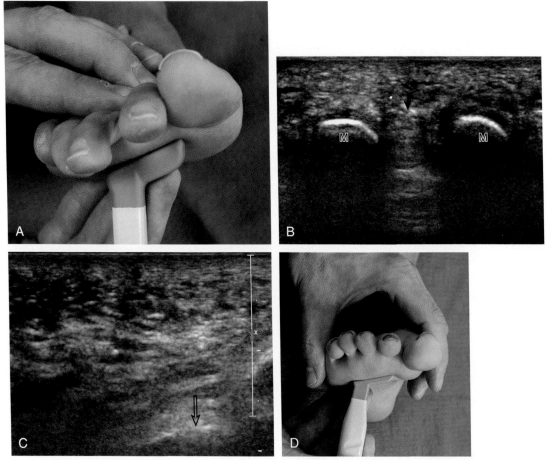

■ **FIGURE 8.26 Forefoot: Morton Neuroma Evaluation.** A, Coronal imaging plantar over the metatarsal heads shows (B) hyperechoic and mildly heterogeneous tissues *(curved arrow)* between the metatarsal heads *(M)*. Sagittal imaging between metatarsal heads shows (C) similar finding *(open arrow, dorsal skin surface and examiner's finger)*. Plantar coronal imaging with Mulder maneuver is shown in (D).

the metatarsal heads from a plantar approach (Fig. 8.26A). The examiner's finger from the other hand is placed at the dorsal aspect of the forefoot over the web space to be evaluated (Fig. 8.26B). This maneuver assists evaluation because the inter-metatarsal space is widened and the soft tissues are compressed, improving visualization, while potentially reproducing the patient's symptoms when a neuroma is present. Evaluation also continues in long axis in the sagittal plane (Fig. 8.26C). A similar long axis image can be obtained with the transducer over the dorsal foot and manual palpation over the plantar aspect. Returning to the plantar short axis approach, dynamic assessment for Morton neuroma can be completed by manually squeezing the metatarsals together from side to side and imaging from a plantar approach (Fig. 8.26D). This maneuver (called the *sonographic Mulder sign*) will cause plantar displacement of a neuroma also producing symptoms.[29] When screening for inflammatory arthritis, the

dorsal recesses of the metatarsophalangeal joints should be assessed, in particular the fifth metatarsal head (dorsal, lateral, and plantar), as well as the first interphalangeal joint in addition to any symptomatic areas to assess for rheumatoid arthritis.[30] The medial first metatarsal head should also be routinely imaged to assess for gout. The plantar plate may also be evaluated in the sagittal plane, normally appearing as a hyperechoic structure attached to the proximal phalanx and superficial to the flexor tendon (Fig. 8.27).[2,31]

■ JOINT AND BURSAL ABNORMALITIES

Joint Effusion and Synovial Hypertrophy: General Comments

Evaluation for joint pathology should focus on relevant joint recesses for effusion and synovial hypertrophy. For the ankle or tibiotalar joint, the

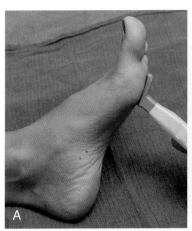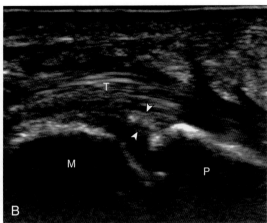

■ FIGURE 8.27 **Forefoot: Plantar Plate Evaluation.** A, Sagittal imaging plantar over the metatarsal heads shows (B) hyperechoic and triangular plantar plate *(arrowheads)*. *M,* Metatarsal head; *P,* proximal phalanx; *T,* flexor tendon.

anterior recess with the foot in slight plantar flexion is the most sensitive position and location to identify joint effusion.[32] Simple fluid distention of a joint is typically anechoic forming a teardrop shape, extending over the talar dome, and possibly extending proximally over the distal tibia displacing the hyperechoic anterior fat pad (Fig. 8.28). The normal hypoechoic hyaline cartilage that covers the talar dome, which measures 1 to 2 mm and is uniform in thickness, should not be mistaken for joint effusion (see Fig. 8.2B). For the foot, dorsal recesses of the intertarsal, metatarsophalangeal, and interphalangeal joints are targeted. With regard to the metatarsophalangeal joints, each dorsal joint recess distends proximally over the metatarsal (Fig. 8.29) as well as over the proximal phalanx when large (see Fig. 8.41). Causes for anechoic joint effusion are many and include infection (Fig. 8.30), trauma, osteoarthritis (Fig. 8.31), and other arthritides (discussed later). Joint fluid within the first metatarsophalangeal joint is often asymptomatic but may relate to early osteoarthritis. Intra-articular bodies from degenerative arthritis and trauma appear hyperechoic with possible shadowing within a joint recess (Fig. 8.32) (Video 8.2). Intra-articular bodies may also migrate to the medial ankle tendon sheaths (see Fig. 8.69B) because communication with the ankle joint is common.

Increased echogenicity of joint fluid can be the result of complex fluid, as seen in infection (Figs. 8.33 and 8.34), hemorrhage (Fig. 8.35) (Video 8.3), and gout (see Fig. 8.49). Echogenic joint fluid also may resemble synovial hypertrophy (Fig. 8.36). To assist in this differentiation, compressibility and internal echo movement with transducer pressure, redistribution with joint movement, and lack of flow on color Doppler imaging suggest complex fluid rather than synovial hypertrophy. Joint recess echogenicity and vascularity do not predict infection, and ultrasound-guided aspiration should be considered if there is concern for infection. In the setting of synovial hypertrophy, adjacent cortical irregularity may be from erosions, which can be seen in inflammatory (see Inflammatory Arthritis in next section; see Chapter 2 for infection) and non-inflammatory conditions, which include pigmented villonodular synovitis[33] (Fig. 8.37) and synovial chondromatosis (Fig. 8.38). In the latter condition, hyperechoic and possibly shadowing foci may be identified.[34] Synovial hypertrophy may also be found in the ankle joint deep to the anterior talofibular ligament in anterolateral impingement syndrome (Fig. 8.39), where echogenic synovial hypertrophy greater than 10 mm is associated with symptoms and adjacent ligament abnormality.[35] Nonspecific mild synovial thickening, usually with little or no flow on color Doppler imaging, can be seen with osteoarthritis and may not correlate with patient symptoms (Fig. 8.40).[36,37]

Inflammatory Arthritis

Important target sites for arthritis evaluation in addition to any focal symptomatic area should include the distal fifth and first metatarsal heads because these are common sites for involvement from rheumatoid arthritis and gout, respectively. With regard to rheumatoid arthritis, ultrasound findings include joint effusion (Fig. 8.41) and synovial hypertrophy, which is usually hypoechoic (Figs. 8.42 and 8.43) (Video 8.4), but is possibly isoechoic (Fig. 8.44) (Video 8.5), compared with subcutaneous fat, with possible increased flow on color Doppler imaging.[38,39] In the presence of

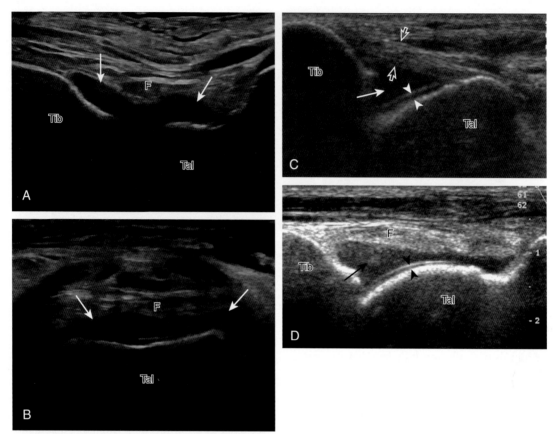

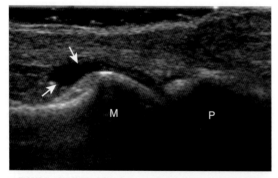

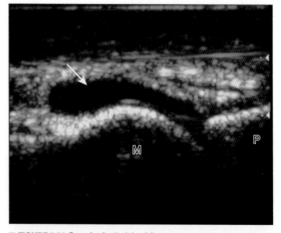

■ FIGURE 8.28 **Joint Effusion: Tibiotalar Joint.** Ultrasound images over the anterior ankle in three patients show (A) sagittal and (B) transverse plane hypoechoic distention of the anterior ankle joint recess *(arrows)*, (C) anechoic distention *(arrow)* anterolateral deep to the anterior talofibular ligament *(open arrows)*, and (D) hypoechoic anterior ankle joint recess distention *(arrow)*. Note displacement of anterior fat pad *(F)* and the interface with hyaline articular cartilage *(arrowheads)*. *Tal,* Talus; *Tib,* tibia.

■ FIGURE 8.29 **Joint Effusion: Metatarsophalangeal Joint.** Ultrasound image in sagittal plane dorsal to metatarsophalangeal joint shows anechoic distention of the dorsal joint recess, which extends proximal *(arrows)* over metatarsal *(M)*.

■ FIGURE 8.30 **Septic Arthritis: Metatarsophalangeal Joint.** Ultrasound image shows anechoic distention *(arrow)* of the dorsal recess of the first metatarsophalangeal joint from infection. *M,* Metatarsal head; *P,* proximal phalanx.

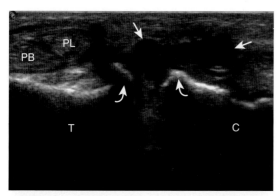

■ FIGURE 8.31 Osteoarthritis: Posterior Subtalar Joint.
Ultrasound image in coronal plane over lateral hindfoot
shows anechoic distention *(arrows)* of joint recess with
adjacent osteophytes *(curved arrows)*. *C,* Calcaneus;
PL, peroneus longus tendon; *PB,* peroneus brevis
tendon; *T,* talus.

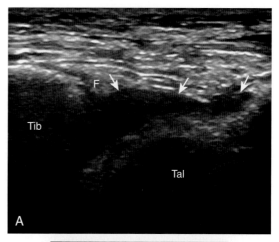

A

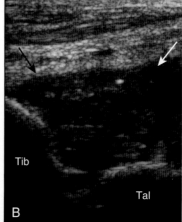

B

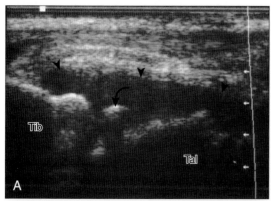

A

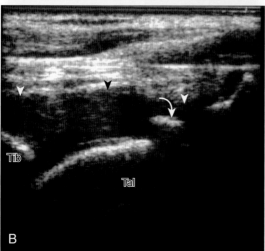

B

■ FIGURE 8.32 Intra-Articular Body: Tibiotalar Joint.
Ultrasound images over the anterior ankle joint recess
show hyperechoic and shadowing intra-articular body
(curved arrow) surrounded by anechoic joint fluid
(arrowheads). Note movement of the intra-articular
body distally within the anterior ankle joint recess
between A and B. *Tal,* Talus; *Tib,* tibia.

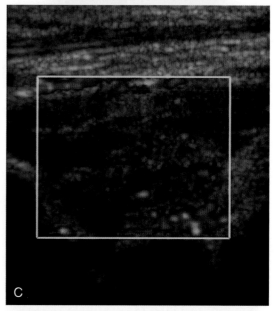

C

■ FIGURE 8.33 Complex Joint Effusion: Infection. Ultrasound images over the anterior ankle with plantar flexion
in two patients show (A) hypoechoic distention and
(B and C) hypoechoic to isoechoic distention *(arrows)*
with peripheral flow on power Doppler imaging. In
each case, swirling of intra-articular contents was noted
with transducer pressure. Note displaced anterior fat
pad *(F)*. *Tal,* Talus; *Tib,* tibia.

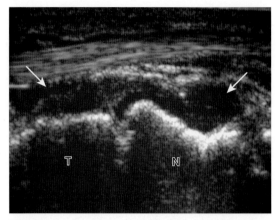

■ FIGURE 8.34 **Complex Joint Effusion: Infection.** Ultrasound image in sagittal plane over dorsal midfoot shows hypoechoic distention *(arrows)* of the talonavicular joint. *N,* Navicular; *T,* talus.

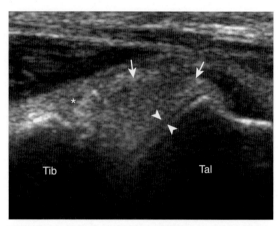

■ FIGURE 8.35 **Complex Joint Effusion: Hemorrhage.** Ultrasound image over the anterior ankle with plantar flexion shows hyperechoic distention *(arrows)* from hemorrhage after ankle trauma. Note displacement of anterior fat pad *(asterisk)* and interface with hyaline articular cartilage *(arrowheads)*. *Tal,* Talus; *Tib,* tibia.

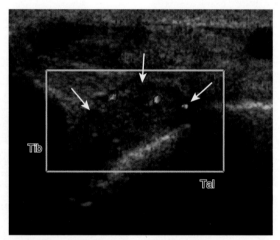

■ 1.   FIGURE 8.36 **Synovial Hypertrophy: Infection.** Ultrasound image over the anterior ankle with plantar flexion shows hypoechoic to isoechoic distention of the anterior ankle joint recess *(arrows)* with internal flow on color Doppler imaging. *Tal,* Talus; *Tib,* tibia.

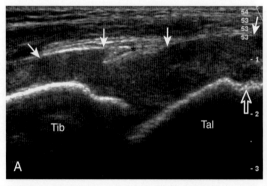

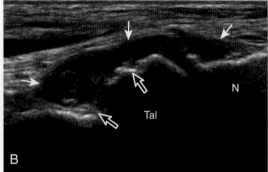

■ FIGURE 8.37 **Pigmented Villonodular Synovitis.** Ultrasound images from two patients show hypoechoic to isoechoic distention *(arrows)* of the (A) anterior ankle recess and (B) talonavicular joint recess. Note bone erosions *(open arrows)* *(asterisk,* fat pad). *N,* Navicular; *Tal,* talus; *Tib,* tibia.

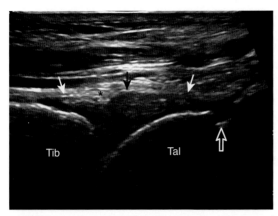

■ **FIGURE 8.38 Synovial Chondromatosis.** Ultrasound image over anterior ankle shows hypoechoic to isoechoic distention *(arrows)* of the anterior ankle recess with bone erosions *(open arrow)* *(asterisk,* fat pad). *Tal,* Talus; *Tib,* tibia.

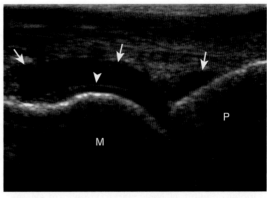

■ **FIGURE 8.41 Rheumatoid Arthritis: Joint Effusion.** Ultrasound image over dorsal metatarsophalangeal joint shows anechoic dorsal joint recess distention *(arrows)* over the distal metatarsal *(M)* and to a lesser extent the proximal phalanx *(P)* *(arrowhead,* cartilage interface).

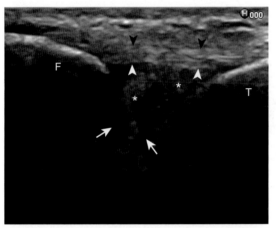

■ **FIGURE 8.39 Anterolateral Impingement Syndrome.** Ultrasound image long axis to normal anterior talofibular ligament *(arrowheads)* shows anechoic fluid *(arrows)* and echogenic synovial hypertrophy *(asterisks). F,* Fibula, *T,* talus.

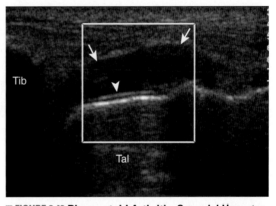

■ **FIGURE 8.42 Rheumatoid Arthritis: Synovial Hypertrophy.** Ultrasound image over the anterior ankle with plantar flexion shows hypoechoic distention *(arrows)* that was noncompressible with no flow on color Doppler imaging and no joint fluid at joint aspiration *(arrowhead,* cartilage interface). *Tal,* Talus; *Tib,* tibia.

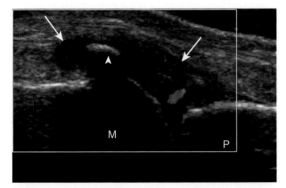

■ **FIGURE 8.40 Osteoarthritis: Metatarsophalangeal Joint.** Ultrasound image dorsal over first metatarsophalangeal joint shows hypoechoic synovial hypertrophy *(arrows)* and osteophyte *(arrowhead)* with mild internal flow on color Doppler imaging. *M,* Metatarsal; *P,* proximal phalanx.

synovial hypertrophy, disruption of the normally smooth bone cortex in two planes indicates erosions. Because the ultrasound findings of rheumatoid arthritis are not specific and resemble other inflammatory conditions, including other systemic arthritides and infection, the distribution of findings is very helpful along with radiographic and serologic correlation. The fifth metatarsal head is the most common site of erosions in rheumatoid arthritis (Fig. 8.45) (Video 8.6), with possible involvement of the other metatarsophalangeal joints and first interphalangeal joint (Fig. 8.46) as other key target sites.[30,40-43] There exist numerous concavities of the distal metatarsal cortex that should not be misinterpreted as erosions.[44] Other manifestations of rheumatoid arthritis in the foot

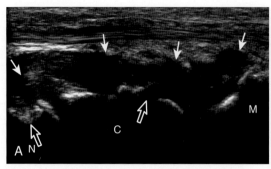
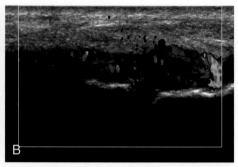

■ **FIGURE 8.43 Rheumatoid Arthritis: Synovial Hypertrophy.** Ultrasound images (A and B) over dorsal recesses of mid-foot show hypoechoic synovial hypertrophy *(arrows)*, erosions *(open arrows)*, and increased flow on color Doppler imaging. *N,* Navicular; *C,* cuneiform; *M,* metatarsal.

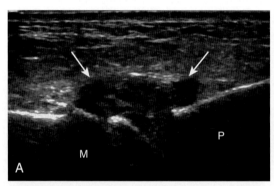
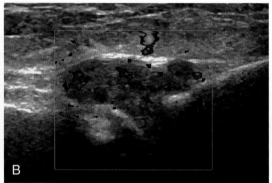

■ **FIGURE 8.44 Rheumatoid Arthritis: Synovial Hypertrophy.** Ultrasound images (A and B) over the second meta-tarsophalangeal joint show hypoechoic to isoechoic distention of the joint recess *(arrows)* with internal flow on power Doppler imaging. *M,* Metatarsal; *P,* proximal phalanx.

and ankle include the retrocalcaneal bursitis with possible erosion (Fig. 8.47) (Video 8.7), adventitious bursae (see Fig. 8.62; Video 8.6), hypoechoic rheumatoid nodules (Fig. 8.48),[32] and abnormalities of the tendons and tendon sheath (see Tendon and Muscle Abnormalities).[38]

With regard to gout, the most common site of involvement is the first metatarsophalangeal joint. Within a joint, one may see effusion, often with hyperechoic foci (representing microtophi) (Fig. 8.49) (Video 8.8), coating of the hyaline cartilage with monosodium urate crystals (called the *double contour sign*) (Fig. 8.50) (Videos 8.9 and 8.10), and synovial hypertrophy (Fig. 8.51).[45] The double contour sign has been shown to disappear when the serum urate level decreases below 6 mg/dL.[46] Imaging at the medial aspect long axis to the distal first metatarsal often shows amorphous hyperechoic tophus with anechoic inflammatory halo, with possible direct extension into a cortical erosion (Fig. 8.52) (Videos 8.11 and 8.12).[47] Tophi may also involve tendon (Fig. 8.53) and tendon sheaths (Fig. 8.54) (Video 8.13), bursae (Fig. 8.55) (Video 8.14), and other joints (Fig. 8.56).

Other inflammatory arthritides include sero-negative spondyloarthropathies, such as reactive arthritis and psoriatic arthritis. The ultrasound findings of this category of inflammatory arthritis include nonspecific intra-articular findings of joint fluid, synovial hypertrophy, and possible erosions; however, the finding of bone proliferation in the form of inflammatory enthesopathy at tendon and ligament attachments is characteristic of sero-negative spondyloarthropathy (Fig. 8.57).[48,49] Because degenerative enthesopathy is common at several sites in the foot and ankle, such as at the Achilles tendon attachment, correlation with radiography and identifying true inflammatory findings at ultrasound are critical.

Bursal Abnormalities

There are two bursae around the distal Achilles tendon: the retrocalcaneal and retro-Achilles bursae. The retrocalcaneal bursa, located between the calcaneus and distal Achilles tendon, may normally contain fluid with anteroposterior distention up to 2.5 mm.[19] Abnormal distention of the

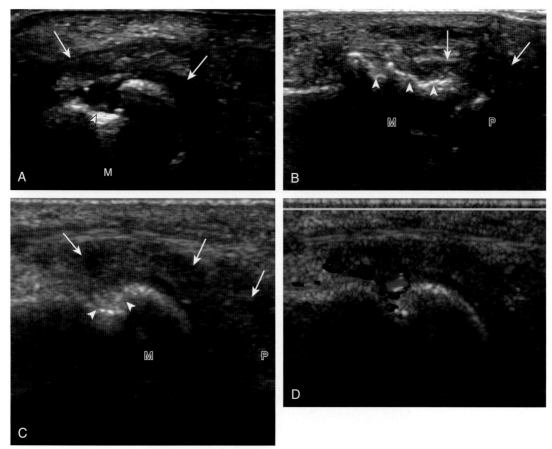

■ FIGURE 8.45 **Rheumatoid Arthritis: Erosions.** Ultrasound images of the fifth metatarsophalangeal joint in three patients (A, B/C, and D) show hypoechoic synovial hypertrophy *(arrows)* and cortical erosions *(arrowheads)* and (D) hyperemia on color Doppler imaging. *M,* Fifth metatarsal head; *P,* proximal phalanx.

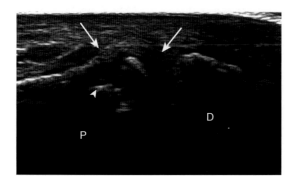

■ FIGURE 8.46 **Rheumatoid Arthritis: First Interphalangeal Joint.** Ultrasound image long axis to medial great toe shows hypoechoic synovial hypertrophy *(arrows)* and cortical erosion *(arrowhead)* of metatarsal head *(M).* *P,* Proximal phalanx; *D,* distal phalanx.

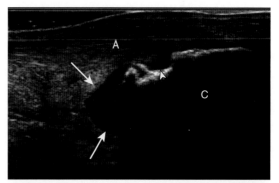

■ FIGURE 8.47 **Rheumatoid Arthritis: Retrocalcaneal Bursitis.** Ultrasound image long axis to distal Achilles tendon *(A)* shows hypoechoic synovial hypertrophy distending the retrocalcaneal bursa *(arrows)* with an erosion *(arrowhead)* of the calcaneus *(C).*

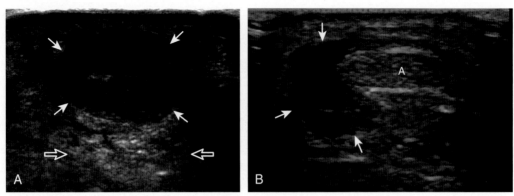

■ FIGURE 8.48 **Rheumatoid Arthritis: Rheumatoid Nodule.** Ultrasound images (A) over lateral foot and (B) short axis to Achilles tendon *(A)* show predominantly hypoechoic nodule *(arrows)* with increased through-transmission in A *(open arrows). (B, Courtesy Brian Robertson, Ann Arbor, Michigan.)*

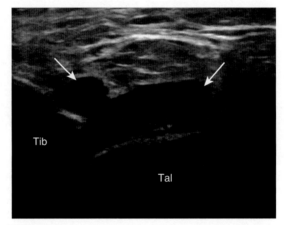

■ FIGURE 8.49 **Gout: Complex Effusion.** Ultrasound image over dorsal ankle shows hypoechoic distention *(arrows)* of anterior ankle joint recess with internal reflective crystals. *Tal,* Talus; *Tib,* tibia.

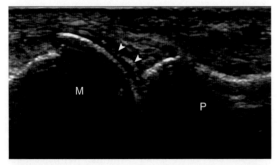

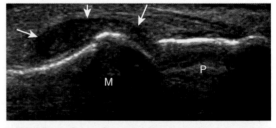

■ FIGURE 8.51 **Gout: Synovial Hypertrophy.** Ultrasound image over dorsal first metatarsophalangeal joint shows hypoechoic synovial hypertrophy *(arrows)* with flow on color Doppler. *M,* Metatarsal; *P,* proximal phalanx.

■ FIGURE 8.50 **Gout: Urate Icing (Double Contour Sign).** Ultrasound image over dorsal first metatarsophalangeal joint shows urate icing of hyaline articular cartilage *(arrowheads). M,* Metatarsal; *P,* proximal phalanx.

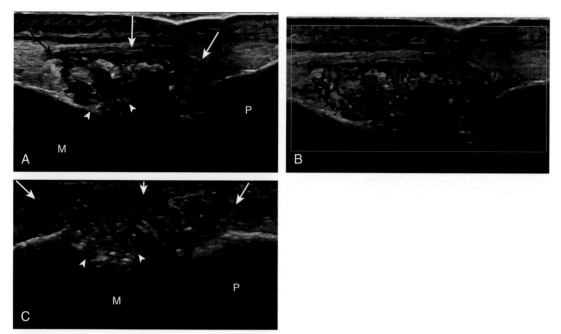

■ **FIGURE 8.52 Gout: Tophus and Erosion.** Ultrasound images in axial plane over medial distal first metatarsal shows cortical erosion *(arrowheads)* and adjacent echogenic tophus *(arrows)* extending from metatarsophalangeal joint with increased flow on color Doppler imaging. *M,* Metatarsal; *P,* proximal phalanx.

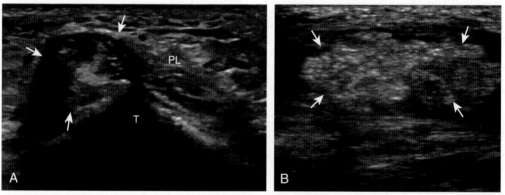

■ **FIGURE 8.53 Gout: Tophus.** Ultrasound images short axis to (A) peroneus brevis and (B) tibialis anterior tendons show hyperechoic tophi with hypoechoic halo *(arrows)*. *PL,* Peroneus longus tendon; *T,* peroneal tubercle of calcaneus.

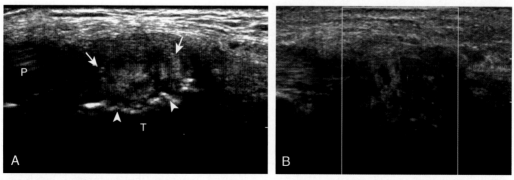

■ **FIGURE 8.54 Gout: Tophus, Erosion.** Ultrasound image (A) over medial ankle shows *(arrows)* hyperechoic tophus associated with tibialis posterior tendon *(P)*. Note erosions *(arrowheads)* of medial talus *(T)* and increased flow on color Doppler (B).

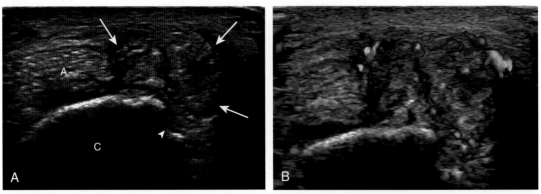

■ FIGURE 8.55 **Gout: Retrocalcaneal Bursa.** Ultrasound images (A and B) in axial plane over the distal Achilles tendon *(A)* shows cortical erosion *(arrowhead)* and adjacent echogenic tophus *(arrows)* with increased flow on color Doppler imaging. *C,* Calcaneus.

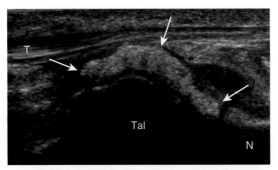

■ FIGURE 8.56 **Gout: Talonavicular Joint.** Ultrasound color Doppler image in sagittal plane over the dorsal midfoot shows hyperechoic tophus *(arrows)* extending from talonavicular joint with adjacent hyperemia. *Tal,* Talus; *N,* navicular; *T,* extensor tendon.

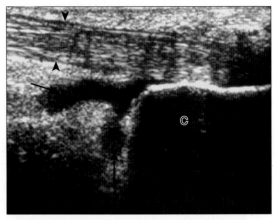

■ FIGURE 8.58 **Retrocalcaneal Bursal Distention.** Ultrasound image in the sagittal plane shows anechoic distention of the retrocalcaneal bursa *(arrows)* *(arrowheads,* Achilles tendon). *C,* Calcaneus.

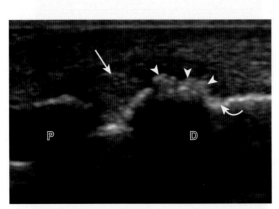

■ FIGURE 8.57 **Psoriatic Arthritis.** Ultrasound image over the interphalangeal joint of the first toe shows bone proliferation *(arrowheads),* erosion *(curved arrow),* and isoechoic to hyperechoic synovial hypertrophy *(arrow).* *D,* Distal phalanx; *P,* proximal phalanx.

retrocalcaneal bursa may be mechanical (Fig. 8.58), from adjacent tendon tear (Fig. 8.59), from primary inflammation as in rheumatoid arthritis (see Fig. 8.47) (see Video 8.7), or related to adjacent Achilles enthesopathy. The retro-Achilles

bursa, located superficial to the distal Achilles tendon, is not normally visualized and is considered an adventitious bursa. Distention of the retro-Achilles bursa may also be mechanical or inflammatory (Fig. 8.60). The presence of an abnormally distended retrocalcaneal bursa and retro-Achilles bursa with adjacent abnormalities of the Achilles tendon and a prominent posterior superior aspect of the calcaneus is described in patients with *Haglund syndrome* (Fig. 8.61).[50]

Bursae may also form around the foot and ankle at sites of pressure, termed *adventitious bursae.*[51] Such bursae are commonly found in the forefoot plantar to the metatarsal heads and calcaneus, particularly in patients with rheumatoid arthritis (Fig. 8.62) (Videos 8.15 and 8.16).[51,52] Another site of an adventitious bursa is superficial to the medial malleolus (Fig. 8.63).[53] Normal bursae are located between the metatarsal heads, called *intermetatarsal bursae,* and are often distended and associated with Morton neuromas but may be an

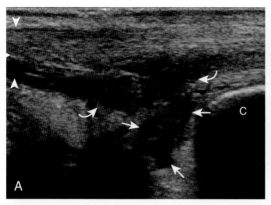

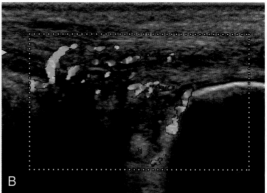

■ FIGURE 8.59 **Retrocalcaneal Bursal Distention and Achilles Tendon Tear.** Ultrasound images (A and B) in the sagittal plane show heterogeneous distention of the retrocalcaneal bursa *(arrows)* with adjacent Achilles tendon partial tear and tendinosis *(curved arrows)* *(arrowheads*, Achilles tendon). *C,* Calcaneus.

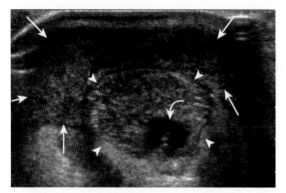

■ FIGURE 8.60 **Retro-Achilles Bursal Infection.** Ultrasound image short axis to the Achilles tendon shows hypoechoic to isoechoic distention of the retro-Achilles bursa *(arrows)*. Note incidental tendinosis *(curved arrow)* of the Achilles tendon *(arrowheads)*.

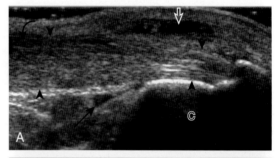

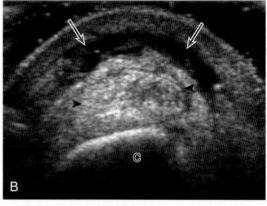

■ FIGURE 8.61 **Haglund Syndrome.** Ultrasound images (A) long axis and (B) short axis to the distal Achilles tendon show anechoic fluid in the retrocalcaneal bursa *(arrow)*, the retro-Achilles bursa *(open arrows)*, and tendinosis *(curved arrow)* of the Achilles tendon *(arrowheads)*. *C,* Calcaneus.

asymptomatic finding if located in the first through third interspaces and less than 3 mm in width (see Fig. 8.151) (Video 8.17).[54] Another bursa at the anterolateral ankle that commonly contains minimal fluid is the *Gruberi bursa*, located between the extensor digitorum longus tendons and the talus (Fig. 8.64) (Videos 8.18 and 8.19).[3] Unlike a ganglion cyst, this bursa is easily compressed with transducer pressure and in a characteristic location deep to the extensor digitorum longus typically without symptoms.

■ TENDON AND MUSCLE ABNORMALITIES

Medial Ankle

TENOSYNOVITIS (MEDIAL ANKLE)

Of the medial tendons, the tibialis posterior tendon is most frequently abnormal, usually at the level of the medial malleolus. Tenosynovitis is characterized by distention of the tendon sheath and may be anechoic if it consists of simple fluid (Fig. 8.65).[55] Tendon sheath distention that is of increased echogenicity may be from complex fluid or synovial hypertrophy; when distention is not anechoic, displacement and internal movement of echoes with transducer pressure as well as absence of internal color flow suggest complex

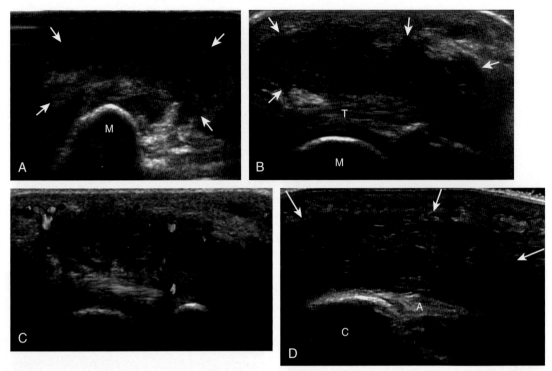

■ **FIGURE 8.62 Adventitious Bursa.** Ultrasound images over the plantar aspect of the foot in three patients (A, B/C, and D) show heterogeneous but predominantly hypoechoic adventitious bursa formation *(arrows)*, which was collapsible with transducer pressure. *M*, Metatarsal; *T*, flexor tendon; *C*, calcaneus; *A*, plantar aponeurosis.

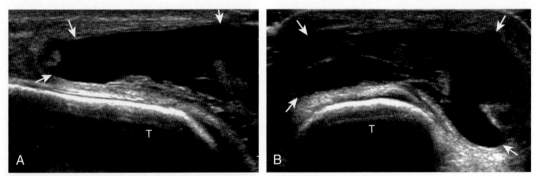

■ **FIGURE 8.63 Medial Malleolus Bursa.** Ultrasound images in the (A) coronal and (B) axial planes over the distal tibia *(T)* show predominantly anechoic distention *(arrows)* with internal septations.

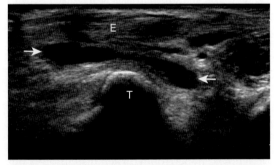

■ **FIGURE 8.64 Gruberi Bursa.** Ultrasound image short axis to extensor digitorum longus tendons *(E)* shows distention of the Gruberi bursa *(arrows)*, which was easily compressible. Note increased through-transmission. *T*, Talus.

fluid (Video 8.20).[56] Up to 4 mm of fluid may normally distend the posterior tibial tendon sheath just beyond the medial malleolus.[19] This normal fluid may be asymmetrical, but a helpful feature is the lack of symptoms with transducer pressure and lack of flow on color Doppler imaging. In addition, the ankle joint can normally communicate with the medial tendon sheaths, especially the flexor hallucis longus tendon. Distention of the posterior tibial tendon sheath greater than 5.8 mm can indicate early posterior tibial tendon dysfunction (Fig. 8.65B).[57] Evaluation for tibialis posterior tendon dysfunction should also include the adjacent spring ligament for abnormalities (see Fig. 8.139).[58]

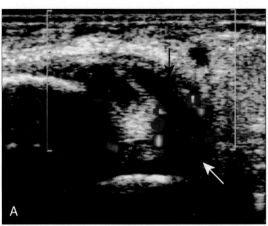
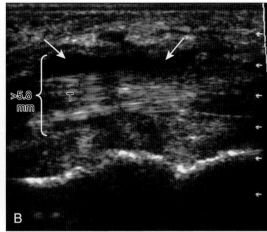

■ FIGURE 8.65 **Tenosynovitis: Tibialis Posterior Tendon.** Ultrasound images from two patients show (A) anechoic distention *(arrows)* with increased peripheral blood flow on color Doppler imaging from mechanical tenosynovitis, and (B) hypoechoic tendon sheath distention *(arrows)* that measures greater than 5.8 mm from posterior tibial tendon dysfunction. *T,* Tibialis posterior tendon.

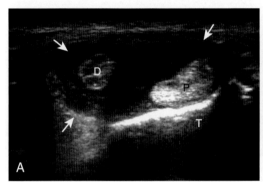
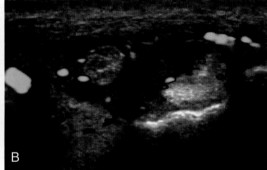

■ FIGURE 8.66 **Tenosynovitis: Ankylosing Spondylitis.** Ultrasound images short axis to the tibialis posterior *(P)* and flexor digitorum longus *(D)* tendons show surrounding mixed hypoechoic synovial hypertrophy *(arrows)* with increased flow on color Doppler imaging. *T,* Tibia.

Tenosynovitis is commonly mechanical or traumatic, potentially associated with an underlying tendon abnormality. Inflammation related to systemic arthritis, such as seronegative spondyloarthropathy (Fig. 8.66) and rheumatoid arthritis (Fig. 8.67) (Video 8.21), is another cause. Uncommonly, infection can involve the tendon sheath as an extension from adjacent soft tissue or bone infection. Regardless of origin, increased flow may be demonstrated on color Doppler imaging. While more commonly hypoechoic, synovial tissue surrounding a tendon may be isoechoic or hyperechoic to tendon; toggling the transducer when imaging the tendon in short axis will differentiate tendon from echogenic synovial hypertrophy in that the latter does not demonstrate anisotropy and will remain hyperechoic adjacent to the hypoechoic tendon (Fig. 8.68).

Tendon sheath distention may also focally involve the flexor hallucis longus tendon at the level of the os trigonum, posterior to the talus in the setting of *os trigonum syndrome.*[59] More distally, tendon sheath distention may also occur where the flexor hallucis longus and flexor digitorum longus tendons cross (the *knot of Henry*) under the mid-foot (Fig. 8.69A). Because of the normal communication between the medial tendon sheaths and the ankle joint, intra-articular bodies may migrate into medial tendon sheaths (Fig. 8.69B). Marked focal distention of medial tendon sheath in the absence of anterior ankle joint recess distention suggests tenosynovitis, rather than communicating ankle joint fluid (Fig. 8.70). Dynamic evaluation of the flexor hallucis longus tendon may show tendon impingement (Video 8.22).

TENDINOSIS (MEDIAL ANKLE)

Tendinosis is characterized by abnormal hypoechogenicity with possible enlargement of the involved tendon but without disruption of tendon fibers (Fig. 8.71).[60] The term *tendinosis* is used rather

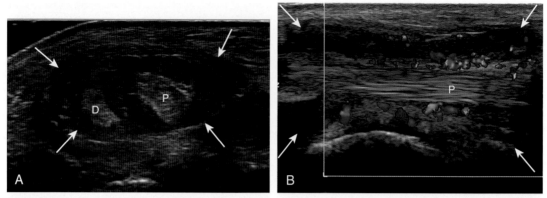

■ **FIGURE 8.67 Tenosynovitis: Rheumatoid Arthritis.** Ultrasound images (A) short axis and (B) long axis to the tibialis posterior *(P)* and flexor digitorum longus *(D)* tendons show surrounding hypoechoic to isoechoic synovial hypertrophy *(arrows)* with increased flow on color Doppler imaging.

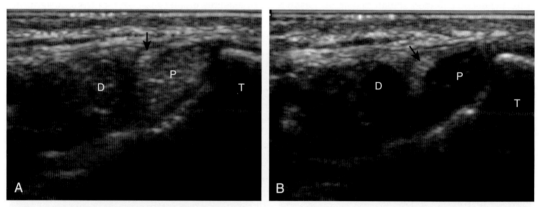

■ **FIGURE 8.68 Synovial Hypertrophy: Pitfall.** Ultrasound images short axis to the tibialis posterior *(P)* and flexor digitorum *(D)* longus tendons show hyperechoic synovial hypertrophy *(arrow)* without (A) and with (B) tendon anisotropy by toggling the transducer. *T,* Tibia.

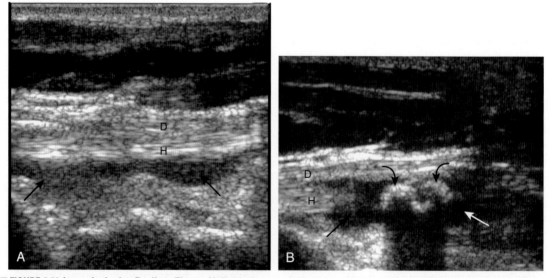

■ **FIGURE 8.69 Intra-Articular Bodies: Flexor Hallucis Longus.** Ultrasound images (A and B) long axis to the flexor hallucis longus *(H)* and flexor digitorum longus *(D)* tendons show anechoic joint fluid *(arrows)* and ossified intra-articular bodies *(curved arrows)* at the knot of Henry from the ankle joint.

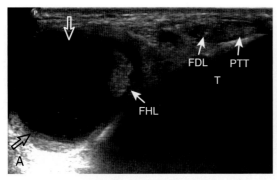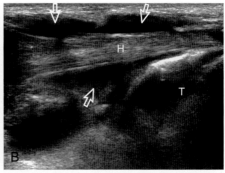

■ FIGURE 8.70 **Tenosynovitis: Flexor Hallucis Longus.** Ultrasound images (A) short and (B) long axis to flexor hallucis longus tendon *(H)* show isolated hypoechoic distention of the tendon sheath *(open arrows)*. *FDL,* Flexor digitorum longus; *FHL,* flexor hallucis longus; *PTT,* tibialis posterior; *T,* tibia.

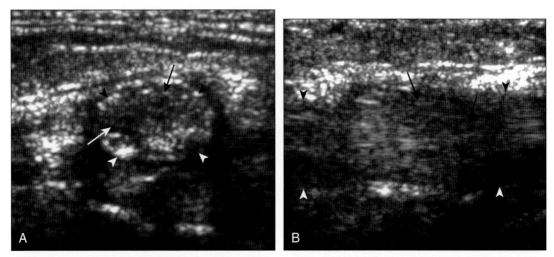

■ FIGURE 8.71 **Tendinosis: Tibialis Posterior Tendon.** Ultrasound images (A) short axis and (B) long axis to the tibialis posterior tendon *(arrowheads)* show hypoechoic swelling *(arrows)* from tendinosis without disruption of tendon fibers.

than *tendinitis* because this condition typically represents a degenerative process and not an inflammatory process. Tendinosis commonly involves a segment of tendon that courses around an osseous structure, such as at the medial malleolus.

PARTIAL-THICKNESS TEAR (MEDIAL ANKLE)

Partial-thickness tears may initially appear as well-defined intra-substance anechoic or hypoechoic areas or clefts that partially disrupt the tendon fibers, often in the setting of underlying tendinosis (Fig. 8.72).[58] It is difficult to differentiate between severe intra-substance tendinosis and interstitial tear in the continuum of a diseased tendon, although the latter is more likely if the abnormality is well defined and anechoic. One type of tear is a longitudinal split, which may

extend to one (Fig. 8.73) or two (Fig. 8.74) tendon surfaces (Video 8.23).[61] This latter type of tear is best visualized with the tendon in short axis, where the normal tendon is split into two bundles separated by an anechoic or hypoechoic cleft. Injury to the adjacent flexor retinaculum appears as hypoechoic thickening (Fig. 8.75) and possible avulsion fragment from the medial malleolus, which may be associated with tendon subluxation or dislocation (Fig. 8.76) (Video 8.24).[62] A tendon may be entrapped or torn when in contact with fixation hardware (Fig. 8.77) or displaced within a fracture (Fig. 8.78).[63]

FULL-THICKNESS TEAR (MEDIAL ANKLE)

Full-thickness complete tears are characterized by full-width fiber disruption, tendon stump retraction, and interposed fluid, hemorrhage, or

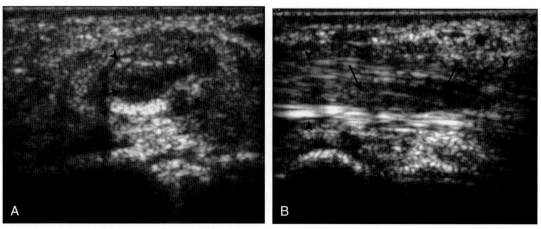

■ **FIGURE 8.72 Intrasubstance Tear: Tibialis Posterior Tendon.** Ultrasound images (A) short axis and (B) long axis to the posterior tibial tendon *(arrowheads)* show well-defined hypoechoic areas *(arrows)* with disruption of tendon fibers.

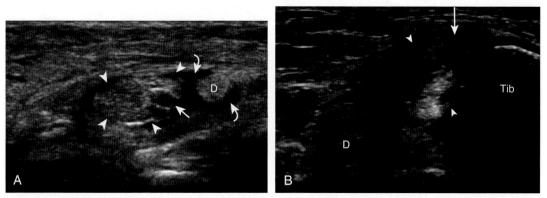

■ **FIGURE 8.73 Longitudinal Tear: Tibialis Posterior Tendon.** Ultrasound images short axis to the tibialis posterior tendon *(arrowheads)* in two patients show a longitudinal cleft *(arrow)* extending to tendon surface. *D,* Flexor digitorum longus tendon; *Tib,* tibia.

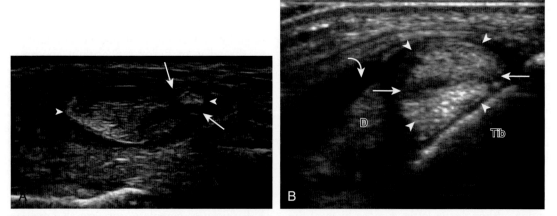

■ **FIGURE 8.74 Longitudinal Tear: Tibialis Posterior Tendon.** Ultrasound images short axis to the tibialis posterior tendon *(arrowheads)* in two patients show a longitudinal cleft *(arrows)* that involves two surfaces of the tendon *(curved arrow,* anechoic fluid in tendon sheath). *D,* Flexor digitorum longus tendon; *Tib,* tibia.

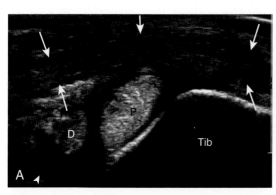
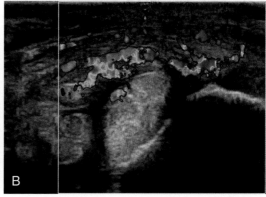

■ FIGURE 8.75 **Flexor Retinaculum Injury.** Ultrasound images show hypoechoic thickening of the flexor retinaculum *(arrows)* and tenosynovitis *(arrowhead)* with hyperemia on color Doppler image. *Tib,* Tibia; *P,* tibial posterior tendon; *D,* flexor digitorum longus tendon.

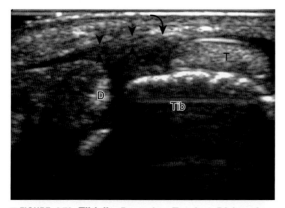

■ FIGURE 8.76 **Tibialis Posterior Tendon Dislocation.** Ultrasound image shows anterior dislocation of the tibialis posterior tendon *(T)* with tibial detachment *(curved arrow)* of the flexor retinaculum *(arrowheads). D,* Flexor digitorum longus tendon.

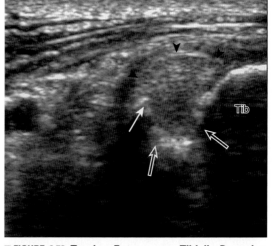

■ FIGURE 8.78 **Tendon Entrapment: Tibialis Posterior.** Ultrasound image short axis to tibialis posterior tendon *(arrowheads)* shows tendon entrapment within a tibial fracture *(open arrows),* where bone partially indents the tendon *(arrow). Tib,* Tibia.

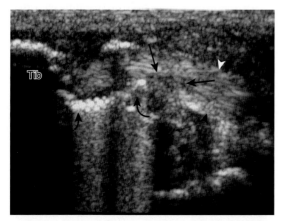

■ FIGURE 8.77 **Partial-Thickness Tear: Tibialis Posterior Tendon, Hardware.** Ultrasound image shows partial tendon disruption *(arrows)* of the tibialis posterior tendon *(arrowheads)* from a protruding metal screw *(curved arrows).* Note reverberation artifact deep to screw. *Tib,* Tibia.

synovial hypertrophy that fills the torn tendon gap (Fig. 8.79).[61] Tear of the tibialis posterior tendon may occur at the level of the medial malleolus. In this setting, an intact flexor digitorum longus tendon should not be mistaken for the tibialis posterior tendon when the latter is torn and retracted from view. The tibialis posterior tendon may also tear distally or avulse a fragment of the navicular bone, especially in diabetic patients, associated with tendon retraction. This must be differentiated from an accessory navicular bone found in an intact tibialis posterior tendon, which is a normal variant that may become symptomatic in some individuals when the synchondrosis between the accessory navicular and the native navicular is injured (Fig. 8.80). Pain

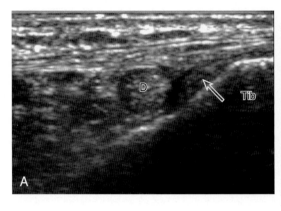
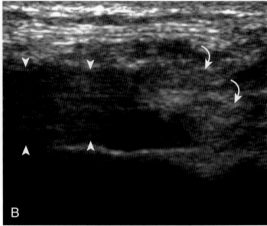

■ **FIGURE 8.79 Full-Thickness Complete Tear: Tibialis Posterior Tendon.** Ultrasound images (A) axial plane at medial malleolus and (B) sagittal plane over distal stump show absence of the tibialis posterior tendon at the medial malleolus *(open arrow)*. Note posterior tibial tendon *(arrowheads)* and retracted tendon stump *(curved arrows)* proximal to medial malleolus. *D,* Flexor digitorum longus tendon; *Tib,* tibia.

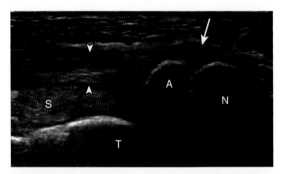

■ **FIGURE 8.80 Symptomatic Accessory Navicular.** Ultrasound image long axis to the distal tibialis posterior tendon *(arrowheads)* shows the accessory navicular *(A)*, adjacent navicular *(N)*, and soft tissue edema *(arrow)*. Note talus *(T)* and superomedial component of spring ligament *(S)*.

induced by focal pressure from the transducer over the accessory navicular synchondrosis is an indirect ultrasound finding of injury.

Lateral Ankle

TENOSYNOVITIS (LATERAL ANKLE)

Tenosynovitis of the peroneal tendons may occur at the level of the lateral malleolus, which appears anechoic from simple fluid (Fig. 8.81) or hypoechoic, isoechoic, or hyperechoic from complex fluid or synovial hypertrophy (Fig. 8.82).[64,65] Synovial tissue, although more commonly hypoechoic, may also appear isoechoic or hyperechoic relative to subcutaneous fat, which may simulate tendon (see Fig. 8.88). The presence of hyperemia on color Doppler imaging suggests that hypoechoic distention is from synovial hypertrophy, rather than from complex fluid.[56]

TENDINOSIS AND LONGITUDINAL TEAR (LATERAL ANKLE)

Tendinosis is also common at the lateral malleolus, appearing as abnormal hypoechogenicity with possible enlargement of the involved tendon, but without tendon fiber disruption (Fig. 8.83).[64,66,67] An enlarged or hypertrophied peroneal tubercle may be associated with peroneal tendon pathology, such as tendinosis (Fig. 8.84).[68,69] Well-defined abnormalities within the substance of the tendon could represent severe tendinosis (Fig. 8.85) or intrasubstance tendon tear (Fig. 8.86).

An abnormal hypoechoic or anechoic cleft that extends to the tendon surface is characteristic of a longitudinal tear (Figs. 8.87 and 8.88).[64,70] In the diagnosis of peroneal tendon tear, ultrasound has been shown to be 100% sensitive and 90% accurate.[66] Although involvement of either peroneal tendon is possible, the peroneus brevis tendon is more commonly torn, in part because of its more common location between the peroneus longus and fibula. Initially, the peroneus brevis tendon appears as a horseshoe shape that encompasses the peroneus longus tendon (see Fig. 8.82).[66] The two segments of peroneus brevis tendon may separate, best appreciated in short axis, and the peroneus longus tendon may be seen to interpose between the two peroneus brevis tendon pieces (Videos 8.25, 8.26, and 8.27).[66] One must not misinterpret echogenic synovial hypertrophy as a separate segment of tendon that would falsely indicate a longitudinal split tear. Toggling the

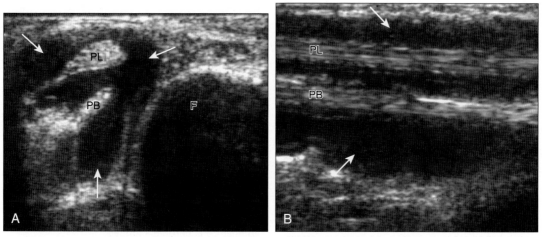

■ FIGURE 8.81 **Tenosynovitis: Peroneal Tendons.** Ultrasound images (A) short axis and (B) long axis to the peroneus longus *(PL)* and peroneus brevis *(PB)* tendons show anechoic and hypoechoic distention *(arrows)* of the tendon sheath. *F,* Fibula.

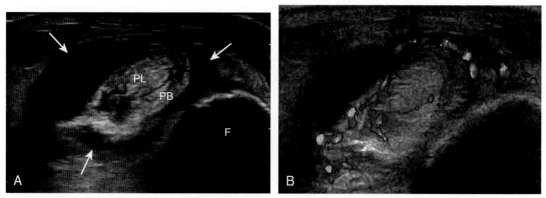

■ FIGURE 8.82 **Tenosynovitis: Peroneal Tendons.** Ultrasound images short axis to the peroneus longus *(PL)* and peroneus brevis *(PB)* tendons show anechoic distention *(arrows)* of the tendon sheath with hyperemia. Note horseshoe-shaped peroneus brevis indicating early longitudinal tear. *F,* Fibula.

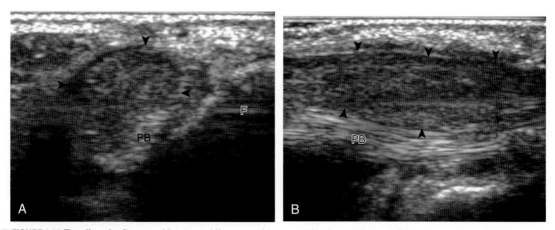

■ FIGURE 8.83 **Tendinosis: Peroneal Longus.** Ultrasound images (A) short axis and (B) long axis to peroneal tendons show hypoechoic enlargement of the peroneus longus *(arrowheads)*. *F,* Fibula; *PB,* peroneus brevis.

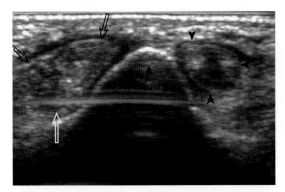

■ FIGURE 8.84 **Tendinosis: Enlarged Peroneal Tubercle.** Ultrasound image short axis to the peroneal tendons shows hypoechoic and swollen tendinosis of the peroneus brevis *(arrowheads)* and peroneus longus *(open arrows)* at an enlarged peroneal tubercle *(curved arrow).*

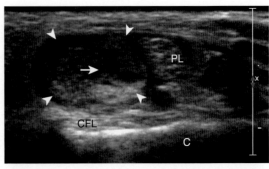

■ FIGURE 8.85 **Tendinosis: Peroneus Brevis Tendon.** Ultrasound image short axis to the enlarged peroneus brevis tendon *(arrowheads)* shows well-defined hypoechoic areas *(arrows)* with possible anechoic intrasubstance tear. *C,* Calcaneus; *CFL,* calcaneofibular ligament; *PL,* peroneus longus.

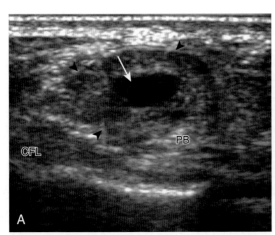

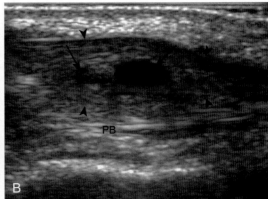

■ FIGURE 8.86 **Tendinosis and Intra-Substance Tear: Peroneal Longus.** Ultrasound images (A) short axis and (B) long axis to the peroneus longus *(arrowheads)* show a well-defined anechoic area *(arrows)* that disrupts the fibers within the peroneus longus tendon. Note coexisting hypoechoic and swollen tendinosis. *CFL,* Calcaneofibular ligament; *PB,* peroneus brevis.

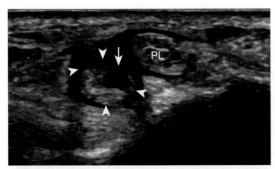

■ FIGURE 8.87 **Longitudinal Tear: Peroneal Brevis Tendon.** Ultrasound image short axis to peroneus brevis tendon *(arrowheads)* shows anechoic cleft that extends to tendon surface *(arrow).* Note mild hypoechoic tenosynovitis. *PL,* Peroneus brevis tendon.

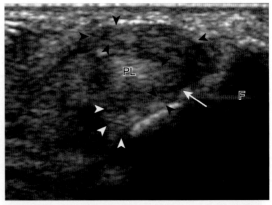

■ FIGURE 8.88 **Longitudinal Split Tear: Peroneal Brevis.** Ultrasound image transverse shows a horseshoe-shaped peroneus brevis tendon *(arrowheads)* with focal discontinuity *(arrow).* *F,* Fibula; *PL,* peroneus longus tendon.

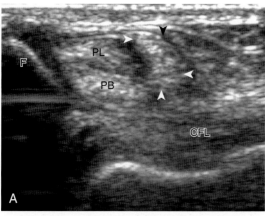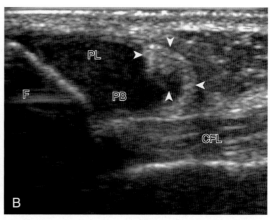

■ **FIGURE 8.89 Hyperechoic Synovial Hypertrophy.** Ultrasound image short axis to the peroneal tendons shows (A) hyperechoic tissue *(arrowheads)* adjacent to the peroneus longus *(PL)* and peroneus brevis *(PB)* tendons that may simulate tendon. Toggling the transducer shows (B) anisotropy of the peroneus longus *(PL)* and peroneus brevis *(PB)* tendons, whereas the hyperechoic synovial tissue *(arrowheads)* does not change in echogenicity thereby excluding a tendon fragment. *CFL,* Calcaneofibular ligament; *F,* fibula.

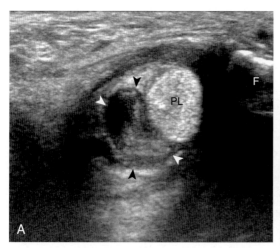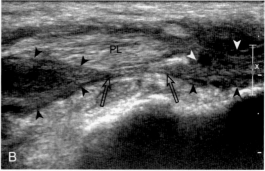

■ **FIGURE 8.90 Full-Thickness Complete Tear: Peroneal Brevis.** Ultrasound images (A) short axis and (B) long axis to the peroneal tendons show focal discontinuity *(open arrows)* of the peroneus brevis tendon *(arrowheads)*. *F,* Fibula; *PL,* peroneus longus.

transducer (see Fig. 1.3) causes the tendon tissue to become hypoechoic from anisotropy, whereas echogenic synovial tissue remains hyperechoic (Fig. 8.89).

COMPLETE TENDON TEAR (LATERAL ANKLE)

Full-thickness complete tears are characterized by full-width tendon fiber disruption, tendon stump retraction, and interposed hemorrhage or fluid in the torn tendon gap.[66] Such tears may occur at the level of the lateral malleolus (Fig. 8.90). More distally, a peroneus longus tendon tear may be associated with fracture of the os peroneum, a normal ossicle within the peroneus longus tendon at the level of the cuboid bone

(Fig. 8.91).[22] Because the normal os peroneum may be bipartite, correlation should be made with symptoms elicited by transducer pressure and degree of retraction of the fractured bone fragments, if present. Os peroneum fragment separation of 6 mm or more suggests os peroneum fracture and a full-thickness peroneus longus tendon tear (Video 8.28).[22] There is often significant proximal retraction of the torn tendon stump and os peroneum fragment, even to the level of the tibiotalar joint (Fig. 8.91C). Avulsion fracture of the base of the fifth metatarsal may also be seen related to plantar aponeurosis and the peroneus brevis tendon (Fig. 8.92).[71] Muscle or tendon injury may occur at any site if in contact with metal hardware (Fig. 8.93) (Video 8.29).

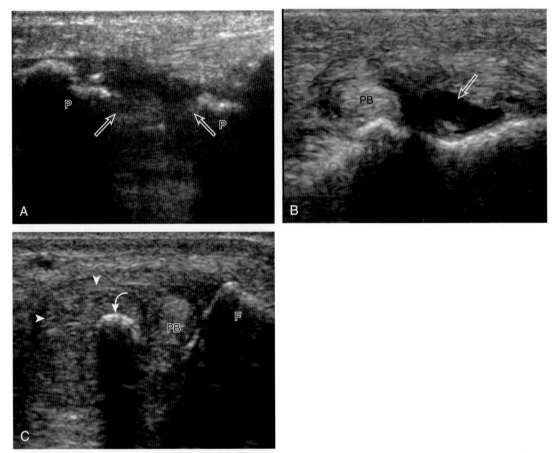

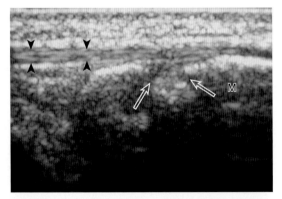

■ FIGURE 8.91 **Full-Thickness Tear: Peroneal Longus and Os Peroneum Fracture.** Ultrasound image (A) long axis to the distal peroneus longus shows fracture *(open arrows)* of the os peroneum *(P)* with distraction and full-thickness peroneus longus tear (left side of image is proximal). Ultrasound image from a different patient (B) short axis to the peroneal tendons over the peroneal tubercle shows absence of the peroneus longus tendon *(open arrow).* C, Proximally at the level of the distal fibula *(F),* the retracted os peroneum fracture fragment *(curved arrow)* and peroneus longus tendon stump *(arrowheads)* are identified. *PB,* Peroneus brevis.

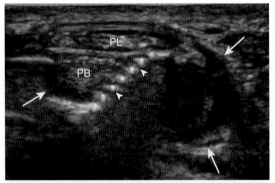

■ FIGURE 8.92 **Avulsion Fracture: Fifth Metatarsal Base.** Ultrasound image long axis to the distal peroneus brevis tendon *(arrowheads)* shows fracture *(open arrows)* at the base of the fifth metatarsal *(M).*

■ FIGURE 8.93 **Peroneus Brevis: Screw Impingement.** Ultrasound image short axis to the peroneus brevis tendon *(PB)* shows a threaded fibular screw *(arrowheads)* penetrating the peroneus brevis muscle *(arrows). PL,* Peroneus longus tendon.

TENDON SUBLUXATION AND DISLOCATION (LATERAL ANKLE)

At its attachment on the fibula, the superior peroneal retinaculum may be injured, which may appear as hypoechoic thickening or complete disruption with associated cortical irregularity (Fig. 8.94).[72] With complete retinaculum discontinuity, subluxation or dislocation of the peroneal tendons may occur, predisposing to tenosynovitis and tendon tear. Because tendon displacement may only occur transiently, dynamic ankle evaluation with dorsiflexion and eversion is often required for diagnosis of tendon displacement.[64,70,73] With peroneal tendon displacement, the superior peroneal retinaculum may be thickened and partially stripped away from the fibula, termed a *type 1 injury* (Fig. 8.95A) (Video 8.30).[8] With peroneal tendon subluxation or dislocation, the retinaculum may be detached, without (Fig. 8.95B) (Video 8.31) or with (Fig. 8.95C and D) a fibular avulsion bone fragment.[8] Intra-sheath peroneal tendon subluxation may also be demonstrated dynamically, which is associated with an abnormal convex posterior contour of the posterior fibula, low-lying peroneus brevis muscle, peroneus quartus, and subsequent tendon tear, but with an intact superior peroneal retinaculum (Fig. 8.96) (Videos 8.32, 8.33, 8.34, 8.35, and 8.36).[73,74] Less commonly, tendon subluxation may occur at the level of the peroneal tubercle.

NORMAL VARIANTS (LATERAL ANKLE)

The peroneus quartus is an accessory tendon found in up to 22% of ankles and is located adjacent to the peroneus brevis and longus tendons (Fig. 8.97).[9] At ultrasound, the peroneus quartus has a variable appearance representing hypoechoic muscle, hyperechoic tendon, or both.[9] If unrecognized, the accessory tendon can be misinterpreted as one of the segments of a peroneal tendon split tear. To differentiate between the two conditions, distal imaging is helpful because a peroneus quartus typically inserts onto the retrotrochlear eminence of the calcaneus, whereas a true longitudinal split follows the direction of the peroneal tendons, and the two tendon pieces eventually

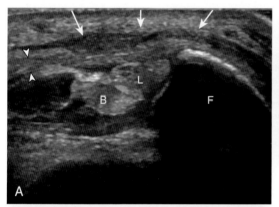

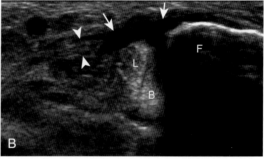

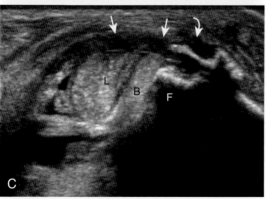

■ **FIGURE 8.94 Superior Peroneal Retinaculum Injury.** Ultrasound images short axis to the peroneal tendons in three patients show (A) hypoechoic thickening *(arrows)* and (B and C) disruption *(arrows)* of the superior peroneal retinaculum *(arrowheads)*. Note cortical irregularity *(curved arrow)* in C. *F,* Fibula; *B,* peroneus brevis; *L,* peroneus longus.

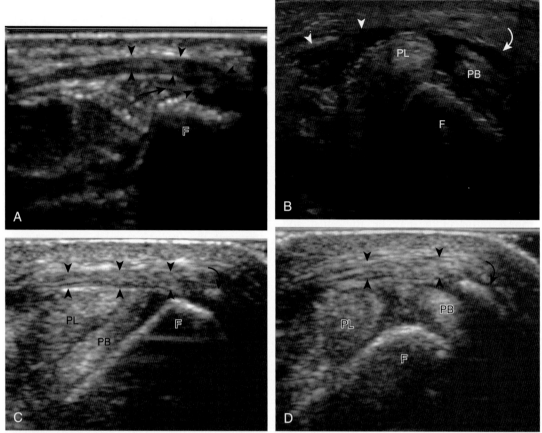

■ **FIGURE 8.95 Subluxation and Dislocation: Peroneal Tendons.** Ultrasound images in three patients short axis to the peroneal tendons show (A) transient peroneal subluxation into a type 1 retinaculum injury pouch *(arrow)* with thickened and hypoechoic superior peroneal retinaculum *(arrowheads)* and bone irregularity of the fibula *(F)*, (B) anterior peroneus longus *(PL)* dislocation and peroneus brevis *(PB)* subluxation with detachment *(curved arrow)* of the superior retinaculum *(arrowheads)* from the fibula *(F)*, and (C and D) superior peroneal retinaculum *(arrowheads)* avulsion fracture *(curved arrows)* from the fibula *(F)* with peroneus brevis dislocation *(PB)*, which is present only at dorsiflexion and eversion (D) (right side of images is anterior).

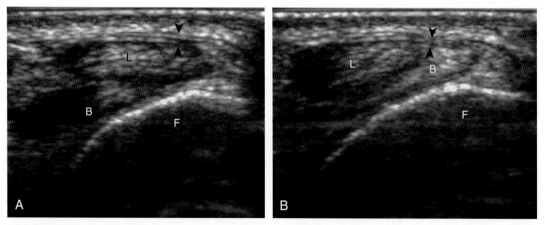

■ **FIGURE 8.96 Intra-Sheath Subluxation: Peroneal Tendons.** Ultrasound images short axis to peroneal tendons show abnormal movement of tendons with dynamic imaging between A and B (*arrowheads,* superior peroneal retinaculum). *B,* Peroneus brevis; *F,* fibula; *L,* peroneus longus.

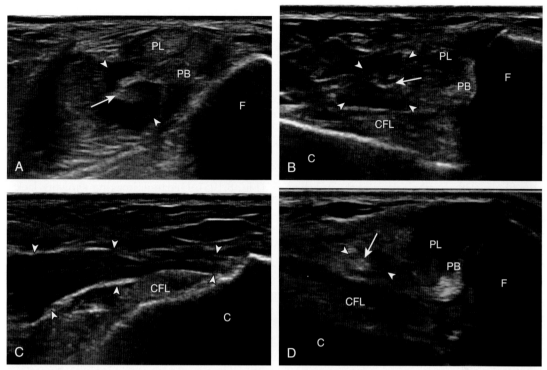

■ FIGURE 8.97 **Peroneus Quartus.** Ultrasound images short axis (A,B) and long axis (C) show the central hyperechoic tendon *(arrow)* and surrounding hypoechoic muscle *(arrowheads)* of the peroneus quartus, which inserts on the retrotrochlear eminence of the calcaneus *(C)*. Ultrasound image from a different patient (D) in short axis shows a similar peroneus quartus. *CFL,* Calcaneofibular ligament.

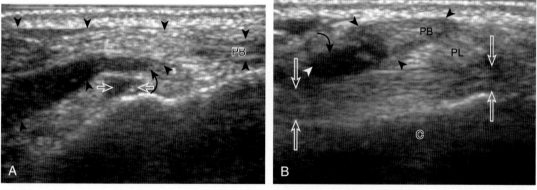

■ FIGURE 8.98 **Low-Lying Muscle Belly of Peroneus Brevis.** Ultrasound images (A) long axis and (B) short axis to peroneal tendons show tapering peroneus brevis *(arrowheads)* to tendon *(PB)* with muscle tissue that extends distally *(curved arrow)* beyond the fibula and over the calcaneofibular ligament *(open arrows). C,* Calcaneus; *PL,* peroneus longus.

reunite to reconstitute a normal peroneal tendon distally. In addition, the hyperechoic tendon is usually surrounded by hypoechoic muscle tissue, unlike a longitudinal split tear of the peroneus brevis. As another normal variant, the presence of a low-lying muscle belly of the peroneus brevis may predispose to peroneus tendon pathology, which is diagnosed when the peroneus brevis

muscle tissue is identified beyond the fibula (Fig. 8.98).[7]

TENDONS AS LIGAMENT RECONSTRUCTION (LATERAL ANKLE)

After injury to the lateral ligaments of the ankle, the peroneal tendons may be used in lateral ligament reconstruction.[75] In general, the peroneus brevis tendon may be surgically rerouted through a tunnel in the fibula and reattached to the fifth metatarsal, the peroneal brevis tendon may be split so that one segment is looped around the fibula and reattached to itself, or the peroneus brevis may be transected above the fibula and used through various tunnels in the fibula and calcaneus while still attached to the fifth metatarsal.[75] At ultrasound, the peroneus brevis split segment may be followed from distal to proximal as it enters into the anterior aspect of the fibula, exits the fibula posteriorly, and then is reattached to itself (Fig. 8.99). The anterior talofibular ligament may also be directly repaired (see Fig. 8.135).

Anterior Ankle and Anterior Lower Leg

TENDON PATHOLOGY (ANTERIOR ANKLE/LOWER LEG)

Pathology of the anterior tendons is less common than of other areas of the ankle, but similar findings of tenosynovitis (Figs. 8.100 and 8.101) (Video 8.37), tendinosis (Fig. 8.102), and tendon tear may occur.[76] With a full-thickness tendon tear, the collapsed tendon sheath distal to a retracted tendon should not be mistaken for intact tendon (Fig. 8.103). Dynamic imaging showing lack of tendon movement excludes partial-thickness tear and confirms a complete tear (Video 8.38). As a possible variation of normal, the distal tibialis

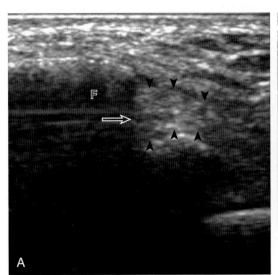

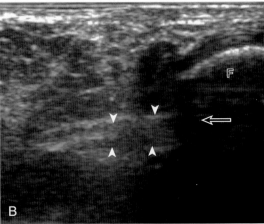

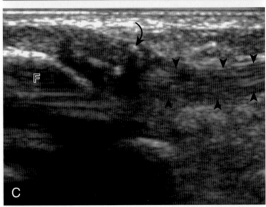

■ **FIGURE 8.99 Lateral Ankle Ligament Reconstruction (Chrisman-Snook Procedure).** Ultrasound image (A) long axis to the peroneus brevis shows the peroneus brevis tendon *(arrowheads),* which enters into a tunnel *(open arrow)* from the anterior aspect of the fibula *(F).* Ultrasound image (B) long axis to the peroneus brevis shows the peroneus brevis tendon *(arrowheads),* which leaves the fibular tunnel *(open arrow)* from the posterior aspect. Ultrasound image (C) long axis to the peroneus brevis shows peroneus brevis tendon with suture material *(curved arrow)* reattached to the native peroneus brevis tendon *(arrowheads).* F, Fibula.

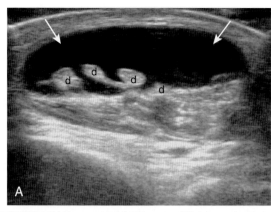

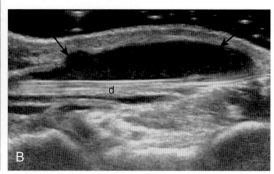

■ FIGURE 8.100 **Tenosynovitis: Extensor Digitorum Longus.** Ultrasound images (A) short and (B) long axis to extensor digitorum *(d)* show hypoechoic complex fluid *(arrows)* distention of the tendon sheath.

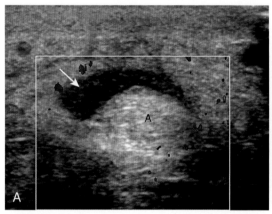

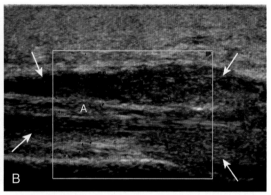

■ FIGURE 8.101 **Septic Tenosynovitis: Tibialis Anterior.** Ultrasound color Doppler images (A) short and (B) long axis to tibialis anterior tibialis show hypoechoic complex fluid *(arrows)* distention of the tendon sheath.

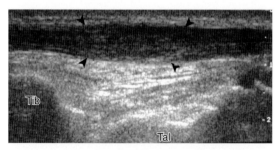

■ FIGURE 8.102 **Tendinosis: Tibialis Anterior.** Ultrasound image long axis to the tibialis anterior tendon shows hypoechoic fusiform enlargement *(arrowheads)* without tendon fiber disruption. *Tal,* Talus; *Tib,* tibia.

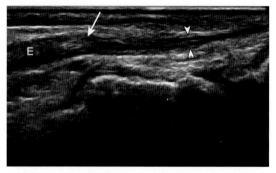

■ FIGURE 8.103 **Full-Thickness Tear: Extensor Hallucis Longus.** Ultrasound image long axis to extensor hallucis tendon *(E)* shows a complete tear with tendon stump retraction *(arrow).* Note collapsed tendon sheath distally *(arrowheads).*

anterior tendon may have a longitudinal split near its insertion.[77] Findings that suggest a tendon tear rather than normal variation include associated symptoms, pain with transducer pressure, and tendon hyperemia on color Doppler imaging. Most tibialis anterior tendon tears occur within 3 cm of its insertion, although full-thickness

tibialis anterior tendon tears may retract significantly and produce a mass-like area at the tendon stump, possibly associated with an avulsion fracture fragment (Fig. 8.104).[77] Other avulsion fractures may occur, such as extensor digitorum brevis

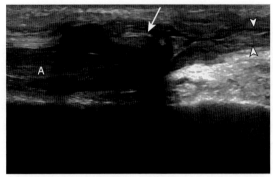

■ **FIGURE 8.104 Full-Thickness Tear and Avulsion: Tibialis Anterior.** Ultrasound image long axis to tibialis anterior tendon *(A)* shows a complete tear with tendon stump retraction containing an avulsion fracture fragment *(arrow)*. Note collapsed tendon sheath distally *(arrowheads)* and shadowing from ossific fragment.

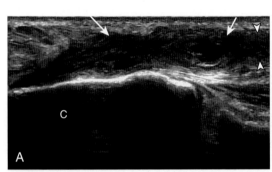

■ **FIGURE 8.105 Tear: Extensor Digitorum Brevis.** Ultrasound images long axis to extensor digitorum *(arrowheads)* in two different patients show (A) hypoechoic tear *(arrows)* and (B) hyperechoic avulsion fracture fragment *(arrow)*. C, Calcaneus.

avulsion from the calcaneus (Fig. 8.105). Tendon abnormalities may also result from abnormal contact between a tendon and fixation hardware (Fig. 8.106) (Video 8.39).[63] An injured superior extensor retinaculum will appear hypoechoic and thickened (Fig. 8.107).[72]

MUSCLE HERNIA (ANTERIOR ANKLE/LOWER LEG)

Other types of anterior compartment disorders include muscle hernias, which most commonly involve the tibialis anterior, although other muscle compartments may be involved (Fig. 8.108). At ultrasound, a muscle hernia is characterized by muscle tissue that extends superficial to and beyond the enveloping fascial layer.[78] A well-defined defect in the thin hyperechoic fascia may be seen, usually at the site of a perforating vessel. A muscle hernia may also occur at a site of intact but thinned fascia.[79] Dynamic imaging with joint movement, muscle contraction, or the patient standing may be needed to demonstrate the muscle hernia, which may be transient and absent at rest (Videos 8.40, 8.41, and 8.42).[78,79]

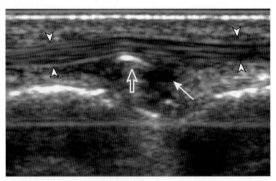

■ **FIGURE 8.106 Tendon Displacement: Hardware.** Ultrasound image shows the extensor hallucis tendon *(arrowheads)* is displaced by protruding screw *(open arrow)* with adjacent edema *(arrow)*.

Posterior Ankle

PARATENDINITIS AND TENDINOSIS (POSTERIOR ANKLE)

Abnormalities of the Achilles tendon may involve the tendon itself or surrounding tissues. Because the Achilles tendon does not possess a true tendon sheath but rather a paratenon, abnormal hypoechoic swelling or anechoic fluid immediately adjacent to the tendon represents paratendinitis (or paratenonitis) (Fig. 8.109).[80] Tendinosis, a degenerative process, appears as abnormal tendon hypoechogenicity but without disruption of the tendon fibers (Figs. 8.110, 8.111, and 8.112).[81] The term *tendinosis* is used rather than *tendinitis* because no true inflammation is present.[81] Tendinosis may be focal within a tendon segment or may diffusely involve the tendon diameter with fusiform

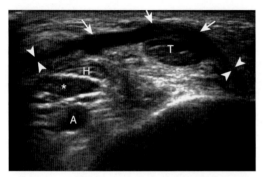

■ FIGURE 8.107 **Superior Extensor Retinaculum Injury.** Ultrasound image short axis to tibialis anterior tendon *(T)* at level of distal tibia shows hypoechoic thickening *(arrows)* of the superior extensor retinaculum *(arrowheads)* (*asterisk,* extensor hallucis longus muscle). *A,* Anterior tibial artery; *H,* extensor hallucis longus tendon.

enlargement.[81] Achilles tendon abnormalities such as tendinosis may demonstrate increased flow on color Doppler imaging (Video 8.43). Not present in normal Achilles tendons, increased blood flow has been shown to represent neovascularity and not inflammation, and is associated with patient symptoms.[82] Power Doppler imaging demonstrates more flow than conventional color Doppler imaging, which originates from the deep or anterior surface of the tendon.[82] When evaluating for Achilles tendon flow, the transducer should be floated on a thick layer of gel as the slightest amount of pressure from the transducer may obliterate visible flow in the Achilles tendon and surrounding soft tissues (Video 8.44). In addition, dorsiflexion at the foot may also obliterate visible blood flow as the Achilles tendon is stretched. When enthesophytes are identified at the distal Achilles tendon, common degenerative enthesopathy should not be confused with inflammatory enthesopathy, the latter of which will show hyperemia, adjacent tendon abnormality, possible erosions, and ill-defined enthesophyte borders at ultrasound and radiography.[83,84]

PARTIAL-THICKNESS ACHILLES TEAR (POSTERIOR ANKLE)

Partial-thickness Achilles tendon tears may initially appear as a more defined hypoechoic or anechoic

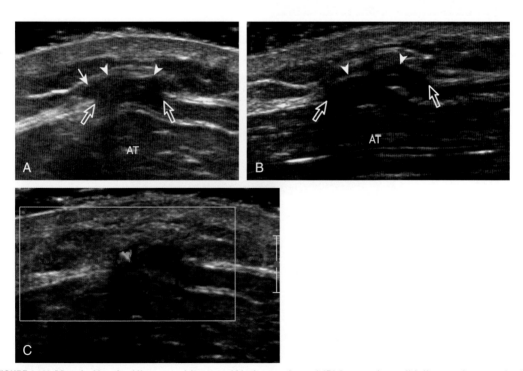

■ FIGURE 8.108 **Muscle Hernia.** Ultrasound images (A) short axis and (B) long axis to tibialis anterior muscle *(AT)* show defect in the fascia *(between open arrows)* and muscle hernia *(arrowheads)*. Note perforating vessel *(arrow)* in A and flow in C.

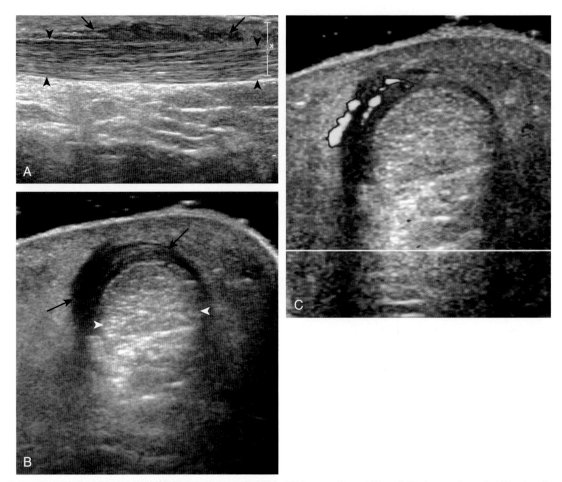

■ **FIGURE 8.109 Achilles Paratendinitis.** Ultrasound images (A) long axis and (B and C) short axis to Achilles tendon *(arrowheads)* show adjacent hypoechoic soft tissue thickening *(arrows)* with increased flow on power Doppler imaging.

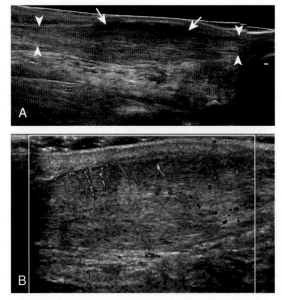

■ **FIGURE 8.110 Tendinosis: Achilles.** Ultrasound (A) gray scale and (B) color Doppler images long axis to the Achilles tendon *(arrowheads)* show hypoechoic swelling *(arrows)* without tendon fiber discontinuity. Note increased blood flow representing neovascularity in B.

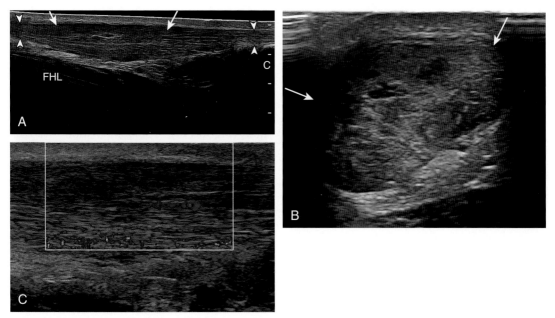

■ **FIGURE 8.111 Tendinosis: Achilles.** Ultrasound images (A) long axis (extended field of view) and (B) short axis to the Achilles tendon *(arrowheads)* show diffuse hypoechoic swelling *(arrows)* without tendon fiber discontinuity. Note neovascularity in (C). *FHL,* Flexor hallucis longus; *C,* calcaneus.

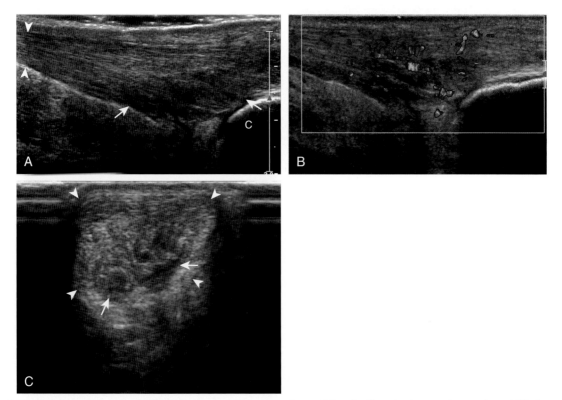

■ **FIGURE 8.112 Tendinosis: Achilles.** Ultrasound (A) gray scale and (B) color Doppler images long axis and (C) short axis to the Achilles tendon *(arrowheads)* show hypoechoic swelling *(arrows)* and increased blood flow from neovascularity without tendon fiber discontinuity. *C,* Calcaneus.

area or cleft within the tendon that partially disrupts tendon fibers (Fig. 8.113);[85] Achilles tendon enlargement greater than 1 cm and significant intrinsic tendon abnormalities indicate a partial-thickness tear in addition to underlying tendinosis.[81] Partial-thickness tears may involve the musculotendinous junction (Fig. 8.114), where

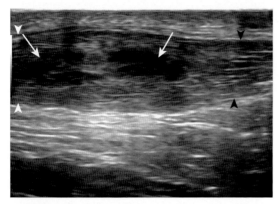

■ **FIGURE 8.113 Partial-Thickness Tear: Mid-Achilles.** Ultrasound image long axis to Achilles tendon *(arrowheads)* shows with fusiform hypoechoic swelling and focal anechoic fiber disruption *(arrows)*.

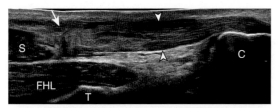

■ **FIGURE 8.114 Partial-Thickness Tear: Proximal Achilles.** Ultrasound image long axis to Achilles tendon shows focal anechoic fiber disruption *(arrows)* at the musculotendinous junction with distal tendinosis *(arrowheads)*. *S,* Soleus; *FHL,* flexor hallucis longus; *T,* tibia; *C,* calcaneus.

dynamic ultrasound evaluation with ankle dorsiflexion and plantar flexion is used to demonstrate tendon fiber continuity to exclude full-thickness tendon tear (Video 8.45). Achilles tendinosis and partial-thickness tears may also involve the distal aspect of the Achilles tendon, often associated with cortical irregularity of the calcaneus and adjacent retrocalcaneal or retro-Achilles bursal fluid (Fig. 8.115). The combination of a distal Achilles tendon abnormality, adjacent bursal distention (retrocalcaneal and retro-Achilles), and prominence of the posterosuperior corner of the calcaneus is termed *Haglund syndrome* (see Fig. 8.61).[50]

FULL-THICKNESS ACHILLES TEAR (POSTERIOR ANKLE)

Full-thickness tears of the Achilles tendon are characterized by complete tendon fiber disruption and tendon retraction, commonly 2 to 6 cm proximal to the calcaneal attachment (Fig. 8.116).[86] The torn tendon ends are hypoechoic with the proximal stump tapered and the distal stump displaced anteriorly toward Kager fat pad. There is often posterior acoustic shadowing from refraction at the tendon stumps, a helpful indirect sign of tear that may be overlooked unless a larger field of view is used.[86] The torn tendon gap may fill with mixed echogenicity fluid or hemorrhage, or possibly a portion of the adjacent hyperechoic fat pad.[87]

One important pitfall in the setting of a full-thickness Achilles tendon tear is the presence of an intact plantaris tendon at the medial aspect of the Achilles tendon that may simulate intact Achilles tendon fibers (Fig. 8.117) (Video 8.46).[86] The plantaris tendon is usually intact in the setting of a full-thickness Achilles tendon tear, which

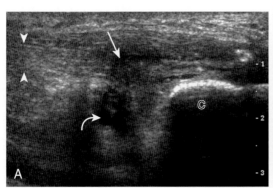

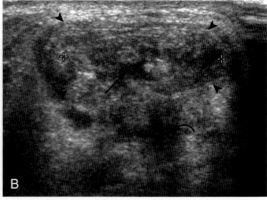

■ **FIGURE 8.115 Partial-Thickness Tear: Distal Achilles.** Ultrasound images (A) long axis and (B) short axis to the Achilles tendon *(arrowheads)* show diffuse fusiform hypoechoic swelling and focal tendon tear anteriorly *(arrows)* *(curved arrow,* retrocalcaneal bursa). *C,* Calcaneus.

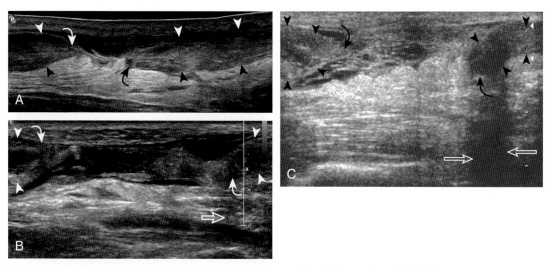

■ FIGURE 8.116 **Full-Thickness Tear: Achilles.** Ultrasound images (A to C) long axis to the Achilles tendon *(arrowheads)* in three patients show full-thickness tear between torn tendon stumps *(curved arrows)* and interposed hemorrhage. Note posterior acoustic shadowing *(open arrows)* deep to the tendon stumps, tapered hypoechoic appearance of the Achilles tendon at the tear, and variable hypoechoic hemorrhage.

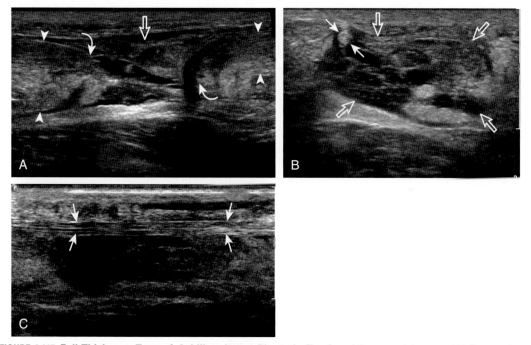

■ FIGURE 8.117 **Full-Thickness Tear of Achilles: Intact Plantaris Tendon.** Ultrasound images (A) long axis and (B) short axis to the Achilles tendon *(arrowheads)* show retracted tendon stumps *(curved arrows)* at site of tear *(open arrows)*. C, Note intact plantaris tendon *(arrows)* in long axis located at medial aspect of tendon tear. Plantaris tendon is also shown in B.

may be related to the fact that the plantaris is a stronger tendon compared to the Achilles.[88] The distal Achilles tendon may also avulse a bone fragment from the calcaneus (Fig. 8.118), which may be large in size in diabetic patients.

With a suspected full-thickness Achilles tendon tear, using dynamic imaging is essential to ensure an accurate diagnosis. With passive ankle dorsi-flexion and plantar flexion, tendon retraction at the tear becomes more obvious because one tendon stump moves without translation of move-ment to the other tendon stump (Videos 8.47 and 8.48). This becomes important in the setting of a subacute or chronic tendon tear, in which

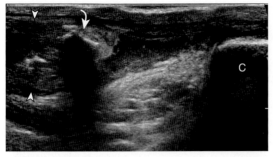

■ **FIGURE 8.118 Achilles Avulsion at Calcaneus.** Ultrasound image long axis to the Achilles tendon *(arrowheads)* shows hyperechoic fracture fragment *(curved arrow)* proximally displaced from the calcaneus *(C)* (right side of image is distal). Note posterior acoustic shadowing deep to ossific fragment.

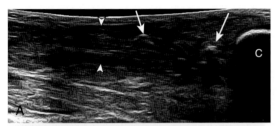

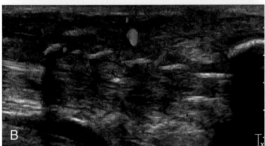

■ **FIGURE 8.119 Achilles Tendon: Primary Repair.** Ultrasound images long axis to the Achilles tendon *(arrowheads)* show hypoechoic and swollen tendon with hyperechoic suture *(arrows)* and neovascularity at site of repair. *C,* Calcaneus.

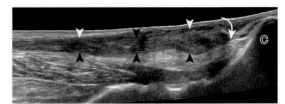

■ **FIGURE 8.120 Achilles Tendon: Re-tear.** Ultrasound extended field of view image long axis to the Achilles tendon *(arrowheads)* shows hypoechoic and swollen tendon with distal full-thickness re-tear *(curved arrow).* *C,* Calcaneus.

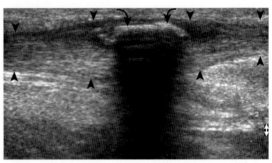

■ **FIGURE 8.121 Achilles Tendon Ossification.** Ultrasound images (A) long axis and (B) short axis to the Achilles tendon *(arrowheads)* show hyperechoic and shadowing ossification *(curved arrows)* within the thickened Achilles tendon.

MISCELLANEOUS ACHILLES PATHOLOGY (POSTERIOR ANKLE)

Other Achilles tendon abnormalities include ossification of the Achilles tendon, associated with prior trauma, surgery, and ankle immobilization (Fig. 8.121).[90] Ultrasound can also identify xanthoma deposition in the Achilles tendon, which represents xanthoma cells, extracellular cholesterol, giant cells, and inflammatory cells, seen in heterozygous familial hypercholesterolemia.[91] Such deposits range from focal hypoechoic nodules to a heterogeneously hypoechoic swollen Achilles tendon (Fig. 8.122).[92]

Calf

MEDIAL GASTROCNEMIUS (CALF)

Proximal to the Achilles tendon, the calf muscles and tendons may be injured. One of the most commonly injured structures is the medial head of the gastrocnemius where it tapers distally over the soleus, also called *tennis leg* (Fig. 8.123).[11,93] At this site, the tendon fibers are disrupted at the aponeurosis with anechoic or hypoechoic fluid or hemorrhage with variable degrees of tendon retraction.[94] The patient can usually indicate the site of injury based on the location of symptoms.

hemorrhage and scar tissue may simulate tendon fibers, and, in fact, partial healing may be present (Video 8.49). If conservative management of a full-thickness Achilles tendon is being considered, the distance of residual distraction at the tendon stumps in neutral and plantar flexion may affect management decisions (Video 8.50).[89] After surgical repair, the intact Achilles tendon may be heterogeneous and hypoechoic with hyperechoic suture material, although tendon fiber continuity should be seen (Fig. 8.119) (Video 8.51). A full-thickness recurrent tear of the Achilles tendon repair typically shows tendon retraction (Fig. 8.120).

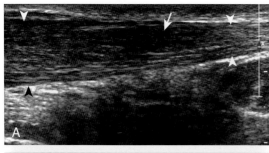

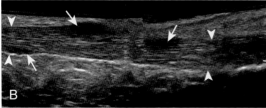

■ **FIGURE 8.122 Xanthoma Deposition: Achilles Tendon.** Ultrasound images from two patients long axis to the Achilles tendon *(arrowheads)* show focal hypoechoic xanthoma deposits *(arrows)*.

A remote injury at this site will show increased echogenicity and distortion of the normal fiber architecture (Fig. 8.124).[95]

PLANTARIS (CALF)

Another calf abnormality is a plantaris tendon injury.[96,97] A partial-thickness tear appears as a hypoechoic and irregular but intact tendon. A complete tear will appear as a tubular anechoic or mixed-echogenicity fluid collection between the muscle bellies of the medial gastrocnemius and soleus with lack of visualization of the plantaris tendon or tendon discontinuity (Fig. 8.125).[96,97] These findings are commonly located more proximally in the calf compared with a medial head of the gastrocnemius tear. Distal medial head of the gastrocnemius and plantaris tears may occur together.

OTHER MUSCLES (CALF)

Injuries to the soleus and lateral gastrocnemius muscles may occur less commonly, often the result of a direct injury (Fig. 8.126).[11] Although a hematoma may occur in this setting or in patients predisposed to bleeding, the finding of an intramuscular hematoma, especially if spontaneous, should raise concern for underlying primary malignancy or metastasis as a cause for the hemorrhage (Fig. 8.127). As a normal variation, an accessory soleus muscle can be identified adjacent to the Achilles tendon in the Kager fat pad, which inserts either on the Achilles or onto the calcaneus

(Fig. 8.128). Although this may present clinically as a mass, its normal muscle echotexture at sonography and characteristic location are diagnostic for accessory soleus muscle.[98,99] Injury to an accessory soleus may also occur (Fig. 8.129).[100]

Plantar Foot
PLANTAR FASCIOPATHY (PLANTAR FOOT)

Abnormalities of the plantar aponeurosis may take several forms.[101] A common abnormality represents hypoechoic thickening (>4 mm) of the proximal plantar fascia at the calcaneal origin, best measured in long axis (Fig. 8.130).[27,102] Although termed *plantar fasciitis*, findings may relate to repetitive microtrauma, repair of microtears, degeneration, or edema.[27,101] An acute injury of the plantar fascia may cause hypoechoic thickening if partially torn (Fig. 8.131) or complete disruption with heterogeneous hemorrhage if a full-thickness tear.

PLANTAR FIBROMATOSIS (PLANTAR FOOT)

Another abnormality that involves the plantar fascia at the central and medial aspect of the foot arch is plantar fibromatosis.[103] This condition represents fibroblastic proliferation, often at multiple sites in the plantar fascia and bilateral. At ultrasound, plantar fibromatosis appears as hypoechoic or isoechoic fusiform nodules or masses that cause thickening of the plantar fascia and may extend in a dorsal or plantar direction from the plantar fascia (Fig. 8.132) (Videos 8.52 and 8.53).[104,105] These nodules uncommonly show significant vascularity.[103] Because the appearance of plantar fibromatosis is not specific for one diagnosis at ultrasound, the location of the abnormality and its multiplicity (seen in up to 26%) or bilaterality (seen in up to 36%) suggests the diagnosis of plantar fibromatosis.[103]

■ LIGAMENT ABNORMALITIES
General Comments

The lateral ankle is a common site for ligament injury. At ultrasound, partial ligament tears are characterized by hypoechoic thickening of the involved ligament, but some continuous ligament fibers are still seen.[106] An acute full-thickness ligament tear is characterized by discontinuity or non-visualization of the ligament and replacement with hypoechoic or heterogeneous tissue that represents the torn ligament and hemorrhage.[106] Osseous avulsions appear as hyperechoic bone fragments with possible shadowing attached to the involved ligament. Depending on the severity, evaluation of a remote ligament tear may show

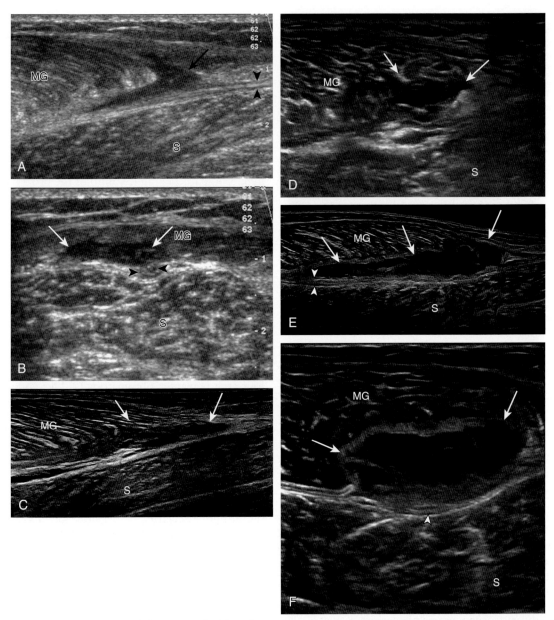

■ **FIGURE 8.123 Medial Head of Gastrocnemius Tear: Acute.** Ultrasound images long axis and short axis to the distal medial head of gastrocnemius *(MG)* in three patients (A/B, C/D, E/F) show mixed echogenicity but predominantly hypoechoic tear *(arrows)* at the aponeurosis with variable retraction (*arrowheads,* plantaris). *S,* Soleus.

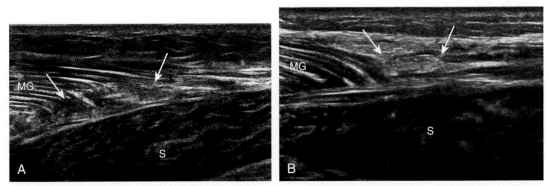

■ **FIGURE 8.124 Medial Head of Gastrocnemius Tear: Remote.** Ultrasound images in two patients long axis to the distal medial head of gastrocnemius *(MG)* show a hyperechoic scar and disorganization *(arrows)* at site of prior tear. *S,* Soleus.

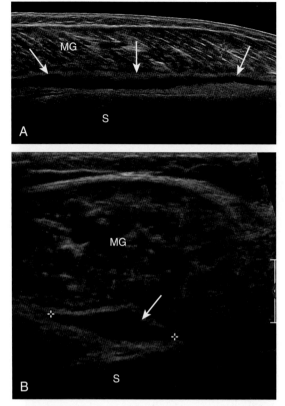

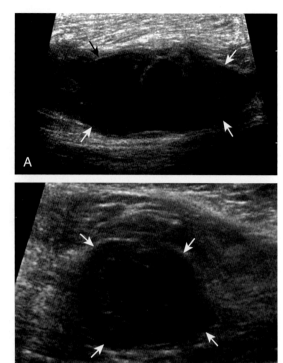

■ FIGURE 8.125 **Plantaris Tear.** Ultrasound images (A) long and (B) short axis to the medial head of gastrocnemius *(MG)* show anechoic fluid *(arrows* and *between cursors* in B) in the expected location of the plantaris tendon. *S,* Soleus.

■ FIGURE 8.127 **Metastasis.** Ultrasound images (A) long axis and (B) short axis to gastrocnemius show heterogeneous but predominantly hypoechoic intra-muscular metastasis *(arrows).*

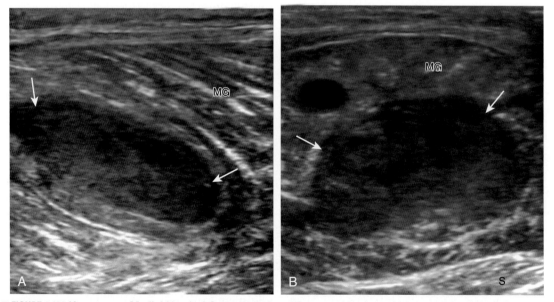

■ FIGURE 8.126 **Hematoma: Medial Head of Gastrocnemius.** Ultrasound images (A) long axis and (B) short axis to the medial head of the gastrocnemius *(MG)* show heterogeneous hypoechoic to isoechoic hemorrhage *(arrows).* *S,* Soleus.

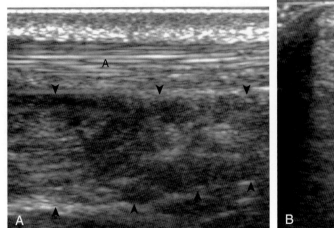
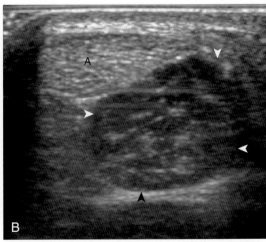

■ **FIGURE 8.128 Accessory Soleus Muscle.** Ultrasound images (A) long axis and (B) short axis to the distal Achilles tendon *(A)* show accessory soleus muscle *(arrowheads).*

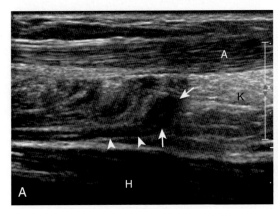
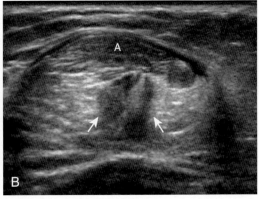

■ **FIGURE 8.129 Injury: Accessory Soleus Muscle.** Ultrasound images (A) long axis and (B) short axis to the accessory soleus muscle *(arrowheads)* show abnormal hypoechogenicity *(arrows). A,* Achilles tendon; *H,* flexor hallucis longus muscle; *K,* Kager fat pad.

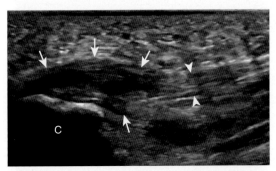

■ **FIGURE 8.130 Plantar Fasciopathy.** Ultrasound image long axis to the proximal plantar aponeurosis *(arrowheads)* shows hypoechoic thickening *(arrows). C,* Calcaneus.

non-visualization or a thickened ligament. Bone fragments may persist, but lack of pain with transducer pressure is a helpful indicator that the injury was remote.

Anterior Talofibular and Calcaneofibular Ligaments

Of the lateral ankle ligaments, the anterior talofibular ligament is most commonly torn, isolated, or in combination with calcaneofibular ligament tear (in up to 70% of patients).[106] Isolated tears of the calcaneofibular ligament are not common, whereas posterior talofibular ligament tears are rare.[106] Ultrasound has been shown to be effective in evaluation for anterior talofibular ligament tears (Fig. 8.133).[107] Dynamic imaging that elicits an anterior drawer sign is helpful in equivocal cases (Video 8.54).[108] This can be

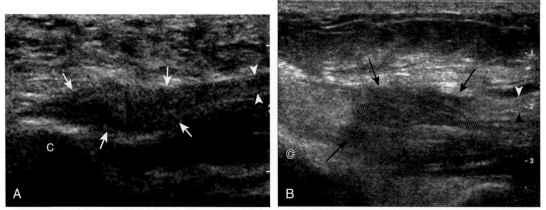

■ FIGURE 8.131 **Plantar Aponeurosis Injury.** Ultrasound images (A and B) long axis to the plantar aponeurosis *(arrowheads)* in two patients show abnormal hypoechoic thickening *(arrows)*. *C,* Calcaneus.

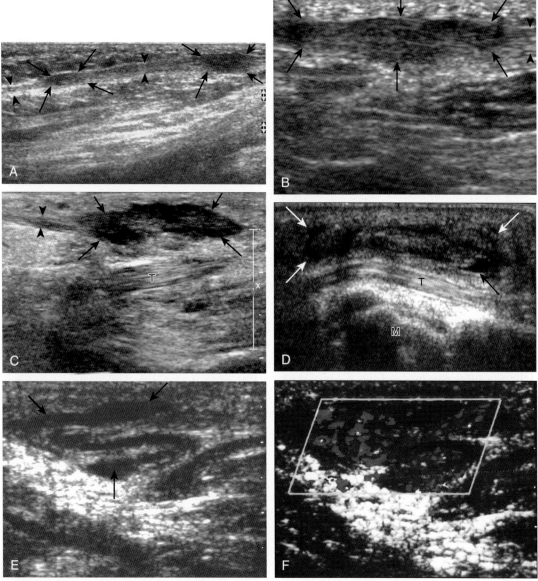

■ FIGURE 8.132 **Plantar Fibromatosis.** Ultrasound images (A–F) from five patients show hypoechoic nodules and masses *(arrows)* of plantar aponeurosis *(arrowheads)*. Note vascular channels and increased blood flow on color Doppler imaging in E and F (same patient). *M,* First metatarsal head; *T,* flexor tendons. *(D: From Pham H, Fessell DP, Femino JE, et al: Sonography and MR imaging of selected benign masses in the ankle and foot. AJR Am J Roentgenol 180:99-107, 2003.)*

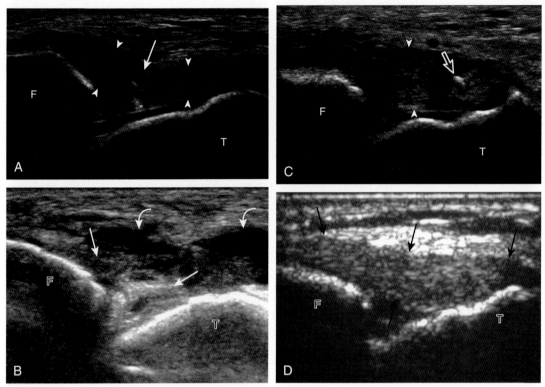

■ **FIGURE 8.133 Anterior Talofibular Ligament: Injury.** Ultrasound images long axis to the anterior talofibular ligament from four patients show (A) discontinuity *(arrow)* of the anterior talofibular ligament *(arrowheads)*, (B) heterogeneous mixed-echogenicity non-visualization *(arrows)* of the anterior talofibular ligament with adjacent hemorrhage *(curved arrows)*, (C) hypoechoic thickening *(arrowheads)* with a hyperechoic avulsion fracture fragment *(open arrow)*, and (D) hypoechoic thickening without ligament discontinuity *(arrows)* or symptoms representing remote injury. *F,* Fibula; *T,* talus.

accomplished with the patient lying prone, placing the transducer long axis to the anterior talofibular ligament, and then manually applying anterior directed stress over the heel and observing asymmetrical anterior translation of the talus relative to the fibula. A calcaneofibular ligament tear typically appears as abnormal hypoechoic swelling at the calcaneal attachment (Fig. 8.134). With dorsiflexion, continued laxity of the calcaneofibular ligament and lack of displacement of the peroneal tendons away from the calcaneus can be an indirect sign of a complete calcaneofibular ligament tear.[109] After ligament injury, lateral ankle ligament surgical reconstruction may involve a direct ligament repair (Fig. 8.135) or the peroneus brevis tendon (see Fig. 8.99).[75]

Anterior Inferior Tibiofibular Ligament

Another important lateral ankle ligament is the anterior inferior tibiofibular ligament. Injury to this ligament resembles other ligament injuries showing abnormal hypoechogenicity and fiber discontinuity (Fig. 8.136).[106] Dynamic imaging with the foot in dorsiflexion and eversion will often show widening between the distal tibia and fibula at the site of the ligament tear.[110] When an anterior inferior tibiofibular ligament tear is present, the interosseous membrane between the tibia and fibula should also be evaluated for tear (Fig. 8.137).[25] Also termed a *high ankle sprain,* this injury is associated with prolonged morbidity if it is not accurately diagnosed and treated.[111] The presence of an anterior inferior tibiofibular ligament tear should raise suspicion for an interosseous membrane injury, while a normal tibiofibular ligament excludes an interosseous membrane injury and predicts a shorter return to play in an athlete.[111] With a high ankle sprain, the superiorly transmitted force may propagate through the interosseous membrane proximally and exit as a high fibular fracture, which is termed a *Maisonneuve fracture* (Fig. 8.137B).[25] The fibular fracture appears as a cortical step-off at ultrasound with focal pain elicited with transducer pressure. This type of injury may also be associated with an isolated posterior or medial malleolus fracture of the tibia and deltoid ligament tear.[112]

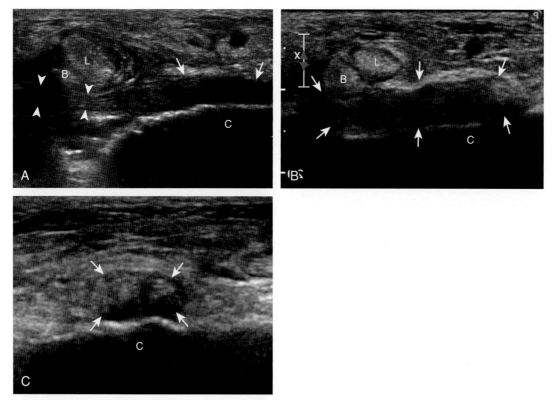

■ FIGURE 8.134 Calcaneofibular Ligament: Injury. Ultrasound image (A) long axis to the calcaneofibular ligament *(arrowheads)* shows hypoechoic thickening of distal calcaneofibular ligament *(arrows)* at calcaneus *(C).* Ultrasound images (B) long axis and (C) short axis to the calcaneofibular ligament in a second patient show diffuse hypoechoic thickening *(arrows).* L, Peroneus longus; B, peroneus brevis.

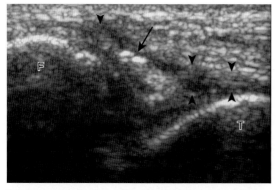

■ FIGURE 8.135 Anterior Talofibular Ligament: Primary Repair (Broström Procedure). Ultrasound image long axis to the anterior talofibular ligament shows echogenic suture *(arrow)* and hypoechoic but continuous anterior talofibular ligament fibers *(arrowheads).* F, Fibula; T, talus.

Deltoid Ligament

Deltoid ligament tears are more difficult to diagnose at ultrasound, largely because this structure represents the confluence of several ligaments with possible variability.[16,113] Although each of the individual components of the deltoid ligament can be evaluated in the normal ankle, deltoid ligament injuries typically produce hypoechoic swelling that involves several components with possible ligament discontinuity and associated hyperechoic avulsion fracture fragments (Fig. 8.138).[106,114] Pain with transducer pressure directly over the deltoid ligament is further evidence to support acute injury. In the presence of distal fibula fracture, ultrasound is an accurate method to identify associated deltoid ligament injury.[115] The spring ligament may also be injured, which can appear as hypoechoic thickening of the superomedial calcaneonavicular ligament, often associated with adjacent tibialis posterior tendon abnormality (Fig. 8.139).[21]

Other Ligaments

Other ligament injuries around the foot and ankle are often manifested by bone avulsion fragments or malalignment of the osseous structures. Although these smaller and less commonly injured ligaments are not routinely evaluated with ultra-

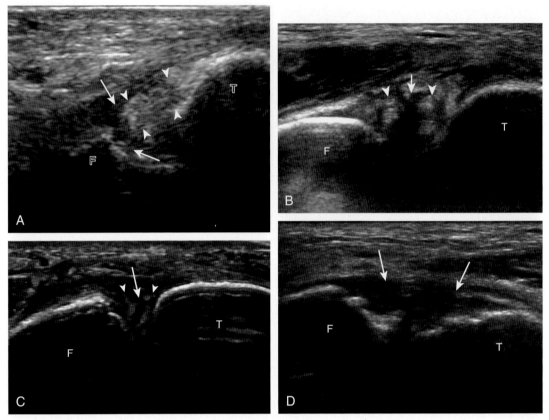

■ FIGURE 8.136 **Anterior Inferior Tibiofibular Ligament: Injury.** Ultrasound images long axis to the anterior inferior tibiofibular ligament from four patients after acute injury show hypoechoic discontinuity *(arrows)* of the anterior inferior tibiofibular ligament *(arrowheads)*. *F,* Fibula; *T,* tibia.

sound, a patient may direct examination to an area of ligament injury based on symptoms. Examples include avulsion of the talonavicular ligament (Fig. 8.140A), calcaneocuboid ligament (Fig. 8.140B), and bifurcate ligament attachment on the anterior process of the calcaneus (Fig. 8.140C), which should not be confused with extensor digitorum brevis avulsion (see Fig. 8.105B).[116] In addition, abnormal widening and hypoechoic hemorrhage between the medial cuneiform and second metatarsal base can indirectly suggest Lisfranc ligament disruption (Fig. 8.141).[117] Tear of the dorsal tarsometatarsal ligament between the medial cuneiform and second metatarsal base, which can be identified at ultrasound, is another indirect sign of a tear of Lisfranc ligament proper.[117] A normal variant os intermetatarsus, located between the first and second metatarsal bases, should not be mistaken for a Lisfranc ligament injury–related fracture fragment (Fig. 8.142). Location of the os intermetatarsus distal to the middle cuneiform and normal tarsometatarsal alignment assists in this

differentiation. Potentially associated with ligament injury of the metatarsophalangeal joint, plantar plate injuries are characterized by abnormal hypoechogenicity or a hypoechoic cleft at the attachment of the plantar plate to the proximal phalanx (Fig. 8.143) (Video 8.55). Subsequent hypoechoic pericapsular fibrosis may result (Fig. 8.144), which should not be mistaken for a Morton neuroma (see Fig. 8.149).

■ FRACTURE

Although it is understood that radiography should be the initial imaging method of choice to evaluate for fracture, it is not uncommon for a radiographically occult fracture to be identified at ultrasound. There are many osseous structures in the ankle and foot, and therefore it is not practical to assess each osseous structure routinely for abnormality. To identify a fracture at ultrasound, one relies on the patient to direct examination based on point tenderness or the focal point of symptoms. It

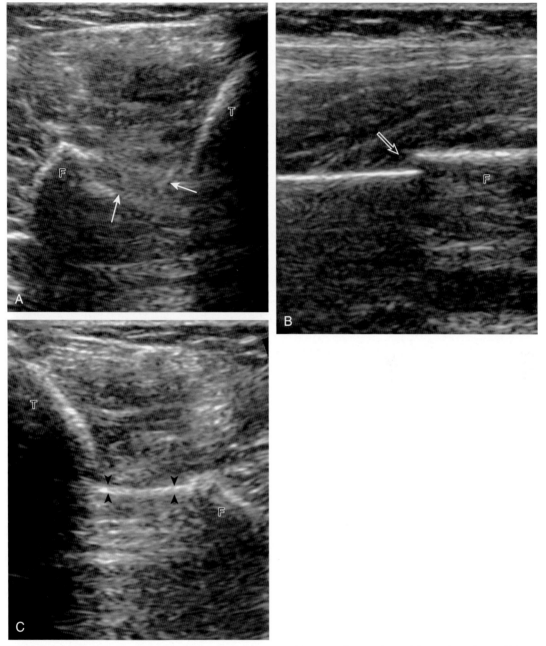

■ FIGURE 8.137 **Maisonneuve Fracture.** Transverse ultrasound image of anterolateral lower leg shows (A) non-visualization of the interosseous membrane *(arrows)*. Coronal ultrasound of proximal lateral fibula shows (B) cortical step-off fracture *(open arrow)*. Transverse ultrasound image of contralateral asymptomatic leg shows (C) normal interosseous membrane *(arrowheads)*. *F,* Fibula; *T,* tibia.

is critical, before completion of an ultrasound examination of the foot or ankle, to ask the patient to indicate any focal site of symptoms. Identification of a cortical step-off of the normally smooth and echogenic cortical surface is diagnostic for fracture, especially if it is associated with pain from transducer pressure.[118] Knowledge of the normal osseous structures and their articulations is essential to not mistake a joint space for a displaced fracture. One may image the normal contralateral foot and ankle for comparison. Stress fractures may also be diagnosed with ultrasound, which can appear as cortical irregularity, thickened periosteum, and hyperemia.[119]

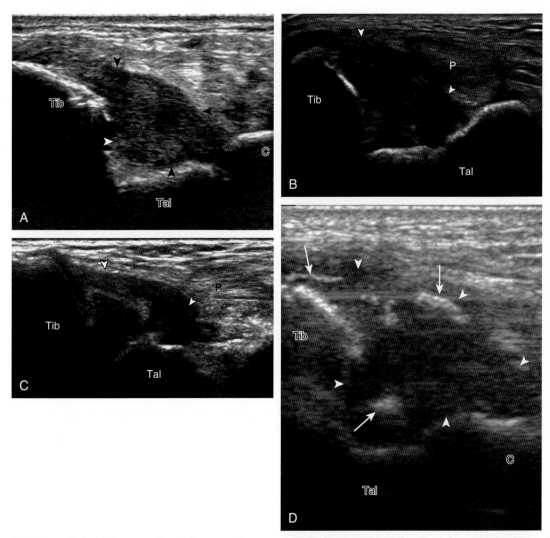

■ **FIGURE 8.138 Deltoid Ligament Tear.** Ultrasound images at the medial malleolus in the coronal or oblique coronal plane from four patients show hypoechoic swelling of the deltoid ligament *(arrowheads)*. Note involvement of the posterior tibiotalar component in (B) and fracture fragments *(arrows)* in (D). *C,* Calcaneus; *Tal,* talus; *Tib,* tibia, *P,* tibialis posterior tendon.

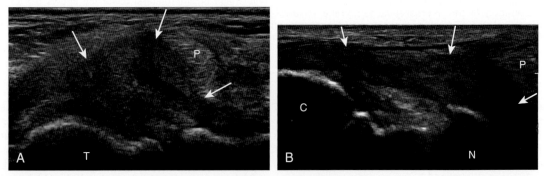

■ **FIGURE 8.139 Spring Ligament: Injury.** Ultrasound images from two patients show hypoechoic thickening *(arrows)* of the superomedial calcaneonavicular ligament. *P,* Tibialis posterior tendon; *T,* talus; *C,* calcaneus.

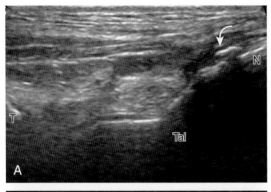

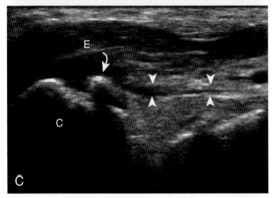

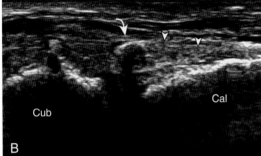

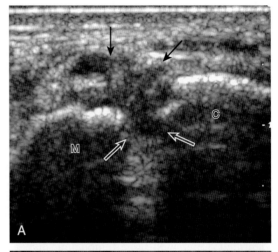

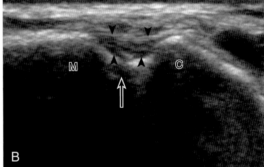

■ FIGURE 8.141 **Lisfranc Ligament Tear.** Ultrasound image in the coronal plane between the medial cuneiform (C) and second metatarsal base (M) shows (A) abnormal widening (open arrows), hypoechoic hemorrhage (arrows), and non-visualization of the dorsal tarso-metatarsal ligament. Asymptomatic comparison shows (B) normal dorsal tarsometatarsal ligament (arrowheads) and normal distance and alignment (open arrow) between medial cuneiform (C) and second metatarsal base (M).

■ FIGURE 8.140 **Other Avulsion Fractures.** Ultrasound sagittal images long axis to each respective ligament (arrowheads) show avulsion fractures (curved arrows) at the (A) talonavicular ligament, (B) calcaneocuboid ligament, and (C) bifurcate ligament. T, Tibia; Tal, talus; N, navicular; Cub, cuboid; Cal, calcaneus; C, anterior process of calcaneus; E, extensor digitorum brevis muscle.

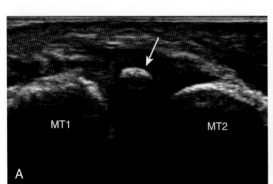

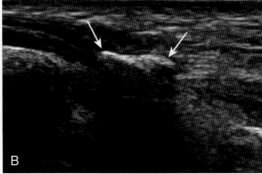

■ FIGURE 8.142 **Os Intermetatarsus.** Ultrasound images in the (A) coronal and (B) sagittal planes between the first (MT1) and second (MT2) metatarsals show the hyperechoic and shadowing os intermetatarsus (arrows).

Acute fractures may occur at tendon or ligament attachments, and these were discussed earlier, in the tendon and ligament sections of this chapter. Besides these locations, acute fractures may occur essentially anywhere in the foot and ankle, related to the mechanism of injury. For example, distal fibular (Fig. 8.145A) and proximal fifth metatarsal (see Fig. 8.92) fractures are associated with inversion ankle injuries.[120] Stress fractures of bone classically involve the metatarsal shafts (Fig. 8.145B and C), the navicular bone (usually in the sagittal plane) (Fig. 8.146A), and the hallux sesamoids (Fig. 8.146B).[121] With stress fractures, early ultrasound findings include focal hypoechogenicity along the cortex from hematoma or periostitis.[122] A step-off deformity or fracture line may also be identified. Later with bone remodeling, hyperechoic callous formation becomes evident (Fig. 8.145C). Ultrasound can also diagnose physeal

injuries in children, which appear as adjacent hypoechoic hemorrhage or edema and possible wide or irregular physis and adjacent subperiosteal hematoma.[123] Although difficult to visualize, cortical irregularity and collapse of the metatarsal head (commonly the second) can indicate Freiberg disease, which is fracture and necrosis of the metatarsal head from repetitive trauma (Fig. 8.147). Ultrasound has been used to assess callous formation after static interlocked nail placement for tibia fracture (Fig. 8.148).[121]

■ PERIPHERAL NERVE ABNORMALITIES

Morton neuroma is a non-neoplastic enlargement of a common plantar digital nerve as a result of nerve entrapment or trauma characterized by perineural fibrosis, vascular proliferation, endoneurium edema, and axonal degeneration.[124] The most common sites for Morton neuroma are the second and third web spaces at the level of the metatarsal heads.[124,125] At ultrasound, Morton neuroma appears as a hypoechoic mass, which is more likely symptomatic when it is greater than 5 mm (Fig. 8.149).[126] In the coronal plane, the neuroma often extends in a plantar direction from between the metatarsal heads with concave borders medial and lateral.[127] In the sagittal plane, identification of the hypoechoic common plantar digital nerve, which enters into the neuroma, ensures the diagnosis.[124] This finding, along with plantar location and non-compressibility of the mass, helps to exclude intermetatarsal bursal distention as a cause for a hypoechoic mass (Video 8.56). Compression of the neuroma between the transducer at the plantar aspect and the examiner's finger over the dorsal aspect of the foot should reproduce the patient's symptoms related to the neuroma. Dynamic evaluation with application

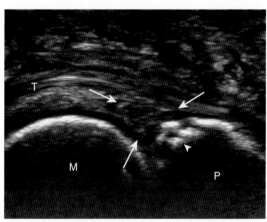

■ **FIGURE 8.143 Plantar Plate: Injury.** Ultrasound image in sagittal plane over plantar foot shows hypoechoic plantar plate *(arrows)* with cortical irregularity *(arrowhead)* at the proximal phalanx *(P)* attachment. *T,* Flexor tendon; *M,* metatarsal head.

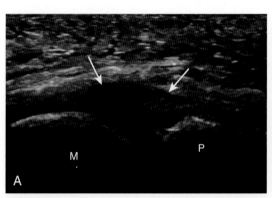
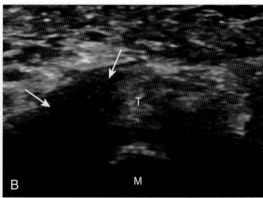

■ **FIGURE 8.144 Pericapsular Fibrosis.** Ultrasound image in parasagittal plane over plantar foot medial to plantar plate shows hypoechoic pericapsular fibrosis *(arrows)*. *M,* Metatarsal head; *P,* proximal phalanx; *T,* flexor tendon.

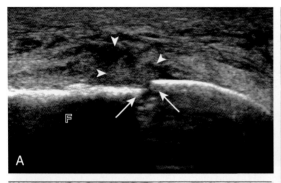

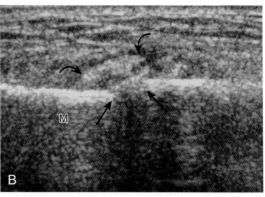

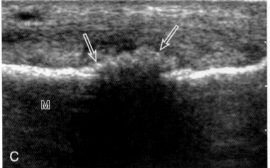

■ **FIGURE 8.145 Fractures: Fibula and Metatarsal.** Ultrasound image (A) of the fibula *(F)* shows fracture step-off deformity *(arrows)* and adjacent hypoechoic and isoechoic hemorrhage *(arrowheads)*. Ultrasound images of the metatarsal shaft *(M)* in two patients show (B) fracture step-off *(arrows)* and hyperechoic callus *(curved arrows)* and (C) bone remodeling and bridging callus *(open arrows)*. *(C: From Craig JG, Jacobson JA, Moed BR: Ultrasound of fracture and bone healing. Radiol Clin North Am 37:737-751, ix, 1999.)*

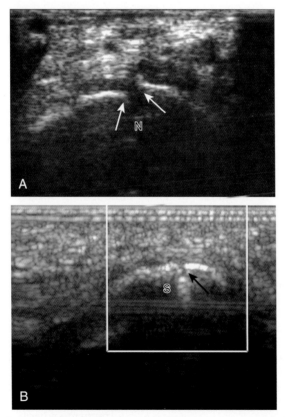

■ **FIGURE 8.146 Fractures: Navicular and Sesamoid.** Ultrasound image in the coronal plane shows (A) step-off and mild displacement *(arrows)* of navicular *(N)* stress fracture. Ultrasound image in the sagittal plane shows (B) fracture *(arrow)* of a hallux sesamoid *(S)*.

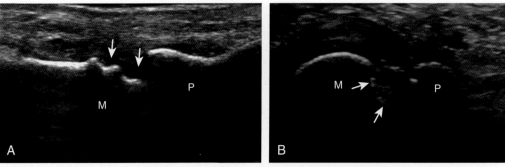

■ **FIGURE 8.147 Freiberg Disease.** Ultrasound images over dorsal (A) and plantar (B) aspects of the second metatarsal head in two patients show cortical irregularity *(arrows)* of the metatarsal head (*M*). *P*, Proximal phalanx.

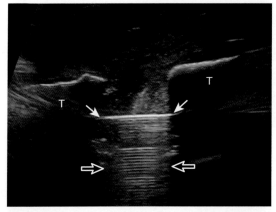

■ **FIGURE 8.148 Tibia Fracture: Non-Union.** Ultrasound image long axis to tibial *(T)* shaft at site of fracture shows visualization of the hyperechoic metal intramedullary nail *(arrows)* with posterior reverberation artifact *(open arrows)* with no overlying callus.

of opposed medial and lateral force to compress the metatarsal heads may displace a neuroma in a plantar direction and cause a palpable click (the sonographic Mulder sign), which can increase diagnostic confidence (Fig. 8.150) (Videos 8.57 and 8.58).[29] This dynamic maneuver can increase sensitivity of ultrasound in diagnosis of an intermetarsal mass from 65% to 100%.[128] It is not uncommon for Morton neuromas to be associated with intermetatarsal bursal distention, which can appear as an adjacent compressible anechoic fluid collection, usually in a more dorsal location.[129] An isolated intermetarsal bursa may be hypoechoic similar to a Morton neuroma but is typically compressible, not associated with the common plantar digital nerve or neuroma-like symptoms (Fig. 8.151), and is usually asymptomatic if located in the first through third interspaces and less than 3 mm in width.[54] Additionally, a Morton neuroma should be differentiated from pericapsular fibrosis associated with a plantar plate injury (see Fig. 8.144).

Another example of nerve entrapment involves the tibial nerve in the tarsal tunnel, which is an enclosed space posterior to the distal tibia bound by the flexor retinaculum that contains the tibial nerve and medial tendons. Tibial nerve entrapment at this site, called *tarsal tunnel syndrome*, may be secondary to a ganglion cyst (Fig. 8.152) (Video 8.59) or varicosities (Fig. 8.153) (Video 8.60), although any space-occupying process can have the same effect.[12,130] Another cause for symptoms related to the tibial nerve is a peripheral nerve sheath tumor (see Fig. 2.58), where its possible eccentric location relative to the nerve, hypoechoic appearance, and increased through-transmission should not be mistaken for a complex ganglion cyst (Fig. 8.154) (Video 8.61).[131] Another site prone to nerve compression is the superficial peroneal nerve where it pierces the crural fascia at an average of 9 cm proximal to the fibular tip.[10] A neuroma can form at this site, appearing swollen and hypoechoic, owing to traction injury, thickened fascia, or muscle hernia (Fig. 8.155) (see Video 8.42).[12,132]

Trauma to a peripheral nerve may cause findings at ultrasound that range from hypoechoic swelling to complete nerve discontinuity with

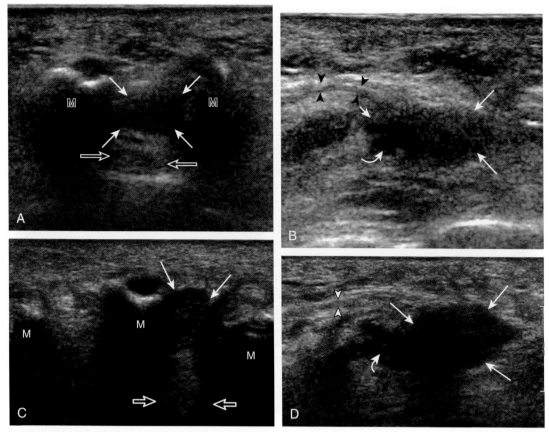

■ **FIGURE 8.149 Morton Neuroma.** Ultrasound images in the coronal and sagittal planes in two patients (A/B and C/D) show hypoechoic Morton neuroma *(arrows)*. Note hypoechoic common plantar digital nerve *(arrowheads)* continuous with the neuroma and increased through-transmission *(open arrows)* and associated anechoic inter-metatarsal bursa *(curved arrow)*. M, Metatarsal heads.

retraction. In the setting of nerve transection, neuroma formation is an expected response as the nerve attempts to regenerate, which appears as hypoechoic swelling of the terminal nerve end (Figs 8.156 and 8.157).[133] Peripheral nerve sheath tumors are discussed in Chapter 2.

■ MASSES AND CYSTS

In evaluation of a foot or ankle mass, the differential diagnosis is largely based on the anatomic location of the mass and if it originates from a joint, from the bone, or from the soft tissues apart from a joint.[129] Most joint processes that may manifest as a mass are synovial proliferative disorders, such as pigmented villonodular synovitis (see Fig. 8.37)[33] or synovial chondromatosis (see Fig. 8.38). Similarly, a well-defined hypoechoic mass arising from a tendon sheath commonly represents a giant cell tumor of the tendon sheath (pigmented villonodular tenosynovitis) (Fig. 8.158).[134] Masses visualized at ultrasound that arise

from bone may be malignant or aggressive (Fig. 8.159) (see Chapter 2) and are best evaluated with radiography and MRI. Regarding other soft tissue masses, ultrasound may differentiate cystic and solid masses and may guide percutaneous biopsy or aspiration.

The most common benign mass in the foot and ankle is a ganglion cyst.[135] Classically, a ganglion cyst is anechoic, with increased through-transmission and no associated mass (Fig. 8.160).[135] However, most ganglion cysts are hypoechoic, multilocular, and lobular. In addition, the viscous nature of the fluid may create low-level echoes within the cyst. Location of a ganglion cyst within the tarsal tunnel may compress the tibial nerve (see Fig. 8.152) (see Video 8.59). Ganglion cysts of the foot and ankle may show communication with adjacent joints or tendon sheaths and involve the sinus tarsi. A ganglion cyst should be differentiated from a bursa, such as the Gruberi bursa between the extensor digitorum longus tendons and the talus (see Fig. 8.64).[3] A fluid collection that is unilocular, compressible, and in the

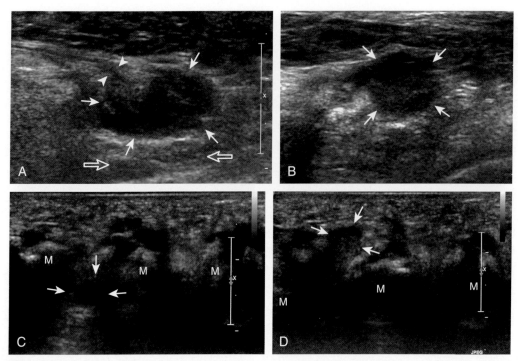

■ **FIGURE 8.150 Morton Neuroma.** Ultrasound images in the sagittal plane scanned from (A) plantar and (B) dorsal show hypoechoic Morton neuroma *(arrows)*. Note hypoechoic common plantar digital nerve *(arrowheads)* continuous with the neuroma and increased through-transmission *(open arrows)*. Ultrasound images in the coronal plane in neutral (C) and with side-to-side compression of metatarsals (D) show plantar displacement of the Morton neuroma *(arrows)*, which produced symptoms. *M, Metatarsal heads.*

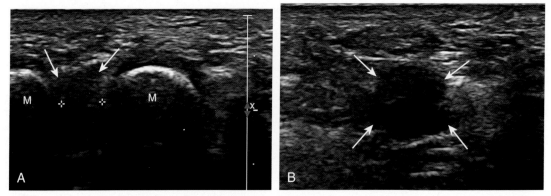

■ **FIGURE 8.151 Intermetatarsal Bursa.** Ultrasound images in the (A) coronal and (B) sagittal planes show hypoechoic intermetarsal bursa *(arrows)*. Note absence of common plantar digital nerve associated with the bursa. *M, Metatarsal heads.*

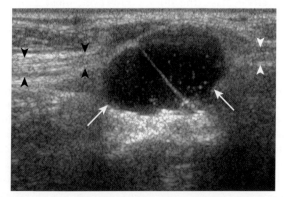

■ **FIGURE 8.152 Tarsal Tunnel Syndrome: Ganglion Cyst.** Ultrasound image long axis to tibial nerve *(arrowheads)* shows ganglion cyst *(arrows)* causing nerve compression. Note internal echoes of cyst and increased through-transmission.

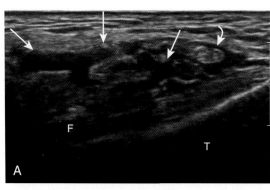

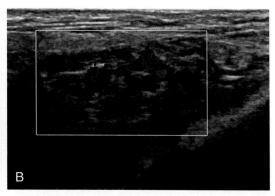

■ FIGURE 8.153 **Tarsal Tunnel Syndrome: Varicosities.** Ultrasound images short axis to tibial nerve *(curved arrow)* shows varicosities *(arrows)* within tarsal tunnel. *F,* Flexor hallucis longus; *T,* tibia.

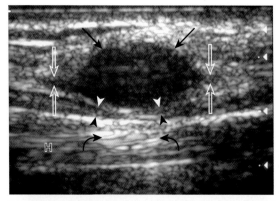

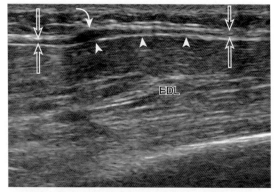

■ FIGURE 8.154 **Schwannoma: Tibial Nerve.** Ultrasound image shows a hypoechoic schwannoma *(arrows)* that originates from a portion of the tibial nerve *(open arrows)* with compression of other tibial nerve fibers *(arrowheads)*. Note increased through-transmission *(curved arrows)*. *H,* Flexor hallucis longus tendon. *(From Reynolds Jr DL, Jacobson JA, Inampudi P, et al: Sonographic characteristics of peripheral nerve sheath tumors. AJR Am J Roentgenol 182:741-744, 2004.)*

■ FIGURE 8.155 **Superficial Peroneal Nerve Neuroma From Muscle Hernia.** Ultrasound image long axis to superficial peroneal nerve *(open arrows)* shows hypoechoic swelling *(curved arrow)* where nerve penetrates fascia at site of a focal muscle hernia *(arrowheads)*, present only during muscle contraction. *EDL,* Extensor digitorum longus.

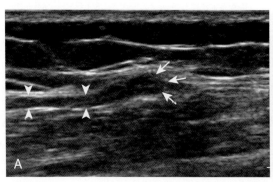

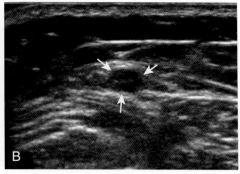

■ FIGURE 8.156 **Traumatic Neuroma: Superficial Peroneal Nerve.** Ultrasound images (A) long and (B) short axis to superficial peroneal nerve *(arrowheads)* show hypoechoic terminal nerve swelling *(arrows)* at transection site.

anatomic location of a bursa indicates bursal etiology, in contrast to a ganglion cyst that is usually non-compressible and multilocular.[3] Ultrasound can be used to guide percutaneous aspiration, in which a large-bore needle is often needed because of the high viscosity of the cyst contents. In evaluation of the lateral ankle, the normal calcaneofibular ligament in cross section

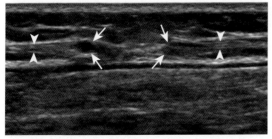

■ **FIGURE 8.157 Traumatic Neuromas: Sural Nerve.** Ultrasound image long axis to sural nerve *(arrowheads)* shows hypoechoic swelling *(arrows)* at the nerve ends at site of transection. Note degree of retraction.

may appear hypoechoic as a result of anisotropy and should not be misinterpreted as a small ganglion cyst (see Fig. 8.18C and D).

Another type of cyst that may involve the foot is an epidermal inclusion cyst, with implantation of epidermis into the dermis or subcutis from trauma proposed as one cause.[136] At ultrasound, an epidermal inclusion cyst typically appears hypoechoic to surrounding tissues but with low-level internal echoes and a hypoechoic rim and increased through-transmission, which at times may simulate a solid mass; internal linear echogenic or dark clefts are a characteristic feature (Fig. 8.161).[137] Increased blood flow on color Doppler imaging and lobulated margins are more likely after cyst rupture.[138] Another soft tissue abnormality to consider when evaluating a plantar mass or potential foreign body is a plantar wart, which characteristically appears hypoechoic with arterial blood flow (Fig. 8.162).[139]

Other benign and malignant masses that are not specific to the foot and ankle are discussed in Chapter 2.[140] Plantar fibromatosis (see Fig. 8.132)

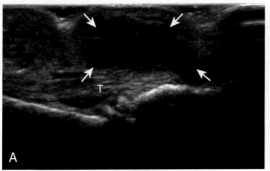
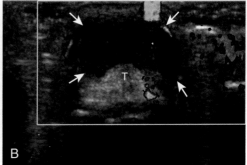

■ **FIGURE 8.158 Giant Cell Tumor of Tendon Sheath.** Ultrasound images (A) long axis and (B) short axis to flexor tendons *(T)* of second toe show hypoechoic mass *(arrows)* in contact with tendon. Note increased through-transmission.

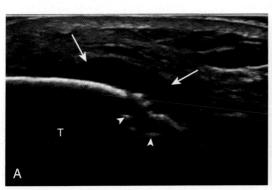
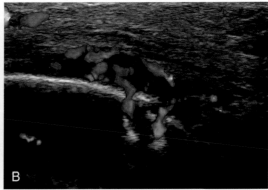

■ **FIGURE 8.159 Osteomyelitis.** Ultrasound images over tibia show hypoechoic periostitis *(arrows)* with hyperemia and cortical disruption *(arrowheads)* representing osteomyelitis.

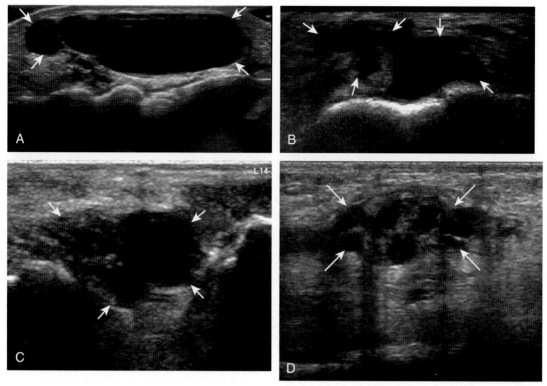

■ **FIGURE 8.160 Ganglion Cysts.** Ultrasound images (A–D) from four patients show anechoic to hypoechoic ganglion cysts *(arrows),* with features of internal echoes, lobulations, multiple locules, septations, and increased through-transmission. Note (C) location of the ganglion cyst in the sinus tarsi.

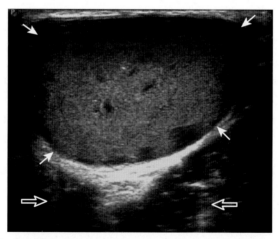

■ **FIGURE 8.161 Epidermal Inclusion Cyst.** Ultrasound image shows heterogeneous hypoechoic cyst with internal low level echoes *(arrows),* vague hypoechoic halo, characteristic internal echogenic and dark clefts, and increased through-transmission *(open arrows).*

was discussed earlier in this chapter. One must also consider the possibility of an inflammatory process that simulates a soft tissue mass, such as a chronic foreign body reaction (see Chapter 2). Other causes for palpable mass include muscle hernia (see Fig. 8.108) and accessory soleus muscle (see Fig. 8.128). Soft tissue masses associated with inflammatory arthritis include rheumatoid nodule (see Fig. 8.48), adventitious bursa (see Fig. 8.62), and gouty tophi (see Fig. 8.53).

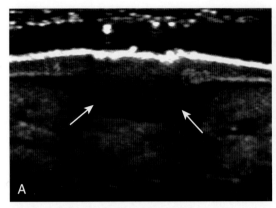
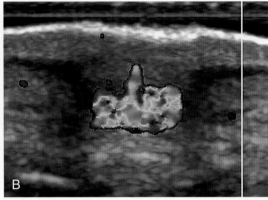

■ **FIGURE 8.162 Plantar Wart.** Ultrasound image shows hypoechoic plantar wart extending deep from dermis *(arrows)* with characteristic arterial flow at base.

SELECT REFERENCES

11. Delgado GJ, Chung CB, Lektrakul N, et al: Tennis leg: clinical US study of 141 patients and anatomic investigation of four cadavers with MR imaging and US. *Radiology* 224(1):112–119, 2002.

12. Martinoli C, Court-Payen M, Michaud J, et al: Imaging of neuropathies about the ankle and foot. *Semin Musculoskelet Radiol* 14(3):344–356, 2010.

16. Campbell KJ, Michalski MP, Wilson KJ, et al: The ligament anatomy of the deltoid complex of the ankle: a qualitative and quantitative anatomical study. *J Bone Joint Surg Am* 96(8):e62, 2014.

20. Sconfienza LM, Orlandi D, Lacelli F, et al: Dynamic high-resolution US of ankle and midfoot ligaments: normal anatomic structure and imaging technique. *Radiographics* 35(1):164–178, 2015.

38. Taljanovic MS, Melville DM, Gimber LH, et al: High-resolution US of rheumatologic diseases. *Radiographics* 35(7):2026–2048, 2015.

45. Thiele RG: Role of ultrasound and other advanced imaging in the diagnosis and management of gout. *Curr Rheumatol Rep* 13(2):146–153, 2011.

49. Kaeley GS: Review of the use of ultrasound for the diagnosis and monitoring of enthesitis in psoriatic arthritis. *Curr Rheumatol Rep* 13(4): 338–345, 2011.

64. Lee SJ, Jacobson JA, Kim SM, et al: Ultrasound and MRI of the peroneal tendons and associated pathology. *Skeletal Radiol* 42(9):1191–1200, 2013.

78. Beggs I: Sonography of muscle hernias. *AJR Am J Roentgenol* 180(2):395–399, 2003.

86. Hartgerink P, Fessell DP, Jacobson JA, et al: Full- versus partial-thickness Achilles tendon tears: sonographic accuracy and characterization in 26 cases with surgical correlation. *Radiology* 220(2): 406–412, 2001.

93. Lee SJ, Kim OH, Choo HJ, et al: Ultrasonographic findings of the various diseases presenting as calf pain. *Clin Imaging* 40(1):1–12, 2016.

106. Peetrons P, Creteur V, Bacq C: Sonography of ankle ligaments. *J Clin Ultrasound* 32(9):491–499, 2004.

121. Craig JG, Jacobson JA, Moed BR: Ultrasound of fracture and bone healing. *Radiol Clin North Am* 37(4):737–751, ix, 1999.

The complete references for this chapter can be found on *www.expertconsult.com.*

INTERVENTIONAL TECHNIQUES

Ultrasound-guided percutaneous procedures have several advantages, including real-time assessment and guidance, in which continuous visualization of a needle is possible throughout the procedure.[1,2] With ultrasound guidance, a needle can be precisely placed in a target while avoiding important structures, such as nerves and blood vessels. This allows very high accuracy and low complication rate, especially compared with blind needle placement. In general, when compared with non-imaging guidance, ultrasound-guided percutaneous needle injections are more accurate, more efficacious, and more cost-effective.[3] Compared with other imaging-guided techniques like computed tomography (CT), ultrasound is especially effective when a target is superficial. In addition, procedure time is typically reduced compared with CT, and ultrasound is not limited to standard imaging planes. Other intrinsic advantages of ultrasound are not specifically related to intervention but include availability, portability, lack of ionizing radiation, and relative low cost.

This chapter first reviews technical considerations when performing an ultrasound-guided procedure. This is followed by topics related to joint, bursal, tendon sheath, tendon, and miscellaneous procedures. Because the procedure that is completed using ultrasound guidance can vary widely (diagnostic or therapeutic injection versus aspiration), the ultrasound guidance aspect is emphasized here, rather than the efficacy of the specific procedure.[3-5] Regardless of the procedure, if one can identify the target and the needle with ultrasound and understand what structures lie in the projected needle path, ultrasound can offer an accurate and safe method for needle guidance for essentially any procedure. Knowledge of anatomy and of normal and abnormal sonographic findings is essential to accurately identify a target. Of note, the photographs in this chapter that show needle and transducer placement are for illustrative purposes only, in that sterile technique and needles were not used. Examples of interventional ultrasound reports are shown in Boxes 9.1 and 9.2.

■ TECHNICAL CONSIDERATIONS
Needle Guidance Overview

When performing a percutaneous needle procedure using ultrasound guidance, there are several techniques that can be used. Generally speaking,

---

 BOX 9.1 Sample Interventional Ultrasound Report

Examination: Ultrasound-Guided Injection of Right Biceps Brachii Long Head Tendon Sheath
    Date of Study: March 11, 2017
    Patient Name: James Murphy
    Registration Number: 8675309
    History: Pain
    Findings: Limited ultrasound over the anterior right shoulder demonstrates minimal joint fluid distending the biceps brachii long head tendon sheath. No evidence for hyperemia or synovial hypertrophy to suggest tenosynovitis. No evidence for biceps brachii long head tendon tear. No tendon subluxation or dislocation with dynamic imaging. No abnormal subacromial-subdeltoid bursal thickening.

After obtaining both written and verbal informed consent discussing potential risks (bleeding, infection, soft tissue injury) and benefits, using sterile technique and local anesthetic injection (provide type and amount), a 22-gauge spinal needle with trocar was inserted into the long head of the biceps brachii tendon sheath. Intra-sheath location of needle tip was confirmed with a small amount of anesthetic injection. This was followed by corticosteroid injection (provide type and amount).

The patient tolerated the procedure well without complications. The patient's pain level changed from 8/10 before procedure to 2/10.
    Impression:
1. Limited diagnostic ultrasound of the anterior shoulder showed minimal joint fluid.
2. Successful long head biceps brachii tendon sheath corticosteroid injection with pain relief as noted above and without complications.

 BOX 9.2 Sample Interventional Ultrasound Report

Examination: Ultrasound-Guided Right Iliopsoas Bursal Injection
    Date of Study: March 11, 2011
    Patient Name: Chazz Reinhold
    Registration Number: 8675309
    History: Pain, evaluate for tendon tear
    Findings: Limited ultrasound over the anterior right hip showed no hip joint effusion and unremarkable anterior hip labrum. The rectus femoris was normal. No evidence for iliopsoas bursal distention. Dynamic imaging showed no evidence for snapping iliopsoas tendon.

After obtaining both written and verbal informed consent discussing potential risks (bleeding, infection, soft tissue injury) and benefits, using sterile technique and local anesthetic injection (provide type and amount), a 20-gauge spinal needle with trocar was directed between the psoas major tendon of the iliopsoas complex and ilium superior to the femoral head. Needle tip location between the tendon and ilium was confirmed with a small amount of anesthetic injection. This was followed by corticosteroid injection (provide type and amount).

The patient tolerated the procedure well without complications. The patient's pain level changed from 8/10 before procedure to 2/10.
    Impression:
1. Limited diagnostic ultrasound of the anterior right hip showed no abnormality.
2. Successful right iliopsoas bursal corticosteroid injection with pain relief as noted above and without complications.

---

ultrasound-guided procedures can be separated into indirect and direct approaches. With the indirect approach, ultrasound is used to identify a target and to determine the depth, and then the skin directly overlying the target is marked. The transducer is removed, and the needle is directed perpendicular to the skin into the target. This approach may work for large superficial targets but is significantly limited because the needle is never directly visualized in the target, and real-time assessment during the procedure is not possible. Therefore, the direct approach, where the needle is visualized with ultrasound within the target, is preferred over the indirect approach to ensure a much higher accuracy and lower complication rate.

There are several techniques that may be employed when using the direct approach, which includes either needle guide or freehand techniques. The use of a needle guide, in which a guide is physically attached to the ultrasound transducer, is not routinely used for musculoskeletal procedures. Because most musculoskeletal procedures are relatively superficial, and given the extra steps required when using a needle guide, a freehand approach is favored.

When using the freehand direct approach, there are two methods to direct a needle relative to the transducer and sound beam: in plane and out of plane. With the in-plane approach, the needle is directed under the long axis of the transducer and sound beam in plane, and the entire needle, including its tip, is visible at all times during the procedure (Fig. 9.1) (Video 9.1). This enables real-time correction of angle and depth while the needle is advanced. The in-plane approach is the preferred method in most situations because continual visualization of the entire needle, including the needle tip and target, minimizes complications and maximizes accuracy when compared with the out-of-plane approach.

With the out-of-plane approach, the needle is passed perpendicular to the transducer so that

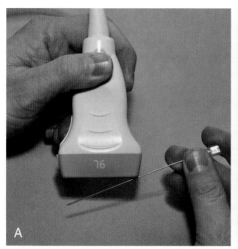

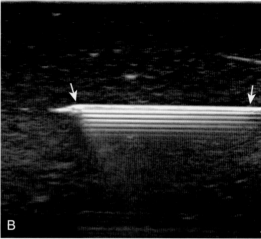

■ **FIGURE 9.1** **Needle Guidance: In Plane.** A, Image shows that needle is parallel to the transducer axis and in plane with sound beam. B, Ultrasound image shows needle *(arrows)* in plane with sound beam. Note posterior reverberation artifact when needle is perpendicular to sound beam.

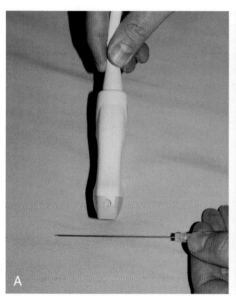

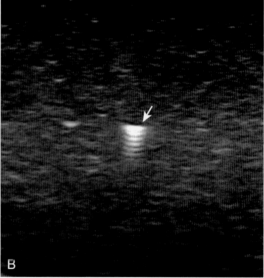

■ **FIGURE 9.2** **Needle Guidance: Out of Plane.** A, Image shows that needle is 90 degrees to transducer axis or crossing the plane of the sound beam, which results in (B) a hyperechoic focus *(arrow)* and reverberation artifact at ultrasound. Note that it is unclear whether B shows the needle tip or shaft.

the needle passes through the plane of the sound beam (Fig. 9.2) (Video 9.2). The disadvantage with this approach is that only a short segment of the needle is seen where the needle passes through the sound beam plane. When using the out-of-plane approach, the needle entrance site is centered over the target, and the needle enters from the side of the transducer (see Fig. 9.13). When inserting the needle, there is some trial and error required as the needle passes through the sound beam, is retracted, and then repeatedly redirected, typically deeper, to eventually get to

the target. Another disadvantage is that one cannot determine what segment of the needle is represented on the ultrasound image, the shaft or tip of the needle, because they look exactly the same as a single bright echo with reverberation artifact. Although the in-plane approach is preferred in most situations, the out-of-plane approach may be used in situations in which the target is very superficial, such as guiding a needle into small joints of the hand and foot. Regardless of the in-plane or out-of-plane approach, once the needle is seen in the target, it is critical that the transducer is turned 90 degrees to confirm accurate location of the needle tip.

Approach, Transducer and Needle Selection, and Ergonomics

The first step in planning an ultrasound-guided procedure (after performing a diagnostic ultrasound to identify the target and pertinent surrounding anatomy) is proper positioning of the patient. I prefer to always have the patient supine when performing any procedure, to avoid the potential for a vasovagal reaction (the patient). Next, the generalized needle approach and transducer plane are planned before marking and cleansing the skin. When performing an extremity procedure, there is often a choice between having the needle enter along the flat surface of the extremity or the curved surface. There are several benefits of having the needle enter along the curved surface, including more room to work in the space next to the extremity rather than directly over the flat surface of an extremity. Another advantage is that the puncture site can be an increased distance from the transducer (Fig. 9.3). This is helpful in that the needle can be more perpendicular to the sound beam (and therefore more conspicuous), and in addition the needle is not directly touching the transducer, which comes into play depending on the level of aseptic technique (see discussion later in the chapter).

Transducer choice should also be considered at this time. In procedures of the extremities involving the elbow, wrist, hand, knee, ankle, and foot, a linear transducer greater than 10 MHz is typically used because the target is usually superficial. A high-frequency transducer provides the highest resolution, and the sound beam projecting in a linear fashion parallel to the transducer face creates an echogenic appearance of the needle (see Fig. 1.1A). A small-footprint transducer is often helpful at the distal extremities; often, a larger footprint transducer does not make contact with the full surface of the skin because of the multiple curvatures of the distal extremities and decreased thickness of soft tissues compared with more proximal joints. An offset to a small-footprint probe (often referred to as a *hockey-stick design*) is not required but is helpful when performing procedures of small parts because the hand holding the transducer is then away from the puncture site, improving visualization at the puncture site (see Fig. 1.1C). When performing procedures of the shoulder and hip, a curvilinear transducer is often selected (see Fig. 1.1B). The benefits of this type of transducer include a larger field of view of deeper structures and a lower frequency, improving sound beam penetration. In addition, the sound beam is emitted in a more radial fashion, which helps to improve conspicuity of a needle that is steeply angled to reach a deep target.

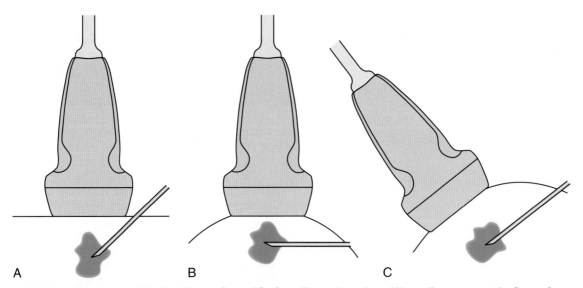

A   B   C

■ FIGURE 9.3 **Needle Entry Site: Flat Versus Curved Surface.** Illustrations show (A) needle entry over the flat surface of an extremity, which results in oblique orientation of needle relative to sound beam. Needle entry (B) over the curved surface allows the puncture site to be farther from the transducer and the needle orientation perpendicular relative to sound beam. A similar arrangement can be obtained (C) by moving the transducer away from the puncture site using heel-toe maneuver to deform the overlying soft tissues. *(Adapted from illustrations by Carolyn Nowak, Ann Arbor, Michigan.)*

With regard to needle selection, in general I prefer a 20-gauge spinal needle (3.5 inches long) for shoulder and knee procedures, and a 22-gauge needle (either 3.5 or 1.5 inches long) for more distal procedures, and a 25-gauge needle for superficial injections. Regardless of needle gauge, a stiffer needle is preferred to avoid bending of the needle. Because the goal of the direct in-plane method is to have the needle aligned with the ultrasound beam, a bent needle would not be fully visible in the ultrasound beam. A needle with a trocar (or stylet) may improve conspicuity at ultrasound and will ensure that the needle easily passes through fascial planes and does not get plugged with tissue as the needle is advanced. There are several disadvantages of using a needle with a trocar. One is that the transducer must be set down so that one's hand is free to remove the trocar and attach a syringe for injection or aspiration. Another disadvantage is that the needle contains air once this trocar is removed. This becomes problematic during an injection in that the air within the needle is initially injected into the soft tissues, which obscures the target. This latter problem can be avoided if the needle advancement stops short of the target, the trocar is removed, and a small amount of saline or anesthetic agent is injected to displace the air from the needle, and then the needle can be advanced to the target so that the definitive injection will contain air. I prefer to only use a trocar when aspirating to simplify the procedure and avoid the extra steps just described.

With regard to ergonomics, it is essential that the operator is comfortable during a procedure. I prefer to have the ultrasound monitor directly beyond or within 45 degrees to either side of the patient to enable full view of the ultrasound image without excessive turning of the head or spine. A wall-mounted accessory monitor with an adjustable arm is very effective. I also prefer to have a stool on wheels to minimize fatigue and maximize mobility. Typically, the operator's dominant hand should hold the needle, and the other hand should hold the transducer, although it is ideal to develop ambidextrous skills. For the in-plane approach the transducer can be positioned on the patient so that the needle is entering from the right or left side, or the transducer and needle may be aligned as though one is looking down a gun site.

Prepping the Site

The first step in the procedure after finding the target, determining the approach, and choosing the transducer is marking the skin. This is completed before cleansing the skin and before sterile conditions. With a direct method of needle guidance, the transducer is placed over the target and the puncture site is determined. A mark is placed at the puncture site (such as an X), and a line is placed at the other end of the transducer to indicate the imaging plane (Fig. 9.4). The use of a surgical marker will help to ensure that the marks are not washed off during cleansing of the skin. If using the indirect method, an opened paper clip passed between the transducer face and the skin can be used to accurately mark the skin directly over a target (Video 9.3).[6]

With regard to sterile technique, the use of a probe cover and preparing a sterile field at the puncture site will minimize the risk of infection. A comprehensive sterile field is essential in that ultrasound gel can act as a conduit for infection from non-cleansed areas, even if the ultrasound gel is itself sterile.[7] Although sterile preparation

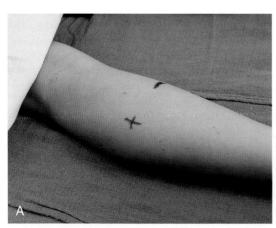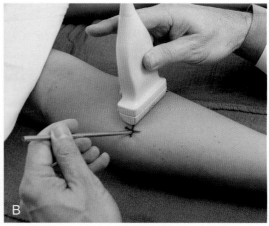

■ FIGURE 9.4 **Skin Marking: Freehand Direct In-Plane Approach.** A and B, Transducer is positioned between the X at site of needle insertion and a line defining the transducer position and imaging plane.

of the site can take variable forms, the following represents the procedure used by this author. First, the sterile procedure tray is opened, and appropriate needles, syringes, and sterile ultrasound probe cover are gently dropped onto the sterile tray. The transducer to be used is placed in the transducer holder of the ultrasound machine (if present), and a thick layer of non-sterile ultrasound gel is placed on the transducer face (Fig. 9.5A). After washing hands, the operator wears sterile gloves and prepares the procedure site with chlorhexidine solution. Sterile drapes or towels are placed around the puncture site covering the areas not washed with chlorhexidine solution. The puncture site is anesthetized with local anesthetic using a 25-gauge needle. The sterile probe cover is then held covering the operator's sterile hand, and the probe cover is placed over the non-sterile probe and gel (Fig. 9.5B and C). The operator then extends the probe cover along the transducer cable (Fig. 9.5D and E) and secures the cover with sterile rubber bands (included with the probe cover). Alternatively, an assistant can fill the inside of the sterile probe cover with non-sterile gel and lower the probe into the sterile probe cover (Fig. 9.5F). Sterile gel that is also included in the sterile probe cover kit is then opened and deposited on one of the sterile drapes near the puncture site. The transducer in the cover is then dipped into the sterile gel and placed between the X and the line to reconfirm the target. The probe is removed from the site, and the procedure needle enters the skin (about 1 cm) at the puncture site. The transducer is returned to the procedure site to visualize the needle. Of note, the transducer is removed from the procedure site until the needle penetrates the skin to avoid inadvertent puncture of the transducer or transducer cover. With a sterile field placed around the procedure site, the operator can easily set the transducer down on the field while exchanging syringes, minimizing contamination.

Needle Visualization

The first critical rule when performing the in-plane method of needle guidance is that the needle should not be advanced unless it is seen in its entirety (when using in plane technique); otherwise, the procedure is essentially blind and not image guided. As stated earlier, the procedure is initiated when the needle is placed through the skin at the puncture site about 1 cm. At this point, the transducer is placed over the projected needle path, and the echogenic needle is identified. This is accomplished by moving the transducer side to side over the needle. Because the sound beam is focused, it is not uncommon to have the needle directly under the transducer but not visible on

the ultrasound image. Side-to-side movement of the transducer should only be 1 mm at a time so as not to move the transducer away from the needle. Moving the probe too fast or abruptly is a common reason why the needle is not visualized. It is often helpful to look down at the procedure site to ensure that the needle is indeed beneath and parallel to the transducer plane. Once again, the needle should not be advanced until seen in its entirety.

Once the needle is visualized in long axis, the target should also be visualized. If the needle is seen but the target is not visible, the transducer can then be rotated to line up the puncture site with the target. By looking down at the new probe direction, the needle can be easily angled into the same transducer plane so that both the needle and target can be seen. This can only be accomplished with the needle in the subcutaneous fat, where needle movement is effortless and without symptoms. This is one reason why the needle and target should both be visualized in the same plane prior to advancing the needle given the flexibility in optimizing transducer, needle, and target alignment. Once the needle enters the deeper muscle tissues and fascial planes, movement of the needle or correction of needle path is limited and often painful.

Another basic concept is that the needle and transducer should not be moved at the same time. The transducer is moved to identify the needle, and the needle is then advanced (see Video 9.1). If the needle is no longer visualized during the procedure, needle advancement is stopped, and the transducer is moved as it was before, until the needle is again visualized and fully in plane. The transducer is then fixed in position as the needle is advanced again.

If a target is very superficial, the procedure may be more difficult; when the needle penetrates the skin the needle tip may already be either in the target or have missed the target. To assist, a sterile gel standoff may be considered (Fig. 9.6). With this technique, one end of the probe is lifted off the skin and sterile gel is placed. The needle can then be visualized within the gel prior to penetrating the skin and then redirected as needed for accurate needle placement within the target.

There are several options to improve conspicuity of the needle with ultrasound. A larger needle with a trocar may help, but a larger needle is not chosen for this reason. Coated or etched needles may be used, making the needle more echogenic (Fig. 9.7).[8] This is helpful when performing a procedure where the target is deep and the needle angle is steep, which decreases needle conspicuity due to needle anisotropy. A very helpful option is to "jiggle" the needle while slowly moving the

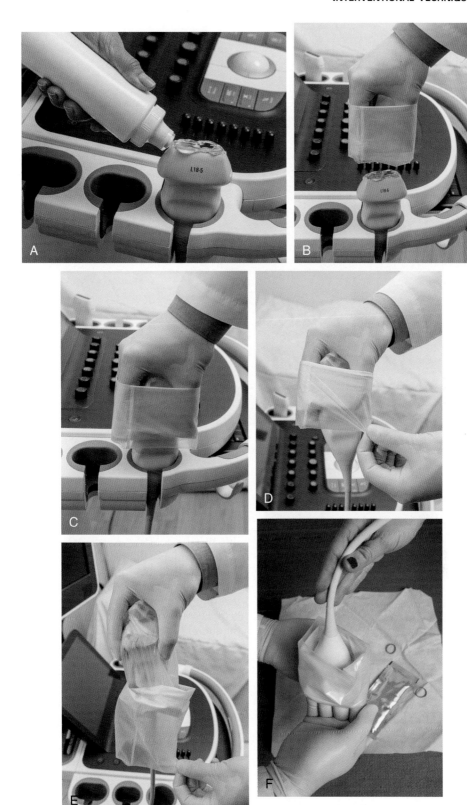

■ **FIGURE 9.5 Sterile Probe Cover.** Non-sterile gel placed on probe (A); sterile probe cover lowered over probe and grasped (B and C); extending probe cover over probe (D and E); alternatively, an assistant may lower non-sterile probe into cover (F).

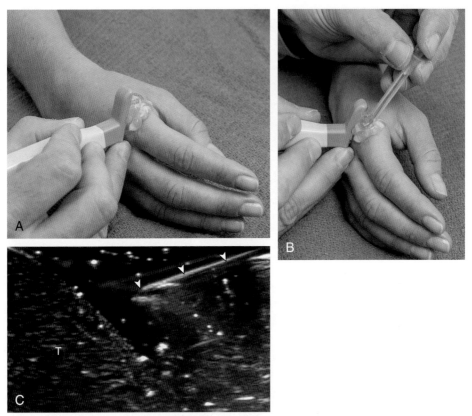

■ FIGURE 9.6 **Sterile Gel Standoff.** A and B, Thick layer of sterile gel is placed between the probe and skin surface to allow (C) visualization of the needle *(arrowheads)* within gel before penetrating the skin and soft tissues *(T)*.

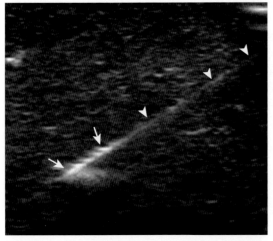

■ FIGURE 9.7 **Echogenic Needle Tip.** Ultrasound image shows needle *(arrowheads)* with increased echogenicity at needle tip *(arrows)*.

transducer over the projected needle path (Video 9.4). With this maneuver, the needle is moved minimally forward and backward along the needle path, similar to needle movement with an intention or caffeinated tremor, which causes movement of the adjacent soft tissue and can help locate the needle. Of note, the needle in this maneuver is not advanced or moved side to side. To identify this distal tip of the needle, the needle can be rotated, which will create an echogenic focus as the bevel becomes more perpendicular to the sound beam (Video 9.4). The most important technique to improve visualization of the needle is to have the needle as close to perpendicular to the sound beam as possible. Similar to anisotropy of tendons, a needle that is oblique to the sound beam will be less echogenic (Fig. 9.8A), whereas a needle that is perpendicular will be very echogenic with a strong reverberation artifact (see Fig. 9.1B) (Video 9.5). A perpendicular alignment between the sound beam and needle can be accomplished by having the puncture site farther removed from the transducer, which is possible when performing a procedure along the curvature of an extremity (see Fig. 9.3B). Another option is to move the transducer or deform the soft tissues with a heel-toe maneuver (see Fig. 9.3C). Many ultrasound machines have the ability to steer the ultrasound beam so that the insonation angle between the needle and the beam is ideally perpendicular to eliminate needle anisotropy (Fig. 9.8B).

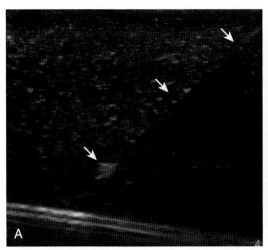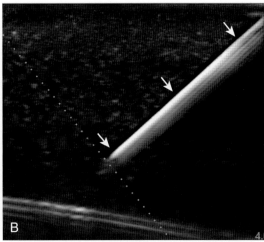

■ FIGURE 9.8 **Needle Anisotropy and Beam Steering.** Ultrasound image with needle oblique to sound beam shows (A) poor visualization of needle *(arrows)* due to anisotropy. The use of beam steering (B) will direct the sound beam perpendicular to needle, eliminating anisotropy and increasing echogenicity of needle *(arrows)*.

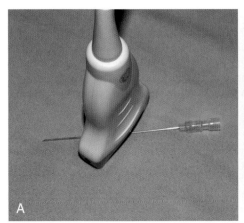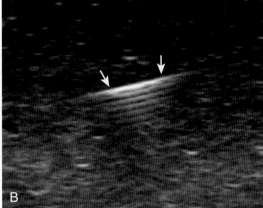

■ FIGURE 9.9 **Oblique Needle Orientation.** Needle oblique to transducer sound beam (A) producing (B) a short segment of the needle *(arrows)* visible at ultrasound.

When attempting to align the needle along the long axis of the sound beam, as in the in-plane approach, only a short segment of the needle may be visualized. This finding indicates that the transducer alignment and needle are not parallel but instead are crossing each other (Fig. 9.9). The longer the visible segment, the more the needle and sound beam are parallel. To correct this, the transducer should be turned clockwise or counterclockwise. If the segment of needle is increasing in length, the rotation is in the correct direction because the needle and sound beam become more parallel (Video 9.6). On the contrary, if the segment of needle becomes shorter, the transducer is being turned in the wrong direction because less of the needle is in the sound beam path. It is easiest to simply look down at the needle

and transducer plane to determine which direction to rotate the probe to achieve parallel planes.

■ JOINT PROCEDURES

Percutaneous joint procedures can include aspiration (for infection or crystal analysis), injection (both diagnostic and therapeutic using anesthetic agents or corticosteroids, or for the purpose of injecting contrast before MRI or CT),[9] or less commonly synovial biopsy. Accuracy of such procedures is improved compared with blind attempt if the needle tip is directly visualized with ultrasound within the target.[5] One key concept is that nearly every synovial joint in the extremity has one recess that preferentially distends with joint fluid and is visible at imaging.[10] These recesses directly communicate with their respective joint articulations so that a joint procedure targets these sites rather than the joint articulations, which would potentially harm fibrocartilage and hyaline cartilage. These distinct joint recesses are assessed for joint fluid or synovial hypertrophy and are targeted for the joint procedure.

When accessing a joint recess for a procedure, the specific recess of a joint is assessed. If there is distention of the recess with fluid, that site would be the ideal target. If the recess is not distended, then the site is still targeted, although injection of a collapsed recess is more difficult. In this situation, intra-articular needle placement should be confirmed prior to the diagnostic or therapeutic injection. This is accomplished with a test injection of local anesthetic or saline. Uncommonly, if a joint recess is not distended, a needle can be directly advanced into a joint articulation, such as accessing the sacroiliac joint or first carpometacarpal joint. Joint injection can be completed with almost any needle gauge, although I prefer a 20- or 22-gauge needle for stiffness. Joint aspiration should be at least 20 or 22 gauge, with 18 gauge considered if joint fluid is heterogeneous. Synovial biopsies may be completed with soft tissue core biopsy guns, whereas 22-gauge needles with short throw (i.e., 1 cm) are preferred given the small sizes of the various joint recesses (Video 9.7). Biopsies of synovial hypertrophy tend to be reserved to evaluate for atypical infection or synovial proliferative disorders (such as pigmented villonodular synovitis); such biopsies in the setting of a systemic inflammatory arthritis often reveal nonspecific inflammation.

Shoulder

Regarding the shoulder joint, joint effusions accumulate within the biceps brachii tendon sheath because this space openly communicates with the glenohumeral joint (in the absence of biceps brachii long head tenosynovitis).[11] Other glenohumeral joint recesses include the axillary recess, the subscapularis recess, and the posterior glenohumeral joint recess (assessed in external rotation).[12] To access the glenohumeral joint, a posterior approach targeting the posterior glenohumeral recess is preferred (Fig. 9.10).[4,13] The transducer is placed long axis to the infraspinatus, and the needle is advanced in plane from lateral to medial (or medial to lateral) until the needle tip is located at the surface of the humeral head hyaline cartilage (see Video 9.7). The joint recess is wider more medial adjacent to the hyperechoic fibrocartilage labrum, especially with external rotation of the shoulder. The biceps brachii tendon

sheath is not typically targeted for glenohumeral joint access because open communication between the biceps sheath and joint may not always be present in the setting of biceps tenosynovitis.

The acromioclavicular joint can be accessed in several different ways. I prefer an in-plane needle approach with the transducer in the coronal plane on the body and the needle passing superficial to the acromion and entering from lateral to medial (Fig. 9.11) (Video 9.8). Another method is an in-plane approach with the transducer in the sagittal plane and the needle entering from anterior to posterior (Fig. 9.12), although this technique may be difficult if the joint space is narrowed. Lastly, an out-of-plane approach may be used with the transducer in the coronal plane on the body (Fig. 9.13). With regard to the sternoclavicular joint, I prefer an in-plane approach from lateral to medial to avoid structure deep to the joint (Fig. 9.14) although an out-of-plane approach can also be used.[14]

Elbow

For the elbow joint, the most sensitive location to identify a joint effusion by ultrasound is the posterior olecranon recess (in the olecranon fossa) with the elbow flexed, where a joint effusion or synovial process displaces the adjacent hyperechoic fat pad posterior and superior.[15] Needle placement is transverse to the extremity, in plane with the transducer, with the needle advanced from lateral to medial (Fig. 9.15) (Video 9.9). Positioning of the elbow in slight extension prior to needle placement may redistribute the joint fluid more superficially, aiding in aspiration.

Wrist and Hand

With regard to the wrist and hand, the dorsal recesses are the typical accessible targets. There are three wrist joints: distal radioulnar, radiocarpal, and midcarpal. For all three of these joint recesses, I prefer the in-plane approach with the transducer in the axial plane on the body and the needle entering from ulnar or radial along the curvature of the extremity (Fig. 9.16) (Video 9.10).[16] The radiocarpal joint may also be accessed in the sagittal plane as well.[17] Aspiration of the small joints of the hand can be more difficult given their superficial location. The dorsal recesses are targeted either with an in-plane approach in the parasagittal (Fig. 9.17A) or transverse plane (Fig. 9.17B), or an out-of-plane approach (Fig. 9.17C). With either approach, the overlying extensor tendon in the sagittal plane and the neurovascular structures at the medial and lateral aspects must be avoided.

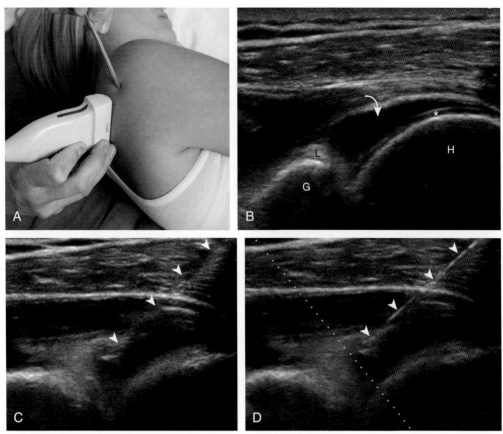

■ **FIGURE 9.10 Shoulder Joint Aspiration: In-Plane Lateral Approach (Infection).** A, Transducer and needle position for simulated posterior glenohumeral joint recess procedure. Ultrasound images show (B) anechoic distention of posterior glenohumeral joint recess *(curved arrow)* before aspiration *(asterisk,* hyaline articular cartilage), (C) needle placement *(arrowheads)* within joint effusion, with (D) improved needle visualization *(arrowheads)* using beam steering. *H,* Humeral head; *G,* glenoid; *L,* labrum.

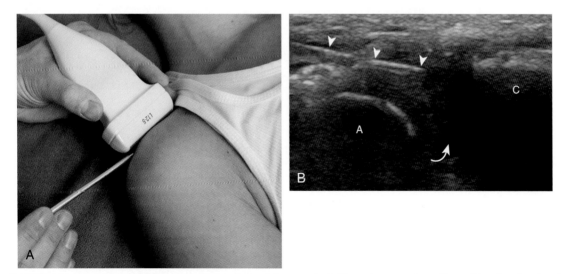

■ **FIGURE 9.11 Acromioclavicular Joint: In-Plane Lateral Approach.** A, Transducer and needle position for simulated acromioclavicular joint procedure. Ultrasound image shows (B) needle *(arrowheads)* within acromioclavicular joint *(curved arrow)*. *A,* Acromion; *C,* clavicle.

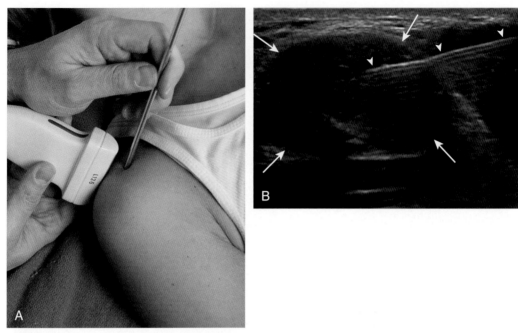

■ **FIGURE 9.12 Acromioclavicular Joint: In-Plane Anterior Approach.** A, Transducer and needle position for simulated acromioclavicular joint procedure. Ultrasound image shows (B) needle *(arrows)* in acromioclavicular joint *(arrowheads).*

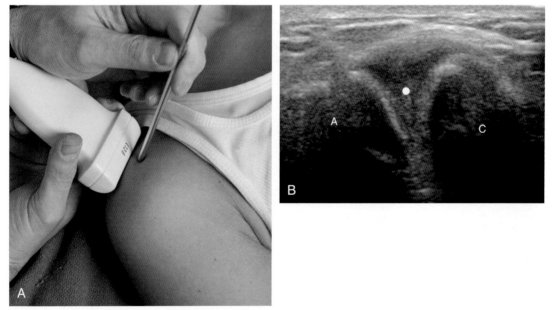

■ **FIGURE 9.13 Acromioclavicular Joint: Out-of-Plane Anterior Approach.** A, Transducer and needle position for simulated acromioclavicular joint procedure. Ultrasound image shows (B) proposed location of needle *(white circle)* between acromion *(A)* and clavicle *(C).*

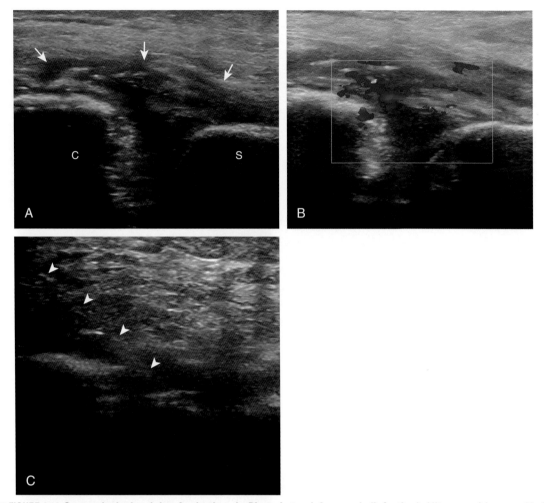

■ FIGURE 9.14 **Sternoclavicular Joint Aspiration: In-Plane Lateral Approach (Infection).** Ultrasound images (A–C) show hypoechoic distention of the sternoclavicular joint *(arrows)* and hyperemia, with needle aspiration *(arrowheads)*. *C,* Clavicle; *S,* sternum.

Hip and Pelvis

For needle placement into the hip joint, the anterior joint recess overlying the femoral neck is the preferred target.[18] Placing the needle over the femoral head is not recommended as this increases likelihood of the injection being extra-articular, and needle placement more superiorly can potentially harm the acetabular labrum.[18] The needle is guided into the anterior hip joint recess with an in-plane approach long axis to the femoral neck in the sagittal-oblique plane (Fig. 9.18) (Video 9.11), although an in-plane lateral to medial approach can also be used.[10,19,20] Because of the depth of the target in many adults, the needle is often quite oblique to the sound beam, which makes the needle less echogenic from anisotropy. The use of a curvilinear transducer is often helpful in this situation. As described earlier, for injecting a collapsed joint recess it is often helpful to first inject local anesthetic to ensure accurate intra-articular needle placement before final injection.[20]

For aspiration or injection of the pubic symphysis, the transducer is placed in the transverse plane, and the needle can enter lateral to medial with an in-plane approach (Fig. 9.19), or an out-of-plane approach may be used. Ultrasound-guided needle placement into the sacroiliac joint typically is in plane with the transducer in the axial plane on the body, with the needle entering from medial to lateral (Fig. 9.20).[21,22] The adjacent sacral neural foramina, which are just medial to the sacroiliac joints, should not be mistaken as the sacroiliac joints. Last, at the superior aspect of the sacroiliac joints where the space between the ilium and sacrum is widened, this is not the true synovial joint articulation, which is located more inferiorly where the joint space is relatively narrow.

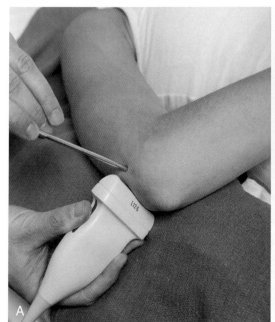

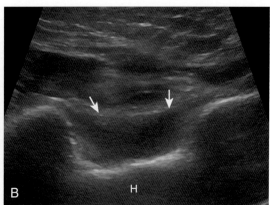

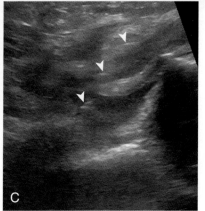

■ FIGURE 9.15 **Elbow Joint Aspiration: In-Plane Lateral Approach (Gout).** A, Transducer and needle position for simulated elbow joint procedure. Ultrasound images show (B) hypoechoic distention of the posterior elbow joint recess *(arrows)* and (C) needle placement *(arrowheads)*. *H,* Humerus.

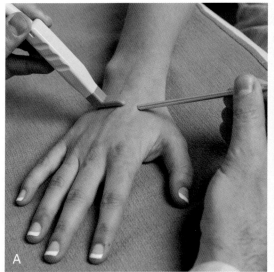

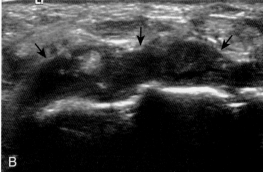

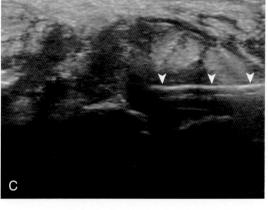

■ FIGURE 9.16 **Midcarpal Joint Aspiration: In-Plane Radial Approach (Pseudogout).** A, Transducer and needle position for simulated midcarpal joint procedure. Ultrasound images show (B) heterogeneous but predominantly hypoechoic distention of the dorsal recess of the midcarpal joint *(arrows)* and (C) needle placement *(arrowheads)*.

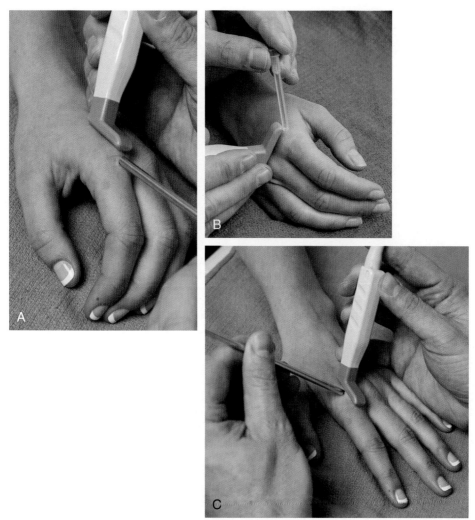

■ **FIGURE 9.17 Metacarpophalangeal Joint Aspiration.** Simulated images of (A) parasagittal in-plane, (B) transverse in-plane, and (C) sagittal out-of-plane approaches.

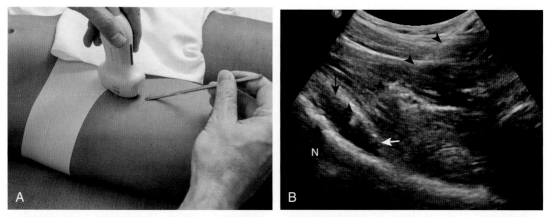

■ **FIGURE 9.18 Hip Joint Aspiration: In-Plane Inferior Approach (Infection).** A, Transducer and needle position for simulated hip joint procedure. Ultrasound image shows (B) needle placement *(arrowheads)* within the anechoic distended anterior hip joint recess *(arrows)*. *N,* Femoral neck.

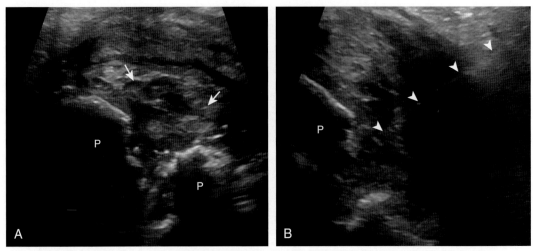

■ FIGURE 9.19 **Symphysis Pubis Aspiration: In-Plane Lateral Approach (Infection).** Ultrasound images show (A) heterogeneous but predominantly hypoechoic distention of the pubic symphysis joint recess *(arrows)* and (B) needle placement *(arrowheads)*. Note erosions of pubis *(P)*.

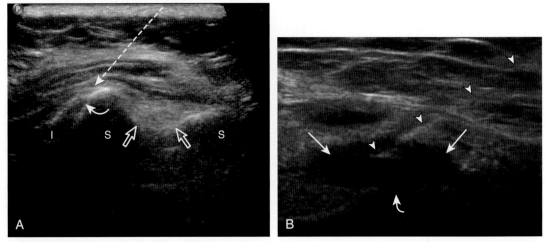

■ FIGURE 9.20 **Sacroiliac Joint: In-Plane Midline Approach.** A, Ultrasound image shows proposed location of needle *(dashed arrow)* to sacroiliac joint *(curved arrow)* (right side of image is midline). Note sacral neural foramen *(open arrows)*. *I,* Ilium; *S,* sacrum. Ultrasound image from a different patient (B) shows needle placement *(arrowheads)* within distended recess *(arrows)* from sacroiliac joint *(curved arrow)*.

Knee

Distention of the knee joint occurs around the patella, commonly superolateral to the patella. Fluid collects in the suprapatellar recess under the quadriceps with the knee in slight flexion, or medial or lateral to the patella under the retinaculum when the knee is extended.[23,24] Given this variability, all three areas around the patella should be assessed for joint recess distention. To access the knee joint, I prefer an in-plane approach with the transducer transverse on the body and the needle entering from lateral to medial along the curvature of the extremity, usually targeting the superolateral aspect of the joint recess (Fig. 9.21) (Video 9.12).[25] To access the proximal tibiofibular joint, the transducer is placed in the transverse plane on the body over the anterior aspect of the joint, and an out-of-plane approach is used (Fig. 9.22) (Video 9.13).[26]

Ankle and Foot

For the ankle joint, the anterior recess is accessed for aspiration or injection.[27] There are two different approaches to consider. The first is an in-plane approach with the transducer in the sagittal plane on the body and the needle entering

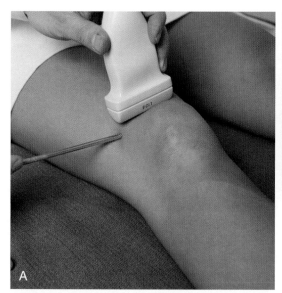

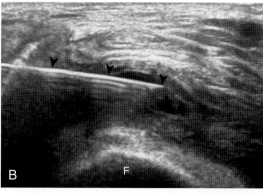

■ **FIGURE 9.21 Knee Joint Aspiration: In-Plane Lateral Approach.** A, Transducer and needle position for simulated knee joint procedure. Ultrasound image shows (B) needle placement *(arrowheads)* within the anechoic distended knee joint recess. *F,* Femur.

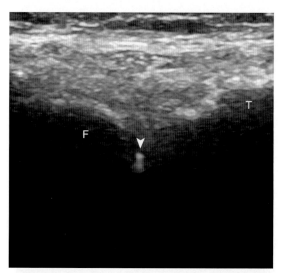

■ **FIGURE 9.22 Proximal Tibiofibular Joint Injection: Out-of-Plane Approach.** Ultrasound image shows needle *(arrowhead)* with posterior reverberation artifact within tibiofibular joint. *F,* Fibula; *T,* tibia.

from inferior to superior, usually between the tibialis anterior and extensor hallucis longus tendons (Fig. 9.23).[28] The other approach is an in-plane approach with the transducer transverse on the body and the needle entering from medial to lateral beneath the tibialis anterior tendon and dorsalis pedis artery (Fig. 9.24) (Video 9.14). For the posterior subtalar joint, there are several approaches that can be considered, including anterolateral (Fig. 9.25) (Video 9.15), posterolateral, posteromedial, as well as via the sinus tarsi.[29,30]

For the metatarsophalangeal and interphalangeal joints, a parasagittal in-plane (Fig. 9.26A and B) (Video 9.16), transverse in-plane (Fig. 9.26C) or out-of-plane (Fig. 9.26D) approach can access the dorsal recesses or joint articulations, similar to what was described for the metacarpophalangeal and interphalangeal joints of the hand.

■ BURSAL PROCEDURES

Bursal injection or aspiration using ultrasound guidance can be more accurate than a blind attempt when the needle tip is accurately identified within the bursa.[4] Regardless, needle placement within a collapsed bursa is more difficult compared with one that is distended. Before attempting injection into a collapsed bursa, a test injection with a small amount of local anesthetic can be used to ensure accurate needle placement in the bursa, which will appear as bursal distention with the injection moving away from the needle tip and low resistance to injection. Knowledge of the various bursae around the body allows differentiation between true bursal distention from a nonspecific soft tissue fluid collection. When guiding a needle into a bursa, the bursal wall is often difficult to penetrate, and frequently the needle tents the wall, which may simulate an intra-bursal location of the needle tip (see Baker Cyst). True intra-bursal location is evident when the needle does not retract on its own and can be easily and freely moved within the bursa. When one anticipates complete aspiration of a bursa,

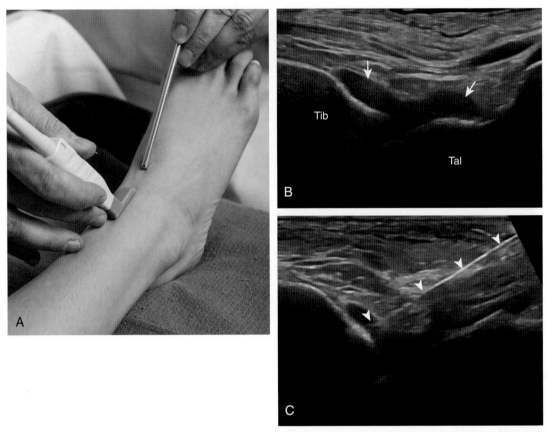

■ **FIGURE 9.23 Ankle Joint Aspiration: In-Plane Anterior Approach.** A, Transducer and needle position for simulated ankle joint procedure. Ultrasound image shows (B) hypoechoic distention of the anterior ankle joint recess *(arrows)* and needle placement *(arrowheads)*. *Tal,* Talus; *Tib,* tibia.

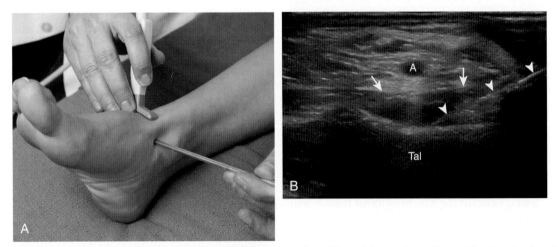

■ **FIGURE 9.24 Ankle Joint Aspiration: In-Plane Medial Approach.** A, Transducer and needle position for simulated ankle joint procedure. Ultrasound image shows (B) hypoechoic distention of the anterior ankle joint recess *(arrows)* and needle placement *(arrowheads)*. *A,* Dorsalis pedis artery; *Tal,* Talus.

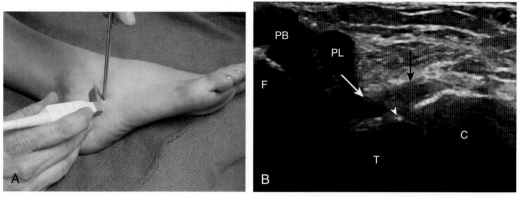

■ **FIGURE 9.25 Posterior Subtalar Joint: Anterolateral Out-of-Plane Approach.** A, Transducer and needle position for simulated posterior subtalar joint procedure. Ultrasound image shows (B) needle *(arrowhead)* and distended posterior subtalar joint *(arrows)*. Note peroneus longus *(PL)* and brevis *(PB)* tendons hypoechoic from anisotropy. *C,* Calcaneus; *T,* talus; *F,* fibula.

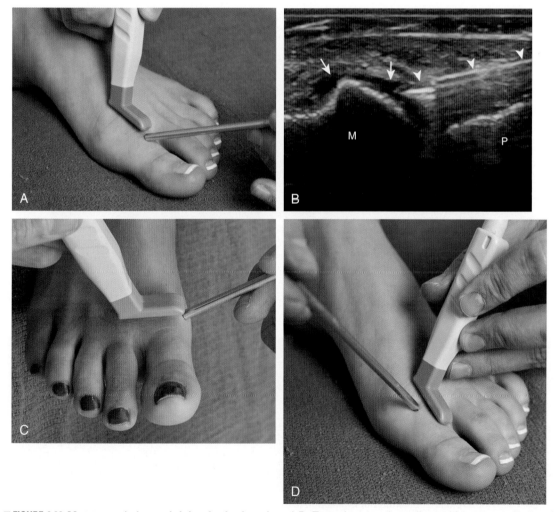

■ **FIGURE 9.26 Metatarsophalangeal Joint Aspiration.** A and B, Transducer and needle position parasagittal and adjacent to the extensor tendon for simulated metatarsophalangeal joint procedure, hypoechoic dorsal recess distention *(arrows)* and needle *(arrowheads)*. *M,* Metatarsal head; *P,* proximal phalanx. C, Simulated transverse in-plane and (D) out-of-plane approaches.

an introducer rather than a standard needle should be considered. With an introducer, the inner trocar or stylet is removed after the needle is in the bursa, and the needle end is relatively blunt, which minimizes trauma and potential bleeding as the opposing wall of the bursa collapses down onto the needle tip. Alternatively, a standard needle can be slowly withdrawn under ultrasound guidance as the bursa is aspirated and collapses as it approaches the needle tip.

Subacromial-Subdeltoid Bursa

One of the more common bursal injections involves the subacromial-subdeltoid bursa. I prefer the in-plane approach with the transducer in the sagittal plane and the needle entering from posterior to anterior, targeting the area of the bursa that is distended (Fig. 9.27). The transducer may also be placed in the coronal plane with the needle entering in-plane from lateral to medial (Fig. 9.28) (Video 9.17). If the bursa is not distended, the needle is directed superficial to the supraspinatus tendon; a test injection with anesthetic agent is completed to confirm bursal location of the needle before corticosteroid injection (Video 9.18). During an intra-bursal injection, there should be low resistance. In addition, one may not directly see filling of the bursa as the initial injection distends a portion of the bursa that is not in the field of view (Video 9.19). If the puncture site is placed several centimeters away

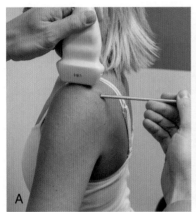
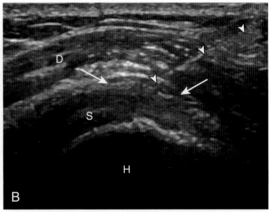

■ FIGURE 9.27 **Subacromial-Subdeltoid Bursa Injection (Posterior In-Plane Approach).** A, Transducer and needle position for simulated subacromial-subdeltoid procedure. Ultrasound image shows (B) focal hypoechoic distention of the subacromial-subdeltoid bursa *(arrows)* and needle placement *(arrowheads)*. D, Deltoid; H, humeral head; S, supraspinatus tendon.

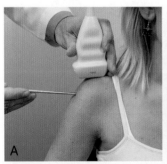
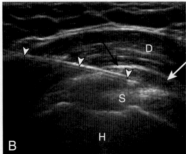
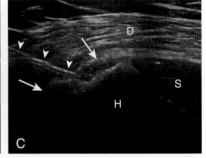

■ FIGURE 9.28 **Subacromial-Subdeltoid Bursa Injection (Lateral In-Plane Approach).** A, Transducer and needle position for simulated subacromial-subdeltoid procedure. Ultrasound image shows (B) focal hypoechoic distention of the subacromial-subdeltoid bursa *(arrows)* and needle placement *(arrowheads)*. Ultrasound image from a different patient shows (C) needle placement in the subacromial-subdeltoid bursa, which is distended distal to the greater tuberosity *(H)*. D, Deltoid; H, humeral head; S, supraspinatus tendon.

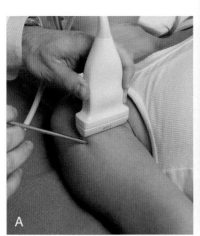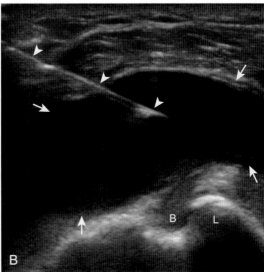

■ **FIGURE 9.29 Subacromial-Subdeltoid Bursa Aspiration (In-Plane Approach).** A, Transducer and needle position for simulated subacromial-subdeltoid procedure. Ultrasound image (B) shows anechoic distention of the subacromial-subdeltoid bursa *(arrows)* and needle placement *(arrowheads)*. *B,* Biceps brachii long head tendon; *L,* lesser tuberosity.

from the end of the transducer down the slope of the skin surface, then the needle can be directed perpendicular to the transducer sound beam, making the needle more conspicuous. The subacromial-subdeltoid bursa extends from under the acromion over the supraspinatus, infraspinatus, subscapularis, and cortex of the proximal humerus, where any site of bursal distention can be a target for aspiration or injection (Fig. 9.29) (Videos 9.20 and 9.21).

Iliopsoas Bursa

Another bursa that may be targeted is the iliopsoas bursa.[31-33] As described in Chapter 6, the iliopsoas bursa is uncommonly distended, and, if distended, it usually relates to a hip joint process because of the potential communication between the two synovial spaces. For needle placement into the iliopsoas bursa, the transducer is placed parallel to the inguinal ligament just at or superior to the level of the femoral head, and an in-plane approach from lateral to medial is used (Fig. 9.30A and B). With a non-distended iliopsoas bursa, the needle is directed deep to the psoas major tendon of the iliopsoas complex.[33] The continuous cortical contour of the ilium is used as a useful bony landmark. Injecting just superior to the level of the femoral head will ensure the injection is not inadvertently within the hip joint. Typically, the injection accumulates between the iliopsoas tendon and the adjacent ilium, lifting the iliopsoas anteriorly (Fig. 9.30C) (Videos 9.22 and 9.23), which indicates filling of the iliopsoas bursa.

Greater Trochanteric Bursae

There are several bursae around the greater trochanter, the largest being the trochanteric (or subgluteus maximus) bursa, located between the posterior facet of the greater trochanter and the gluteus maximus, although a distended trochanteric bursa can extend anterior over the gluteus medius tendon.[34] Similar to the iliopsoas bursa, the trochanteric bursa is uncommonly distended and rarely inflamed as an isolated cause of symptoms, but rather is associated with adjacent gluteus tendon abnormalities in the setting of greater trochanteric pain syndrome. To aspirate or inject a distended trochanteric bursa using ultrasound guidance, the patient is rolled decubitus, the transducer is placed in the transverse plane on the body, and the needle is directed in plane with the transducer from posterior to anterior (Fig. 9.31).

Baker Cyst

Another common bursal aspiration is the gastrocnemio-semimembranosus bursa, when distended it is termed a *popliteal* or *Baker cyst.* Injection or aspiration can be completed with the needle in plane with the transducer. I prefer the needle either entering from inferior to superior (Fig. 9.32) (Videos 9.24 and 9.25), although other approaches such as a medial or lateral approach may be considered (Fig. 9.33). Because approximately 50% of Baker cysts communicate to the knee joint in patients older than 50 years, the

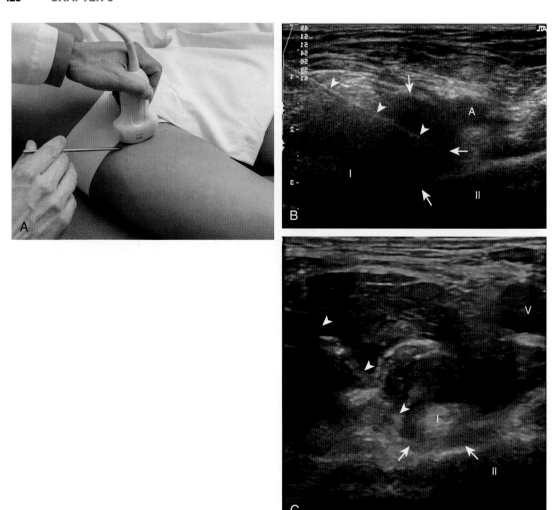

■ **FIGURE 9.30 Iliopsoas Bursa Aspiration and Injection.** A, Transducer and needle position for simulated iliopsoas bursa procedure. Ultrasound image shows (B) hypoechoic iliopsoas bursa distention *(arrows)* medial to iliopsoas *(I)* and needle *(arrowheads)*. *A,* External iliac artery; *II,* ilium. Ultrasound image from a different patient (C) shows needle *(arrowheads)* positioned between the psoas major tendon *(I)* and ilium *(II)* with hypoechoic injection *(arrows)*. *V,* External iliac vein.

knee joint should be aspirated first if distended before aspiration and injection of a Baker cyst.[35] Failure to do so can result in immediate re-accumulation of joint fluid within the Baker cyst (Fig. 9.33D). Aspiration of a Baker cyst may be followed with a direct corticosteroid injection, which has been shown to be more effective compared to intra-articular corticosteroid injection following Baker cyst aspiration.[36]

Other Bursae

Among the various other bursae throughout the body, those that are very superficial, including the olecranon (Fig. 9.34) and prepatellar bursae (Fig. 9.35), are often aspirated blindly, with

ultrasound guidance used only when blind aspiration attempt has failed or bursal injection is required. Virtually any bursae, such as the ischial (or ischiogluteal) (Fig. 9.36),[37] semimembranosus-tibial collateral ligament (Fig. 9.37),[38] pes anserinus (Fig. 9.38),[39] and retrocalcaneal (Fig. 9.39) bursae, to name a few, can be targeted with ultrasound guidance.

■ TENDON SHEATH PROCEDURES

Ultrasound is also an ideal method to guide tendon sheath injections or aspirations. When performing such procedures, an area of tendon sheath disten-tion is an optimal target and preferred over an

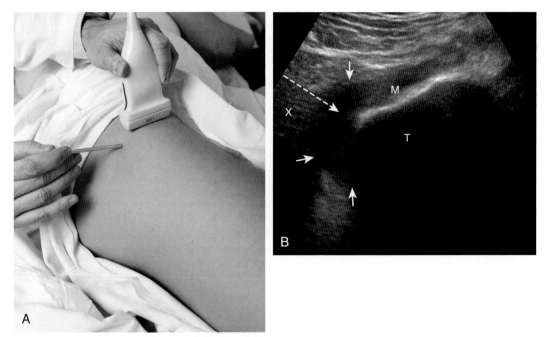

■ FIGURE 9.31 **Trochanteric Bursa.** A, Transducer and needle position for simulated trochanteric bursa procedure. Ultrasound image shows (B) hypoechoic distended trochanteric bursa *(arrows)* and location of needle *(dashed arrow)* (left side of image is posterior). *T,* Posterior facet of greater trochanter; *X,* gluteus maximus.

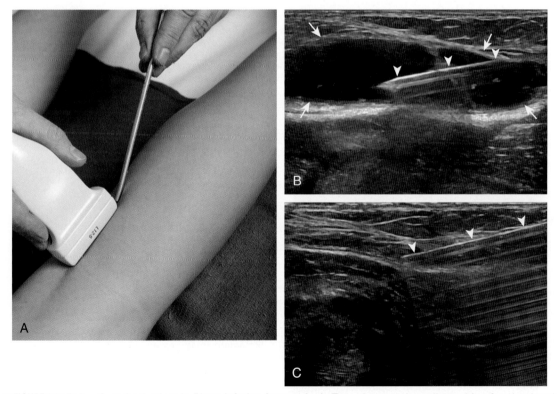

■ FIGURE 9.32 **Baker Cyst Aspiration: In-Plane Inferior Approach.** A, Transducer and needle position for simulated Baker cyst procedure (right side of image is distal). Ultrasound images show (B) predominantly anechoic distention of a Baker cyst *(arrows)* with needle placement *(arrowheads)* successfully aspirated in C.

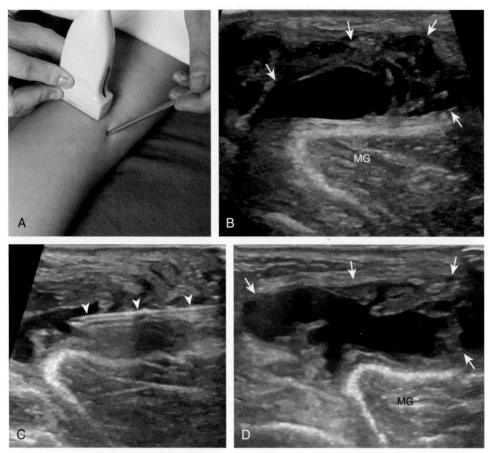

■ FIGURE 9.33 **Baker Cyst Aspiration: In-Plane Medial and Lateral Approach With Reaccumulation.** A, Transducer and needle position using medial approach for simulated Baker cyst procedure. Ultrasound images show (B) predominantly anechoic but heterogeneous distention of a Baker cyst *(arrows)* and (C) needle placement *(arrowheads)* using lateral approach. After successful and complete aspiration, the patient immediately returned (D) because joint was not aspirated first and Baker cyst fluid had reaccumulated from the knee joint. *MG,* Medial head of gastrocnemius.

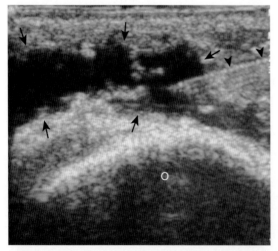

■ FIGURE 9.34 **Olecranon Bursa Aspiration (Aseptic).** Ultrasound image over olecranon process *(O)* shows in plane needle placement *(arrowheads)* within the anechoic distended olecranon bursa *(arrows).*

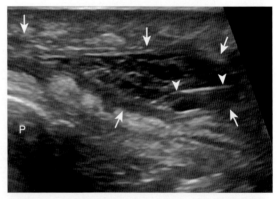

■ FIGURE 9.35 **Prepatellar Bursa Aspiration (Infection).** Ultrasound image shows in-plane needle placement *(arrowheads)* within the hypoechoic and heterogeneous distended prepatellar bursa *(arrows). P,* Patella.

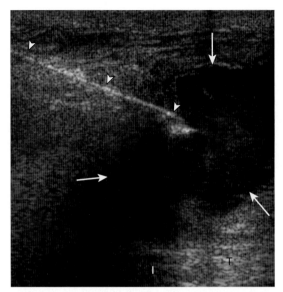

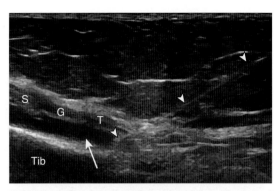

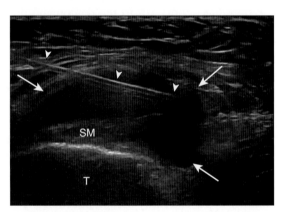

FIGURE 9.36 **Ischiogluteal Bursa Aspiration.** Ultrasound image over ischial tuberosity *(I)* shows in-plane needle placement *(arrowheads)* within the hypoechoic and heterogeneous distended ischiogluteal bursa *(arrows)*. *T,* Hamstring tendons.

FIGURE 9.38 **Pes Anserinus Bursa Aspiration.** Ultrasound image shows in-plane needle placement *(arrowheads)* within the hypoechoic distended pes anserinus bursa *(arrows)*. *S,* Sartorius; *G,* gracilis; *T,* semitendinosus; *Tib,* tibia.

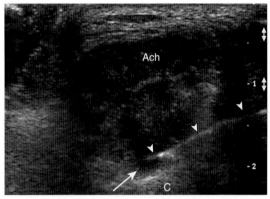

FIGURE 9.37 **Semimembranosus-Tibial Collateral Ligament Bursa Aspiration.** Ultrasound image shows in-plane needle placement *(arrowheads)* within the hypoechoic distended semimembranosus-tibial collateral ligament bursa *(arrows)*. *SM,* Semimembranosus; *T,* tibia.

FIGURE 9.39 **Retrocalcaneal Bursa Injection.** Ultrasound image short axis to Achilles tendon *(Ach)* shows in plane needle placement *(arrowheads)* with hypoechoic distention of the retrocalcaneal bursa *(arrow)*. *C,* Calcaneus. *(Courtesy C. Yablon, MD, Ann Arbor, Michigan.)*

attempt to place a needle in a collapsed tendon sheath. When attempting to inject into a non-distended tendon sheath, a test injection with a small amount of local anesthetic can be used to ensure accurate placement of the needle tip where the injection will flow freely away from the needle in the tendon sheath with low resistance.

There are two approaches to guiding a needle into a tendon sheath: short axis and long axis relative to the tendon. I prefer the short axis for several reasons. First, when approaching a tendon sheath in short axis to the tendon, the needle tip can be placed superficial to the tendon, next to the tendon, or deep to the tendon (Fig. 9.40). In long axis, the needle can only be placed superficial to the tendon. The flexibility in using the short axis method enables one to target fluid distention of the tendon sheath that may only be located deep to the tendon. In addition, when injecting corticosteroids, I prefer to inject deep to the tendon rather than superficially adjacent to the subcutaneous fat, to minimize the risk for fat atrophy. The other reason that short axis is ideal is that the needle is typically introduced along the curvature of the extremity, which decreases the obliquity of the needle relative to the sound beam and increasing needle conspicuity. When injecting corticosteroids, the needle should be flushed with local anesthetic or saline before withdrawing it to avoid corticosteroid deposition in the subcutaneous tissues, which may cause skin atrophy and depigmentation.[40]

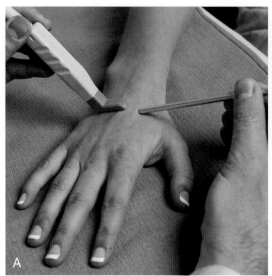
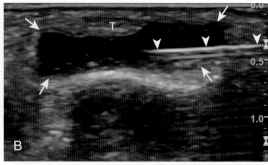

■ FIGURE 9.40 **Extensor Digitorum Tendon Sheath Aspiration.** A, Transducer and needle position for simulated wrist tendon sheath procedure. Ultrasound image shows (B) anechoic distention of the tendon sheath *(arrows)*. Note needle placement *(arrowheads)* deep to tendon *(T)*.

Many peritendon injections may not be targeting the tendon sheath but rather an overlying bursa, such as the subgluteus maximus (or trochanteric) bursa superficial to the gluteus medius, or ischial (or ischiogluteal) bursa superficial to the hamstring tendons.[41,42] Other peritendon injections may simply be infiltrating tissue planes over a tendon, such as an injection superficial to the common extensor tendon at the elbow. The use of corticosteroids in such procedures injected superficial to tendinosis often reduces pain, although the symptom relief is temporary and the underlying tendon condition is not effectively treated.[43,44]

Other peritendon procedures have been described using ultrasound guidance, which include hydrodissection or scraping to strip soft tissues away from tendon, as well as injection of sclerosis agents for ablation of entering neovascularity.[45-47] Ultrasound-guided procedures may also involve the pulleys of the hand, where the tendon sheath may be targeted with an injection or fenestration.[48-50] The plantar aponeurosis may also be targeted, where I prefer guiding a needle in plane from medial to lateral.[51] Injection of steroid into the plantar aponeurosis is associated with a 2% risk of rupture, while injection deep to aponeurosis will affect the inferior calcaneal nerve.[52,53]

Biceps Brachii Long Head

The biceps brachii long head tendon sheath is a common injection that is more accurate using ultrasound guidance compared with blind attempt.[54] I prefer an in-plane approach, with the transducer short axis to the tendon and the needle entering from lateral to medial (Fig. 9.41) (Video 9.26). The projected needle path should be assessed with color Doppler because the anterior circumflex humeral artery and its branches are routinely seen and may be in the needle path (Fig. 9.41C). An injection volume of 5 mL or greater within the biceps brachii long head tendon sheath will be expected to enter into the glenohumeral joint given this normal anatomic communication.[11]

De Quervain Tenosynovitis

Another upper extremity tendon injection site is the first extensor wrist compartment for de Quervain tenosynovitis (Fig. 9.42). I prefer an in-plane approach, with the transducer in short axis to the tendons and the needle entering from ulnar to radial at the dorsal wrist (Video 9.27).[55] The needle is advanced between the extensor pollicis brevis tendon and the adjacent radius for injection. Because subcompartmentalization of the first extensor compartment is frequent, the needle can be advanced deep to the extensor pollicis brevis into the abductor pollicis longus tendon sheath if diffuse filling around each tendon is not noted at the initial injection.[56,57] This is another advantage of the short axis approach for this procedure. Positioning the needle deep to the extensor pollicis brevis also avoids contact with the superficial branch of the radial nerve overlying the tendons and minimizes skin atrophy or depigmentation if corticosteroids leak into the adjacent tissues. The needle is typically flushed

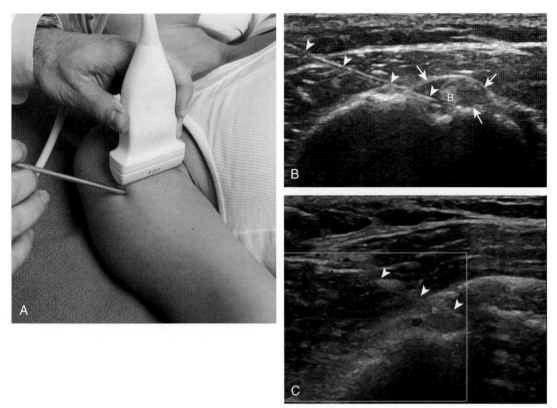

■ FIGURE 9.41 **Biceps Brachii Long Head Tendon Sheath Injection.** A, Transducer and needle position for simulated biceps brachii long head tendon sheath procedure. Ultrasound image shows (B) needle placement *(arrowheads)* with hypoechoic distention of tendon sheath *(arrows)* (left side of image is lateral). Note flow in adjacent branch of the anterior circumflex humeral artery in C. *B,* Long head of biceps brachii tendon.

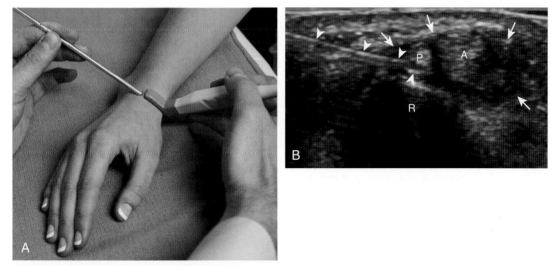

■ FIGURE 9.42 **De Quervain Tenosynovitis Injection.** A, Transducer and needle position for simulated first dorsal wrist compartment procedure. Ultrasound image shows (B) needle *(arrowheads)* positioned between extensor pollicis brevis tendon *(P)* and radius *(R)*. Note filling of both extensor pollicis brevis and abductor pollicis longus *(A)* tendon sheaths *(arrows)*.

with local anesthetic or saline after injecting corticosteroids before removing the needle to avoid deposition of corticosteroids along the exiting needle track.

Piriformis

Ultrasound can guide injection of the piriformis, where it has been reported that the use of ultrasound guidance improves accuracy over fluoroscopic guidance.[58] For this technique, the piriformis is first identified in long axis with the transducer in the oblique-axial plane on the body just inferior to the sacroiliac joint and greater sciatic notch. A curvilinear transducer of frequency lower than 10 MHz helps to ensure depth penetration and a large field of view. Passive internal and external hip rotation during imaging is also helpful in that movement of the piriformis during this maneuver makes it more conspicuous. A needle can then be guided as a peritendon injection, or intramuscular if desired, using an in-plane approach in long axis to the piriformis from either a lateral or medial approach (Fig. 9.43). If the segment of piriformis over the ilium is targeted, then the ilium can be used as a backstop for safety measures if the needle visualization is difficult.

■ TENDON PROCEDURES
Calcific Tendinosis Lavage and Aspiration

Treatment of calcific tendinosis can be carried out with a single puncture of a 20-gauge needle with a trocar (or stylet) using an in-plane approach (Figs. 9.44 and 9.45) (Video 9.28).[59] The use of a trocar helps to ensure that the needle does not get plugged with calcification while entering the calcific deposit. If the calcification is associated

with shadowing, one cannot visualize the needle after it enters into the calcification, so care should be taken not to advance the needle through the other side of the calcification. When the needle is in place within the center of the calcification, the trocar is removed, and a syringe with 2 to 5 mL of anesthetic agent or saline is connected to the needle. The procedure begins with lavage of the calcification with a minimal pulsed injection. Typically, the calcification is quite thick, and there will be much resistance to injection. As the syringe plunger is released, the backpressure from inside the calcific deposit will bring the calcifications into the needle. The one puncture technique is used for this purpose so that the increased pressure forces the calcification back into the needle and syringe. Alternatively, a two needle approach has

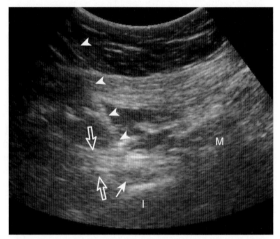

■ FIGURE 9.43 **Piriformis Peritendon Injection.** Ultrasound image shows needle *(arrowheads)* with hypoechoic injection *(arrow)* around piriformis tendon *(open arrows)* (left side of image is lateral). *I,* Ilium; *M,* piriformis muscle.

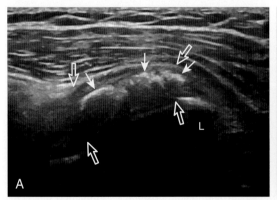
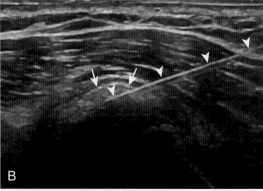

■ FIGURE 9.44 **Calcific Tendinosis Lavage and Aspiration: Subscapularis.** Ultrasound images long axis to the subscapularis tendon *(open arrows)* show (A) echogenic and partially shadowing calcifications *(arrows)*. Note needle placement *(arrowheads)* and decreased shadowing as calcification is aspirated in B. *L,* Lesser tuberosity.

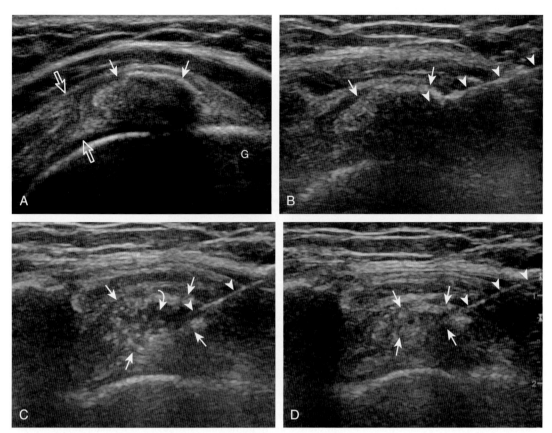

■ FIGURE 9.45 **Calcific Tendinosis Lavage and Aspiration: Supraspinatus.** Ultrasound images long axis to the supraspinatus tendon *(open arrows)* show (A) echogenic and partially shadowing calcification *(arrows)*. Note (B) needle placement *(arrowheads)* within calcification. With continued lavage and aspiration, (C) the central aspect is more hypoechoic *(curved arrow)* with decreased shadowing and decreased size in D. *G,* Greater tuberosity.

been described for continuous lavage and aspiration.[60] The maneuver of short pulsed injection with aspiration from spontaneous backpressure is repeated. When there is minimal shadowing, one will see swirling of the calcification and decreasing echogenicity as the calcium is diluted and aspirated (Videos 9.29 and 9.30). During the aspiration, echogenic calcifications are often seen moving within the needle (Video 9.31). When the syringe becomes slightly opaque from calcification, a new syringe is connected, and the process is repeated. This continues with a third syringe. Positioning of the syringe dependent relative to the targeted tendon calcification will allow the more dependent calcifications to collect in the syringe instead of being reinjected. In the situation in which the original calcification is amorphous without shadowing, the procedure is complete when the calcification decreases in amount or echogenicity and the syringes contain calcification. When the calcification is echogenic with shadowing, progressive dilution of the tendon calcification is not visible because of the shadowing, so one

relies on visualization of the calcification within the syringes to indicate completion (Video 9.32). In this latter situation, there may be little or no change when comparing the calcification before and after the procedure; however, a dramatic interval change with delayed resorption of calcification can still be seen weeks after the procedure (Fig. 9.46).

At the completion of the lavage and aspiration of rotator cuff calcific tendinosis, the needle is withdrawn into the adjacent subacromial-subdeltoid bursa for corticosteroid and anesthetic injection (see Video 9.32). This latter procedure is essential because patients can develop a calcific bursitis after the procedure. Lavage and aspiration usually result in immediate improvement of symptoms, although transient increase in symptoms may occur about 15 weeks after the procedure.[61] Improved symptoms correlate with reduction in size of the calcification.[62] Although patients treated with lavage and aspiration had better outcomes 1 year after the procedure than those who were not treated, outcomes at 5 and

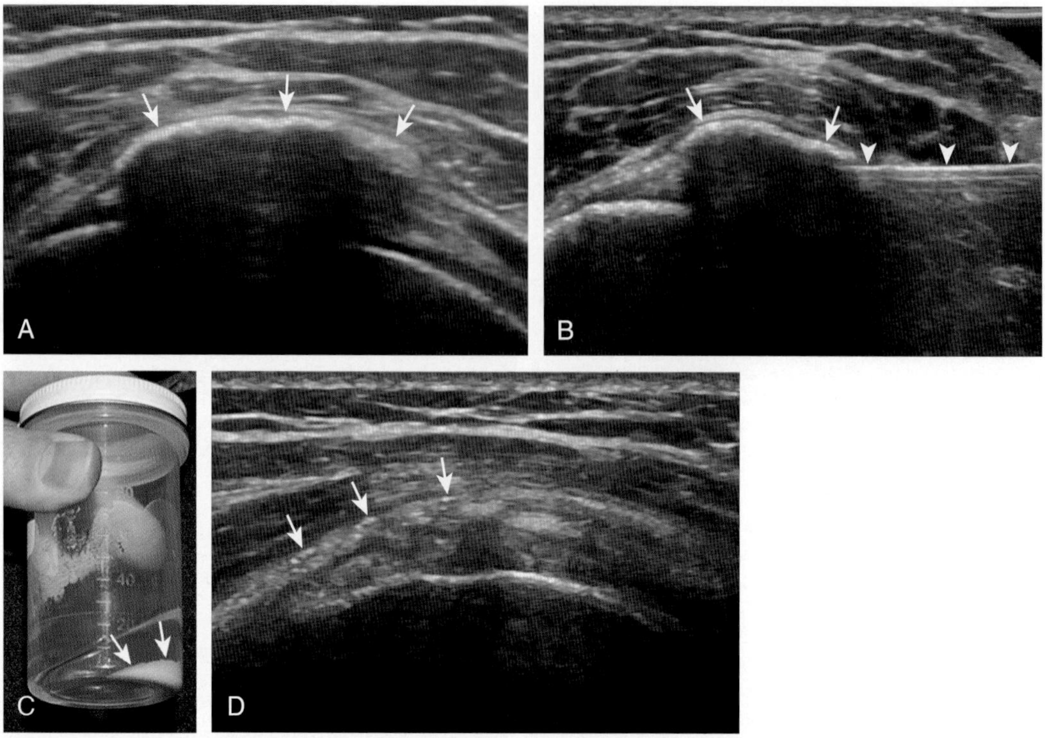

■ FIGURE 9.46 **Calcific Tendinosis Lavage and Aspiration: Supraspinatus.** Ultrasound images short axis to the supraspinatus tendon show (A) echogenic and shadowing large calcification *(arrows)*. Note (B) needle placement *(arrowheads)* within calcification. After lavage and aspiration, specimen jar (C) shows calcification dependent within the local anesthetic *(arrows)*. Although there was no immediate change in the ultrasound appearance of the calcification at the end of the lavage and aspiration, repeat ultrasound 3 weeks after the procedure showed (D) nearly complete resorption of the calcifications, several of which were found in the subacromial-subdeltoid bursa *(arrows)*.

10 years were similar.[63] Lavage and aspiration of calcium may be completed in any accessible tendon, such as the gluteal tendons at the greater trochanter, and also can be considered for treatment of calcific bursitis at the resorptive phase of calcific tendinitis.

Tendon Fenestration (Tenotomy or Dry Needling)

When a tendon shows tendinosis or partial tear, a needle can be guided into the affected tendon segment using ultrasound guidance as an effective method to disrupt tendon degeneration and stimulate healing.[44] Common sites for this procedure include the common extensor tendon of the elbow (Fig. 9.47) (Video 9.33),[64,65] the gluteus minimus and medius tendons (Fig. 9.48) (Videos 9.34 and 9.35),[66] the hamstring tendons (Fig. 9.49) (Videos 9.36 and 9.37), the patellar tendon (Fig. 9.50) (Videos 9.38 and 9.39),[41] and the Achilles tendon (Fig. 9.51) (Videos 9.40 and 9.41), although other tendons have been treated with success.[44,67] By repeatedly passing the needle into the abnormal

tendon, healing can be stimulated by disruption of the degenerative area and by causing local bleeding, which releases growth factors.[44] The procedure is completed with a 20- or 22-gauge needle using an in-plane technique relative to the transducer and sound beam and the needle entering along the long axis of the tendon. The needle is placed through the skin, and a small amount of anesthetic agent is placed at the surface of the abnormal tendon. The needle is then repeatedly inserted into the abnormal tendon segment; the needle is withdrawn just out of the tendon, redirected and advanced to an adjacent area, and repeated. The procedure continues until the entire segment of abnormal tendon is treated and softens, confirmed in both short axis and long axis dimensions. This typically involves passing the needle 20–30 times, but this varies depending on the size of the tendon abnormality. If the tendon abnormality is adjacent to bone at the enthesis, the needle is also directed to the bone surface. If there is hyperemia on color or power Doppler imaging in the abnormal tendon segment before the fenestration, one will often see increased

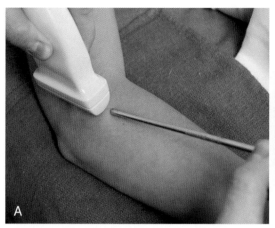

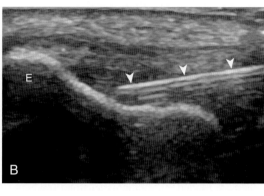

■ **FIGURE 9.47 Tendon Fenestration: Common Extensor Tendon of Elbow.** A, Transducer and needle position for simulated common extensor tendon procedure. Ultrasound image shows (B) needle *(arrowheads)* long axis to common extensor tendon with distal tip located within hypoechoic tendinosis. *E,* Lateral epicondyle of humerus.

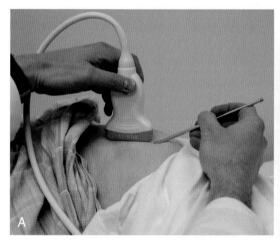

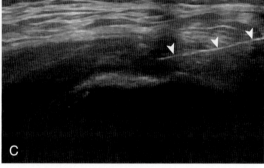

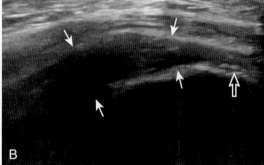

■ **FIGURE 9.48 Tendon Fenestration: Gluteus Medius Tendon.** A, Transducer and needle entry site for simulated gluteus medius procedure. Ultrasound images (B and C) show hypoechoic tendon swelling *(arrows)* with cortical irregularity of greater trochanter *(open arrow).* Note (C) needle position *(arrowheads)*

echogenicity from bleeding. The patient should reduce activity related to the tendon for several weeks, with possible bracing if Achilles tendon if treated. Patients are also instructed to avoid ice and non-steroidal anti-inflammatory drugs for 2 weeks after the procedure so that inflammation as the essential first step in tissue healing is not inhibited.

Platelet-Rich Plasma, Whole Blood, and Other Injections

Although a discussion regarding the complexity and relative effectiveness of tendon injections is beyond the scope of this chapter, several topics related to ultrasound-guided injection deserve comment.[68] The use of ultrasound guidance can

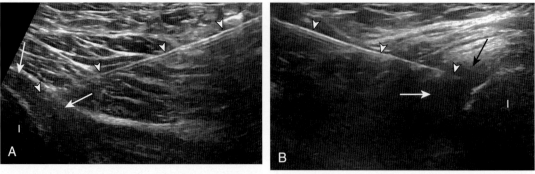

■ **FIGURE 9.49 Tendon Fenestration: Hamstring Tendons.** Ultrasound images in two different patients show hypoechoic proximal hamstring tendinosis *(arrows)* and fenestration (A) long axis to hamstrings with needle *(arrowheads)* entering from distal to proximal and (B) short axis to hamstrings with needle *(arrowheads)* entering from lateral to medial. *I,* Ischial tuberosity.

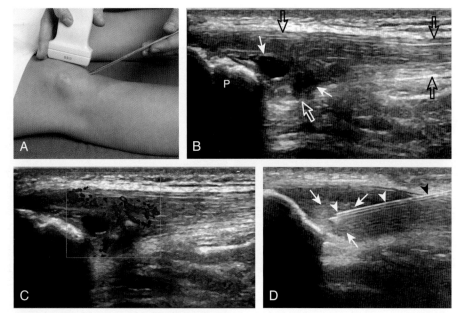

■ **FIGURE 9.50 Tendon Fenestration: Patellar Tendon.** A, Transducer and needle position for simulated proximal patellar tendon procedure. Ultrasound images (B and C) show abnormal hypoechogenicity *(arrows)* of the patellar tendon *(open arrows)* with increased through transmission, cortical irregularity of the patella *(P),* and neovascularity in C. During tendon fenestration procedure (D), no fluid could be aspirated. Note needle *(arrowheads)* and increased echogenicity at the fenestration site from hemorrhage *(arrows).*

ensure that platelet-rich plasma (Fig. 9.52) (Videos 9.42, 9.43, and 9.44), whole blood (Fig. 9.53) (Video 9.45), and other injections are accurate while minimizing complications as for any other percutaneous ultrasound-guided procedure. Similar to other procedures, an in-plane approach relative to the transducer is most accurate. Typically, platelet-rich plasma or whole blood injection into a tendon occurs in conjunction with tendon fenestration. Injection of hyperosmolar dextrose and other irritants have also been described as

potential tendon treatments, which has been termed *prolotherapy.*[69]

■ MISCELLANEOUS PROCEDURES
Cyst Aspiration

Two general categories of cysts that may be aspirated using ultrasound guidance are ganglion cysts and cysts associated with fibrocartilage tears (meniscus and labrum).[70] In both settings, the

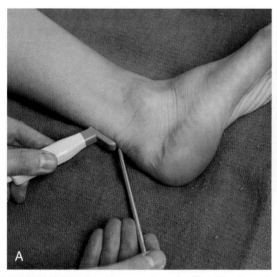
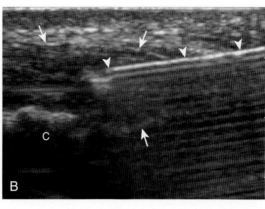

■ **FIGURE 9.51 Tendon Fenestration: Achilles Tendon.** A, Transducer and needle position for simulated Achilles tendon procedure. Ultrasound image (B) shows needle placement *(arrowheads)* within abnormal hypoechoic swollen distal Achilles tendon *(arrows)*. C, Calcaneus.

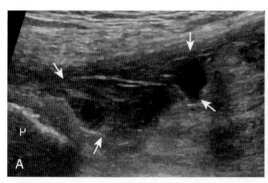
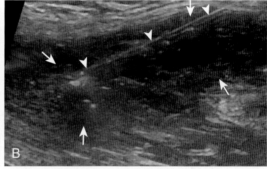

■ **FIGURE 9.52 Autologous Platelet-Rich Plasma Injection: Adductor Longus Tendon.** Ultrasound images long axis to the adductor longus show (A) predominantly hypoechoic heterogeneous tear of the proximal adductor longus tendon *(arrows)* with (B) subsequent needle placement *(arrowheads)* and platelet-rich plasma injection *(arrows)*. P, Pubis.

fluid in the cyst is often viscous, and the cyst is often multilocular, which can limit the success of the aspiration (Fig. 9.54). Typically, a large-gauge (16-gauge) needle is used, and cyst lavage may improve aspiration (Fig. 9.55) (Video 9.46). Ganglion cysts may recur after aspiration and injection because a connection or neck to a joint or tendon sheath is usually present. Ganglion cyst aspiration may also be followed by corticosteroid injection.[71] Cysts associated with fibrocartilage often recur as well, because the cyst originates from the tear of the meniscus or labrum (shoulder or hip) (Fig. 9.56) (Video 9.47).

Peripheral Nerve

Injections adjacent to a peripheral nerve are carried out with an in-plane approach with the transducer short axis to the peripheral nerve. This approach allows the injection to be instilled at least partially circumferential to the nerve, which increases the effectiveness of a sensory block.[72] The characteristic appearance of a peripheral nerve is best appreciated in short axis, and adjacent vascular structures are also easily seen. For injection of the carpal tunnel, the needle is in plane with the transducer and sound beam, with the transducer

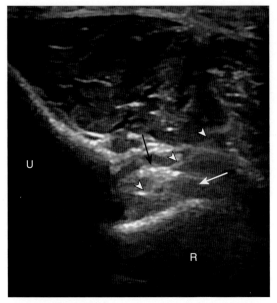

FIGURE 9.53 Autologous Whole Blood Injection: Distal Biceps Brachii Tendon. Ultrasound image long axis to the distal biceps brachii tendon in elbow flexion and hyperpronation shows needle placement *(arrowheads)* within the hypoechoic tendinosis *(arrows)* from a dorsal approach. *R,* Radial tuberosity; *U,* ulna.

in short axis to the median nerve, and the needle enters from ulnar to radial over the volar aspect of the wrist.[73] Injection of the lateral femoral cutaneous nerve should target the segment of nerve that is hypoechoic and enlarged, typically where the nerve passes beneath the inguinal ligament (Fig. 9.57).[74,75] With regard to the tibial nerve in the tarsal tunnel, the needle is in plane with the transducer in short axis to the tibial nerve, and the needle enters from posterior to anterior next to the Achilles tendon and over the flexor hallucis longus tendon. Injection of an amputation neuroma may be completed either short axis (Fig. 9.58) or long axis to the affected nerve.[76] Injection of a Morton neuroma is typically long axis to the affected nerve with the needle entering from the dorsal aspect of the web space (Fig. 9.59) (Video 9.48).[77,78]

Biopsy

Although a full discussion of ultrasound-guided biopsy is beyond the scope of this chapter, a few fundamentals will be mentioned.[79] The first is that a biopsy of a suspected mass or malignancy should be performed at a hospital or institution where

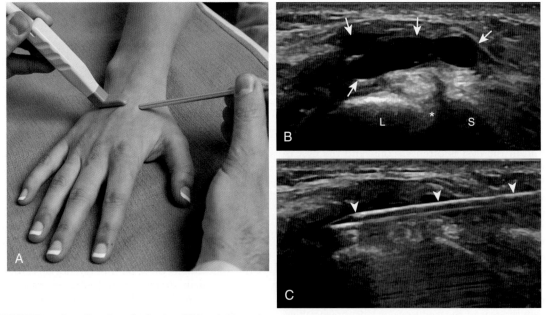

FIGURE 9.54 Ganglion Cyst Aspiration: Wrist. A, Transducer and needle position for simulated dorsal wrist ganglion procedure. Ultrasound images show (B) anechoic and lobular dorsal ganglion cyst *(arrows)* and (C) subsequent needle placement *(arrowheads)* for aspiration *(asterisk,* scapholunate ligament). *L,* Lunate; *S,* scaphoid.

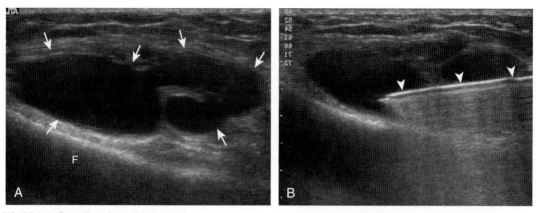

■ **FIGURE 9.55 Ganglion Cyst Aspiration: Knee.** Ultrasound images show (A) anechoic and lobular ganglion cyst *(arrows)* and (B) subsequent needle placement *(arrowheads)* for aspiration. *F,* Femur.

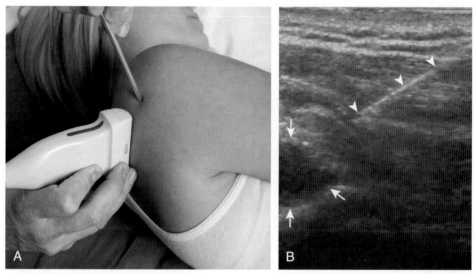

■ **FIGURE 9.56 Paralabral Cyst Aspiration: Shoulder.** A, Transducer and needle position for simulated posterior shoulder paralabral procedure. Ultrasound image shows (B) needle *(arrowheads)* approaching hypoechoic paralabral cyst *(arrows)*. Right side of ultrasound image is lateral.

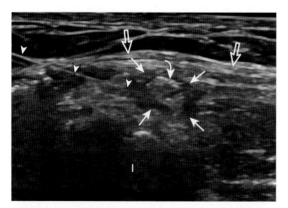

■ **FIGURE 9.57 Lateral Femoral Cutaneous Nerve: Injection.** Ultrasound image shows needle *(arrowheads)* with hypoechoic injection *(arrows)* surrounding the lateral femoral cutaneous nerve *(curved arrow)*. Note inguinal ligament *(open arrows)*. *I,* Ilium.

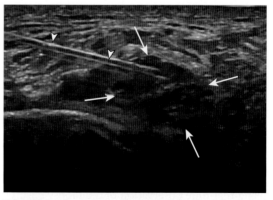

■ **FIGURE 9.58 Amputation Neuroma: Injection.** Ultrasound image shows needle *(arrowheads)* at neuroma *(arrows)*.

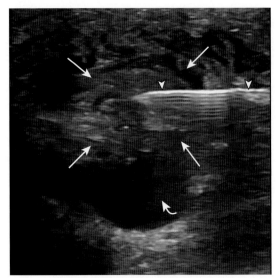

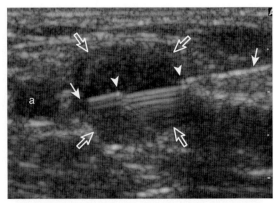

■ **FIGURE 9.61 Lymph Node Biopsy: Lymphoma.** Ultrasound image shows the entire length of the needle *(arrows)*, including the distal tip, visible in the long axis of the transducer. Note the opening in needle surface for biopsy *(arrowheads)* with reverberation artifact and needle placement within an axillary lymph node *(open arrows)*. Biopsy revealed a B-cell lymphoma. *a,* Artery.

■ **FIGURE 9.59 Morton Neuroma: Injection.** Ultrasound image shows needle *(arrowheads)* within Morton neuroma *(arrows)*. Note filling of adjacent intermetatarsal bursa *(curved arrow)*.

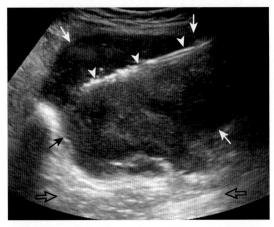

■ **FIGURE 9.60 Soft Tissue Mass Biopsy: Lymphoma.** Ultrasound images shows hyperechoic biopsy needle *(arrowheads)* within hypoechoic mass *(arrows)*. Note increased through-transmission *(open arrows)*.

the tumor will be treated. This allows an open communication between the physician performing the procedure and the surgical oncologist. Because the surgeon resects the tumor along the biopsy needle path, this planning is critical. Using ultrasound guidance, several biopsy specimens are taken from various areas of the soft tissue tumor to ensure thorough sampling (Fig. 9.60).[80,81] Guiding the biopsy needle with an in-plane approach and using real-time observation of the biopsy ensures accurate sampling (Videos 9.49 and 9.50). In addition, seeding of adjacent compartments, such as neurovascular structures and an adjacent joint, should be avoided (Fig. 9.61).

SELECT REFERENCES

3. Finnoff JT, Hall MM, Adams E, et al: American Medical Society for Sports Medicine (AMSSM) position statement: interventional musculoskeletal ultrasound in sports medicine. *Br J Sports Med* 49(3):145–150, 2015.

4. Daley EL, Bajaj S, Bisson LJ, et al: Improving injection accuracy of the elbow, knee, and shoulder: does injection site and imaging make a difference? A systematic review. *Am J Sports Med* 39(3):656–662, 2011.

10. Fessell DP, Jacobson JA, Craig J, et al: Using sonography to reveal and aspirate joint effusions. *AJR Am J Roentgenol* 174(5):1353–1362, 2000.

19. Rowbotham EL, Grainger AJ: Ultrasound-guided intervention around the hip joint. *AJR Am J Roentgenol* 197(1):W122–W127, 2011.

23. Fenn S, Datir A, Saifuddin A: Synovial recesses of the knee: MR imaging review of anatomical and pathological features. *Skeletal Radiol* 38(4):317–328, 2009.

32. Blankenbaker DG, De Smet AA, Keene JS: Sonography of the iliopsoas tendon and injection of the iliopsoas bursa for diagnosis and management of the painful snapping hip. *Skeletal Radiol* 35(8):565–571, 2006.

34. Pfirrmann CW, Chung CB, Theumann NH, et al: Greater trochanter of the hip: attachment of the abductor mechanism and a complex of three bursae—MR imaging and MR bursography in cadavers and MR imaging in asymptomatic volunteers. *Radiology* 221(2):469–477, 2001.

35. Ward EE, Jacobson JA, Fessell DP, et al: Sonographic detection of Baker's cysts: comparison with MR imaging. *AJR Am J Roentgenol* 176(2):373–380, 2001.

40. MacMahon PJ, Eustace SJ, Kavanagh EC: Injectable corticosteroid and local anesthetic preparations: a

review for radiologists. *Radiology* 252(3):647–661, 2009.

43. Coombes BK, Bisset L, Vicenzino B: Efficacy and safety of corticosteroid injections and other injections for management of tendinopathy: a systematic review of randomised controlled trials. *Lancet* 376(9754):1751–1767, 2010.

44. Chiavaras MM, Jacobson JA: Ultrasound-guided tendon fenestration. *Semin Musculoskelet Radiol* 17(1):85–90, 2013.

59. Lee KS, Rosas HG: Musculoskeletal ultrasound: how to treat calcific tendinitis of the rotator cuff by ultrasound-guided single-needle lavage technique. *AJR Am J Roentgenol* 195(3):638, 2010.

66. Jacobson JA, Rubin J, Yablon CM, et al: Ultrasound-guided fenestration of tendons about the hip and pelvis: clinical outcomes. *J Ultrasound Med* 34(11): 2029–2035, 2015.

68. Sheth U, Simunovic N, Klein G, et al: Efficacy of autologous platelet-rich plasma use for orthopaedic indications: a meta-analysis. *J Bone Joint Surg Am* 94(4):298–307, 2012.

The complete references for this chapter can be found on *www.expertconsult.com.*

Sample Diagnostic Ultrasound Reports

 BOX 3.1 Sample Diagnostic Shoulder Ultrasound Report: Normal, Complete

Examination: Ultrasound of the Shoulder
Date of Study: March 11, 2017
Patient Name: Juan Atkins
Registration Number: 8675309
History: Shoulder pain, evaluate for rotator cuff abnormality
Findings: No evidence of joint effusion. The biceps brachii long head tendon is normal without tendinosis, tear, tenosynovitis, or subluxation/dislocation. The supraspinatus, infraspinatus, subscapularis, and teres minor tendons are also normal. No subacromial-subdeltoid bursal abnormality and no sonographic evidence for subacromial impingement with dynamic maneuvers. The posterior labrum is unremarkable. Additional focused evaluation at site of maximal symptoms was unrevealing.
Impression: Unremarkable ultrasound examination of the shoulder. No rotator cuff abnormality.

 BOX 3.2 Sample Diagnostic Shoulder Ultrasound Report: Abnormal, Complete

Examination: Ultrasound of the Shoulder
Date of Study: March 11, 2017
Patient Name: Chazz Michael Michaels
Registration Number: 8675309
History: Shoulder pain, evaluate for rotator cuff abnormality
Findings: There is a focal anechoic tear of the anterior, distal aspect of the supraspinatus tendon measuring 1 cm short axis by 1.5 cm long axis. The anterior margin of the tear is adjacent to the rotator interval. There is no involvement of the subscapularis, infraspinatus, or rotator interval. A moderate amount of infraspinatus and supraspinatus fatty degeneration is present. There is a small joint effusion distending the biceps brachii tendon sheath and moderate distention of the subacromial-subdeltoid bursa. No biceps brachii long head tendon abnormality and no subluxation/dislocation. Mild osteoarthritis of the acromioclavicular joint. Additional focused evaluation at site of maximal symptoms was unrevealing.
Impression: Focal or incomplete full-thickness tear of the supraspinatus tendon with infraspinatus and supraspinatus muscle atrophy.

BOX 4.1 Sample Diagnostic Elbow Ultrasound Report: Normal, Complete

Examination: Ultrasound of the Elbow
Date of Study: March 11, 2011
Patient Name: Kevin Saunderson
Registration Number: 8675309
History: Elbow pain, evaluate for tendon abnormality
Findings: No evidence of joint effusion or synovial process. The biceps brachii and brachialis are normal. The common flexor and extensor tendons are also normal. No significant triceps brachii abnormality. The anterior bundle of the ulnar collateral ligament and lateral collateral ligament complex are normal. The ulnar nerve, radial nerve, and median nerve at the elbow are unremarkable. No abnormality in the cubital tunnel region with dynamic imaging. Additional focused evaluation at site of maximal symptoms was unrevealing.
Impression: Unremarkable ultrasound examination of the elbow.

BOX 4.2 Sample Diagnostic Elbow Ultrasound Report: Abnormal, Complete

Examination: Ultrasound of the Elbow
Date of Study: March 11, 2011
Patient Name: Ricky Bobby
Registration Number: 8675309
History: Elbow pain, evaluate for tendon abnormality
Findings: There is a partial-thickness tear of the distal biceps brachii tendon involving the superficial short head tendon with approximately 2 cm of retraction but with intact long head. Dynamic evaluation shows continuity of the long head excluding full-thickness tear. No joint effusion. The triceps brachii, common extensor, and common flexor tendons are normal. The ulnar, radial, and median nerves are unremarkable, including dynamic evaluation of the ulnar nerve. Unremarkable ulnar and lateral collateral ligaments. No bursal distention.
Impression: Partial-thickness tear of the distal biceps brachii tendon.

BOX 5.1 Sample Diagnostic Wrist Ultrasound Report: Normal, Complete

Examination: Ultrasound of the Wrist
Date of Study: March 11, 2011
Patient Name: Derrick May
Registration Number: 8675309
History: Numbness, evaluate for carpal tunnel syndrome
Findings: The median nerve is unremarkable in appearance, measuring 8 mm^2 at the wrist crease and 7 mm^2 at the pronator quadratus. No evidence of tenosynovitis. The radiocarpal, midcarpal, and distal radioulnar joints are normal without effusion or synovial hypertrophy. The wrist tendons are normal without tear or tenosynovitis. Normal dorsal component of the scapholunate ligament. No dorsal or volar ganglion cyst. Unremarkable Guyon canal. Additional focused evaluation at site of maximal symptoms was unrevealing.
Impression: Unremarkable ultrasound examination of the wrist.

BOX 5.2 Sample Diagnostic Wrist Ultrasound Report: Abnormal, Complete

Examination: Ultrasound of the Wrist
Date of Study: March 11, 2011
Patient Name: Jacobim Mugatu
Registration Number: 8675309
History: Numbness, evaluate for carpal tunnel syndrome
Findings: The median nerve is hypoechoic and enlarged, measuring 15 mm^2 at the wrist crease and 7 mm^2 at the pronator quadratus. No evidence of tenosynovitis. The radiocarpal, midcarpal, and distal radioulnar joints are normal without effusion or synovial hypertrophy. The wrist tendons are normal without tear or tenosynovitis. Normal dorsal component of the scapholunate ligament. No dorsal ganglion cyst. A 7-mm volar ganglion cyst is noted between the radial artery and flexor carpi radialis tendon. Unremarkable Guyon canal. Additional focused evaluation at site of maximal symptoms was unrevealing.
Impression:
1. Ultrasound findings compatible with carpal tunnel syndrome.
2. A 7-mm volar ganglion cyst.

BOX 6.1 Sample Diagnostic Hip Ultrasound Report: Normal, Complete

Examination: Ultrasound of the Right Hip
Date of Study: March 11, 2016
Patient Name: Jack White
Registration Number: 8675309
History: Hip pain, evaluate for bursitis
Findings: The hip joint is normal without effusion or synovial hypertrophy. Limited evaluation of the anterior labrum is unremarkable. No evidence of iliopsoas bursal distention or snapping iliopsoas tendon with dynamic imaging. The remaining anterior tendons, including the rectus femoris and sartorius, as well as the adductors, are normal.

Evaluation of the lateral hip is normal. No evidence of abnormal bursal distention around the greater trochanter. The gluteus minimus and medius tendons are normal. No abnormal snapping with dynamic evaluation.
Impression: Unremarkable ultrasound examination of the hip.

BOX 6.2 Sample Diagnostic Hip Ultrasound Report: Abnormal, Complete

Examination: Ultrasound of the Right Hip
Date of Study: March 11, 2016
Patient Name: Brennan Huff
Registration Number: 8675309
History: Hip pain, evaluate for tendon tear
Findings: There is a partial tear of the adductor longus origin at the pubis. No evidence of full-thickness tear or tendon retraction. The common aponeurosis and rectus abdominis tendon are normal, as is the pubic symphysis.

The hip joint is normal without effusion or synovial hypertrophy. There is a possible tear of the anterior labrum. No paralabral cyst. No evidence of iliopsoas bursal distention or snapping iliopsoas tendon with dynamic imaging.

Evaluation of the lateral hip is normal. No evidence of abnormal bursal distention around the greater trochanter. The gluteus minimus and medius tendons are normal. No abnormal snapping with dynamic evaluation.
Impression:
1. Partial-thickness tear of the proximal adductor longus.
2. Possible anterior labral tear. Consider MR arthrography if indicated.

BOX 7.1 Sample Diagnostic Knee Ultrasound Report: Normal, Complete

Examination: Ultrasound of the Right Knee
Date of Study: March 11, 2016
Patient Name: Meg White
Registration Number: 8675309
History: Trauma
Findings: The extensor mechanism, including the quadriceps tendon, patella, and patellar tendon, is normal without bursal abnormalities. No significant joint effusion or synovial hypertrophy. The medial collateral and lateral collateral ligaments are normal. Unremarkable iliotibial tract, biceps femoris, popliteus tendon, and common peroneal nerve. No Baker cyst. Limited evaluation of the menisci is unremarkable.
Impression: Unremarkable ultrasound examination of the right knee.

BOX 7.2 Sample Diagnostic Knee Ultrasound Report: Abnormal, Complete

Examination: Ultrasound of the Right Knee
Date of Study: March 11, 2016
Patient Name: Frank Ricard
Registration Number: 8675309
History: Pain, evaluate for cyst
Findings: The extensor mechanism, including the quadriceps tendon, patella, and patellar tendon, is normal. There is a moderate-sized joint effusion and no synovial hypertrophy or intra-articular body. The medial and lateral collateral ligaments are normal, as is the iliotibial tract, biceps femoris, popliteus tendon, and common peroneal nerve. There is medial compartment joint space narrowing and osteophyte formation with mild extrusion of the body of the medial meniscus, which is abnormally hypoechoic. No parameniscal cyst. There is a Baker cyst measuring 2 × 2 × 6 cm. Abnormal hypoechogenicity is noted at the inferior margin of the Baker cyst. There is also a hypoechoic cleft involving the posterior horn of the medial meniscus, which extends to the articular surface.
Impression:
1. Baker cyst with evidence for rupture.
2. Medial compartment osteoarthritis with moderate joint effusion.
3. Suspect posterior horn medial meniscal tear. Consider MRI for confirmation if indicated.

BOX 8.1 Sample Diagnostic Ankle Ultrasound Report: Normal, Complete

Examination: Ultrasound of the Right Ankle
Date of Study: March 11, 2017
Patient Name: John Mayer
Registration Number: 8675309
History: Pain, evaluate for tendon tear
Findings: No evidence of ankle joint effusion. Anteriorly, the tibialis anterior, extensor hallucis longus, and extensor digitorum longus are normal. Medially, the tibialis posterior, flexor digitorum longus, flexor hallucis longus, tibial nerve, and deltoid ligament are normal. Laterally, the peroneus brevis and longus are normal, as are the anterior talofibular, calcaneofibular ligament, and anterior tibiofibular ligaments. Posteriorly, the Achilles tendon and plantar fascia are normal. Focused ultrasound examination directed by patient symptoms over the lateral ankle revealed no abnormality.
Impression: Unremarkable ultrasound examination of the right ankle. No tendon abnormality.

BOX 8.2 Sample Diagnostic Ankle Ultrasound Report: Abnormal, Complete

Examination: Ultrasound of the Right Ankle
Date of Study: March 11, 2017
Patient Name: Ron Burgundy
Registration Number: 8675309
History: Pain, evaluate for tendon tear
Findings: There is a small ankle joint effusion. No synovial hypertrophy. Laterally, there is abnormal anechoic fluid and hypoechoic synovial hypertrophy surrounding the peroneal tendons at the level of the distal fibula. A longitudinal tear is seen in the peroneus brevis. The superior peroneal retinaculum is torn at the fibula, and peroneal tendon dislocation occurs with dynamic evaluation in ankle dorsiflexion and eversion. No low-lying peroneus brevis muscle. Otherwise, the anterior talofibular, calcaneofibular ligament, and anterior tibiofibular ligaments are normal.

Anteriorly, the tibialis anterior, extensor hallucis longus, and extensor digitorum longus are normal. Medially, the tibialis posterior, flexor digitorum longus, flexor hallucis longus, tibial nerve, and deltoid ligament are normal.

Posteriorly, the Achilles tendon and plantar fascia are normal. Focused ultrasound examination directed by patient symptoms over the lateral ankle corresponded to the peroneal tendon tear.
Impression:
1. Longitudinal split tear of the peroneus brevis and tenosynovitis.
2. Superior peroneal retinaculum tear and transient anterolateral dislocation of the peroneal tendons with dynamic imaging.
3. Small ankle joint effusion.

BOX 9.1 Sample Interventional Ultrasound Report

Examination: Ultrasound-Guided Injection of Right Biceps Brachii Long Head Tendon Sheath
Date of Study: March 11, 2017
Patient Name: James Murphy
Registration Number: 8675309
History: Pain
Findings: Limited ultrasound over the anterior right shoulder demonstrates minimal joint fluid distending the biceps brachii long head tendon sheath. No evidence for hyperemia or synovial hypertrophy to suggest tenosynovitis. No evidence for biceps brachii long head tendon tear. No tendon subluxation or dislocation with dynamic imaging. No abnormal subacromial-subdeltoid bursal thickening.

> After obtaining both written and verbal informed consent discussing potential risks (bleeding, infection, soft tissue injury) and benefits, using sterile technique and local anesthetic injection (provide type and amount), a 22-gauge spinal needle with trocar was inserted into the long head of the biceps brachii tendon sheath. Intra-sheath location of needle tip was confirmed with a small amount of anesthetic injection. This was followed by corticosteroid injection (provide type and amount).

> The patient tolerated the procedure well without complications. The patient's pain level changed from 8/10 before procedure to 2/10.

Impression:
1. Limited diagnostic ultrasound of the anterior shoulder showed minimal joint fluid.
2. Successful long head biceps brachii tendon sheath corticosteroid injection with pain relief as noted above and without complications.

BOX 9.2 Sample Interventional Ultrasound Report

Examination: Ultrasound-Guided Right Iliopsoas Bursal Injection
Date of Study: March 11, 2011
Patient Name: Chazz Reinhold
Registration Number: 8675309
History: Pain, evaluate for tendon tear
Findings: Limited ultrasound over the anterior right hip showed no hip joint effusion and unremarkable anterior hip labrum. The rectus femoris was normal. No evidence for iliopsoas bursal distention. Dynamic imaging showed no evidence for snapping iliopsoas tendon.

> After obtaining both written and verbal informed consent discussing potential risks (bleeding, infection, soft tissue injury) and benefits, using sterile technique and local anesthetic injection (provide type and amount), a 20-gauge spinal needle with trocar was directed between the psoas major tendon of the iliopsoas complex and ilium superior to the femoral head. Needle tip location between the tendon and ilium was confirmed with a small amount of anesthetic injection. This was followed by corticosteroid injection (provide type and amount).

> The patient tolerated the procedure well without complications. The patient's pain level changed from 8/10 before procedure to 2/10.

Impression:
1. Limited diagnostic ultrasound of the anterior right hip showed no abnormality.
2. Successful right iliopsoas bursal corticosteroid injection with pain relief as noted above and without complications.

Note: Page numbers followed by "f" refer to illustrations; page numbers followed by "t" refer to tables; page numbers followed by "b" refer to boxes.